LEADING AND MANAGING IN CANADIAN NURSING

LEADING AND MANAGING IN CANADIAN NURSING

First Canadian Edition

Patricia S. Yoder-Wise, RN, EdD, NEA-BC, ANEF, FAAN
Dean Emerita and Professor Emerita
Texas Tech University Health Sciences Center
Lubbock, Texas

Canadian Editor

Lyle G. Grant, RN, BComm, BSN, MSN, JD, PhD
Coordinator, Institute for Nursing Scholarship
Saskatchewan Polytechnic
Saskatoon, Saskatchewan;
Adjunct Professor
School of Nursing
University of Regina
Regina, Saskatchewan

Assistant Editor

Sandra Regan, RN, BScN, MScN, MA, PhD
Assistant Professor
Arthur Labatt Family School of Nursing
Western University
London, Ontario

ELSEVIER

ELSEVIER
MOSBY

LEADING AND MANAGING IN CANADIAN NURSING, FIRST CANADIAN EDITION

Notices

Knowledge and best practice in this field are constantly changing. As new research and experience broaden our understanding, changes in research methods, professional practices, or medical treatment may become necessary.

Practitioners and researchers must always rely on their own experience and knowledge in evaluating and using any information, methods, compounds, or experiments described herein. In using such information or methods, they should be mindful of their own safety and the safety of others, including parties for whom they have a professional responsibility.

With respect to any drug or pharmaceutical products identified, readers are advised to check the most current information provided (i) on procedures featured or (ii) by the manufacturer of each product to be administered, to verify the recommended dose or formula, the method and duration of administration, and contraindications. It is the responsibility of practitioners, relying on their own experience and knowledge of their patients, to make diagnoses, to determine dosages and the best treatment for each individual patient, and to take all appropriate safety precautions.

To the fullest extent of the law, neither the Publisher nor the authors, contributors, or editors, assume any liability for any injury and/or damage to persons or property as a matter of products liability, negligence or otherwise, or from any use or operation of any methods, products, instructions, or ideas contained in the material herein.

The Publisher

Library and Archives Canada Cataloguing in Publication

Yoder-Wise, Patricia S., 1941-, author
    Leading and managing in Canadian nursing / Patricia S. Yoder-Wise, RN, EdD, NEA-BC, ANEF, FAAN, Dean Emerita and Professor Emerita, Texas Tech University Health Sciences Center, Lubbock, Texas ; Canadian editor, Lyle G. Grant, RN, BComm, BSN, MSN, JD, PhD, Coordinator, Institute for Nursing Scholarship, Saskatchewan Polytechnic, Saskatoon, Saskatchewan, Adjunct Professor, School of Nursing, University of Regina, Regina, Saskatchewan ; assistant editor, Sandra Regan, RN, BScN, MScN, MA, PhD, Assistant Professor, Arthur Labatt Family School of Nursing, Western University, London, Ontario.
-- First Canadian edition.

ISBN 978-1-926648-61-3 (pbk.)

    1. Nursing services--Canada--Administration. 2. Leadership--Canada.
I. Grant, Lyle G., editor II. Regan, Sandra, editor III. Title.

RT89.Y63 2014	362.17'3	C2014-903617-5

Vice President, Publishing: Ann Millar
Managing Editor: Roberta A. Spinosa-Millman
Publishing Services Manager: Jeffrey Patterson
Project Manager: Jeanne Genz
Copy Editor: Claudia Forgas
Proofreader: Wendy Thomas
Cover Design: Brett J. Miller, BJM Graphic Design & Communications
Cover Image: Datacraft
Book Designer: Ashley Miner
Photography: Dennis Scanio, Florissant, Missouri
Typesetting and Assembly: Toppan Best-set Premedia Limited

Elsevier Canada
555 Richmond Street West, Suite 1100, Toronto, ON, Canada M5V 3B1
Phone: 1-866-896-3331
Fax: 1-416-255-5456

1 2 3 4 5 18 17 16 15 14

E-book ISBN: 978-1-926648-62-0

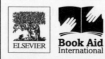

This book is dedicated to the families and friends who supported us as
we created it; to the faculty who are dedicated to producing the nursing
service leaders for the ever changing health care services; to the learners
who have committed to an exciting career in nursing administration;
and to the nurse leaders who face the incredible issues of health care
every day, who do their best in leading important changes in practice,
and who remain committed to the glory of nursing: the care we deliver
to patients.

Lead on! ¡Adelante!

—Patricia S. Yoder-Wise

I dedicate this book to those who share a vision and the courage
to lead and inspire others to create positive changes in nursing
for the benefit of those we serve.

—Lyle G. Grant

ACKNOWLEDGEMENTS

I am delighted to present the first Canadian edition of *Leading and Managing in Canadian Nursing*. The completed work is a culmination of the efforts of many. All contributors were fortunate to be working from the 5th edition of *Leading and Managing in Nursing* in creating a Canadian edition. The 5th edition has many strengths and features on which we built. Adaptation is filled with both challenges and opportunities, and those who worked with me were generous with their expertise, suggestions, and commitment to producing a Canadian edition of the finest quality. I take this opportunity to thank and acknowledge the work and dedication of many for their tremendous contributions.

First, I extend heartfelt thanks to the 25 contributing authors who did the writing for the Canadian edition. All contributors were challenged to write and include material that is relevant to nurses across Canada, regardless of nursing credential and location. Of the many challenges to writing, we sought geographical balance in the content and directed our attention to the pedagogical challenges of writing to varied student audiences who may consider this material at various stages during their respective nursing education program. Through the applied efforts of the contributors and our editorial team, we have a product that has strong application and relevancy to multiple student audiences with content suited to a variety of nursing programs. It was particularly gratifying and humbling for me to work with so many experts in nursing leadership and management from across Canada. The process of working with our contributors was somewhat selfishly enriching for me, as I learned much from each author and was able to converse with some people I respect but had not previously met. I am so pleased that we have been able to compile, present, and share this wealth of Canadian knowledge with other nurses, teachers, and learners. I am honoured to have helped curate the wealth of knowledge our authors bring to the text. The diversity in our authorship demonstrates to students the richness of perspectives available, and I hope the pool of talent gathered for this edition inspires students to find a role model and mentor in advancing their own ambitions for nursing leadership and management.

The writing, reviewing, and production elements required of me during the development and production of the text ultimately required the joint effort of my household. I am particularly grateful for the support, sacrifices, and endurance shared by my spouse, Wanderley Grant. We ultimately share a vision for constant improvement in nursing and to creating positive differences in the lives of those nursing touches.

I felt honoured to work with and so appreciated the efforts of Roberta A. Spinosa-Millman, the managing editor. Her tireless work, resourcefulness, ability to share in a laugh, readiness to listen, and unfailing support were amazing. I also extend thanks to the many others at Elsevier who worked so hard to support completion of the text. I especially acknowledge the support of Ann Millar, vice-president, Publishing, and Claudia Forgas, our copy editor. I was constantly amazed by the pool of talent assembled at Elsevier to support the publication of this text.

Special thanks and acknowledgement go to my assistant editor, Sandra Regan, for her contributions and continued support. Her abilities and willingness to help where and when needed and her willingness to assist me so capably through a variety of processes made her contributions invaluable. I also thank Madeline Press and Sarah Hanson for their assistance with matters of content research, preparing manuscripts, proofing, providing comments on manuscripts in progress, and acting as my sounding board when required.

On behalf of all of the production team and the contributors, I thank those who participated as peer-reviewers, including our student reviewers. Peer review was a critical piece to refining the content and relevance of the writing. All participating reviewers provided thoughtful, considered, and thorough review and comments that we applied to improving the text.

Nursing leadership and management in Canada hold exciting challenges and opportunities for nurses. During current times of transition in health care delivery, there is critical need for nursing to lead in health care management, administration, and service delivery. Nursing needs to share a perspective of caring within evidence-informed approaches to improve health care and the workplaces and environments that support the delivery of health services in Canada. We must all find the best ways and times to lead and follow to improve outcomes for patients, families, and communities. Change is the known constant in nursing and health care and can sometimes wear heavy if its opportunities get lost. Be inspired, hold onto a positive vision, remain patient centred in meeting challenges, and keep focused on how to contribute to making improvements.

Lyle G. Grant
RN, BComm, BSN, MSN, JD, PhD
Saskatchewan Polytechnic
Saskatoon, Saskatchewan;
University of Regina
Regina, Saskatchewan

CONTRIBUTORS

CANADIAN CONTRIBUTORS

Yolanda Babenko-Mould, RN, BScN, MScN, PhD

Assistant Professor
Arthur Labatt Family School of Nursing
Western University
London, Ontario

Judy Boychuk Duchscher, RN, BScN, MN, PhD

Assistant Professor
Faculty of Nursing
University of Calgary
Calgary, Alberta

Barbara Campbell, RN, BN, MN, PhD

Associate Professor
School of Nursing
Director of International Relations
University of Prince Edward Island
Charlottetown, Prince Edward Island

Shelley L. Cobbett, RN, BN, GnT, MN, EdD

Adjunct Assistant Professor
School of Nursing
Dalhousie University
Halifax, Nova Scotia

Susan M. Duncan, RN, BScN, MScN, PhD

Associate Professor
School of Nursing
Thompson Rivers University
Kamloops, British Columbia

Wendy A. Gifford, RN, PhD

Assistant Professor
Faculty of Health Sciences, School of Nursing
University of Ottawa
Ottawa, Ontario;
Research Associate
Saint Elizabeth Health Care
Markham, Ontario

Angela J. Gillis, RN, PhD

Professor
School of Nursing
St. Francis Xavier University
Antigonish, Nova Scotia

Deb A. Gordon, RN, BScN, MBA, CHE

Vice President and Chief Health Operations Officer,
    Northern Alberta
(Acting) Vice President Collaborative Practice,
    Nursing and Health Professions
Alberta Health Services
Edmonton, Alberta

Lyle G. Grant, RN, BComm, BSN, MSN, JD, PhD

Coordinator, Institute for Nursing Scholarship
Saskatchewan Polytechnic
Saskatoon, Saskatchewan
Adjunct Professor
School of Nursing
University of Regina
Regina, Saskatchewan

Sarah E. Hanson, RPN, BA, MScN(c)

Sessional Instructor
School of Nursing
University of Northern British Columbia
Prince George, British Columbia

Kandis Harris, RN, BScN, MN(s)

Instructor
Faculty of Nursing—Moncton Campus
University of New Brunswick
Moncton, New Brunswick

Ena L. Howse, RN, PhD

Associate Professor (Retired)
School of Nursing
Queen's University
Kingston, Ontario

Suzanne Johnston, RN, BN, MN, PhD

Vice President Clinical Programs and Chief Nursing
  Officer
Northern Health British Columbia
Prince George, British Columbia
Adjunct Professor
School of Nursing
University of Northern British Columbia
Prince George, British Columbia;
Adjunct Professor
School of Nursing
University of British Columbia
Vancouver, British Columbia

Arden Krystal, BScN, MHA, CNE

Executive Vice President and Chief Operating Officer
Provincial Health Services Authority
Vancouver, British Columbia

Nancy Lefebre, RN, BScN, MScN, FCCHSE

Senior Vice President, Knowledge and Practice, and
  Chief Clinical Executive
Saint Elizabeth Health Care
Markham, Ontario

Heather MacMillan, RN, BSc, MSc(A)

Instructor
Faculty of Health Sciences—Nursing
Douglas College
Coquitlam, British Columbia

Maura MacPhee, RN, PhD

Associate Professor
School of Nursing
University of British Columbia
Vancouver, British Columbia

Jayne Naylen McChesney, RN, BScN, MHS

Nursing Advisor
Saskatchewan Collaborative Bachelor of Science in
  Nursing (SCBScN) and Nursing Education Pro-
  gram of Saskatchewan (NEPS)
Saskatchewan Polytechnic
Regina, Saskatchewan;
Adjunct Professor
School of Nursing
University of Regina
Regina, Saskatchewan

Colleen A. McKey, RN, BScN, MScHSA, PhD, CHE, FACHE

Assistant Dean, School of Nursing, and Director,
  Leadership and Management Program
Faculty of Health Sciences
McMaster University
Hamilton, Ontario

Sandra A. Pike-MacDonald, RN, BN, MN, PhD

Professor
School of Nursing
Memorial University of Newfoundland
St. John's, Newfoundland and Labrador

Sandra Regan, RN, BScN, MScN, MA, PhD

Assistant Professor
Arthur Labatt Family School of Nursing
Western University
London, Ontario

Selvi Roy, MSW, PhD(c)

Sessional Instructor and Research Assistant
Faculty of Education
University of Prince Edward Island
Charlottetown, Prince Edward Island

Kathy L. Rush, BSN, MSc, PhD

Associate Professor
School of Nursing—Okanagan
University of British Columbia
Kelowna, British Columbia

Erin Wilson, MScN-NP(F), PhD(c)

Assistant Professor
University of Northern British Columbia
Prince George, British Columbia

Heather D. Wilson, RN, BA, MSN

Professor
Faculty of Health and Human Services
Vancouver Island University
Nanaimo, British Columbia

Carol A. Wong, RN, BScN, MScN, PhD

Associate Professor
Arthur Labatt Family School of Nursing
Western University
London, Ontario

U.S. CONTRIBUTORS

Mary Ellen Clyne, NEA-BC, RN, MSN

Executive Director
Clara Maass Medical Center
Belleville, New Jersey

Mary Ann T. Donohue, NEA-BC, APN, RN, PhD

Vice President of Clinical Care Services
Jersey Shore University Medical Center
Neptune, New Jersey

Karen A. Esquibel, RN, PhD

Assistant Professor
Anita Thigpen Perry School of Nursing
Texas Tech University Health Sciences Center
Lubbock, Texas

Michael L. Evans, FAAN, FACHE, NEA-BC, RN, PhD

Dean and Professor
Goldfarb School of Nursing at Barnes-Jewish College
St. Louis, Missouri

Victoria N. Folse, LCPC, PMHCNS-BC, APN, PhD

Director and Associate Professor
School of Nursing
Illinois Wesleyan University
Bloomington, Illinois

Debra Hagler, ANEF, CNE, ACNS-BC, RN, PhD

Clinical Professor and Coordinator for Teaching
    Excellence
College of Nursing & Health Innovation
Arizona State University
Phoenix, Arizona

Catherine A. Hill, CS, RN, MSN

Director of Quality
Texas Health Resources
Dallas, Texas

Cheri Hunt, NEA-BC, RN, MHA

Vice President for Nursing and Chief Nursing Officer
The Children's Mercy Hospital
Kansas City, Missouri

Karren Kowalski, FAAN, NEA-BC, RN, PhD

Professor
Anita Thigpen Perry School of Nursing
Texas Tech University Health Sciences Center
Lubbock, Texas
Grant and Project Director
Colorado Center for Nursing Excellence
Denver, Colorado

Mary E. Mancini, FAAN, FAHA, NE-BC, RN, PhD

Professor and Associate Dean
College of Nursing—Arlington
The University of Texas
Arlington, Texas

Dorothy A. Otto, ANEF, RN, MSN, EdD

Associate Professor
School of Nursing
University of Texas Health Science Center
Houston, Texas

Janis B. Smith, DNP, RN

Director, Clinical Information Systems
The Children's Mercy Hospital
Kansas City, Missouri

Susan Sportsman, RN, PhD

Dean
College of Health Sciences and Human Services
Midwestern State University
Wichita Falls, Texas

Trudi B. Stafford, RN, PhD

Vice President and Chief Nursing Officer
Baylor All Saints Medical Center
Fort Worth, Texas

Angela L. Stalbaum, NE-BC, RN, MSN

Chief Nursing Officer
Seton Family of Hospitals—Seton Medical Center
    Austin
Austin, Texas

Diane M. Twedell, CENP, RN, DNP

Nurse Administrator
Mayo Clinic
Rochester, Minnesota

Ana M. Valadez, FAAN, NEA-BC, EdD, RN

Professor Emerita
Anita Thigpen School of Nursing
Texas Tech University Health Sciences Center
Lubbock, Texas

Patricia S. Yoder-Wise, RN, EdD, NEA-BC, ANEF, FAAN

Dean Emerita and Professor Emerita
Texas Tech University Health Sciences Center
Lubbock, Texas

Margarete Lieb Zalon, ACNS-BC, RN, PhD

Professor
Department of Nursing
University of Scranton
Scranton, Pennsylvania

REVIEWERS

CANADIAN REVIEWERS

Peer review is critical to the quality and utility of scholarly and practice informing publications. Through the efforts of expert peers, knowledge is tested for its veracity and completeness and questions are asked that improve and refine our thinking and writing. Peer review is also important to the development of best practices, best evidence, and continuous development of the nursing profession, so is welcomed and appreciated. Our peer reviewers provided insightful comments and suggestions that helped refine the presentation of the material in this textbook. The end result of their efforts, as in any peer review process, is a stronger presentation of information for the readership. We are grateful to the masked reviewers of this publication. Thank you!

Catherine Aquino-Russell, RN, BScN, MN, PhD

Professor and Bachelor of Nursing Program Director
Faculty of Nursing—Moncton Campus
University of New Brunswick
Moncton, New Brunswick

Andrea Bodnar, BSN, BA, RN, CNCC, MSN/Ed

Lecturer
Applied Health Sciences—Nursing
Brock University
St. Catharines, Ontario

Stephanie Buckingham, RN, BSN, MALT

Professor
Faculty of Health and Human Services
Vancouver Island University
Nanaimo, British Columbia

Pasquale Fiore, RN, BScN, MSc Health Adm, Cert Ed

Faculty
Department of Nursing
Camosun College;
Instructor
School of Nursing
University of Victoria
Victoria, British Columbia

Sandra Gessler, RN, MPA

Coordinator, Clinical Practice & Baccalaureate
    Program for Registered Nurses
Faculty of Nursing
University of Manitoba
Winnipeg, Manitoba

Elizabeth Haugh, BA, RN, MScN (Admin.)

Adjunct Assistant Professor
Faculty of Nursing
University of Windsor
Windsor, Ontario

Diane Hemmings, RN, MSc, MA, PhD

Sessional Lecturer
Community Health Sciences and Humanities
    Departments
Brock University
St. Catharines, Ontario

Mitzi Grace Mitchell, RN, GNC, BScN, BA, MHSc, MN, DNS, PhD (Public Health)

Professor
Seneca College of Applied Arts and Technology
Toronto, Ontario

Mary Ellen Nicholson, RN, BScN, MHSc, CPHN, CCBS, CHE, PhD(c)

Faculty
Faculty of Health Science
School of Nursing
McMaster University
Hamilton, Ontario

Bukola Salami, RN, MN, PhD

Assistant Professor
Lawrence S. Bloomberg Faculty of Nursing
University of Toronto
Toronto, Ontario

Cindy Smith, RN, BScN, MN
Associate Dean of Nursing
Saskatchewan Polytechnic—Wascana Campus
Regina, Saskatchewan

Landa Terblanche, RN, PhD
Associate Professor
School of Nursing
Trinity Western University
Langley, British Columbia

Molly Westland, RN, BScN, MN
Chair, School of Community Development and
  Health
Sir Sandford Fleming College
Peterborough, Ontario

STUDENT REVIEWERS

Understanding that students are the most important group of users of this textbook, we sought to involve students directly in the review process. We believe our processes were unique to textbook development and ones that we will repeat. Students contributed insightful and professional reviews and raised new matters from their perspectives that we applied to the final product. A special thank you to the following University of Northern British Columbia nursing students:

Diana Almeida
Renee Beauchamp
Connie-Lynn Fiola
Stephanie Friesen
Elisa Hall
Megan Holland
Sarah A. Lymburner
Ranveeer Minhas
Annick McIntosh
Jayde Neufeld
Daniel N. Polysou
Chad Ridsdale

PREFACE

PREFACE TO THE INSTRUCTOR

Leading and managing are two essential expectations of all professional nurses and are more important than ever in today's rapidly changing health care system. To lead and manage successfully, nurses must possess not only knowledge and skills but also a caring and compassionate attitude. After all, leading and managing are both about people.

Volumes of information on leadership and management principles can be found in nursing, health care administration, business, and general literature. The numerous journals in each of these fields offer research and opinion articles focused on improving leaders' and managers' abilities. The previous US editions of this text demonstrated that learners, faculty, and nurses in practice found that a text that synthesized applicable knowledge and related it to contemporary practice was useful. Whereas clinical nursing textbooks offer exercises and assignments designed to provide opportunities for learners to apply theory to patients, nursing leadership and management textbooks traditionally offered limited opportunities of this type. We changed that tradition by incorporating application exercises within the text and linking this text to a Web site (*Evolve*) where resources such as case studies exemplify a chapter's point. A chapter on patient safety was included because of the critical importance it has in the way leaders and managers must make decisions. Protecting the patient is an obligation of all who engage in patient care. A chapter on workplace violence and incivility was included because of their prevalence in the workplace and their threat to patient safety, personnel safety, retention, and recruitment.

This book results from our continued strong belief in the need for a text that focuses in a distinctive way on the nursing leadership and management issues of today and tomorrow. We continue to find that we are not alone in this belief. We took seriously the various comments by faculty and learners offered in person or heard from by e-mail. This first Canadian edition conveys important and timely information to users as they focus on the critical roles of leading, managing, and following.

CONCEPT AND PRACTICE COMBINED

Innovative in both content and presentation, *Leading and Managing in Canadian Nursing* merges theory, research, and practical application in key leadership and management areas. Our overriding concern in this edition remains to create a text that, while well-grounded in theory and concept, presents the content in a way that is real. Wherever possible, we use real-world examples from the continuum of today's health care settings to illustrate the concepts. Because each chapter contributor focuses on synthesizing the assigned content, you will find no lengthy quotations in these chapters. We have made every effort to make the content as engaging, inviting, and interesting as possible. Reflecting our view of the real world of nursing leadership and management today, the following themes pervade the text:

- Every role within nursing has the basic concern for safe, effective care for the people we exist for—our patients and clients.
- The focus of health care is shifting from the hospital to the community.
- Patients and the health care workforce are becoming increasingly culturally diverse.
- Today, virtually every nurse leads, manages, and follows, regardless of title or position.
- The patient plays a central role in the delivery of nursing and health care.
- Communication, collaboration, team building, and other interpersonal skills form the foundation of effective nursing leadership and management.
- Change continues at a rapid pace in health care and society in general.
- Movement toward evidence-based and evidence-informed practices is critical to the delivery of effective nursing care and is long overdue.
- An anticipation of health care delivery over the next several years will rely on the above themes for nurses.

DIVERSITY OF PERSPECTIVES

Contributors are recruited from diverse settings, roles, and geographical areas, enabling them to offer a broad perspective on the critical elements of nursing leadership and management roles. To help bridge the gap often found between nursing education and nursing practice, some contributors were recruited from academia and others from practice settings. This blend not only contributes to the richness of this text but also conveys a sense of oneness in nursing. The historical "gap" between education and service must become a sense of a continuum and not a chasm.

AUDIENCE

This book is primarily designed for undergraduate learners in nursing leadership and management courses. Because of the text's strong Canadian content, portions of the text may inform nurses engaged in graduate studies. In addition, we know that nurses in practice, who had not anticipated formal leadership and management roles in their careers, use this text to capitalize on their own real-life experiences as a way to develop greater understanding about leading and managing and the important role of following. Because today's learners are more visually oriented than past learners, we have incorporated illustrations, boxes, and a functional full-colour design to stimulate interest and maximize learning. In addition, numerous examples and A Challenge at the outset of each chapter provide relevance to the real world of nursing.

ORGANIZATION

We have organized this text around issues that are key to the success of professional nurses in today's constantly changing health care environment.

First, it is important to understand the core concepts of leading and managing and how the theories and foci differ from each other. For example, headship (holding a formal position or title) does not always mean that person is demonstrating leadership. Next, nurses should understand key concepts as they relate to leading and managing. You will find key organizational information that ranges from our chief concern of patient centredness to a basic understanding about the types of organizations delivering care to the changing demands for quality, technology, and cost-effectiveness. Patient relationships influence how to deliver care and relationships with staff. Cultural diversity does not focus so much on understanding diversities of patients (appropriate for clinical textbooks) as it does on understanding and valuing diversities in employees (critical to leading and managing) and the influence of diverse staff on diversities of patients. The text then transitions from the critical elements of teams and how they interact to accomplish work to the individual expectations and influences we must have throughout our careers.

Because repetition plays a crucial role in how well learners learn and retain new content, some topics appear in more than one chapter and in more than one section. For example, several of the chapters in this text address the issue of disruption in the workplace. The issue of workplace disruptions or violence are so prevalent in today's health care world that we have devoted a chapter to the issue to pull several key points together. We have also made an effort to express a variety of different views on some topics, as is true in the real world of nursing. This diversity of views in the real world presents a constant challenge to leaders and managers, who address the critical tasks of creating positive workplaces so that those who provide direct care thrive and continuously improve the patient experience.

DESIGN

The functional full-colour design is used to emphasize and identify the text's many teaching and learning strategies, which are featured to enhance learning. Full-colour photographs not only add visual interest but also provide visual reinforcement of concepts, such as body language and the changes occurring in contemporary health care settings. Figures elucidate and depict concepts and activities described in the text graphically.

TEACHING AND LEARNING STRATEGIES

The numerous teaching and learning strategies featured in this text are designed both to stimulate learners' interest and to provide constant reinforcement throughout the learning process. In addition, the visually appealing, full-colour design itself serves a learning purpose. Colour is used consistently throughout the text to help the reader identify the various chapter elements described in the following sections.

CHAPTER OPENER ELEMENTS

- The introductory paragraph briefly describes the purpose and scope of the chapter.
- *Objectives* articulate the chapter's learning goals, typically at the application level or higher.
- *A Challenge* presents a contemporary nurse's real-world concern related to the chapter's focus.

ELEMENTS WITHIN THE CHAPTERS

Glossary Terms appear in colour type in each chapter. Definitions appear in the Glossary at the end of the text.

Exercises stimulate learners to think critically about how to apply chapter content to the workplace and other real-world situations. They provide experiential reinforcement of key leading and managing skills. Exercises are highlighted within a full-colour box and are numbered sequentially within each chapter to facilitate using them as assignments or activities.

Research Perspectives and *Literature Perspectives* illustrate the relevance and applicability of current scholarship to practice. Research Perspectives always appear in boxes with a "magnifying lens" icon in the upper left corner. Literature Perspectives always appear in boxes with a "book" icon in the upper left corner.

Theory Boxes provide a brief description of relevant theory and key concepts. Theory Boxes always appear with a "thought bubble" icon in the upper left corner.

Numbered boxes contain lists, tools such as forms and work sheets, and other information relevant to chapter content that learners will find useful and interesting.

END-OF-CHAPTER ELEMENTS

A Solution provides an effective method to handle the real-life situations set forth in *A Challenge*.

The Evidence contains one example of evidence related to the chapter's content or it contains a summary of what the literature shows to be evidence related to the topic.

Need to Know Now summarizes the most critical key points for new graduates in preparation for their transition to the workforce.

Chapter Checklists summarize key concepts from the chapter in both paragraph and itemized list form.

Tips offer practical guidelines for learners to follow in applying some aspect of the information presented in each chapter.

References provide the learner with a list of key sources for further reading on topics found in the chapter.

OTHER TEACHING AND LEARNING STRATEGIES

The *Glossary* contains a comprehensive list of definitions of all boldfaced terms used in the chapters.

COMPLETE TEACHING AND LEARNING PACKAGE

In addition to the text *Leading and Managing in Canadian Nursing*, Instructor Resources are provided online through *Evolve* (http://evolve.elsevier.com/Canada/Yoder-Wise/leading/). These resources are designed to help instructors present the material in this text. They include the following assets:

- **PowerPoint Slides** for each chapter with lecture notes where applicable (over 600 slides total)
- **ExamView Test Bank** with over 750 multiple-choice questions.

Rationales are based on NCLEX Competencies. Answers and text page reference(s) are also provided.

- **Instructor's Manual**
  - Chapter Objectives
  - Chapter Outline
  - Terms to Know
  - Teaching Suggestions
  - Instructions for Text Chapter Exercises
  - Skills Checklist
  - Discussion/Essay Questions
  - Experiential Exercises and Learning Activities
  - Suggested Guest Speakers
- **Application Activities and Answers** for each chapter
- **Case Studies** for each chapter
- **Questions to Consider** for each chapter
- **Exercise Answers** for each chapter
- **Image Collection** (over 50 images)

Student Resources can also be found online through *Evolve* (http://evolve.elsevier.com/Canada/Yoder-Wise/leading/). These resources provide students with additional tools for learning and include the following assets:

- **Sample Cover Letters and Résumés**
- **Suggested Readings and Internet Resources**

As a professional nurse in today's changing health care system, you will need strong leadership and management skills more than ever, regardless of your specific role. You will also need to be an independent, dependable follower. The first edition of *Leading and Managing in Canadian Nursing* not only provides the conceptual knowledge you will need but also offers practical strategies to help you hone the various skills so vital to your success as a leader and manager.

Because repetition is a key strategy in learning and retaining new information, you will find many topics discussed in more than one chapter. In addition, as in the real world of nursing, you will often find several different views expressed on a single topic. This repetition reinforces ideas and illustrates how one concept has multiple applications. Rather than referring you to another portion of the text, the key information is provided within the specific chapter, but perhaps in less depth. Because leading and managing are skills that require specific situation considerations, you can see why such a diversity of views exists.

To help you make the most of your learning experience, try the following strategy. Read the opening paragraph of each chapter. This preview should create a context for your reading. The *Objectives* suggest what your accomplishments should be by the time you conclude the chapter. Look at the end of the chapter for the checklist of the key points. *A Challenge* allows you to "hear" a real-life situation and always asks what you think you would do if you were the nurse (*A Solution*, at the end of the chapter, examines what the nurse did in the situation and asks you to think about how that fits for you and why). The introduction and subsequent content, like any text, provide critical information. For some learners, it is useful to skim those headings and the box content to gain an overall sense of the concepts inherent in the chapter. For others, reading and reflecting from the beginning of the chapter to the end might be useful. The material in boxes (boxes, tables, *Research Perspectives*, *Literature Perspectives*, and *Theory Boxes*) is designed to augment understanding of the content in the text narrative. *The Evidence* at the end of the chapters highlights what we know in at least one case about the topic. The checklist at the end of each chapter highlights the key points the chapter presented, and tips illustrate ways to apply the content just studied. After you complete each chapter, stop and think about what the chapter conveyed. What does it mean for you as a leader, follower, and manager? How do the chapter's content and your interaction with it relate to the other chapters you have already completed? How might you briefly synthesize the content for a non-nurse friend? Reading the chapter, restating its key points in your own words, and completing the text exercises and online activities will go far to help you make the content truly your own.

We think you will find leading and managing to be an exciting, challenging field of study, and we have made every attempt to reflect that belief in the design and approach of this edition.

LEARNING AIDS

The first edition of *Leading and Managing in Canadian Nursing* incorporates important tools to help you learn about leading and managing and apply your new knowledge to the real world. The next few pages graphically point out how to use these study aids to your best advantage.

The vivid full-colour chapter opener *photographs* and other photographs throughout the text help convey each chapter's key message while providing a glimpse into the real world of leading and managing in nursing.

The *introductory paragraph* tells you what you can expect to find in the chapter. To help set the stage for your study of the chapter, read it first and then summarize in your own words what you expect to gain from the chapter.

The list of *Objectives* helps you focus on the key information you should be able to apply after having studied the chapter.

In *A Challenge*, practising nurse leaders or managers offer their real-world views of a concern related to the chapter. Has a nurse you know had similar or dissimilar challenges?

A CHALLENGE

Ann, a nurse manager at Seaview Home Health Care, had previously worked in a large urban hospital system as a staff nurse. When Ann moved to Seaview, she took a staff nurse position in home health care and was promoted to nurse manager within the first year. On her team, care provision was disjointed and ineffective, and client and nurse satisfaction levels were low. Moreover, issues were evident in the areas of delegation and support for health care assistants, and family support and teaching were not consistently a part of nursing practice. After several months of assessing how nurses worked and learning which resources were available to support their practice,

Ann determined that it would be beneficial to redesign how care was delivered. Patient-centred care was a model of care that Ann was familiar with at the large city hospital where she had previously worked, but is was not a model that had been used at Seaview. Ann wondered if she could adapt the model used in the hospital to make positive differences in client outcomes and the delivery of care in home health care nursing.

What do you think you would do if you were Ann?

Most chapters contain at least one *Research Perspective* or *Literature Perspective* box that you can identify by the respective "magnifying glass" or "book" icon in the upper left corner. These boxes summarize articles of interest and point out their relevance and applicability to practice. Check the journal that the article came from to find a list of indexing terms to help you locate additional and even more recent articles on the same topic.

RESEARCH PERSPECTIVE

Resource: Klein, C., Granados, D., Salas, E., et al. (2009). Does team building work? *Small Group Research, 40,* 191–222. doi:10.1177/1046496408328821

The authors undertook an extensive meta-analysis of team-building research that focused on four specific components of teams: goal setting, interpersonal relationships, problem solving, and role clarification. The meta-analysis included 103 articles published between 1950 and 2007 and expanded the original work conducted in 1999. The outcomes measured were cognitive, affective, process, and performance based. The results suggested that team-building activities have a moderately positive effect across all team outcomes, whereas the strongest effect existed for goal setting and role clarification. The size of the team can also be important, and teams of 10 or fewer members seem to have more success.

These findings indicated that most work teams need to be limited in size (with 10 or fewer members per group) and that the focus when forming the team is on clarifying the goals of the team and the role of each team member.

Implications for Practice
The implications of this meta-analysis are important for nursing practice. How often do we find ourselves in teams of more than 10 individuals? Is this really a team or a group of individuals who have come together to address or provide input on an issue? Often, when a team is formed, we look to people we like to work with, who think the same way we do, and who have a similar set of skills that we do. A team should be formed based on the knowledge and skills required to address the issue. When a team has varying skills and backgrounds, it is very helpful to take the time to clarify roles, set team goals, and use tools that help with problem solving. Try these strategies (or suggest to the leader to try these strategies) the next time you are asked to be part of a team.

LITERATURE PERSPECTIVE

Resource: Kouzes, J. M., & Posner, B. Z. (2007). *The leadership challenge* (4th ed.). San Francisco, CA: Jossey-Bass, John Wiley & Sons.

Kouzes and Posner's (2007) Leadership Practices Framework focuses on how leaders—whether formal or informal—can mobilize people to get extraordinary things done. For example, informal leaders such as novice nurses can guide others along pioneering journeys to phenomenal accomplishments. The research and work that Kouzes and Posner have done establish relationships as the core of leading any change or initiative. Five key aspects of establishing and maintaining relationships constitute the heart of this leadership model:

- **Model the way:** Credibility is the foundation of leadership. It is established by consistently *doing what you say you will do* or by *setting the example* for the other team members.
- **Inspire a shared vision:** Imagine exciting and ennobling possibilities, and enlist others in these dreams through positive attitude, excitement, and hard work.
- **Challenge the process:** Seek innovative ways to change, grow, and improve—experiment and take risks.

- **Enable others to act:** Foster collaboration by promoting cooperation and building trust. Create a sense of reciprocity or give and take. Establish a sense of "We're all in this together."
- **Encourage the heart:** Novice leaders encourage their constituents to carry on. They keep hope and determination alive, recognize contributions, and celebrate victories.

When nurses use this model to approach leadership, they can strengthen their skills. Each of the examples above provides a way for new, emerging, and established leaders to remain committed to the team with which they work.

Implications for Practice
Each of us has leadership qualities that we bring to every encounter. Think about using the strategies for each of the practices in dealing with patients, families, peers, co-workers, and the team. If each of us consciously engages in "doing what we say we will do" and "setting examples," imagine the positive impact this would have on ourselves and others. The five leadership practices speak to the core of the profession of nursing.

Most chapters contain a *Theory Box* to highlight and summarize pertinent theoretical concepts.

THEORY BOX
Theory X/Theory Y

THEORY/CONTRIBUTOR	KEY IDEA	APPLICATION TO PRACTICE
McGregor (1960)	**Theory X:** Authoritarian • People do not like to work. • People need to have the threat of punishment. • People want to be told what to do.	This style might be useful when quick action or critical decisions must be made in which everyone must perform in the same way. In general, it is ineffective with professionals and creates workplace issues. However, in situations such as violence, this strategy may be necessary.
	Theory Y: Participative • Work is natural, and people like to work. • People use self-control. • People accept responsibility. • People like to solve problems.	This style might be useful when sufficient time is available or when the group must agree to a plan. In general, this approach is effective in health care and helps reinforce the concept of team. It is especially effective when a group is dealing with a quality initiative.

Every chapter contains numbered *Exercises* that challenge you to think critically about concepts in the text and apply them to real-life situations.

Key terms appear in boldface type throughout the chapter. (A list of all key terms used in the chapter appears at the start of the chapter and the *Glossary* at the end of the text contains a list of their definitions.)

The *boxes* in every chapter highlight key information such as lists and contain forms, work sheets, and self-assessments to help reinforce chapter content.

BOX 23-1   ASSESSING THE DEGREE OF CONFLICT RESOLUTION

1. Quality of decisions?
   a. How creative are resulting plans?
   b. How practical and realistic are they?
   c. How well were intended goals achieved?
   d. What surprising results were achieved?
2. Quality of relationships?
   a. How much understanding has been created?
   b. How willing are people to work together?
   c. How much mutual respect, empathy, concern, and cooperation has been generated?

The *tables* that appear throughout the text provide convenient capsules of information for your reference.

TABLE 15-2   NURSING STAFF MIX DECISION-MAKING FRAMEWORK

COMPONENT	SELECTED CRITERIA
Patient factors	Complexity of care needs Predictability of outcomes Risk of negative outcomes
Care provider competencies	Education Experience Expertise
Practice environments	Availability of and access to resources including support for nurses, policies, procedures, care pathways and protocols to guide clinical decision-making

The numerous full-colour *illustrations* visually reinforce key concepts.

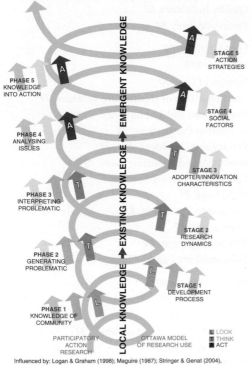

Influenced by: Logan & Graham (1998); Maguire (1987); Stringer & Genat (2004), © 2006 by Campbell

Each chapter ends with these features:

A Solution provides an effective method to handle the situation presented in *A Challenge*.

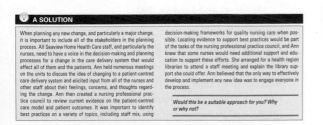

A SOLUTION

When planning any new change, and particularly a major change, it is important to include all of the stakeholders in the planning process. All Seaview Home Health Care staff, and particularly the nurses, need to have a voice in the decision-making and planning processes for a change in the care delivery system that would affect all of them and the patients. Ann held numerous meetings on the units to discuss the idea of changing to a patient-centred care delivery system and elicited input from all of the nurses and other staff about their feelings, concerns, and thoughts regarding the change. Ann then created a nursing professional practice council to review current evidence on the patient-centred care model and patient outcomes. It was important to identify best practices on a variety of topics, including staff mix, using decision-making frameworks for quality nursing care when possible. Locating evidence to support best practices would be part of the tasks of the nursing professional practice council, and Ann knew that some nurses would need additional support and education to support these efforts. She arranged for a health region librarian to attend a staff meeting and explain the library support she could offer. Ann believed that the only way to effectively develop and implement any new idea was to engage everyone in the process.

Would this be a suitable approach for you? Why or why not?

The Evidence identifies and discusses evidence-based research or best practices related to material in the chapter.

THE EVIDENCE

· Nurses who are involved in collective action and who work in organizations where shared governance is practised describe greater job satisfaction and empowerment.

· Nurses who experience a sense of empowerment in the workplace consider that their organization provides a higher quality of care and are more satisfied with the quality of their nursing practice.

Need to Know Now is designed to summarize what the authors think is expected of most new graduates in their first professional positions.

The *Chapter Checklist* provides a quick summary of key points in the chapter. To help you keep in mind the broad themes of the chapter, read it immediately *before* you start reading the chapter. Reading it afterward reinforces the key points.

The *Tips* offer guidelines to follow for each chapter before applying the information presented in the chapter.

NEED TO KNOW NOW

■ Understand and respect the individual needs of the different generations of nurses currently working together in health care settings.
■ Engage in a unit-based, shared-governance council inclusive of staff, allowing for empowerment.

■ Provide professional development opportunities and support for furthering education.
■ Encourage, support, and model the use of evidence-informed practice.
■ Participate in the rewarding and recognition of nursing staff.

CHAPTER CHECKLIST

The role of the nurse manager is multi-faceted and complex. Integrating clinical concerns with management functions, synthesizing leadership abilities with management requirements, and addressing human concerns while maintaining efficiency are the challenges facing the nurse manager. Thus, the nurse manager's role is to ensure effective operation of a defined area, contribute to the overall mission of the organization, and create an environment that supports quality of care for patients.
· The five basic functions of a manager are as follows:
  · Establishes and communicates goals and objectives

· Organizes, analyzes, and divides work into tasks
· Motivates and communicates
· Analyzes, appraises, and interprets performance and measurements
· Develops people, including self
· A nurse manager is responsible for the following:
  · Relationships with those above themselves, peers, and staff for whom they are accountable
  · Professionalism
  · Management of resources

TIPS FOR IMPLEMENTING THE ROLE OF NURSE MANAGER

· Aspects of the role of the nurse manager include being a leader as well as a follower. To be effective in the role, the nurse manager must be dedicated to the following:
  · A management philosophy that values people

· A commitment to patient-focused quality of care outcomes that include both evidence-informed processes and patient health outcomes
· The desire for ongoing learning about health care change and its effect on the nurse manager's role and functions

The *Glossary* at the end of the text lists in alphabetical order all the terms that are boldfaced blue in the text.

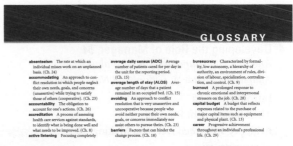

GLOSSARY

absenteeism The rate at which an individual misses work on an unplanned basis. (Ch. 24)
accommodating An approach to conflict resolution in which people neglect their own needs, goals, and concerns (unassertive) while trying to satisfy those of others (cooperative). (Ch. 23)
accountability The obligation to account for one's actions. (Ch. 26)
accreditation A process of assessing health care services against standards, to identify what is being done well and what needs to be improved. (Ch. 8)
active listening Focusing completely

average daily census (ADC) Average number of patients cared for per day in the unit for the reporting period. (Ch. 15)
average length of stay (ALOS) Average number of days that a patient remained in an occupied bed. (Ch. 15)
avoiding An approach to conflict resolution that is very unassertive and uncooperative because people who avoid neither pursue their own needs, goals, or concerns immediately nor assist others to pursue theirs. (Ch. 23)
barriers Factors that can hinder the change process. (Ch. 18)

bureaucracy Characterized by formality, low autonomy, a hierarchy of authority, an environment of rules, division of labour, specialization, centralization, and control. (Ch. 9)
burnout A prolonged response to chronic emotional and interpersonal stressors on the job. (Ch. 28)
capital budget A budget that reflects expenses related to the purchase of major capital items such as equipment and physical plant. (Ch. 13)
career Progressive achievement throughout an individual's professional life. (Ch. 29)

Each of these sections is designed to help learners transfer the words of the text into a personal understanding about what leading, managing, and following mean. Achieving success in those roles helps nurses to be effective team members and to contribute to positive patient care outcomes.

CONTENTS

PART 1: CORE CONCEPTS

1 Leading, Managing, and Following, *3*
Maura MacPhee

Introduction, *4*
Personal Attributes Needed to Lead, Manage, and Follow, *7*
Theory Development in Leading, Managing, and Following, *9*
The Promise of Complexity Science, *12*
Leading, Following, and Managing Competencies, *14*
Leading, Managing, and Following During Complex Times, *17*
Conclusion, *18*

2 Patient Focus, *23*
Sandra Regan and Lyle G. Grant

Safe, Competent, and Ethical Practice, *24*
Patient-Centered Care, *25*
Patient Safety, *26*
Nursing-Sensitive Outcomes, *30*
Conclusion, *31*

3 Developing the Role of Leader, *36*
Michael L. Evans
Adapted by Angela J. Gillis

What Is a Leader?, *37*
The Practice of Leadership, *39*
Leadership Development, *42*
Developing Leaders in the Emerging Workforce, *44*
Surviving and Thriving as a Leader, *46*
The Nurse as Leader, *47*

4 Developing the Role of Manager, *54*
Angela L. Stalbaum and Ana M. Valadez
Adapted by Wendy A. Gifford and Nancy Lefebre

Introduction, *55*
The Management Role, *56*
Evidence-Informed Decision Making, *58*
Mentoring, *59*
Organizational Culture, *59*
Day-to-Day Management Challenges, *59*
Managing Health Care Settings, *60*
Managing Resources, *62*
Informatics, *62*
Budgets, *63*

Quality Indicators, *63*
Professionalism, *64*

5 Legal Issues, *69*
Lyle G. Grant

Sources of Law, *70*
The Regulation of Health Care Workers, *71*
Implications and Liability, *72*
Leadership Perspectives, *74*
Privacy and Confidentiality, *77*
Protective and Reporting Laws, *79*
Labour and Employment, *80*
Drug Laws, *81*
Consent to Treatment, *82*
Malpractice, *82*
Risk Management, *84*
Distinguishing Law and Ethics, *85*

6 Ethical Issues, *90*
Sandra A. Pike-MacDonald

Introduction, *91*
The Relational Context of Ethics, *91*
Relational Ethics, *92*
The Principles of Bioethics, *93*
Code of Ethics for Nurses, *96*
The Interdependent Environment of Nursing, *97*
Defining Ethical Problems for Nurse Managers, *98*
Ethics Committees, *99*
A Model for Ethical Decision Making for Nurse Managers and Leaders, *100*
Conclusion, *101*

7 Making Decisions and Solving Problems, *105*
Ena L. Howse

Introduction, *106*
Problem Solving and Decision Making, *106*
Intellectual Processing in Problem Solving and Decision Making, *107*
Factors That Affect the Quality of Decisions, *109*
Appling the Problem-Solving Process, *110*
Decision-Making Models, *112*
Group Decision Making, *115*
Conclusion, *120*

8 Health Care Organizations, *125*
Ena L. Howse and Lyle G. Grant

Introduction, *126*
The Canadian Health Care System, *126*
Health Care Services Funding, *127*
Organizing the Delivery of Care, *129*
Approaches to Delivering Care, *130*
Types and Classifications of Health Care Services, *132*
A Theoretical Perspective, *136*
Internal Forces Influencing Health Care Organizations, *137*
External Forces Influencing Health Care Organizations, *137*
Health Human Resources, *142*
Conclusion, *144*

9 Understanding and Designing Organizational
Structures, *149*
Mary E. Mancini
Adapted by Carol A. Wong

Introduction, *150*
Mission, *150*
Vision, *152*
Philosophy, *152*
Organizational Culture, *152*
Factors Influencing Organizational Development, *154*
Characteristics of Organizational Structures, *155*
Bureaucracy, *157*
Types of Organizational Structures, *159*
Analyzing Organizations, *164*
Emerging Fluid Relationships, *164*

10 Cultural Diversity in Health Care, *170*
Karen A. Esquibel and Dorothy A. Otto
Adapted by Yolanda Babenko-Mould

Introduction: Concepts and Principles, *171*
Cultural Diversity in Health Care Organizations, *173*
Cultural Diversity and Prejudice, *175*
Culture and Theoretical Models, *176*
Individual and Societal Factors, *178*
Dealing Effectively with Cultural Diversity, *179*
Conclusion, *180*

11 Power, Politics, and Influence, *185*
Maura MacPhee

Introduction, *186*
Key Powerful Canadian Nurse Leaders, *187*
Types of Power, *187*
Empowerment Theories and Nursing, *189*
Power Strategies, *194*
Exercising Power and Influence: Policy and Politics, *195*
Policy Advocacy and Nursing, *199*

PART 2: MANAGING RESOURCES

12 Caring, Communicating, and Managing
with Technology, *207*
Janis B. Smith and Cheri Hunt
Adapted by Kathy L. Rush

Introduction, *208*
Types of Technologies, *209*
Information Systems, *213*
Communication Technology, *217*
Informatics, *218*
Evidence-Informed Practice, *221*
Patient Safety, *222*
Impact of Clinical Information Systems, *223*
Successfully Implementing Health Information
    Technology, *225*
Future Trends and Professional Issues, *226*
Summary, *233*

13 Managing Costs and Budgets, *238*
Trudi B. Stafford
Adapted by Arden Krystal

Introduction, *239*
What Escalates Health Care Costs?, *239*
How Is Health Care Financed?, *240*
Approaches to Health Care Financing, *241*
Using Activity to Inform the Budget, *242*
The Changing Heath Care Economic Environment, *242*
Bending the Cost Curve, *243*
What Does the Health Care Economic Environment
    Mean for Nursing Practice?, *243*
Cost-Conscious Nursing Practices, *243*
Budgets, *247*
The Budgeting Process, *250*
Managing the Unit-Level Budget, *251*

14 Care Delivery Strategies, *256*
Susan Sportsman
Adapted by Heather MacMillan

Introduction, *257*
Case Method (Total Patient Care), *257*
Functional Nursing, *258*
Team Nursing, *260*
Primary Nursing, *262*
Nursing Case Management, *266*
Care Strategies That Influence Care Delivery, *268*
Conclusion, *272*

15 Staffing and Scheduling, *279*
Susan Sportsman
Adapted by Deb A. Gordon

Introduction, *280*
The Staffing Process, *280*
Forecasting Unit Staffing Requirements, *292*
Scheduling, *294*
Evaluating Unit Staffing and Productivity, *295*
Conclusion, *298*

16 Selecting, Developing, and Evaluating Staff, *302*
Diane M. Twedell
Adapted by Arden Krystal

Introduction, *303*
Role Concepts and the Position Description, *303*
Selecting Staff, *304*
Developing Staff, *306*
Performance Appraisals, *307*
Performance Appraisal Tools, *309*

PART 3: CHANGING THE STATUS QUO

17 Strategic Planning and Goal Setting, *319*
Mary Ellen Clyne
Adapted by Sandra Regan

Introduction, *320*
Strategic Planning, *320*

18 Leading Change, *331*
Mary Ann T. Donohue
Adapted by Suzanne Johnston

Introduction, *332*
Context of the Change Environment, *332*
Planned Change Using Linear Approaches, *334*
Nonlinear Change: Chaos Theory and Learning
    Organization Theory, *336*
Major Change Management Functions, *337*
Responses to Change, *340*
Strategies, *342*
Roles and Functions of Change Agents, *344*
Principles, *346*
Conclusion, *347*

19 Building Teams Through Communication and
    Partnerships, *351*
Karren Kowalski
Adapted by Colleen A. McKey

Introduction, *352*
Groups and Teams, *352*
Team Development, *355*

Qualities of a Team Member, *357*
Creating Synergy, *358*
Generational Differences Among Team Members, *359*
The Value of Team Building, *359*
Conflict and Teams, *360*
Communication, *362*
Managing Emotions, *368*
Reflective Practice, *369*
The Role of Leadership in Team Success, *369*

20 Collective Nursing Advocacy, *374*
Susan M. Duncan

Introduction, *375*
Defining Collective Action and Advocacy, *375*
Nursing Organizations and Collective Action, *378*
Nursing Governance, *383*
Conclusion, *387*

21 Managing Quality and Risk, *391*
Victoria N. Folse
Adapted by Carol A. Wong

Introduction, *392*
Quality Management in Health Care, *392*
Benefits of Quality Management, *392*
Planning for Quality Management, *393*
Evolution of Quality Management, *393*
Quality Management and Quality Improvement
    Principles, *394*
The Quality Improvement Process, *396*
Quality Assurance, *403*
Risk Management, *404*
Conclusion, *407*

22 Translating Research into Practice, *411*
Margarete Lieb Zalon
*Adapted by Barbara Campbell, with contributions from
    Selvi Roy*

Introduction, *412*
Research Utilization, *414*
Evidence-Based Practice, *417*
Diffusion of Innovations, *421*
Translating Research into Practice, *423*
Evaluation of Evidence, *425*
Organizational Strategies, *428*
Issues for Nurse Managers and Leaders, *429*

PART 4: INTERPERSONAL AND PERSONAL SKILLS

Interpersonal

23 Understanding and Resolving Conflict, *439*
Victoria N. Folse
Adapted by Jayne Naylen McChesney and Heather D. Wilson

Introduction, *440*
Types of Conflict, *441*
Stages of Conflict, *442*
Categories of Conflict, *443*
Approaches to Conflict Resolution, *444*
Differences of Conflict-Handling Styles Among Nurses, *449*
The Role of the Leader, *450*
Mediation, *452*
Managing Lateral Violence and Bullying, *452*

24 Managing Personal/Personnel Problems, *457*
Karren Kowalski
Adapted by Jayne Naylen McChesney and Heather D. Wilson

Introduction, *458*
Personal/Personnel Problems, *458*
Documentation, *467*
Progressive Discipline, *468*
Termination, *468*
Conclusion, *469*

25 Workplace Violence and Incivility, *474*
Yolanda Babenko-Mould

Introduction, *475*
Defining Workplace Violence and Incivility, *475*
Prevention Strategies, *478*
Horizontal Violence: The Threat from Within, *480*
Conclusion, *482*

26 Practising and Leading in Interdisciplinary Settings, *486*
Erin Wilson

Introduction, *487*
Concepts and Definitions, *487*
The Rise of Distinct Disciplines, *488*
Scope of Practice, *488*
A Framework for Interprofessional Collaboration, *489*
Moving Forward in Collaborative Practice, *491*
Leading Interdisciplinary or Interprofessional Teams, *493*
Working "With" Versus "Alongside" Others, *495*
Conclusion, *495*

Personal

27 Role Transition, *499*
Diane M. Twedell
Adapted by Judy Boychuk Duchscher and Kandis Harris

Introduction, *500*
Types of Role Transitions, *501*
Roles: The ABCS of Understanding Roles, *504*
Role Transition Process, *505*
Strategies to Promote Role Transition, *505*
Conclusion, *511*

28 Self-Management: Stress and Time, *514*
Catherine A. Hill
Adapted by Shelley L. Cobbett

Introduction, *515*
Understanding Stress, *515*
Sources of Job Stress, *516*
Stress Management, *519*
Resolution of Stress, *523*
Time Management, *525*
Meeting Management, *530*
Conclusion, *531*

29 Managing Your Career, *535*
Debra Hagler
Adapted by Lyle G. Grant and Sarah E. Hanson

Introduction, *536*
A Framework, *536*
Career Development, *540*
Career Marketing Strategies, *541*
Data Assembly for Professional Portfolios, *546*
The Interview, *546*
Professional Development, *548*
Academic and Continuing Education, *549*
Certification, *551*
Professional Associations, *551*
A Model for Involvement, *552*
Conclusion, *555*

Future

30 Thriving for the Future, *558*
Patricia S. Yoder-Wise
Adapted by Sandra Regan and Lyle G. Grant

Introduction, *559*
Leadership Demands for the Future, *559*
Leadership Strengths for the Future, *560*
Visioning, *561*
Shared Vision, *562*
Projections for the Future, *563*
Nursing: Preparing for the Future, *564*
Implications, *565*
Conclusion, *565*

Core Concepts

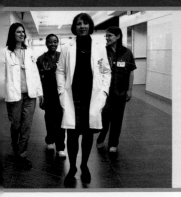

Leading, Managing, and Following

Maura MacPhee

Leading, managing, and following are integral to professional nursing practice. By engaging in constructive behaviours associated with these concepts, nurses can positively influence patient-care and organizational outcomes, regardless of their position title. By understanding the leadership competencies related to leading, managing, and following, the professional nurse can positively influence the quality of health care delivery.

OBJECTIVES

- Link leadership, management, and followership to key theories from a variety of disciplines, including psychology, sociology, management science, and organizational development.
- Identify key competencies associated with effective leadership, management, and followership.
- Examine practical applications associated with leadership, management, and followership.
- Relate personal attributes, such as emotional intelligence and appreciative inquiry, to the capacity of professional nurses to lead, manage, and follow.
- Recognize the challenges associated with leading, managing, and following in complex health care environments, such as those undergoing restructuring.

TERMS TO KNOW

appreciative inquiry (AI)	leadership	strengths-based leadership
authentic leadership	management	transactional leaders
complexity science	patient-centred care	transformational leadership
emotional intelligence (EI)	quality work environment	
followership	restructuring	

❓ A CHALLENGE

After Terry completed her graduate studies in nursing, she realized that she had a real interest in leadership. Terry had also done a graduate project on quality and safety that made her want to do more to ensure safe, quality-care delivery for her patients. This goal led Terry to a conversation with her supervisor, which led her to apply for her current position as nurse leader. Terry's current position was specifically created to address quality and safety in the workplace. Within six months of taking on the new leadership role, several changes to the hospital management structure affected her duties and responsibilities. The hospital went from three program coordinators to two. Terry became responsible for six change management initiatives within one year. The nurses told Terry, "There is too much for us to do. We don't know what is safe to do anymore."

What do you think you would do if you were this nurse leader?

INTRODUCTION

The Canadian Health Care System

The Canadian health care system is based on a vision of health care promotion, primary health care, and community-based care in home settings. The *Canada Health Act* is Canada's federal health legislation for publicly funded health insurance (medicare); it ensures that all Canadians have access to necessary hospitalization and physician care. The Act sets out five criteria for the delivery of insured health services: public administration, comprehensiveness, universality, portability, and accessibility (Health Canada, 2010). Canadians are proud of their public medicare system; in fact, the values underlying our single-payer health care system have become a symbol of our society's strong belief in universal access for all—regardless of ability to pay.

Another important aspect of Canada's approach to health care is our recognition that social determinants of health (such as education, justice, housing, and transit) influence quality of life. Canadians' desire to support social services, such as public housing, is perhaps a barometer of how we define quality of life (Canadian Health Services Research Foundation [CHSRF], 2012). A lack of food and housing, for instance, are strongly associated with health inequalities. Health is also influenced by *social exclusion*, a form of alienation experienced by particular groups (such as Aboriginal people). In Canada, nurses play an important role in helping people, particularly members of socially excluded groups, access the social determinants of health. Community health nurses, in particular, identify practices that decrease health and social inequalities as core competencies. Through advocacy, policy analysis, and political activities, all Canadian nurses can make a positive difference in the health of Canadians (CHSRF, 2012).

Although efforts have been made by a number of groups (e.g., governments, advocacy groups) to shift health care to the community and the home, the majority of health care funding and resources continues to be committed to hospital-based care. At the same time, public health coverage for services such as home care, long-term care, eye care, dentistry, and pharmaceuticals is sorely lacking (Simpson, 2012). Change is necessary. According to Jeffrey Simpson, a Canadian public policy journalist, we need to recognize that "a healthcare system that costs about $200 million a year in public and private money cannot continue as it is... the system is inadequately structured for an aging population and has costs that grow faster than government revenues" (Simpson, 2012, p. 3).

Despite our vision for a healthy and vibrant society, our health care system has problems. Among 30 Organisation for Economic Cooperation and Development (OECD) countries, Canada ranks twenty-third on some health care systems performance indicators. Our health care system lags behind with respect to timeliness of care delivery, the wait time to see family physicians and specialists, and the wait time in emergency departments. Among seven wealthy OECD countries (Australia, Canada, Germany, the Netherlands, New Zealand, the United Kingdom, and the United States), the Commonwealth Fund 2010 International Health Policy Survey showed that our health care system ranks second highest in cost and second last in performance (Canadian Nurses Association [CNA], 2013). Canada has been slowly slipping in its rankings, suggesting that our system is suffering from the "boiling frog" phenomenon. We need to truly examine our system to see where the problems lie—and nursing

TABLE 1-1 STRENGTHS-BASED NURSING LEADERSHIP PRINCIPLES

STRENGTHS-BASED NURSING LEADERSHIP PRINCIPLE	RELATED CONTENT
Strengths-based nursing leaders understand the whole system and the interrelationships among its parts.	Chapter 1: Complexity science
Strengths-based nursing leaders honour the uniqueness of individuals, teams, systems, and organizations.	Chapter 1: Emotional intelligence
Strengths-based nursing leaders create work environments that promote nurses' health and facilitate nurses' development.	Chapter 1: Quality work environments
Strengths-based nursing leaders understand the significance of appreciating multiple perspectives and striving for win-win collaboration.	Chapter 1: Collaborative leadership
Strengths-based nursing leaders recognize that people function best in environments that match their values and beliefs.	Chapter 1: Authentic leadership
Strengths-based nursing leaders understand that knowledge is power.	Chapter 11: Power and empowerment

can lead the charge to achieve the vision of health care promotion and community-based care. According to John G. Abbott, chief executive officer for the Health Council of Canada, "Canada's challenge ahead is to adjust priorities appropriately, ensuring our funding follows the needs of those who require care at home and in the community" (CNA, 2013, p. 2).

Strong nurse leadership is needed from the front line to the executive boardroom in all sectors (e.g., acute care, community, long-term care) to improve the quality and efficiency of health care (Needleman & Hassmiller, 2009). A recent article described "strengths-based" nursing leadership as the type of leadership most needed to shepherd systems transformation in the twenty-first century (Gottlieb, Gottlieb, & Shamian, 2012). According to the article's authors, this type of leadership is needed to "put people and communities at the centre of healthcare" and to promote "strong inter-professionalism and higher-quality, effective and efficient, cost-effective care with better health outcomes" (p. 39). Strengths-based leadership complements other, contemporary leadership styles that will be discussed throughout this book, such as transformational leadership. The premise of strengths-based leadership is that people are more productive when they build on their strengths rather than their weaknesses (Gottlieb, 2012). Nurse leaders, in particular, can exercise strengths-based leadership by creating and maintaining quality practice environments where nurses feel valued and supported by their organizations (MacPhee, Skelton-Green, Bouthillette, et al., 2011; O'Brien-Pallas, Tomblin Murphy, Shamian, et al., 2010). A summary of key strengths-based nursing leadership principles and links to related content in this chapter and Chapter 11 appear in Table 1-1.

Nursing in Canada

The nursing profession constitutes the backbone of the health care system, both in numbers and in its span of influence across the clinical spectrum. Bearing the responsibility of keeping patients safe requires vigilance, acute observation, knowledge of health care delivery processes, and a willingness to act—to engage with patients and families as well as other nurses, health disciplines, and agencies. This willingness and the way one engages in these actions constitute leading, managing, and following (Mendes & Stander, 2011; Riggio, Chaleff, & Lipman-Bluman, 2008).

As important as it is for nurses to ensure that patients have safe passage through the health care system maze, the functions they perform beyond the bedside also require nursing knowledge and values. For instance, nurses develop evidence-informed clinical protocols and design care delivery systems through initiatives such as Transforming Care at the Bedside (TCAB) (Chaboyer, McMurray, Johnson, et al., 2009). They also adapt to ever-changing shifts in human resources. As well, nurses influence policy related to health reform and lead social change movements. These activities expand the depth and breadth of nursing work, demanding even more sophisticated knowledge of ways to lead, manage, and follow.

At the heart of patient safety, care delivery design, policy development, and point-of-care clinical performance is a central tenet: nurses must apply critical thinking to critical actions in complex health care settings to achieve positive patient and organizational outcomes. Typically, nurses make decisions with others to collectively influence constructive change. The core work of nurses is making decisions and taking corresponding actions in engagement with others. This core work demands that nurses be leaders, managers, and followers at the point-of-care, unit, institutional, and even societal levels.

Too often, nurses new to the profession believe their ability to perform clinical procedures is what makes them appear professional to those receiving care, to their peers, or to the public. They might also believe that leadership is only for those holding management positions or that following means blindly adhering to the direction of others. These nurses fail to realize that their professional nursing image and success depend equally on their poise and influence on decision making as well as their ability to engage with others. These professional behaviours are the first lens through which patients, families, supervisors, and other health care providers view them and gain confidence in their abilities.

The way nurses lead, manage, and follow has changed over time. Formerly, nurses took direction unquestioningly from physicians or senior nurses (such as "head" or "charge" nurses). Today, the expectation has shifted from nurses being told what to do to a model of shared decision making and action in collaboration with others. Knowledge and the array of treatment interventions available to patients have grown beyond what a command-and-control model can accommodate in traditional hierarchical organizations. Moreover, patient acuity requires immediate and autonomous responses that are often different from responses that can be pre-assigned. Health care is now delivered in a collaborative and, often, an interdisciplinary manner, with select leadership and management roles (e.g., first-line nurse leaders) serving as information and care-coordination conduits. In clinical settings where technology is available, knowledge management, decision support, and social networking tools are used to reach beyond the confines of tradition-bound organizations and link professionals in different locations to solve complex care and health care system problems. Social networking, as used here, relates to webs of relationships supported by technology that can rapidly transmit and receive information. Social networking tools also provide a means for professional nurses to create a common voice and engage in collective action related to their areas of interest (MacPhee, Suryaprakash, & Jackson, 2009).

The study of leadership, management, and followership behaviour has never been more important to patients (who face making complex health decisions) and to the nursing discipline in an era of major health reform. Each nurse—from point-of-care nurses to those in expanded roles—is accountable for making the best use of scarce nursing resources. Professional nurses are expected to meet their organization's mission and goals, efficiently manage limited health care resources, avert medical errors, achieve patient satisfaction, and ensure positive patient outcomes. In addition, organizations expect nurses to contain costs when delivering patient care, contribute to quality improvement and change initiatives, and interact with other health care team members to resolve clinical and organizational problems. These expectations mean that each nurse must be effective in leading, managing, and following.

This chapter presents various perspectives on the concepts of leading (leadership), managing (management), and following (followership). These concepts are integrated, which means that nurses lead, manage, and follow concurrently. Leading, managing, and following are not activities that are bound to certain types of nursing roles only—all nurses lead, manage, and follow. Before we examine each concept more closely to highlight their differences, we begin with the operational definitions for *leadership*, *management*, and *followership*.

- **Leadership** is the process of engaging and influencing others (Yukl, 2006). Strong leaders are associated with words such as visionary, energetic, inspirational, and innovative: they go beyond the status quo to make a difference for others. The Canadian Nurses Association's position statement on nursing leadership (2009) states that leadership "is about critical thinking, action and advocacy—and it happens in all roles and domains of nursing practice" (p. 1). Any nurse can be a nurse leader, no matter the personality type, gender, ethnicity, or age.
- **Management** is about getting the job done and ensuring that people have the necessary resources to get the job done (Yukl, 2006). Effective managers are able to set goals and objectives and ensure that they are met within established timelines and budgets. Management is traditionally associated with formal authority positions within organizations, but key management competencies, such as deciding how to allocate scarce resources, is important for all levels of nursing.

- Followership involves engaging with others who are leading or managing by contributing to the work that needs to be done (Yukl, 2006). Followers can promote team effectiveness, for instance, by maintaining collaborative work relationships, offering constructive criticism, and sharing leadership and management responsibilities. Effective followers know how to manage themselves (self-management), and they work well with others, particularly in today's complex health care environments where the emphasis is on interdisciplinary teamwork. According to Yukl (2006), important followership guidelines include the following: "Find out what you are expected to do; take the initiative to deal with problems; show appreciation and provide recognition when appropriate; and challenge flawed plans and proposals" (p. 138).

The collective behaviours that reflect leading, managing, and following enhance one another. All interdisciplinary health care providers, including professional nurses, experience situations each day in which they must lead, manage, and follow. Some formal nursing positions, such as charge nurse or nurse manager, require an advanced set of leading and managing know-how to establish organizational goals and objectives, oversee human resources, provide staff with performance feedback, facilitate change, and manage conflict to meet patient-care and organizational requirements. Other nursing positions demand the ability to shift between leading, managing, and following, almost on a moment-by-moment basis. For instance, nurses lead, manage, and follow in daily clinical practice through assignment making, patient and family problem solving, discharge planning, patient education, and coaching and mentoring staff.

EXERCISE 1-1

Using the definitions of *leadership*, *management*, and *followership*, imagine that you are faced with a critically ill patient whose family members are spread throughout the country. Some family members are holding vigil at the patient's side, whereas others are calling the patient-care unit incessantly, taking nurses away from other patient-care responsibilities. You recognize the family's concerns and you want to move from a reactive stance to a proactive position. How would you engage in solving this problem in a leader role? A manager role? A follower role? In which role would you be most comfortable? Least comfortable? Which role would lead to the best outcomes in this situation?

PERSONAL ATTRIBUTES NEEDED TO LEAD, MANAGE, AND FOLLOW

Strong leadership, management, and followership are associated with certain key personal attributes, such as ethical responsibility. A Canadian code of ethics document for registered nurses (CNA, 2008) articulates nursing values and the ethical responsibilities that apply to nurse interactions with patients and their families, the public, and other health care providers. Ethical individuals are not coercive or manipulative, and they collaborate with others. Nurses need to value the six fundamental ethical principles of beneficence, autonomy, truthfulness, confidentiality, justice, and integrity (Yeo, Moorhouse, Khan, et al., 2010).

Ethical leadership is based on a willingness to identify and act on complex problems in an ethical manner. Leadership can be misused when coercive relationships form and information and true goals are withheld. See Chapter 6 for an in-depth discussion on ethics.

An important attribute is how the nurse is in a relationship with the patient. Although members of health care organizations must always consider clinical and organizational goals and priorities, the underlying philosophy associated with excellent health care delivery is patient-centred care (Hobbs, 2009). This type of care includes patients and their family members in the design and delivery of health care at all levels. In one research study in Ontario, nurses in an orthopedic surgery and rheumatology unit adopted a patient-centred philosophy. Over a 24-month period, they gradually transformed their unit's culture and learned the following: "We cannot always fix situations for people, but we can be very helpful by how we are with people and by listening. . . . Our clinical care has improved because we know how to be with people while we are completing the tasks and assessments" (Mitchell, Bournes, & Hollett, 2006, p. 221). The Registered Nurses' Association of Ontario (RNAO, 2002) includes Best Practice Guidelines on its website (http://rnao.ca) that are based on "client/patient centred care." Patient focus and related concepts are discussed in Chapter 2.

Emotional intelligence (EI) is a key attribute closely aligned with individuals' capacity to know themselves and others. Some research has shown that emotionally intelligent leaders—possessing social skills, interpersonal competence, psychological maturity, and emotional awareness that help people harmonize to increase their value in the workplace—can influence staff retention and quality of care delivery (Smith, Profetto-McGrath, & Cummings, 2009). However, one Canadian study demonstrated that even high-EI leaders cannot offset the detrimental effects of **restructuring** (fundamental changes to an organization to achieve greater efficiency or profit) when they have too great a span of control. *Span of control* refers to the number of staff that directly reports to a leader. A large span of control impairs a leader's capacity to form close working relationships with staff (Lucas, Laschinger, & Wong, 2008). Neurobehavioural research involving the limbic system indicates that EI can be learned through educational programs and coaching that help individuals increase their self-awareness and better regulate their emotions (Feather, 2009). Although measuring EI has proven to be challenging, EI is considered "a potential new construct for nursing leadership as well as successful performance in health care settings" (Akerjordet & Severinsson, 2010, p. 363).

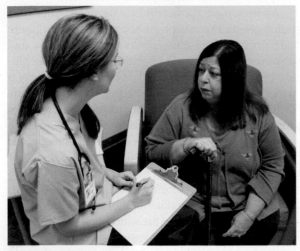

Being empathetic and showing sensitivity to the experiences of others helps nurse leaders develop their emotional intelligence.

Another key attribute is **appreciative inquiry (AI)**, which is associated with how we question and problem solve. AI arose from a field of study known as *positive organizational scholarship (POS)* (Whitney & Trosten-Bloom, 2010). AI is used at all levels (e.g., individual, group, and organizational) to engage people in identifying and accentuating positives within a context, such as a practice environment. Specifically, instead of focusing on the negative (i.e., seeing the glass as half empty), AI emphasizes the positive (i.e., seeing the glass as half full). Stefaniak (2007) described how an AI project in one children's hospital was used to create a practice environment of "nursing excellence." A US nursing study used AI to improve the patient hand-off process (Shendell-Falik, Feinson, & Mohr, 2007). Hand-offs occur between nurses when patients are transferred from one practice setting to another. Communication breakdown during transfer reports or hand-offs have been associated with adverse events. In the US nursing study, the researchers transformed the hand-off process using the 5-D cycle of AI: (1) definition, (2) discovery, (3) dream, (4) design, and (5) destiny. This cycle is similar to project planning or change management, but it uses a positive approach for engaging everybody in the project. "Using a strengths-based improvement process enabled nursing leaders to leverage the staff's ideas. Patient safety was enhanced and an empowered, exceptional work environment was created" (p. 103).

EXERCISE 1-2

1. You are a staff nurse, and your nurse leader has asked you to take part in a change management process involving shift-to-shift reporting. As a nurse with high emotional intelligence (EI), how will you lead, manage, and follow on this project? How will AI assist you?

2. In a private place at work, gather together a circle of colleagues. To promote EI (self-awareness and awareness of others), go around the circle in an open and honest fashion. Everybody needs a turn to speak. Ask the following AI questions:
   a. What does an excellent practice environment look like to you?
   b. What is working well for us in our practice environment?
   c. What can each of us do better to contribute to an excellent practice environment?
   d. What can we do together as a team to contribute to an excellent practice environment?

3. Prepare a sociogram. Make a list of all the individuals and relationships that are important to you at work (e.g., peers, leaders, patients, physicians). Start with your top ten. Using a Likert-like scale of 0 to 10 (0 = not at all; 10 = all the time), indicate how much support you provide on a regular basis. Support includes informational support, emotional support, physical support, and spiritual support. After filling out your list and noting levels of support for each individual and relationship, think about how you can raise your level of support for those individuals who are important to you. You can also fill out the Likert-like scale with respect to how much support you receive from these individuals. This exercise may be a stepping stone for team discussion with respect to workplace supports.

THEORY DEVELOPMENT IN LEADING, MANAGING, AND FOLLOWING

Theories have several important functions for the nursing profession. They propose relationships among concepts that can be scientifically tested. They also serve as analytic tools for understanding, explaining, and predicting phenomena of importance to professional nursing. They can add to our body of professional nursing knowledge and contribute to evidence-informed practices as well (Chinn & Kramer, 2007). Although leadership, management, and followership are intertwined concepts, distinct theories are associated with each of them. Our knowledge of these concepts is continuously evolving as the complexity of health care organizations grows. Many of the theories associated with these concepts originated from other disciplines, such as psychology, sociology, management science, and organizational development. Earlier theory-based research was often classified by its theoretical emphasis on either leader and manager characteristics, follower characteristics, or environmental and situational characteristics. More recently, complex research designs and statistical methods have resulted in theoretical frameworks that test the relationships among multiple characteristics (see Literature Perspective for an example). Leadership, management, and followership theories can also be classified based on interactional levels (e.g., dyadic, team, organizational) and power dynamics (e.g., empowerment theories). Nurse researchers are building on these theories to better understand how nurses can effectively lead, manage, and follow within complex health care environments. The sections that follow will discuss key theories of leadership, management, and followership. As mentioned, in many instances, the three concepts are closely connected.

LITERATURE PERSPECTIVE

Resource: Squires, M., Tourangeau, A., Laschinger, H., et al. (2010). The link between leadership and safety outcomes in hospitals. *Journal of Nursing Management, 18,* 914–925. http://dx.doi.org/10.1111/j.1365-2834.2010.01181.x

The purpose of this Canadian nursing study was to test and refine a theoretical model with proposed relationships among leadership, the quality of the work environment, the safety climate, interactional justice, and nurse and patient safety outcomes. The proposed model was based on social exchange theory and leader–member exchange theory. According to social exchange theory, if an individual receives something of value from another, the individual feels obligated to reciprocate in a manner of similar or greater value. Leader–member exchange theory is based on social exchange theory, but this theory focuses specifically on leader–follower exchange relationships. The model predicts that the quality of leader–follower exchanges is predictive of individual, group, and organizational outcomes. The research hypothesis of this study was that staff nurse perceptions of justice (synonymous with *fairness*) and resonant leadership styles would enhance the quality of the leader–nurse relationship, in turn positively influencing nurses' perceptions of the quality of the work environment and safety climate. *Resonant leadership* was defined as the behaviour of leaders who demonstrate high levels of emotional intelligence, govern their own emotions, and use empathy to build relationships. The researchers also defined quality work environment according to the Canadian Quality Worklife—Quality Healthcare Collaborative (2007). As cited in the study article, "a quality (healthy) work environment provides physical, cultural, psychosocial and work design conditions that maximize health and wellbeing" (p. 917). The nurse researchers used a tool that asked nurses to rate the quality of their work environments according to adequate staffing, communications, participation in decision making, clinical autonomy, scheduling flexibility, and professional development opportunities. Safety climate was defined and measured as nurses' perceptions of safety policies, practices, and procedures. Over 200 Ontario nurses completed the study surveys, and sophisticated data analyses provided support for the hypothesized model: interactional justice and resonant leadership style enhanced the quality of leader–follower relationships that in turn influenced nurses' perceptions of a safe, quality, work environment for staff and patients.

Implications for Practice

The study findings emphasized the importance of strong leader–follower relationships. By fostering relationships with staff that are perceived by staff as fair and emotionally astute, leaders can promote quality and healthy workplaces associated with best possible safety outcomes for nurses and staff. The researchers concluded: "To advocate for safe patient care, interactional justice needs to be part of leadership practices and decisions. This along with incorporating resonant skills of empathy, relating, listening and responding to concerns, will create an atmosphere of trust and respect which facilitates open dialogue and improves relationships between nurse leaders and their subordinates" (p. 922).

Leadership Theories

The Theory Box provides an overview of key leadership theories: from trait theories of the early 1900s to current transformational leadership theories and authentic leadership. Transformational leadership theories, such as full-range theory (Avolio & Yammarino, 2013), represent a shift in thinking about leadership and management. Research has shown that effective managers have characteristics similar to transactional leaders (also known as *contingent reward leaders*), one of the leadership styles within the full-range theory. In many health care organizations, management titles have been replaced with leadership titles. Trends in titles and terminology are being accompanied by concern for collaborative decision making, open communications, and other processes associated with safe, quality work environments. A joint position statement from the Canadian Nurses Association and the Canadian Federation of Nurses Unions (2006) stated the importance of a new vision for nursing leadership: "Nurses who are employers have a direct impact on nurses' work environments, but nurses who act as collaborators, communicators, mentors, role models, visionaries and advocates for quality care also play a leadership role" (p. 2).

THEORY BOX

Key Leadership Theories

THEORY/CONTRIBUTOR	KEY IDEA	APPLICATION TO PRACTICE
Trait Theories Trait theories were studied from 1900 to 1950. These theories are sometimes referred to as the *Great Man Theory*, from Aristotle's philosophy extolling the virtue of being "born" with leadership traits. Stogdill (1948) is usually credited as the pioneer of this school of thought.	Leaders have a certain set of physical and emotional characteristics that are crucial for inspiring others toward a common goal. Some theorists believe that traits are innate and cannot be learned; others believe that leadership traits can be developed in each individual.	Self-awareness of traits is useful for assessing personal strengths (such as drive, motivation, integrity, confidence, cognitive ability) and matching those strengths to types of employment.
Style Theories Instead of focusing on traits, style theories consider how leaders behave. Three main lines of research were the Ohio State University and University of Michigan studies in the 1950s and the Blake and Mouton managerial grid (Blake et al., 1964).	All style theories are based on two types of behaviour: task and relationship behaviours. The combination of these two types of behaviours has been extensively studied to determine the most effective leadership styles. The assumption is that styles can be learned and cultivated.	According to the Blake and Mouton managerial grid (Blake, Mouton, Barnes, et al., 1964), "high-high" leaders are ideal leaders—they have high concern for accomplishing task objectives and high concern for building and maintaining collaborative relationships. Leaders need to develop both types of competencies.
Situational-Contingency Theories Situational-contingency theory emerged in the 1960s and 1970s. It proposed that leadership effectiveness depends on any given situation. Situational variables are research-tested variables that are related to leadership effectiveness in different situations. Outcomes are "contingent" on situational factors. Examples of this type of theory include Fiedler's (1967) contingency model, Vroom and Yetton's (1973) normative decision-making model, House and Mitchell's (1974) path-goal theory, and Hersey and Blanchard's situational leadership theory (1977).	**Path-goal theory:** There are four types of leader behaviours: supportive, directive, participative, and achievement oriented. Leader behaviour should be contingent on task and follower characteristics. Stressful tasks, for instance, require supportive leaders to lower follower anxiety. **Situational leadership theory:** The level of follower maturity influences the appropriate mix of task characteristics and leader behaviour. With novice followers (those who are new at a task), leaders should be directive.	Nurses and leaders must assess each situation as unique and determine appropriate actions accordingly. Leaders must adapt their styles to complement the specific issue faced.

THEORY BOX—cont'd

Key Leadership Theories

THEORY/CONTRIBUTOR	KEY IDEA	APPLICATION TO PRACTICE
Transformational Theories		
Burns (1978) originally introduced the concepts of transformational and transactional leadership. *Transactional leadership* is based on a leader–follower exchange, where the follower expects rewards in exchange for effort. Transactional leaders are similar to managers: they manage the status quo or day-to-day operations. *Transformational leadership* is a process whereby leaders and followers set higher goals and work together to achieve them. Burns felt that this style of leadership was connected with higher moral values. Avolio and Bass (1991) developed a full-range leadership theory with three typologies: transformational, transactional, and laissez-faire. They also developed an accompanying assessment tool, the Multifactor Leadership Questionnaire (MLQ), which has been used extensively in research. See Avolio and Yammarino (2013) for an update on research related to the original full-range theory.	Transformational leaders are known for the four *I*s: idealized influence, intellectual stimulation, individualized consideration, and inspirational motivation. There are three types of transactional leaders: *contingent reward leaders* focus on role clarification and ensuring followers receive appropriate supports to do their work; *management-by-exception active leaders* are vigilant and only intervene when a problem starts to arise; *management-by-exception passive leaders* only intervene after mistakes have occurred. Laissez-faire leaders avoid making decisions and abdicate responsibility.	Cummings, MacGregor, Davey, et al. (2010) examined relationships between types of nurse leaders and follower outcomes. Transformational nurse leaders were associated with positive outcomes such as nurse retention, group cohesion, role clarity, and effectiveness. McGuire and Kennerly (2006) found that transformational nurse leaders were more influential, but important manager characteristics (e.g., goal setting, providing direction) were associated with contingent reward transactional behaviours. Effective nurse leaders need to possess transformational and transactional qualities to succeed in complex health care environments.
Authentic Leadership		
Authentic leadership arises from the positive psychology tradition (Avolio & Gardner, 2005). Authentic leaders are aware of their own values and moral convictions and are constantly realigning their actions to match their values.	Authentic leaders are aware of themselves—authenticity does not involve consideration of others. These leaders are transparent and truthful. Followers are inspired by these leaders and trust them based on perceived congruence between their values and the leaders' values. Moral awareness is a key leadership virtue. An assumption is that followers' moral awareness will be heightened through their trust in authentic leaders.	Some evidence indicates that authentic leadership is associated with emotional intelligence (Klenke, 2005). Authentic leadership begins with self-awareness. Shirey (2006) expanded the original theoretical model to explore how authentic leadership contributes to quality work environments. Authentic leaders can instill hope and trust in followers, which influences follower behaviours such as engagement and satisfaction and results in a more positive work environment. Nurses should assess the congruence between their values and those of their leaders: quality work environments are more apt to arise when leaders and followers share values.

Management Theories

Although distinctions are blurred between leadership and management, a plethora of undergraduate, graduate, and doctoral management programs exist across Canada and internationally. A quick online search of prominent management programs reveals that new course offerings incorporate modern technology, such as computer-simulation modelling of health care systems and operations, and management information systems. Numerous conceptual models and theoretical frameworks support this burgeoning science. Management science has come a long way from the early 1900s when Taylor (1947) became the founder of "scientific management" and the "efficiency movement." Taylor introduced concepts such as labour division and specialization; systematic analysis of the relationship between workers and their assigned tasks; written, standardized procedures; close supervision; rewards for output; worker selection based on the right skills for the right task at the right time; shared manager–worker responsibility for goal achievement; and quality control. Many concepts associated with contemporary leadership, management, and followership are embedded in Taylor's early management theory (Anderson, Sweeney, Williams, et al., 2012).

Henry Mintzberg, a Canadian academic in business and management, has written extensively on organizational structures and processes, contributing to our knowledge of early management theory (Mintzberg, 1990). He proposed coordination mechanisms to accomplish complex tasks, including the standardization of work processes, outputs, worker skills and knowledge, and organizational norms (or beliefs about the nature of work within the organization). Mintzberg also defined ten management roles that fall within three categories: informational, interpersonal, and decisional. For example, the leader role, which falls in the interpersonal category, involves directing, motivating, training, advising, and influencing subordinates.

Followership Theories

Our understanding of followership is evolving along with our understanding of leadership and management. In the literature, the trend has been to replace follower terms with team terms due to the importance of effective teamwork within complex health care environments. However, a small body of followership theory literature exists, distinct from the leadership and management theory literature. According to Baker (2007), social sciences research on followership began in the 1950s, although most research concentrated on leaders and managers. The field of followership enjoyed a renaissance in the 1980s. At that time, Steger, Manners, and Zimmerer (1982) proposed a followership theory based on followers' desire for self-enhancement and self-protection or both. They proposed nine followership styles based on high, medium, or low combinations of these dimensions. Steger et al. (1982) were also interested in the influence of power on follower behaviours. The publication of Kelley's (1988) article "In Praise of Followers" in the *Harvard Business Review* also drew attention to how followers actively contribute to organizational success. Key conclusions drawn from followership research are as follows: a follower is a role rather than a person with inherent characteristics; effective followers are active, not passive; effective followers share the same goals

and purpose as leaders; and an effective relationship between followers and leaders is based on interdependency, mutual trust, and respect (Baker, 2007).

THE PROMISE OF COMPLEXITY SCIENCE

New theories are continually being created, tested, and put into practice—a function carried out by nurse scientists and others. Complexity science is the study of complex systems: "the patterns of relationships within them, how they are sustained, how they self-organize, and how outcomes emerge" (Zimmerman, Lindberg, & Plsek, 2001). Complexity science began with chaos theory and the physical and mathematical sciences. Since then, the social sciences and health care have adopted complexity science principles to better understand the nature of relationships in complex social systems, such as complex health care environments.

Classic science developed theories that used reductionist approaches to understand systems; for example, the study of machines and the human body have focused mainly on the "parts." Complexity science views systems holistically; it considers the whole to be greater than the sum of its parts. The world is full of systems within systems that interact and adapt through relationships. The interactions may appear to be random, but patterns emerge over time. Complexity science offers nurses a new way of understanding complex patient and family dynamics, teamwork within organizations, and even health and well-being (Clancy, Effken, & Pesut, 2008; Plsek & Wilson, 2001).

An important premise of complexity science is that human systems can adapt well to complex situations, often finding their own creative solutions to problems when controls are relaxed. "Creative progress towards a difficult goal can emerge from a few, flexible simple rules, or so called minimum specifications" (Plsek & Wilson, 2001, p. 747). Complexity science thinking stands in sharp contrast to traditional systems thinking, which focuses on developing elaborate plans and specific details on what must be done at every level of an organization. In organizations that follow a complexity science approach, traditional organizational hierarchy plays a less significant role in determining which staff are "keepers of high-level knowledge." It is replaced with decision making distributed among the human assets within an organization without regard to hierarchy. At the practice level, for instance, complexity science encourages health care providers to loosen their control over patients and families. Every voice counts, and every encounter between and among patients and staff contributes to effective decision making (Wilson, Holt, & Greenhalgh, 2001).

Complexity science has borrowed a number of terms from other disciplines (e.g., physics, chemistry, and ecology), such as *strange attractors, tags, emergence, self-organization, chunking, shadow systems, creative tension,* and *complex adaptive systems (CAS)*.

Marion and Uhl-Bien (2001) identified a number of ways in which complexity science encourages individuals to lead, manage, and follow (nursing examples have been added by the chapter author).

Develop Networks. A network is any related group with common involvement in an area of focus or concern. Social networks are found within organizations but also beyond organizational boundaries. For example, nurses can network within their organizations or with professional groups and associations outside their workplace, such as with nurses at a Canadian Nurses Association conference.

Encourage Non-hierarchical "Bottom-up" Interaction Among Workers. As noted earlier, those who lead, manage, and follow are not considered to be within the traditional hierarchy (e.g., where one person is "in charge" and directing others). Shared governance is an example of decision making in which nurses at different organizational levels engage in shaping policy and practices.

Become a Leadership "Tag." The term *tag* references the philosophic, patient-centred, and values-driven characteristics that give an organization its personality, sometimes called *attractors* or *hallmarks of culture*. Although the performance of procedures and functions may be similar in health care settings, an intangible "caring" attractor may exemplify the quality of care delivery in one organization, while cost efficiencies may be the attractor of another organization. The term *tag* refers to these distinctions.

Focus on Emergence. The concept of emergence addresses how individuals in positions of responsibility engage with and discover, through active organizational involvement, those networks that are best suited to respond to problems in creative, surprising, and artful ways—or thinking "outside the box." Nurse staff meetings can be organized to encourage participative decision making, tapping into everyone's creative energy.

Think of the "Big Picture." To have a broader sense of an issue, it's important to think systematically. Nurses think of the big picture when they look past their assignment's needs in relation to the needs of all units of the hospital; focus on the needs of both their patients and all residents in the long-term care facility; or include the community when addressing the problem of emergency department overcrowding.

Recognize the Dynamic, Complex, and Interdependent Nature of Systems. Everything is connected to everything else. Nurses are connected to patients. Patients are connected to families and friends. All together, they are connected to communities and cultures. Communities and cultures make up the fabric of society. The cost of health care is linked to local economies, and local businesses are connected to global industries. Identifying and understanding these relationships help solve problems with full recognition that small decisions can have a large impact.

How has complexity science influenced our understanding of leadership, management, and followership? Leaders do not need to have hypervigilant control over all events but do need to engage with people and the environment. Managers are concerned with ensuring quality, safe care delivery. There are many safety risk factors in health care settings where managers can promote the use of evidence-informed policies and procedures, such as preoperative checklists for surgery patients. Followers are team players full of ideas, stories, and lessons to be learned and shared. When followers recognize safety concerns, they voice their concerns with managers, document unsafe situations (e.g., by filling out an incident report), or both. In complexity science, each individual has the capacity to lead, manage, or follow as needed. The flow among these roles fosters an empowering environment that diminishes fear and organizational silence on matters that are critical to patients, staff, and organizational outcomes.

EXERCISE 1-3
Read the article in the following Research Perspective. It includes a discussion of multiple patient/simultaneity complexity (MP/SC) situations. Now think of an MP/SC situation you experienced as a student. Write down a description of the situation. How did you feel in this situation? Who helped you prioritize and make decisions? If you could go back to this situation and do it all over again, who would you engage in creative problem solving? Remember that the patients and families should be engaged as partners in decision making whenever possible.

RESEARCH PERSPECTIVE

Resource: Kramer, M., Brewer, B., Halfer, D., et al. (2013). Changing our lens: Seeing the chaos of professional practice as complexity. *Journal of Nursing Management, 21*(4), 690–704.

In an interview study conducted with newly licensed registered nurses (RNs), experienced RNs, and managers and educators from 20 Magnet™ hospitals in the United States, the "chaos" of the work environment was most often cited as the major adaptation difficulty for new graduates transitioning into practice. "Getting work done" was a particular concern for new RNs. The purpose of this study was to identify barriers to work effectiveness for new RNs, and to identify management practices to best support new RNs' capacity to safely and effectively complete their work.

A major barrier for new RNs was their inability to coordinate care for multiple patients with multiple simultaneous needs—what the authors call "multiple patient/simultaneity complexity" or MP/SC. To assist new RNs with a safe transition to MP/SC care provision, a complexity science education intervention was piloted with nine volunteer hospitals. New RNs were given MP/SC cases to study prior to their class. Each participant was asked to anonymously describe what he or she would do in this situation, and to indicate comfort or discomfort with the decision. After completing their preassessments of MP/SC dilemmas, the new RNs attended an interactive class with educators and peers to discuss alternative, valid solutions. Complex systems principles were reinforced throughout the class discussion. In a complex system, the many elements or agents in a system can interact in multiple ways, leading to myriad possible courses of action and outcomes. Best solutions for each patient emerged over time, requiring careful observation and continuous assessment of the patient and system (Sturmberg, O'Halloran, & Martin, 2012). After participating in this class, new RNs shifted their thinking from a "one solution" approach to an appreciation for thoughtful RN surveillance and the possibility of multiple, potential right answers. The class also helped new RNs feel more at ease with the unpredictability of MP/SC work environments.

Implications for Practice

This study took place in US Magnet™ hospitals. Magnet™ hospitals are considered the "gold standard" for nursing work environments, and they act as a magnet to recruit and retain nurses. Hospitals must undergo a rigorous accreditation process to receive Magnet™ certification. Magnet™ hospitals typically offer new graduate internships and orientation programs to ease the transition process. This study found that even new RNs in Magnet™ hospitals require extra learning supports to help them gain comfort with MP/SC situations (Kramer, Maguire, Halfer, et al., 2013).

Kramer et al. (2013) found that MP/SC case-based learning and peer discussion are important strategies for nurses to learn from one another. In complex adaptive systems (CAS), individuals adapt and learn together. Another example of CAS, mentioned in the Kramer et al. article, is "inter-assignment rounding" between two nurses and the physicians responsible for those nurses' patients. This rounding format is ideal for facilitating collaboration, problem solving, and more effective, efficient development of joint plans of care. Porter O'Grady, Clark, and Wiggins (2010) contend that complexity science education should be included in nursing education programs and continuing education opportunities.

LEADING, FOLLOWING, AND MANAGING COMPETENCIES

When dealing with theories and concepts, it is easy to lose sight of how to put these ideas into practice. The following sections review important competencies for leaders, managers, and followers. Competencies comprise knowledge, skills, and attitudes, and they are often arranged in checklists or frameworks for self-assessment. Competencies are influenced by the practice setting and the formal level of authority (e.g., front-line nurse leader, departmental manager, and executive director) (Jennings, Scalzi, Rodgers, et al., 2007).

Leading and Managing

Jennings et al. (2007) conducted a focused search of the health care literature from 2000 to 2004, and they identified and critically reviewed 140 articles related to leadership and management competencies. They found that leadership competencies were more commonly addressed in the literature than management competencies. They felt this was due to increased interest in leadership and research evidence that ties effective leadership to enhanced staff, patient, and work environment outcomes. Since their 2007 review, the literature continues to focus on leadership and its significant influence on nursing staff (Laschinger, Finegan, & Wilk, 2009; Weberg, 2010), patient outcomes (Richardson & Storr, 2010), and the work environment (Cummings et al., 2010).

Jennings et al. (2007) found significant overlap in the literature between leadership and management competencies. They identified 36 competency categories, and 23 of them were common to both management and leadership. Ten competency categories accounted for 85% of the competency examples. See Table 1-2.

TABLE 1-2	TOP TEN COMPETENCY CATEGORIES FOR LEADERSHIP AND MANAGEMENT	
RANK	**LEADERSHIP**	**MANAGEMENT**
1	Personal qualities	Interpersonal skills
2	Interpersonal skills	Personal qualities
3	Thinking skills	Thinking skills
4	Setting the vision*	Management skills (Planning, organizing)
5	Communicating	Communicating
6	Initiating change (Championing change/innovation projects)	Business skills (Finance, marketing)
7	Developing people* (Coaching, mentoring, succession planning)	Health care knowledge (Clinical, technical, business)
8	Health care knowledge (Clinical, technical, business)	Human resources management* (Pay scales, benefits)
9	Management skills (Planning, organizing)	Initiating change (Championing change/innovation projects)
10	Business skills (Finance, marketing)	Information management* (Databases, software programs)

*Indicates categories unique to either leadership or management.
Data reprinted from Jennings, B., Scalzi, C., Rodgers, J., & Keane, A., "Differentiating nursing leadership and management competencies," *Nursing Outlook 55*(4):169-175, 2007, with permission from Elsevier.

The top-two competency categories for leadership and management are *personal qualities* and *interpersonal skills*. The *personal qualities* category contains a total of 77 characteristics, including courage, creativity, and confidence. The researchers felt that personal qualities reflect the importance of knowing oneself and developing a "diverse and fluid repertoire" for dealing with people in complex systems (Jennings et al., 2007, p. 171). *Interpersonal skills* are those actions needed to engage others, such as conflict resolution and team-building skills.

Jennings et al. (2007) concluded that clear distinctions between leadership and management are becoming more difficult to ascertain within the literature—and they may not exist in health care settings where both sets of competencies are needed to function effectively within complex health care environments. Although we still distinguish between leadership and management by associating leaders with relational skills and managers with operational skills, these skills sets become fused in reality—distinctions between them are no doubt arbitrary (MacPhee & Suryaprakash, 2012). Ultimately, individuals need to be "prepared with skills appropriate to the care delivery setting, societal demands, and their career stage" (Jennings et al., 2007, p. 174).

EXERCISE 1-4
In your clinical setting, arrange a shadow experience with the front-line nurse leader. Create a table with the top ten competency categories for leadership and management from Table 1-2, and observe the nurse leader during a typical shift. Leave space in your table for note-taking. What competencies does the leader use or display? For instance, what personal qualities does he or she use when interacting with staff, patients, and other health care providers? What interpersonal skills does he or she use? What types of information does he or she communicate to others, and how does he or she communicate it?

Alternatively, arrange an interview with the front-line nurse leader on your student clinical unit. You can conduct the interview by yourself or arrange the interview between your clinical group and the nurse leader. Go through the list of leadership and management competencies and ask the leader how he or she demonstrates the use of the common and unique competencies. Share and discuss your notes in class. Do you have a clear idea of what leaders do and what managers do?

Following

Typically, followers are considered to be passive, uninspired, and waiting for direction. However, just the opposite is true. Followership is an understudied area in the leadership literature, but interest is growing in the ways in which members of a group or team organize themselves into leader–follower

TABLE 1-3   EFFECTIVE FOLLOWER CHARACTERISTICS

CHARACTERISTIC	DESCRIPTION
Interpersonal skills	"The ability to connect with others easily in an adequate period of time" (Antelo et al., 2010, p. 3)
Team player	"An adequate level of comfort when working in a team" (p. 4)
Competent	"Possesses a necessary job-related background and is equipped with required skills and abilities appropriate to the job" (p. 4)
Willing to learn	"[Can] analyze the information given to them, meticulously evaluate situations and actions, and make judgments" (p. 5)
Willing to change and innovate	"Followers are innovative, creative and eagerly open to new ideas" (p. 5)
Effective communicator	"Ability to deliver both positive and negative news (to both supervisors and team members) in the most appropriate way is not an easy task and requires experiences, courage and skills" (p. 6)
Reliable	"Good followers trust and work effectively with others" (p. 6)
Active participant	"Being able to act as a cohesive member of the group and being able to fairly contribute to the overall assignment of the group makes a follower a respected and a welcomed member of the group" (p. 6)
Emotionally intelligent	Followers are "self-aware"; they can control their own behaviours and "express themselves in a graceful manner" (p. 6)
Supportive of others	Followers are able to provide emotional support and support others' innovative ideas and creativity.
Flexible	"Followers are expected to adapt to changing circumstances at the workplace and be able to quickly reanalyze and adjust their behavior according to the situation at hand" (p. 6)
Motivated for goal accomplishment	Followers are self-motivated or intrinsically motivated—they do not require external reinforcement to contribute to teamwork

Data from Antelo, A., Prilipko, E., & Sheridan-Pereira, M. (2010). Assessing effective attributes of followers in a leadership process. *Contemporary Issues in Education Research, 3*(10), 1–12.

relationships that synergize outcomes for the group or team. In effective leader–follower relationships, followers play an important role in sharing and discussing relevant information that informs the leader's decisions (Antelo, Prilipko, & Sheridan-Pereira, 2010). Van Vugt (2009) proposed that our capacity to organize into leader–follower relationships is a group coordination behaviour that evolved in social species, such as humans, over time. Van Vugt, Hogan, and Kaiser (2008) described follower-ship as coordination of one's goals and actions with those of the leader. Some psychologists who study effective teamwork believe that followers have the responsibility to speak up and share critical information with the leader and team when problems or concerns are noted by them. Since leadership is defined as influencing others (Yukl, 2006), followers assume an informal leadership role by actively intervening and "influencing" the actions of others when they recognize the need for intervention to keep the team on course. Followers should be encouraged to act as informal leaders at any time that they have information to share or concerns to raise—to ensure

EXERCISE 1-5

Think about what happens on a typical nursing unit. In an ideal situation, the nurse leader collaboratively makes staffing assignments with the nursing staff, taking into consideration patient needs, the work environment, and the competencies and experience of the nursing staff. The nursing staff needs to play an active role in staffing assignment decisions to ensure effective team performance and safe staffing assignments.

In your clinical unit, observe interactions between the nurse leader and the staff around the change of shift. Are there interactions and discussions between the leader and staff about patient needs? Is the leader soliciting staff ideas? Is the staff offering information and advice?

The change-of-shift observation is an example of just one leader–follower exchange. During the shift, note the quality of leader–follower interactions. Based on what you know about leaders and followers from this chapter, critique the overall quality of leader–follower relationships. Would you want to work on this unit? Why or why not?

best possible outcomes for the team. In this way, the leader–follower relationship is closely intertwined (Hollander, 2009). Teams are considered a basic, functional unit within complex health care systems. Team members, followers, and leaders must know their roles and responsibilities to ensure effective team performance. Regardless of the complexity of the work environment, team members know who to follow for direction and how they can contribute to team success (DeRue, 2011). Table 1-3 provides a summary of key characteristics that Antelo et al. (2010) have used to describe effective followers. Some of these characteristics are very similar to the top ten competency categories for leadership and management that appear in Table 1-2.

LEADING, MANAGING, AND FOLLOWING DURING COMPLEX TIMES

The health care industry is spiralling through unparalleled change, often away from the traditional industrial models that reigned throughout the twentieth century. Most health care organizations today have ethnically diverse staff; have an expansive educational chasm, from non–high school graduates to clinicians with PhDs; have multiple generations of workers with varying values and expectations of the workplace; involve the use of technology to support all aspects of service functioning; and challenge providers, patients, families, and communities environmentally with medical waste, antibiotic-resistant strains of microorganisms, and other risks.

The complexity of the health care system is marred with chronic problems, including information imbalance (sometimes too much, sometimes not enough), an abundance of job roles that challenge resource allocation, intense work that makes examining patterns of practice difficult, increased consumer and regulatory demands, and worker fatigue from constant change.

These problems and other variables make leading, managing, and following increasingly challenging. For example, leaders must address the needs of the diverse community of those seeking care, but language and cultural barriers create the opportunity for misunderstanding. Moreover, those who manage the systems and processes of care may find a temporary workforce—individuals unfamiliar with organizational standards of care and practice—as their primary resource. As well, followers may have leaders from other generations with values different from their own, which makes the opportunity for conflict omnipresent.

The relationship between followers, leaders, and managers is complex. Burns (2000) states, "It would seem so simple at first glance—that leaders lead and followers follow. When the leader dreams the dream or takes the initiative or issues the call, does the follower even hear the leader?" (p. 11).

By developing the leading, managing, and following competencies discussed in this chapter, professional nurses will be better able to adapt to and accept differences and changes in their daily work life as positive rather than negative forces. It is rewarding to be an innovative and inspirational leader, an efficient and effective manager, and an active follower—achieving the best possible safe, quality care delivery within complex health care systems.

Leadership Development and Succession Planning

Many successful professional development programs include a mentorship component and hands-on, relevant leadership and management experiences within health care settings (MacPhee & Bouthillette, 2008; Skelton-Green, Simpson, & Scott, 2007).

In addition to educational opportunities and supports for current staff, health care leadership needs to systematically plan for the future. Succession planning includes the identification of nurses with leadership interests and potential. Canadian nurse researchers conducted an integrative review of health care succession planning that identified a number of strategies, including finding and mentoring potential succession candidates and allocating sufficient time and energy to the planning process (Carriere, Muise, Cummings, et al., 2009). An ongoing problem has been nurses' negative perceptions of leadership and management positions.

Nurses need exposure to positive role models to develop an appreciation for the importance of effective nurse leaders in formal positions of authority within health care organizations. Nurses often consider that few rewards are associated with formal leadership and management positions, particularly when such positions involve workload stressors and increased spans of control related to restructuring (Merrill, Pepper, & Blegen, 2013). Some restructuring, for instance, eliminated mid-level leadership positions, increasing the workloads of first-line nurse leaders (Duffield, Roche, Blay, et al., 2010). However, first-line nurse leaders serve as vital connections between direct care staff and upper levels of administration: they represent staff and advocate for their concerns. One Canadian study showed that first-line nurse leaders can positively influence staff perceptions of the work environment and, in turn, improve nurse retention rates and job satisfaction (Laschinger et al., 2009). First-line nurse leaders are typically recruited directly from staff nurse positions, emphasizing the importance of systematically recruiting, educating, and supporting staff nurses to fulfill these critical positions. The following Research Perspective indicates that empowerment-based leadership can be taught and is important to leadership development.

RESEARCH PERSPECTIVE

Resource: MacPhee, M., Dahinten, V., Hejazi, S., Laschinger, H., Kazanjian, A., McCutcheon, A., & Skelton-Green, J. (2014). Testing the effects of an empowerment-based leadership development programme: Part 1—leader outcomes. *Journal of Nursing Management, 22*(1), 4–15.

A nursing leadership development program for front-line nurse leaders was developed and tested over a 4-year period (2006–2010) in British Columbia (MacPhee & Bouthillette, 2008). An empowerment framework was used to teach self-empowerment and staff empowerment behaviours to novice leaders with less than 3 years' experience (MacPhee et al., 2011). Leaders who participated in the program were asked to complete a survey at the start of the program and 1 year later; their responses were compared with those of a similar group of novice leaders who filled out surveys but did not attend the program. Leaders who attended the program reported the use of significantly more leader-empowering behaviours than those leaders who did not attend the program. This study showed that empowerment strategies are teachable.

Implications for Practice

Other research has shown that leaders' use of empowering behaviours is associated with more engaged staff and healthier work environments (Greco , Laschinger, & Wong, 2006). Since empowerment strategies are teachable, organizations should invest in leadership development programs that use these successful, evidence-informed approaches. Empowerment is discussed in more detail in Chapter 11. One nurse researcher, Dr. Heather Laschinger, has devoted her research career to studying workplace empowerment and the importance of empowerment to leader, staff, and patient outcomes. Visit her website at http://publish.uwo.ca/~hkl. In addition to teachable strategies, some researchers believe that the quality of leader–follower relationships is associated with workplace empowerment. This area of research needs further exploration.

CONCLUSION

This chapter has covered the key theories related to leadership, management, and followership. It has elucidated the many styles, attributes, and competencies associated with strong, effective nurse leaders, managers, and followers. This chapter began with a focus on the strengths and unique assets of our Canadian health care system, as well as the notion of strengths-based leadership. Deficits and inequalities exist in Canada's health care system, but we must build on our societal strengths, such as the *Canada Health Act*; our vision for preventive, community-based care for all; the promotion of the social determinants of health; and the desire to eradicate social exclusion. Strengths-based leadership principles, tied to other concepts in this chapter and other chapters, are a good starting point. Periodically, go back to Table 1-1 and remind yourself of how strong leaders can make a positive difference to the quality and safety of health care delivery in Canada.

A SOLUTION

Terry addressed the nurses' work environment concerns with her supervisor, who said that the changes were mandatory and directed from the executive level. Reflecting on her leadership position, Terry realized that she needed to support the nurses. She began educating them about the changes and working with them to brainstorm strategies to make things work better for everyone. Terry also listened to the nurses. She took the time to be there for them and hear their concerns. Although the changes that were already in the works could not be stopped, Terry could acknowledge what these changes mean to the nurses, particularly those at the front line. Terry also encouraged staff to get more involved, speak up, and take action by joining committees, participating on councils, and volunteering for nurse-related project work. It has been a slow start, but some nurses are getting engaged with change initiatives, and Terry can see a gradual positive difference. This process is not easy, but it is better to be positive about changes than to ignore them or focus on the negatives.

Would this be a suitable approach for you? Why or why not?

THE EVIDENCE

- The use of top-down-only organizational structures is no longer sustainable in creating change. It must be complemented with change led from the bottom up and from networks of interested and committed individuals who form teams.
- Collaboration requires a set of special conditions between leaders, managers, and followers. These conditions include equal representation of every voice, and necessary resources and supports for innovation to occur.
- Complexity science does not refer to the complexity of the decision to be made or to the work environment in isolation but, rather, to examining how systems adapt and function where many possible ideas and actions unfold in a non-prescriptive manner.

NEED TO KNOW NOW

- Know your own values (self-awareness).
- Know the values of the organization. As an employee of the organization, you need to uphold and respect your organization's mission and vision.
- Develop trust early with your teammates, leader, and manager through recognition and sharing of common values.
- Recognize that organizational functioning and safe, quality care delivery depend on trust and respect among leaders, managers, and interdisciplinary teams.
- Remember that followership employs its own unique set of competencies, particularly the willingness to support your leader and team whenever possible.
- Acknowledge the positives—don't dwell on the negatives.
- Contribute to solutions, not problems.
- Seek out strong leader role models and formal leadership development opportunities: they are important components to becoming a strong leader.

CHAPTER CHECKLIST

This chapter presents the case that professional nurses require the competencies, knowledge, skill, and abilities to move in and out of leader, manager, and follower roles with ease, whether in clinical or administrative positions.

- Emotional intelligence is about knowing one's own and others' feelings and emotions, and the argument is made that emotional intelligence is as critical to professional practice as are cognitive and technical skills.
- Health care organizations are experiencing major restructuring that can be stressful to staff and patients without effective leadership, management, and followership.
- Multiple theories are used in today's health care system to address emerging organizational and clinical care needs. We need transformational and transactional leaders in complex health care environments.
- Transformational leaders motivate people to think creatively and to go beyond the status quo: they are visionaries.
- Transactional leaders are synonymous with effective managers. They are concerned with having resources and supports available so that nurses and others can effectively provide safe, quality care.
- Authentic leaders know themselves, model their values, and are open and trustworthy. They inspire trust and respect in others and raise value awareness of those around them.
- Active followers make significant contributions to organizations by working collaboratively with their leaders, managers, and teams. Followers are not passive.
- Complexity science is an amalgamation of concepts from other disciplines that emphasizes the importance of flexibility, adaptability, and the quality of systems interactions and relationships.
- Systematic succession planning and formal leadership development opportunities are critical to the future of nursing leadership.

▌TIPS FOR LEADING, MANAGING, AND FOLLOWING

- Competency frameworks, when available, can be useful tools for determining whether you have the knowledge, skills, and attitudes associated with certain roles and responsibilities. You can use the leader, manager, and follower competencies and attributes in this chapter to create your own checklist. Look for these behaviours in others, and use these competencies to guide your own leader, manager, and follower self-development.

- Basic knowledge of theory and supporting research provides a better appreciation of leading, managing, and following within complex health care contexts.
- Leadership effectiveness is enhanced by professional development opportunities, mentorship, and organizational supports to develop leader and manager competencies.

⊖volve WEBSITE

Visit the Evolve website for Suggested Readings, Internet Resources, and additional resources related to the content in this chapter: http://evolve.elsevier.com/Canada/Yoder-Wise/leading/.

REFERENCES

Akerjordet, K., & Severinsson, E. (2010). The state of science of emotional intelligence related to nursing leadership: An integrative review. *Journal of Nursing Management, 18*(4), 363–382. doi:10.1111/j.1365-2834.2010.01087.x

Anderson, D., Sweeney, D., Williams, T., et al. (2012). *An introduction to management science, quantitative approaches to decision making.* London, UK: Cengage Learning.

Antelo, A., Prilipko, E., & Sheridan-Pereira, M. (2010). Assessing effective attributes of followers in a leadership process. *Contemporary Issues in Education Research, 3*(10), 1–12.

Avolio, B., & Bass, B. (1991). *The full range leadership development programs: Basic and advanced manuals.* Binghamton, NY: Bass, Avolio, & Associates.

Avolio, B., & Gardner, W. (2005). Authentic leadership: Getting to the root of positive forms of leadership. *The Leadership Quarterly, 16*(3), 315–338.

Avolio, B., & Yammarino, F. G. (Eds.). (2013). *Transformational and charismatic leadership: The road ahead* (2nd ed.). West Yorkshire, UK: Emerald.

Baker, S. (2007). Followership: The theoretical foundation of a contemporary construct. *Journal of Leadership & Organizational Studies, 14*(1), 50–61.

Blake, R., Mouton, J., Barnes, L., et al. (1964). Breakthrough in organization development. *Harvard Business Review, 42*(6), 133–155.

Burns, J. (1978). *Leadership.* New York, NY: Harper & Row.

Burns, J. M. (2000). Leadership and followership: Complicated relationships. In B. Kellerman & L. R. Matusak (Eds.), *Cutting edge: Leadership 2000* (n.p.). College Park, MD: The James MacGregor Burns Academy of Leadership.

Canadian Health Services Research Foundation. (2012). Better health. Retrieved from http://www.cfhi-fcass.ca/Libraries/Commissioned_Research_Reports/Muntaner-BetterCare-EN.sflb.ashx.

Canadian Nurses Association. (2008). Code of ethics for registered nurses. Retrieved from http://buydownload.cna-aiic.ca/shopex d.asp?id=4.

Canadian Nurses Association. (2009). Position statement: Nursing leadership. Retrieved from http://www.cna-aiic.ca/CNA/docum ents/pdf/publications/PS110_Leadership_2009_e.pdf.

Canadian Nurses Association. (2013). A nursing call to action. Retrieved from http://www.cna-aiic.ca/en/on-the-issues/national-expert-commission/report-and-recommendations.

Canadian Nurses Association and the Canadian Federation of Nurses Unions. (2006). Joint position statement: Practice environments: Maximizing patients, nurse and system outcomes. http://www.cna-aiic.ca/~/media/cna/page%20content/pdf%20 en/2013/09/04/16/27/2%20-%20ps88-practice-environments-e.pdf.

Carriere, B., Muise, M., Cummings, G., et al. (2009). Healthcare succession planning: An integrative review. *Journal of Nursing Administration, 39*(12), 548–555.

Chaboyer, W., McMurray, A., Johnson, J., et al. (2009). Bedside handover: Quality improvement strategy to "transform care at the bedside." *Journal of Nursing Care Quality, 24*(2), 136–142.

Chinn, P., & Kramer, M. (2007). *Integrated knowledge development in nursing* (7th ed.). St. Louis, MO: Mosby.

Clancy, T., Effken, J., & Pesut, D. (2008). Applications of complex systems theory in nursing education, research and practice. *Nursing Outlook, 56,* 248–256.

Cummings, G., MacGregor, T., Davey, M., et al. (2010). Distinctive outcome patterns by leadership style for the nursing workforce and work environments: A systematic review. *International Journal of Nursing Studies, 47*(3), 363–385. doi:10.1016/j.ijnurstu.2009.08.006.

DeRue, D. S. (2011). Adaptive leadership theory: Leading and following as a complex adaptive process. *Research in Organizational Behavior, 31*, 125–150. doi:10.1016/j.riob.2011.09.007

Duffield, C., Roche, M., Blay, N., et al. (2010). Nursing unit managers, staff retention and the work environment. *Journal of Clinical Nursing, 20*, 23–33.

Feather, R. (2009). Emotional intelligence in relation to nursing leadership: Does it matter? *Journal of Nursing Management, 17*, 376–382.

Fiedler, F. A. (1967). *A theory of leadership effectiveness.* New York, NY: McGraw-Hill.

Gottlieb, L. (2012). *Strengths-based nursing care: Health and healing for person and family.* New York, NY: Springer.

Gottlieb, L., Gottlieb, B., & Shamian, J. (2012). Principles of strengths-based leadership for strengths-based nursing care: A new paradigm for nursing and healthcare for the 21st century. *Canadian Journal of Nursing Leadership, 25*(2), 38–50.

Greco, P., Laschinger, H. K. S., & Wong, C. (2006). Leader empowering behaviours, staff nurse empowerment and work engagement/burnout. *Canadian Journal of Nursing Leadership, 19*(4), 41–56.

Health Canada. (2010). Health care system. Retrieved from http://www.hc-sc.gc.ca/hcs-sss/index-eng.php.

Hersey, P., & Blanchard, K. (1977). *The management of organizational behavior* (3rd ed.). Englewood Cliffs, NJ: Prentice Hall.

Hobbs, J. (2009). A dimensional analysis of patient-centered care. *Nursing Research, 58*(1), 52–62.

Hollander, E. (2009). *Inclusive leadership: The essential leader-follower relationship.* New York, NY: Routledge/Taylor & Francis Group.

House, R. J., & Mitchell, T. R. (1974, Autumn). Path-goal theory of leadership. *Journal of Contemporary Business, 3*, 81–97.

Jennings, B., Scalzi, C., Rodgers, J., et al. (2007). Differentiating nursing leadership and management competencies. *Nursing Outlook, 55*, 169–175. doi:10.1016/j.outlook.2006.10.002

Kelley, R. (1988). In praise of followers. *Harvard Business Review, 66*, 142–148.

Klenke, K. (2005). The internal theater of the authentic leader: Integrating cognitive, affective, conative, and spiritual facets of authentic leadership. In W. L. Gardner, B. J. Avolio, & F. O. Walumba (Eds.), *Authentic leadership theory and practice: Origins, effects, and development* (pp. 155–182). Oxford, UK: Elsevier.

Kramer, M., Brewer, B., Halfer, D., et al. (2013). Changing our lens: Seeing the chaos of professional practice as complexity. *Journal of Nursing Management, 21*(4), 690–704.

Kramer, M., Maguire, P., Halfer, D., et al. (2013). Nurse residency programs: Components and strategies effective in professional socialization of newly licensed registered nurses. *Western Journal of Nursing Research, 35*(4), 459–496.

Laschinger, H., Finegan, J., & Wilk, P. (2009). Context matters: The impact of unit leadership and empowerment on nurses' organizational commitment. *Journal of Nursing Administration, 39*(2), 228–235.

Lucas, V., Laschinger, H., & Wong, C. (2008). The impact of emotional intelligent leadership on staff nurse empowerment: The moderating effect of span of control. *Journal of Nursing Management, 16*, 964–973. doi:10.1111/j.1365-2834.2008.0856.x

MacPhee, M., & Bouthillette, F. (2008). Developing leadership in nurse managers: The British Columbia Nursing Leadership Institute. *Canadian Journal of Nursing Leadership, 21*(3), 64–75.

MacPhee, M., Dahinten, V., Hejazi, S., et al. (2014). Testing the effects of an empowerment-based leadership development programme: Part 1—leader outcomes. *Journal of Nursing Management, 22*(1), 4–15.

MacPhee, M., Skelton-Green, J., Bouthillette, F., et al. (2011). An empowerment framework for nursing leadership development: Supporting evidence. *Journal of Advanced Nursing, 68*(1), 159–169. doi:10.1111/j.1365-2648.2011.05746.x

MacPhee, M., & Suryaprakash, N. (2012). First-line nurse leaders' change management initiatives. *Journal of Nursing Management, 20*(2), 249–259.

MacPhee, M., Suryaprakash, N., & Jackson, C. (2009). Online knowledge networking: What leaders need to know. *Journal of Nursing Administration, 39*(10), 415–422.

Marion, R., & Uhl-Bien, M. (2001). Leadership in complex organizations. *The Leadership Quarterly, 12*, 389–418.

McGuire, E., & Kennerly, S. (2006). Nurse managers as transformational and transactional leaders. *Nursing Economics, 24*(4), 179–186.

Mendes, F., & Stander, M. (2011). Positive organization: The role of leader behavior in work engagement and retention. *SA Journal of Industrial Psychology, 37*(1), 29–41.

Merrill, K., Pepper, G., & Blegen, M. (2013). Managerial span of control: A pilot study comparing departmental complexity and number of direct reports. *Canadian Journal of Nursing Leadership, 26*(3), 53–67.

Mintzberg, H. (1990, March). The manager's job: Folklore and fact. *Harvard Business Review*, 1–13.

Mitchell, G., Bournes, D., & Hollett, J. (2006). Human becoming-guided patient-centered care: A new model transforms nursing practice. *Nursing Science Quarterly, 19*(3), 218–224. doi:10.1177/0894318406289488

Needleman, J., & Hassmiller, S. (2009). The role of nurses in improving hospital quality and efficiency: Real-world results. *Health Affairs, 28*(4), w625–w633.

O'Brien-Pallas, L., Tomblin Murphy, G., Shamian, J., et al. (2010). Impact and determinants of nurse turnover: A pan-Canadian study. *Journal of Nursing Management, 18*, 1073–1086.

Plsek, P. E., & Wilson, T. (2001). Complexity, leadership, and management in healthcare organisations. *British Medical Journal, 323*, 746–749.

Porter-O'Grady, T., Clark, S., & Wiggins, M. (2010). The case for clinical nurse leaders: Guiding nursing practice into the 21st century. *Nurse Leader, 8*(1), 37–41.

Quality Worklife—Quality Healthcare Collaborative. (2007). *Within our grasp: A healthy workplace action strategy for success and sustainability in Canada's healthcare system.* Ottawa, ON: Canadian Council on Health Services Accreditation. Retrieved from http://www.qwqhc.ca/docs/2007QWQHCWithin Grasp.pdf.

Registered Nurses Association of Ontario (RNAO). (2002). C centred care. Retrieved from http://rnao.ca/sites/rnao-ca/f Client_Centred_Care_0.pdf.

Richardson, A., & Storr, J. (2010). Patient safety: A literature review on the impact of nursing empowerment, leadership and collaboration. *International Nursing Review, 57*, 12–21.

Riggio, R., Chaleff, I., & Lipman-Bluman, J. (2008). *How great followers create great leaders and organizations.* San Francisco, CA: Jossey-Bass.

Shendell-Falik, N., Fienson, M., & Mohr, B. (2007). Enhancing patient safety: Improving the patient handoff process through appreciative inquiry. *Journal of Nursing Administration, 37*(2), 95–104.

Shirey, M. (2006). Authentic leaders creating healthy work environments for nursing practice. *American Journal of Critical Care, 15*(3), 256–267.

Simpson, J. (2012). *Chronic condition: Why Canada's health-care system needs to be dragged into the 21st century.* Toronto, ON: Penguin.

Skelton-Green, J., Simpson, B., & Scott, J. (2007). An integrated approach to change leadership. *Canadian Journal of Nursing Leadership, 20*(3). Online special issue. Retrieved from http://www.longwoods.com/content/19277.

Smith, K.B., Profetto-McGrath, J., & Cummings, G. (2009). Emotional intelligence and nursing: An integrative literature review. *International Journal of Nursing Studies, 46*, 1624–1636.

Squires, M., Tourangeau, A., Laschinger, H., et al. (2010). The link between leadership and safety outcomes in hospitals. *Journal of Nursing Management, 18*, 914–925. doi:10.1111/j.1365-2834.2010.01181.x

Stefaniak, K. (2007). Discovering nursing excellence through appreciative inquiry. *Nurse Leader, 5*(2), 42–46. doi:10.1016/j.mnl.2007.01.010

Steger, J., Manners, G., & Zimmerer, T. (1982). Following the leader: How to link management style to subordinate personalities. *Management Review, 71*, 22–28, 49–51.

Stogdill, R. M. (1948). Personal factors associated with leadership: A survey of the literature. *Journal of Psychology, 25*, 35–71.

Sturmberg, J., O'Halloran, D., & Martin, C. (2012). Understanding health system reform—A complex adaptive systems perspective. *Journal of Evaluation in Clinical Practice, 18*, 202–208.

Taylor, F. (1947). *Management science.* New York, NY: Harper and Row.

Van Vugt, M. (2009). Despotism, democracy, and the evolutionary dynamics of leadership and followship. *American Psychologist, 64*(1), 54–56. doi:10.1037/a0014178

Van Vugt, M., Hogan, R., & Kaiser, R. (2008). Leadership, followership and evolution. *American Psychologist, 63*(3), 182–196. doi:10.1037/0003-066X.63.3.182

Vroom, V., & Yetton, P. (1973). *Leadership and decision-making.* Pittsburgh, PA: University of Pittsburgh Press.

Weberg, D. (2010). Transformational leadership and staff retention: An evidence review with implications for healthcare systems. *Nursing Administration Quarterly, 34*(3), 246–258.

Whitney, D. K., & Trosten-Bloom, A. (2010). *The power of appreciative inquiry.* San Francisco, CA: Berrett-Koehler.

Wilson, T., Holt, T., & Greenhalgh, T. (2001). Complexity science: Complexity and clinical care. *British Medical Journal, 323*, 685–688.

Yeo, M., Moorhouse, A., Khan, P., et al. (2010). *Concepts and cases in nursing ethics* (3rd ed.). Peterborough, ON: Broadview Press.

Yukl, G. (2006). *Leadership in organizations* (6th ed.). Upper Saddle River, NJ: Pearson Education.

Zimmerman, B., Lindberg, C., & Plsek, P. (2001). *Edgeware: Insights from complexity science for health care leaders.* Irving, TX: TVA.

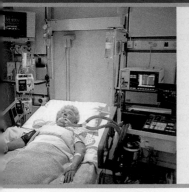

Patient Focus

Sandra Regan and Lyle G. Grant

Patient focus is a broad concept. In this chapter, patient is broadly defined to include any and all those who are interacting with nurses to receive nursing care. Patients include individuals, families, non-professional caregivers, communities, and populations. To meet the public mandate of nursing, nurses in all roles must maintain a focus on patients and patient care. In its simplest form, nursing must work to the benefit of patients. In its more complex form, nursing must focus on patients by applying professional standards to patient-centred care, patient safety, and patient outcomes. Patient focus is also central to effective nursing leadership and management initiatives.

OBJECTIVES

- Understand how nursing professional standards and codes of ethics guide nurses' practice.
- Identify key values of patient-centred care.
- Understand how nurse leadership and management can implement initiatives that promote patient-centred care.
- Describe nursing's role in patient safety and a culture of safety.
- Identify the key organizations and resources that support a patient focus.
- Understand how nursing-sensitive outcomes are used to enhance a patient focus.
- Apply various resources to analyze a patient-safety situation.

TERMS TO KNOW

adverse event	nursing-sensitive outcomes	patient safety
code of ethics	patient- or client-centred care	professional standard
culture of safety		

? A CHALLENGE

Jack is the nurse manager of a medical unit in a regional hospital. The unit has recently undergone staff mixture changes to increase the use of care aides and practical nurses (PNs) and reduce the number of registered nurses (RNs) working at any one time. Although teamwork is encouraged, it is not the reality. PNs have also been asked to assume an expanded scope of practice because of the decrease in RNs and are feeling overwhelmed. RNs are regularly seen admonishing PNs and care aides for decision making about care. Care aides and PNs have responded to the negative attitudes of selected RNs by avoiding working closely with them.

What advantages might there be to building a stronger patient focus in this medical unit, and what advice might you have for Jack?

SAFE, COMPETENT, AND ETHICAL PRACTICE

As members of a regulated profession, nurses are accountable to the public. Provincial and territorial governments have delegated to their respective nursing regulatory bodies the responsibility to regulate the profession in the public interest. One means for the nursing profession to achieve accountability is through the provision of safe, competent, and ethical nursing care. Details of the regulatory frameworks affecting nursing practices are further outlined in Chapters 5 and 20. Nursing regulatory bodies, among their various duties, are responsible for establishing, monitoring, and enforcing the professional standards that govern the practice of nursing. A **professional standard** is an "authoritative statement that sets out the legal and professional basis of nursing practice" (College of Nurses of Ontario, 2009, p. 3). "The primary purpose of standards is to identify for nurses, the public, government, and other stakeholders the desired and achievable level of performance expected of nurses in their practice, against which actual performance can be measured" (Association of Registered Nurses of Newfoundland and Labrador, 2007, p. 2).

While each provincial and territorial nursing regulatory body has developed its own professional standards, standards from one jurisdiction to another share many similarities. For example, standards commonly include statements regarding accountability and responsibility,

the competent application of knowledge, continuing competence, ethics, nurse–patient relationships, and interdisciplinary collaboration. In addition to defining standards, nursing regulatory bodies set out indicators that describe how nurses demonstrate they have met each standard. In some cases, indicators have been developed that are relevant to nurses working in particular domains of practice, such as administration and education. See Box 2-1 for an example of a professional standard and its associated indicators for nurses working in administration.

Patient focus is also integrated in the entry-level competencies for nurses that guide nursing education programs. These entry-level competencies are developed through collaboration among nursing regulatory bodies in Canada. The competencies are grounded in a standards-based conceptual framework—professional responsibility and accountability, knowledge-based practice, ethical practice, service to the public, and self-regulation—with the patient central to the framework (Black, Allen, Redfern, et al., 2008). If you are not already familiar with the entry-level competencies for registered, practical, or psychiatric nurses in your province or territory, you can access them on your nursing regulatory body's website (see the table at the end of this chapter for a list of nursing regulatory bodies).

In addition to professional standards, nurses have codes of ethics that guide their practice. A code of ethics is a statement of a set of values that help guide nurses in ethical practice. The Canadian Nurses Association (CNA) has developed and periodically revises its *Code of Ethics for Registered Nurses*. Practical nurses and psychiatric nurses can find codes of ethics at their provincial association websites. The most universally adopted nursing code in Canada, the CNA's *Code of Ethics for Registered Nurses*, is divided into two parts: Part One sets out the nursing values and core ethical responsibilities, and Part Two describes ethical endeavours that are meant to guide nurses in addressing societal issues such as inequity (Canadian Nurses Association [CNA], 2008). Provincial and territorial registered nursing regulatory bodies have incorporated the CNA's code of ethics in one form or another, and Part One is usually found in their professional standards. A summary of Part One of the CNA's *Code of Ethics for Registered Nurses* appears in Box 2-2.

BOX 2-1   EXAMPLE OF A PROFESSIONAL STANDARD AND INDICATORS FOR NURSES IN AN ADMINISTRATIVE ROLE

The College of Registered Nurses of British Columbia provides indicators to demonstrate how each of its professional standards is applied in four areas of practice. Standard three and its indicators for administration appear here.

Standard 3: Client-Focused Provision of Service

Provides nursing services and works with others to provide health care services in the best interest of clients.

Indicators for Administration

1. Communicates, collaborates and consults with nurses and other members of the health care team about the provision of health care services.
2. Educates others about the nurse's role in the coordination of client care.
3. Develops policies that outline the responsibility and accountability for all involved in appropriate assignment of clients and client care activities.
4. Develops policies that provide direction for nurses on appropriate delegation of nursing activities to other members of the health care team.
5. Develops supporting policies for appropriate regulatory supervision.
6. Guides, directs and seeks feedback from staff and others involved in the planning, delivery and evaluation of health care services as appropriate.
7. Directs and participates in changes to improve client care and administrative practice.
8. Takes appropriate action or reports unsafe practice or professional misconduct to appropriate person or body.
9. Understands and communicates the role of nursing in the health of clients.
10. Assists patients, colleagues, students and others to learn about nursing practice and health care services.

College of Registered Nurses of British Columbia. (2012). *Professional standards for registered nurses and nurse practitioners*. Vancouver, BC: Author.

BOX 2-2   CANADIAN NURSES ASSOCIATION'S CODE OF ETHICS FOR REGISTERED NURSES

The Canadian Nurses Association's Code of Ethics for Registered Nurses (2008) sets out the following nursing values and ethical responsibilities:

1. *Providing safe, compassionate, competent and ethical care*. Nurses provide safe, compassionate, competent, and ethical care.
2. *Promoting health and well-being*. Nurses work with people to enable them to attain their highest possible level of health and well-being.
3. *Promoting and respecting informed decision making*. Nurses recognize, respect, and promote a person's right to be informed and make decisions.
4. *Preserving dignity*. Nurses recognize and respect the intrinsic worth of each person.
5. *Maintaining privacy and confidentiality*. Nurses recognize the importance of privacy and confidentiality and safeguard personal, family, and community information obtained in the context of a professional relationship.
6. *Promoting justice*. Nurses uphold principles of justice by safeguarding human rights, equity, and fairness and by promoting the public good.
7. *Being accountable*. Nurses are accountable for their actions and answerable for their practice.

Nurses in all domains of practice bear the ethical responsibilities identified under each of the seven primary nursing values.

Canadian Nurses Association [CNA]. (2008). Code of Ethics for Registered Nurses (2008 Centennial Edition). Toronto, ON: Author. © Canadian Nurses Association. Reprinted with permission. Further reproduction prohibited.

EXERCISE 2-1

Familiarize yourself with the professional standards and code of ethics set out by the relevant nursing regulatory body in your province and territory. You can also review the entry-level competencies for registered nurses, practical nurses, or psychiatric nurses. A list of the provincial and territorial nursing regulatory bodies can be found at the end of this chapter. How do these standards, entry-level competencies, and codes of ethics inform your role as a nurse? As a future leader? As a follower? How do they guide how you view the patient?

PATIENT-CENTRED CARE

The focus of nursing practice has always been the patient, which includes striving for excellence in patient care. However, historically the needs of the organization or even those of health care providers, including nurses, have at times been placed above those of the patient in decision making about care. Workplace examples include interdisciplinary non-cooperation or competition, communication breakdown, adversarial staff, fear of reprisal for taking opposing views, inflexibility, job dissatisfaction, and emphasis on workplace issues that are not associated with improving patient care and patient participation. Often attitudes affecting patient care are entrenched in organizational cultures and become part of the unstated organizational philosophy of care. Nurses play an important role in influencing these philosophies for the benefit of patients and positive patient outcomes. They also maintain responsibility for identifying and changing systemic factors that hinder patient-centred care. Collaborating with patients and their families in respectful and meaningful ways may require shifting how organizations and health care providers view the patient. Finding effective ways within an organization to promote a philosophy of patient-centred care is an important strategy for maintaining focus or refocusing on the patient and his or her family.

Patient- or client-centred care is an approach in which the patient is viewed as a whole person; it is not just about delivering services and involves advocacy, empowerment, and respecting the patient's autonomy, voice, self-determination, and participation in decision making (Registered Nurses' Association of Ontario [RNAO], 2002, p. 12). The Registered Nurses' Association of Ontario (RNAO) identified eight values that form the foundation of patient- or client-centred care: respect; human dignity; clients are experts for their own lives; clients as leaders; clients' goals coordinate care of the heath care team; continuity and consistency of care and caregiver; timeliness; and responsiveness and universal access. These eight values are discussed in Box 2-3.

Lewis (2009) suggested that managers and governors (board of directors) must make patient-centred care a priority in their two main roles of making policies and ensuring system accountability. A number of activities can be implemented to enact these two roles, and nurses can support or implement many of them. For example, nurses can lead changes that promote team-based and collaborative care, create a culture that discourages behaviours that do not put patients first, and identify and change policies to align with values such as those identified by RNAO (2002). Other areas that governance and management must focus on to enable patient-centred care appear in Box 2-4.

BOX 2-3   THE VALUES OF PATIENT- OR CLIENT-CENTRED CARE

1. *Respect:* Respect clients' wishes, concerns, values, priorities, perspectives, and strengths.
2. *Human Dignity:* Care for clients as whole and unique human beings, not as problems or diagnoses.
3. *Clients Are Experts for Their Own Lives:* Clients know themselves the best.
4. *Clients as Leaders:* Follow the lead of clients with respect to information giving, decision making, care in general and involvement of others.
5. *Clients' Goals Coordinate Care of the Health Care Team:* Clients define the goals that coordinate the practices of the health care team. All members of the team work toward facilitating the achievement of these goals.
6. *Continuity and Consistency of Care and Caregiver:* Continuity and consistency of care and caregiver provides a foundation for client centred care.
7. *Timeliness:* The needs of clients and communities deserve a prompt response.
8. *Responsiveness & Universal Access:* Care that is offered to clients is universally accessible and responsive to their wishes, values, priorities, perspectives, and concerns.

Registered Nurses Association of Ontario (2002). Client Centred Care. Toronto, Canada: Registered Nurses Association of Ontario.

PATIENT SAFETY

When patients come into contact with the health care system, they place a great deal of trust in those providing care to them. They expect the provision of safe care and have a reasonable expectation that they will not be harmed in the process. In 2000, the Institute of Medicine [IOM], a US-based organization, released *To Err Is Human: Building a Safer Health System.* The IOM report stated that in the United States, nearly 100 000 hospital deaths annually were attributed to adverse events. According to the Canadian Patient Safety Institute (n.d.b) online glossary of terms, an adverse event is "an event that results in unintended harm to the patient and is related to the care and services provided to the patient rather than to the patient's underlying condition." The outcome of an adverse event might be disability, extended length of stay, or even death.

Baker, Norton, Flintoft, et al. (2004) conducted the first Canadian study of adverse events (The Canadian Adverse Events Study). They conducted a chart review in 20 randomly selected Canadian hospitals in British

BOX 2-4	GOVERNANCE AND MANAGEMENT ACTIVITIES THAT SUPPORT PATIENT-CENTRED CARE

For managers and governors to support patient-centred care, they must focus on the following:

1. Indicators that capture patient-centredness accurately and comprehensively.
2. Health science education programs that build patient-centred care into the core of their curricula and the formative apprenticeship experiences.
3. Explicit goals and targets for achieving various elements of patient-centred care.
4. Regular patient surveys to monitor the evolution of patient-centred care and identify strengths and weaknesses.
5. Regular provider surveys to monitor their attitudes, expectations, and behaviours.
6. Organizational changes that promote systems thinking, collective accountability, and team-based care.
7. E-health and other technologies that facilitate communication, efficiency, and convenience.
8. Investments in system re-engineering that advance patient-centred care.
9. Progressively more robust policies to spread patient-centred care successes, e.g., mandatory open access scheduling, patient-driven e-health initiatives, transparent reporting of patient-centred care performance, etc.
10. A culture of patient-centred care that refuses to tolerate behaviours that do not put patients first.
11. Incorporating important patient-centred care criteria and measures into accreditation and regulatory employer standards and processes.

Adapted from Lewis, S. (2009). Patient-centred care: An introduction to what it is and how to achieve it: A discussion paper for the Saskatchewan Ministry of Health. Saskatoon, SK: The Change Foundation. Retrieved from http://www.southeastlhin.on.ca/uploadedFiles/Public_Community/Board_of_Directors/Board_Committee/Collaborative_Governance_and_Community_Engagement/Ppatient-Centred-Care%20Steven%20Lewis%202009.pdf.

Columbia, Alberta, Ontario, Quebec, and Nova Scotia in 2000 to provide a national estimate of the incidence of adverse events. They found that the adverse events rate was 7.5 per 100 hospital admissions. This means that an adverse event was experienced in 7.5% of hospital admissions. They further estimated that 36% of the adverse events were preventable and approximately 9250 to 23 750 of the adverse events that ended in death were preventable. It's essential to keep in mind that nursing's mandate to provide safe, competent, and ethical care carries with it an expectation that nurses will contribute to patient safety.

The World Health Organization (n.d.) defines patient safety as "the absence of preventable harm to a patient during the process of health care." Research on adverse events has highlighted the importance of safety in health care organizations and led health care leaders in the United States and Canada to have a more progressive approach to quality and patient safety. Health care organizations typically monitor adverse events through incident reporting systems. These reporting systems permit the identification of trends and patterns in adverse events, which can in turn lead to activities that foster improvements in the health care facility. Quality improvement is discussed further in Chapter 21. The Canadian Institute for Health Information (CIHI) tracks medication and intravenous fluid incidents through the National System for Incident Reporting (NSIR). The NSIR is a secure and anonymous tracking system that supports local regional, provincial, and national efforts to understand how to improve the health care system. You can visit CIHI's website (http://www.CIHI.ca) for more information (the site includes a video on the NSIR). In addition to incident reporting, many health care facilities have created specific roles and departments charged with leading initiatives on patient safety and creating a culture of safety. Creating a culture of safety is essential to reducing adverse events in the Canadian health care system. Wiseman and Kaprielian (2005) suggest that "in a culture of safety the focus is on effective systems and teamwork to accomplish the mutual goal of safe, high-quality performance. When something goes wrong, the focus is on what [or how], rather than who, is the problem. The intent is to bring process failures and system issues to light, and to solve them in a non-biased non-threatening way" (para. 1).

What does a culture of safety look like? In their review of the literature on safety culture, Halligan and Zecevic (2011) list the following attributes as common features of a culture of safety:

- leadership commitment to safety
- open communication founded on trust

- organizational learning
- a non-punitive approach to adverse event reporting and analysis
- teamwork
- shared belief in the importance of safety (p. 340)

Studies have found that when health care facilities create a culture of safety, their staff are more willing to report adverse events (Vogus, Sutcliffe, & Weick, 2010). This is because they understand that the focus is on addressing issues in the system and not blaming individuals. The CNA (2009) position statement on patient safety is as follows: "Although individual competency may be a contributing factor, and individuals remain accountable for their own actions, it is increasingly evident that system competency plays a major role in patient safety. Only when adverse events and near misses are disclosed can they be analyzed in a collaborative manner by the health-care team and other stakeholders to identify and address problems in the system" (p. 2). The position statement goes on to suggest that "strong leadership across the nursing profession is essential to moving forward cultural reform required to ensure the delivery of safe, quality care in professional environments" (p. 2). Whether nurses are front-line staff (followers and leaders) or hold formal leadership positions, all have a role in achieving a culture of safety. Some examples of activities health care organizations can implement to support a culture of safety include establishing Quality Improvement (QI) teams, having regular team "huddles" on the unit, debriefing adverse events when they occur, and requiring completion of a surgical safety checklist. See the Literature Perspective for more on how health care organizations can create a culture of safety.

Nurses are in a unique position to lead and manage patient safety; they are with the patient 24 hours a day, 7 days a week. Few health care providers are positioned with such a patient focus. Nurses in follower and leadership roles can identify safety issues originating at the unit or patient level and give voice to these issues at the organizational level (Thompson, 2000; Tregunno, Jeffs, McGillis Hall, et al., 2009). Creating a culture attuned to patient safety requires a number of leadership skills, such as understanding change processes, being able to manage conflict, and having an understanding of quality and patient safety practices. However, nurse leaders need support and

LITERATURE PERSPECTIVE

Resource: Fleming, M., & Wentzell, N. (2008). Patient Safety Culture Improvement Tool: Development and guidelines for use. *Healthcare Quarterly, 11*(Sp), 10–15.

How can health care organizations improve their culture of patient safety? The authors reported on the early development of the Patient Safety Culture Improvement Tool (PSCIT), which can help health care organizations assess the state of their patient safety culture. Based on a safety culture maturity model, the PSCIT identifies key elements of patient safety: patient safety leadership (patient safety education and training, and patient safety performance evaluation); risk analysis; workload and fatigue management; sharing and learning (organizational learning, incident reporting, and disclosure); and resource management (teamwork training). These elements are rated on a scale of 0 to 4, with 0 indicating no systems in place to promote a positive safety culture and 4 indicating that the positive safety culture is central to the mission of the organization. These elements are assessed for senior leaders, physician leaders, middle managers, and front-line managers. Through this assessment, organizations can understand where they are in implementing a positive patient safety culture and identify areas for improvement. The complete PSCIT is available as an appendix in the published article.

Implications for Practice

Nurses can contribute to creating a culture of patient safety by identifying areas for improvement and leading or managing change. Tools such as the PSCIT can provide evidence to help identify strategies or policies that ensure accountability to the public.

EXERCISE 2-2

Reflect on a recent clinical experience you have had in your nursing education program. Based on what you have read about attributes of a culture of safety, how do these attributes align with your clinical experience? Were you aware of how to report an adverse event? Did you encounter any activities that promote the ideal of a culture of safety? How is patient safety discussed in the mission, vision, or mandate of the organization? Is there a specific role or department in the organization responsible for patient safety?

---

resources to take up this important role. The CNA and the Canadian Patient Safety Institute (CPSI) have developed a number of resources that can be used to support leadership in and management of patient safety. Box 2-5 lists patient safety topics on which the CNA has created a searchable database of references.

BOX 2-5   CANADIAN NURSES ASSOCIATION'S PATIENT SAFETY RESOURCE GUIDE

The Canadian Nurses Association (CNA) has created a searchable database of references related to patient safety that covers the following topics:

- Nurse staffing and skill mix
- Adverse events
- Reporting, data management, and assessment
- New safety practices

- Culture of safety
- Environmental factors
- Quality of care
- Education initiatives and tools
- System restructuring
- Regulation, legislation, and policy
- Major reports

Canadian Nurses Association [CNA]. (2011). Patient Safety Resource Guide. Retrieved from http://www.cna-nurses.ca/CNA/practice/environment/safety/guide/default_e.aspx. © Canadian Nurses Association. Reprinted with permission. Further reproduction prohibited.

Canadian Patient Safety Institute

The Canadian Patient Safety Institute (CPSI) was established in 2003 by Health Canada to support improvements in patient safety and quality. CPSI's vision, "safe healthcare for all Canadians," is supported by the following strategic priorities:

- Improve the safety of patient care in Canada through learning, sharing, and implementing interventions that are known to reduce avoidable harm.
- Build governance capability.
- Support networks.
- Increase capacity through evidence-informed resources and tools.

(Canadian Patient Safety Institute. http://www.patientsafetyinstitute.ca)

The CPSI website is a rich resource for health care organizations as well as practitioners. CPSI's flagship program Safer Healthcare Now! supports front-line health care providers and the delivery system to improve the safety of patient care throughout Canada by implementing interventions known to reduce avoidable harm. The Safer Healthcare Now! website (http://www.saferhealthcarenow.ca) has resources for front-line health care providers and others who want to improve patient safety. The tools and resources at the CPSI website (http://www.patientsafetyinstitute.ca) are free and can be customized to an organization's needs. By incorporating safety competencies in their educational programs and professional development activities, health care leaders can ensure their staff have the knowledge, skills, and attitude to create a culture consistent with quality and patient safety. The CPSI's safety competencies appear in Box 2-6.

The CPSI's Effective Governance for Quality and Patient Safety: A Toolkit for Healthcare Board Members and Senior Leaders provides information on the drivers of quality and patient safety, references (including Canadian studies), and stories from health care organizations. Important drivers of quality and patient safety include access to information, evidence and research, and relevant measures. The drivers for effective governance for quality and patient safety appear in Figure 2-1. Nurses can use this toolkit in their own workplace to ensure patient safety.

BOX 2-6   CANADIAN PATIENT SAFETY INSTITUTE'S SAFETY COMPETENCIES

The Canadian Patient Safety Institute (CPSI) created safety competencies that include six core competency domains:

Domain 1: Contribute to a Culture of Patient Safety—A commitment to applying core patient safety knowledge, skills, and attitudes to everyday work.

Domain 2: Work in Teams for Patient Safety—Working within interprofessional teams to optimize patient safety and quality of care.

Domain 3: Communicate Effectively for Patient Safety—Promoting patient safety through effective health care communication.

Domain 4: Manage Safety Risks—Anticipating, recognizing, and managing situations that place patients at risk.

Domain 5: Optimize Human and Environmental Factors—Managing the relationship between individual and environmental characteristics in order to optimize patient safety.

Domain 6: Recognize, Respond to, and Disclose Adverse Events—Recognizing the occurrence of an adverse event or close call and responding effectively to mitigate harm to the patient, ensure disclosure, and prevent recurrence.

Canadian Patient Safety Institute. (2011). The safety competencies. Retrieved from http://www.patientsafetyinstitute.ca/English/toolsResources/safetyCompetencies/Pages/default.aspx.

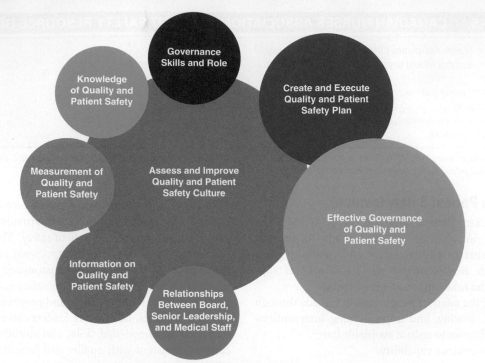

FIGURE 2-1 Drivers for effective governance for quality and patient safety.

EXERCISE 2-3

Visit the CPSI website (http://www.patientsafetyinstitute.ca) and explore the Tools & Resources section. Using information found on the CPSI website, answer the following questions.

1. What was the most frequent type of adverse event reported in the 2004 Canadian Adverse Events Study?
2. On what US initiative was Safer Healthcare Now! modelled?
3. What do 220 000 Canadians develop each year and about 8000 die from annually?
4. What practice by health care workers can reduce the number of health care associated infections by 50%?
5. What type of clinicians brings critical-care expertise to the patient's bedside (or wherever it is needed)?

Adapted from Canadian Patient Safety Institute. (2010). Canadian Patient Safety Week—tools and resources. Retrieved from http://www.patientsafety institute.ca/English/news/cpsw/Pages/ToolsResources.aspx.

NURSING-SENSITIVE OUTCOMES

How do you know if what you are doing is making a difference for the patients you provide care for? How do health care organizations measure nursing's contribution to quality care? While nurses have long been interested in understanding how nursing practice influences patient outcomes, it is in the last decade that a growing body of research in Canada and elsewhere has begun to answer this question. Nursing-sensitive outcomes is the phrase used to describe patient outcomes that are sensitive to nursing practice or interventions. They are measured by indicators that reflect information on patient outcomes. Specifically, information is collected from patient charts or other sources, such as nurse staffing complements and discharge data. This information is entered into a database and is then categorized to provide data on patient outcomes. Several broad categories of patient outcomes were identified by Doran (2011):

- *Functional status:* patients' perceptions of their day-to-day functioning. Examples: activities of daily living.
- *Self-care:* patients' perceptions and abilities to manage their care. Examples: medication administration, healthy eating.
- *Symptom management:* how well symptoms are managed. Examples: pain, fatigue.
- *Adverse patient outcomes:* occurrence and types of adverse events. Examples: hospital-acquired infections, patient falls, readmission to hospital, medication errors.

- *Patient satisfaction:* patient satisfaction with nursing care.
- *Mortality rates:* rates of death for specific, often preventable, causes. Examples: 30-day mortality rates, hospital standardized mortality ratio (pp. 1–18).

When information on patient outcomes is available, nurses can use it in a variety of ways at the individual, unit, and organization level. Patient outcome information is important for patient safety. Doran, Harrison, Laschinger, et al. (2004) suggested the following uses for nurse-sensitive outcomes:

- Develop treatment plans for individual patients.
- Evaluate different approaches to patient care.
- Inform best practices.
- Improve the quality of nursing care.
- Improve patient outcomes.
- Inform staffing policies and decisions.
- Assist organizations to balance the competing demands of access, cost, and quality (p. 3).

Nurse managers might use information about patient outcomes on a particular unit to design specific strategies or change policies to decrease an occurrence of an event such as hospital-acquired infections. Or they might advocate for resources that support patient satisfaction or staffing to optimize patient functional status. Front-line nurses can use information about patient outcomes to design care plans for patients or evaluate interventions. Information about patient outcomes becomes an invaluable tool for nurses to support a patient focus and advocate for nursing resources to improve care delivery. See the Research Perspective for a study on patient-centred care and patient outcomes.

Various sources of information on patient outcomes exist, including the health care organization itself. Health care organizations collect a great deal of information about the patients admitted for care and use this information to assess how well they are doing. Another source of information is the Canadian Institute of Health Information (CIHI). CIHI collects and analyzes information on the health care system, including that collected by health care organizations, to support decisions that will improve the health system. CIHI is able to identify trends and patterns that provide information on how well the health system is performing in a number of respects, including patient safety and some nurse-sensitive outcomes. You can have a look at the variety of information available on Canada's health care system at the CIHI website (http://www.cihi.ca).

RESEARCH PERSPECTIVE

Resource: Sidani, S. (2008). Effects of patient-centered care on patient outcomes: An evaluation. *Research and Theory for Nursing Practice, 22*(1), 24–37.

In this study, the researcher examined the extent to which acute care nurse practitioners (ACNPs) provided patient-centred care and explored the effects of patient-centred care on the patient outcomes of functional status, self-care ability, and satisfaction with care. They were particularly interested in two components of patient-centred care: individualization of care and patient participation in care. A non-experimental design was used and data were collected on patient outcomes at three different times: at admission, 1 week prior to discharge, and 6 to 8 weeks post-discharge. The sample included 320 patients with acute medical or surgical conditions assigned to the care of an ACNP and admitted to one of eight hospitals in southern Ontario. Findings from the study indicated that patients perceived that ACNPs provided patient-centred care; specifically, they encouraged patients to participate in care and individualized patient care to a moderate extent. Patients who were encouraged to participate in their care perceived that they could manage their care. Implementation of individualized care and patient participation in their care were also associated with patient satisfaction with care.

Implications for Practice

Incorporating the values of patient-centred care can positively impact patient outcomes.

CONCLUSION

As you read this book, keep in mind that nurses need to maintain a patient focus. Some means of maintaining a patient focus include asking yourself questions about how power and responsibility are shared with the patient; how input is actively encouraged from the patient and how communication is shared; whether a patient's individuality, cultural needs, values, and life issues have been taken into account; what efforts are being made to include patients who are not presenting for care at the expected care points; and what is being done to enhance prevention and health promotion. All nurses, including those in leadership and administrative roles, need to stay patient focused. They also need to actively engage with patients across the continuum of care in care planning, coordination, and implementation—respecting patient values and preferences—to enhance the impact and quality of care while acting ethically. Nurse managers and other leaders need to facilitate a change in practice whereby nurses are accountable to patients. Health care delivery systems in Canada must emphasize patient centredness and create a culture of safety. Nurses must respond positively and adapt to these changes. Even organizationally focused goals must ultimately address patient needs (the raison d'être of all health care organizations).

A SOLUTION

Staff mixture changes are a reality in the Canadian context. Care and due process in introducing these changes can help make the transition easier. Nurturing philosophies of care that are patient focused and patient centred help ensure that staffing conflicts and tensions do not adversely affect the care the public receives. Patient-centred care helps direct staff energy in productive ways, and patient-centred care combined with appreciative inquiry helps shift the focus on abilities and away from deficits. This situation clearly requires manager involvement. Team building is required. Asking staff to express their concerns using reference to *the patient* rather than *I* is one means of shifting the focus. Asking individuals to "walk in another's shoes" and consider what it is like to be the other person and to identify what skills and abilities the other person brings to the unit is another technique. Jack and his staff should look for ways to modify the culture of care in the medical unit to foster patient centredness, appreciative inquiry, and a culture of safety.

What other techniques might you suggest for improving patient focus and a culture of care in this work environment?

PROVINCIAL AND TERRITORIAL NURSING REGULATORY BODIES

PROVINCE/ TERRITORY	REGISTERED NURSES	LICENSED/REGISTERED PRACTICE NURSES	REGISTERED PSYCHIATRIC NURSES (BRITISH COLUMBIA, ALBERTA, SASKATCHEWAN, AND MANITOBA)
British Columbia	College of Registered Nurses of British Columbia http://www.crnbc.ca	College of Licensed Practical Nurses of British Columbia http://www.clpnbc.org	College of Registered Psychiatric Nurses of British Columbia http://www.crpnbc.ca
Alberta	College and Association of Registered Nurses of Alberta http://www.nurses.ab.ca	College of Licensed Practical Nurses of Alberta http://www.clpna.com	College of Registered Psychiatric Nurses of Alberta http://www.crpna.ab.ca
Saskatchewan	Saskatchewan Registered Nurses' Association http://www.srna.org	Saskatchewan Association of Licensed Practical Nurses http://www.salpn.com	Registered Psychiatric Nurses Association of Saskatchewan http://www.rpnas.com
Manitoba	College of Registered Nurses of Manitoba http://www.crnm.mb.ca	College of Licensed Practical Nurses of Manitoba http://www.clpnm.ca	College of Registered Psychiatric Nurses of Manitoba http://www.crpnm.mb.ca
Ontario	College of Nurses of Ontario http://www.cno.org	College of Nurses of Ontario http://www.cno.org	
Quebec	Ordre des infirmières et infirmiers du Québec http://www.oiiq.org	Ordre des infirmieres et infirmiers auxiliares du Quebec http://www.oiiaq.org	
New Brunswick	Nurses Association of New Brunswick http://www.nanb.nb.ca	Association of New Brunswick Licensed Practical Nurses http://www.anblpn.ca	
Nova Scotia	College of Registered Nurses of Nova Scotia http://www.crnns.ca	College of Licensed Practical Nurses of Nova Scotia http://www.clpnns.ca	

PROVINCIAL AND TERRITORIAL NURSING REGULATORY BODIES—cont'd

PROVINCE/ TERRITORY	REGISTERED NURSES	LICENSED/REGISTERED PRACTICE NURSES	REGISTERED PSYCHIATRIC NURSES (BRITISH COLUMBIA, ALBERTA, SASKATCHEWAN, AND MANITOBA)
Prince Edward Island	Association of Registered Nurses of Prince Edward Island http://www.arnpei.ca	Licensed Practical Nurses Association of Prince Edward Island http://www.lpna.ca	
Newfoundland and Labrador	Association of Registered Nurses of Newfoundland And Labrador http://www.arnnl.ca	College of Licensed Practical Nurses of Newfoundland & Labrador http://www.clpnnl.ca	
Northwest Territories	Registered Nurses Association of Northwest Territories and Nunavut http://www.rnantnu.ca		
Yukon	Yukon Registered Nurses Association http://www.yrna.ca		

THE EVIDENCE

Nurses have an integral role in promoting patient safety. In 2007, the symposium Advancing Nursing Leadership for a Safer Healthcare System was held in Toronto. Jeffs, MacMillan, McKey, et al. (2009) summarized the themes emerging from the research presented at this symposium. They identified four future directions for nursing, including focusing on the patient in patient safety, broadening the knowledge base on patient safety beyond acute care, linking healthy work environments and a culture of patient safety, and bridging evidence-informed research and practice.

NEED TO KNOW NOW

- Know how and where to access resources related to patient- or client-centred care, patient safety, and patient outcomes.
- Contribute to an organization that is accountable to patients and their families.
- Understand how evidence regarding nursing-sensitive outcomes can be used to advocate for patient-centred care and patient safety.
- Know and apply the eight values forming the foundation of patient-centred care in nursing.
- Know and apply the six safety competencies in your nursing practice.

CHAPTER CHECKLIST

Through a philosophy of patient centredness, creating a culture of patient safety, and attending to patient outcomes, nurse leadership and management can advocate for a patient focus and support all nurses to practise in a safe, competent, and ethical manner.

- Nurses in all roles must maintain a patient focus. Foundational to the patient focus, nurse leaders and followers must practise according to the professional standards and code of ethics.
- Nurse leaders and followers play an important role in influencing organizational culture for the benefit

of patients and positive patient outcomes. They also maintain responsibility for identifying and changing systemic factors that hinder patient-centred care.

- Nurse leaders and followers play an important role in identifying potential safety issues and raising awareness of these issues to ensure early intervention and avoid significant and negative outcomes.

- Nurse leaders can use the safety competencies set out by the Canadian Patient Safety Institute to develop educational activities for staff; followers can use the safety competencies to identify gaps in their practice that need to be addressed.
- Organizations that offer support for the creation of a culture of patient safety include the following:
  - Canadian Patient Safety Institute
  - Canadian Nurses Association

TIPS FOR PATIENT-FOCUSED LEADERSHIP

- Review the RNAO Best Practice Guideline titled *Client Centred Care* and identify areas where your unit aligns with the values of patient-centred care and areas for improvement.

- Be aware of the strategies your organization is focusing on to address patient safety.
- Know what patient outcomes are collected and reported for your unit.

evolve WEBSITE

Visit the Evolve website for Suggested Readings, Internet Resources, and additional resources related to the content in this chapter: http://evolve.elsevier.com/Canada/Yoder-Wise/leading/.

REFERENCES

Association of Registered Nurses of Newfoundland and Labrador. (2007). *Standards for nursing practice*. St. John's, NL: Author. Retrieved from http://www.arnnl.ca.

Baker, G. R., Norton, P., Flintoft, et al. (2004). The Canadian Adverse Events Study: The incidence of adverse events among hospital patients in Canada. *Canadian Medical Association Journal, 170*, 1678–1686. doi:10.1503/cmaj.1040498

Black, J., Allen, D., Redfern, L., et al. (2008). Competencies in the context of entry-level registered nurses practice: A collaborative project in Canada. *International Nursing Review, 55*, 171–178.

Canadian Nurses Association. (2008). *Code of ethics for registered nurses (2008 centennial edition)*. Toronto, ON: Author.

Canadian Nurses Association. (2009). Position statement: Patient safety. Retrieved from http://www.cna-aiic.ca/~/media/cna/page%20content/pdf%20fr/2013/07/26/10/48/ps102_patient_safety_e.pdf.

Canadian Nurses Association. (2011). Patient safety resource guide. Retrieved from http://www.cna-nurses.ca/CNA/practice/environment/safety/guide/default_e.aspx.

Canadian Patient Safety Institute. (n.d.a). About CPSI. Retrieved from http://www.patientsafetyinstitute.ca/english/about/pages/default.aspx.

Canadian Patient Safety Institute. (n.d.b). Adverse event. Retrieved from http://www.patientsafetyinstitute.ca/english/toolsresources/governancepatientsafety/pages/glossaryofterms.aspx.

Canadian Patient Safety Institute. (2010). Canadian Patient Safety Week—tools and resources. Retrieved from http://www.patientsafetyinstitute.ca/English/news/cpsw/Pages/ToolsResources.aspx.

Canadian Patient Safety Institute. (2011). The safety competencies. Retrieved from http://www.patientsafetyinstitute.ca/English/toolsResources/safetyCompetencies/Pages/default.aspx.

College of Nurses of Ontario. (2009). *Professional standards, revised 2009*. Toronto, ON: Author.

College of Registered Nurses of British Columbia. (2008). *Professional standards for registered nurses and nurse practitioners*. Vancouver, BC: Author.

Doran, D. (2011). Nursing outcomes: The state of the science (2nd ed.). Sudbury, MA: Jones and Barlett Learning.

Doran, D., Harrison, M. B., Laschinger, H., et al. (2004). *Collecting data on nursing-sensitive outcomes in different care settings: Can it be done? What are the benefits? Report of the nursing and health outcomes feasibility study*. Toronto, ON: University of Toronto.

Fleming, M., & Wentzell, N. (2008). Patient Safety Culture Improvement Tool: Development and guidelines for use. *Healthcare Quarterly, 11*(Sp), 10–15.

Halligan, M., & Zecevic, A. (2011). Safety culture in healthcare: A review of concepts, dimensions, measures and progress. *BMJ Quality and Safety, 20*(4), 338–343. doi:10.1136/bmjqs.2010.040964

Institute of Medicine. (2000). *To err is human: Building a safer health system*. Washington, DC: National Academy Press.

Jeffs, L., MacMillan, K., McKey, C., et al. (2009). Nursing leaders' accountability to narrow the safety chasm: Insights and implications from the collective evidence based on healthcare safety. *Canadian Journal of Nursing Leadership, 22*(1), 86–98.

Lewis, S. (2009). *Patient-centered care: An introduction to what it is and how to achieve it: A discussion paper for the Saskatchewan Ministry of Health*. Saskatoon, SK: The Change Foundation. Retrieved from http://www.changefoundation.ca/docs/patient-centred-care-intro.pdf.

Registered Nurses' Association of Ontario. (2002). Client centred care. Toronto, ON: Author.

Royal College of Physicians and Surgeons of Canada. (2003). *The Canadian patient safety dictionary*. Retrieved from http://rcpsc.medical.org/publications/PatientSafety Dictionary_e.pdf.

Sidani S. (2008). Effects of patient-centered care on patient outcomes: an evaluation. *Research and Theory for Nursing Practice, 22*(1), 24–37. doi:http://dx.doi.org/10.1891/0889-7182.22.1.24

Thompson, P. A. (2000). Patient safety: Pieces of the puzzle. *Journal of Nursing Administration, 30*(11), 509.

Tregunno, D., Jeffs, L., McGillis Hall, L., et al. (2009). On the ball: Leadership for patient safety and learning in critical care. *Journal of Nursing Administration, 39*(7–8), 334–339. doi:10.1097/NNA.0b013e3181ae9653

Vogus, T. J., Sutcliffe, K. M., & Weick, K. E. (2010). Doing no harm: Enabling, enacting, and elaborating a culture of safety in health care. *Academy of Management Perspectives, 24*(4), 60–76. doi:10.5465/AMP.2010.55206385

Wiseman, B., & Kaprielian, V. S. (2005). What do we mean by a culture of safety? Retrieved from http://patientsafetyed.duhs.duke.edu/module_c/what_do_we_mean.html.

World Health Organization. (n.d.). Patient safety. Retrieved from http://www.who.int/patientsafety/about/en/.

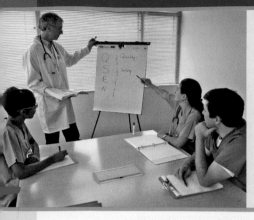

Developing the Role of Leader

Michael L. Evans
Adapted by Angela J. Gillis

This chapter focuses on leadership and its value in advancing the profession of nursing. Leadership development is explained with examples of how to thrive in a leadership position. The differences between the emerging and entrenched workforce generations are explored, and the desired characteristics of a leader for the emerging workforce are described. Leadership is described in a variety of situations, such as clinical settings, community venues, organizations, and political situations. This chapter introduces the opportunities, challenges, and rewards of leadership.

OBJECTIVES

- Analyze the role of leadership in creating a satisfying working environment for nurses.
- Evaluate transactional and transformational leadership techniques for effectiveness and potential for positive outcomes.
- Value the leadership challenges in dealing with generational differences.
- Compare and contrast leadership and management roles and responsibilities.
- Describe leadership development strategies and how they can promote leadership skills acquisition.
- Analyze leadership opportunities and responsibilities in a variety of venues.
- Explore strategies for making the leadership opportunity positive for both leaders and followers.

TERMS TO KNOW

clinical nurse leader (CNL)	leadership	mentor
emerging workforce	learning organization	transactional leadership
entrenched workforce	management	transformational leadership

The nurse manager of the critical care unit at a rural regional hospital is responsible for everything, from the quality of patient care to staff recruitment and retention. The nurse manager has noticed that Lauren, a recently hired and newly graduated nurse, has used almost all of her sick time and allowed the quality of her work to decrease significantly. To understand what is happening, the nurse manager calls Lauren into his office for a conversation. Lauren is forthcoming with information about her feelings for her co-workers and the treatment she is receiving from them. She explains that she is feeling isolated and unwelcome on the floor as the other nurses are continuously ignoring and belittling her to the point where her questions are deemed "stupid" and inappropriate. The unrealistic expectations the staff have of Lauren are contributing to their negative perception of her, and they see Lauren's

questions as a weakness and an excuse to roll their eyes and gossip. Lauren describes a situation where another nurse directly humiliated her by pointing out her faults to the whole staff. Since she was new to the floor and unfamiliar with certain policies, she felt like a child who had been shamed and reprimanded. This treatment just validated her feelings of rejection by the staff. She proceeded to explain the stress she experiences before, during, and after her shifts and how the treatment she is receiving has contributed to her sick time as she feels physically and emotionally drained.

As the leader on this unit, how should the nurse manager deal with this situation?

WHAT IS A LEADER?

Canada's health care system requires a steady supply of visionary nurse leaders who are bold, confident, and courageous, and who can inspire others to support excellence in nursing practice (Canadian Nurses Association [CNA], 2009). Leadership encompasses a range of definitions. A leader is an individual who works with others to develop a vision of the preferred future and to make that vision happen. Alimo-Metcalfe and Alban-Metcalfe (2008) call that type of leadership *engaged leadership*, or the ability to foster a culture where new ways of thinking and change are encouraged, and where people are inspired to bring a shared vision into reality. Leaders bring out the best in people.

The Canadian Nurses Association, or CNA (2009), defines *nursing leadership* as a process that involves critical thinking, action, and advocacy. It happens in all domains of nursing practice. Nursing leadership is about nurses who understand that the development of leaders must begin in nursing schools and continue throughout the career of every nurse. In this context, leadership involves helping nurses at every level visualize their practice as not only a series of scientific caring acts that can change individual lives but also as a lifelong commitment to political action for social change.

Great leaders have been responsible for helping society move forward and for articulating and accomplishing one vision after another throughout time. Dr. Martin Luther King Jr. called his vision a *dream*, and

it was developed because of the input and lived experiences of countless others. Mother Teresa called her vision a *calling*, and it was developed because of the suffering of others. Pierre Elliott Trudeau called his vision a *just society*, which was enacted through the *Canadian Charter of Rights and Freedoms*. Florence Nightingale called her vision *nursing*, and it was developed because people were experiencing a void that was a barrier to their health.

Rush (2011) asserts that leaders work in a relational process with others. An individual can have an impressive title, but that title does not make that person a leader. No matter what the person with that title does, he or she can never be successful without having the ability to inspire the commitment of others to follow. Successful nurse leaders are interdependent upon the actions and accomplishments of many within health care organizations (Kean, Haycock-Stewart, Baggaley, et al., 2011).

Covey (1992) identifies eight characteristics of effective leaders (Box 3-1). These qualities are timeless and when practised consistently can change your view of leadership.

EXERCISE 3-1

List Covey's eight characteristics of effective leaders on the left side of a piece of paper. Next to each characteristic, list any examples of your activities or attributes that reflect the characteristic. Some areas may be blank; others will be full. Think about what this means for you personally.

BOX 3-1   COVEY'S EIGHT CHARACTERISTICS OF EFFECTIVE LEADERS

1. Engage in lifelong learning
2. Are service-oriented
3. Are concerned with the common good
4. Radiate positive energy
5. Believe in other people
6. Lead balanced lives and see life as an adventure
7. Are synergistic; that is, they see things as greater than the sum of the parts
8. Engage themselves in self-renewal

Covey, S. R. (1992). *Principle-centered leadership.* New York, NY: Simon and Schuster.

Health care organizations are complex. Continual learning is essential to stay abreast of new knowledge, to keep the organization moving forward, and to continue delivering the best possible care. A current trend is for organizations to become learning organizations. A learning organization is one that is continually expanding its capacity to create its future and provide opportunities and incentives for its members to learn continuously over time (Senge, 2006). Leaders are responsible for building organizations in which people continually expand their ability to understand complexity and to clarify and improve a shared vision of the future—"that is, they are responsible for learning" (Senge, 2006, p. 340).

The roles of manager and leader are often considered interchangeable; in Chapter 1, aspects of the similarities and differences of these roles were outlined in some detail. The manager may be a leader, but the manager is not required to have leadership skills within the context of moving a group of people toward a vision. The term *manager* is a designated formal position that is assigned to an individual in the organization. In contrast, *leadership* is an achieved and informal role based on abilities. Management involves the activities needed to plan, organize, motivate, and control the human and material resources required to achieve outcomes consistent with the organization's mission and purpose. Management can be taught and learned using traditional teaching techniques. Similarly, leadership is a learnable set of practices that requires continued opportunity for application and feedback. Leadership involves a persistent desire to lead and make a positive difference. It is usually a reflection of rich personal experiences and influence, and it is most effective when followers share the leader's vision.

The challenge facing many health care organizations today is that managers are in place but nurse leaders are missing. We can teach new managers, but our leaders are developed over time and through experience. Thus, it is important that we value, support, and provide our leaders with the one thing vital for good leadership—good followers. Leadership is a social process involving leaders and followers who interact to provide excellence in health care delivery. Followers need three qualities from their leaders: honesty, trust, and integrity (Hader, 2011). Trust is reciprocal. Leaders who trust their followers are, in turn, trusted by them.

Managers are concerned with doing things correctly in the present. The manager's role is important in work organizations because managers ensure that operations run smoothly and that well-developed formulas are applied to staffing situations, economic decisions, and other daily operations. Managers are concerned less with developing creative solutions to problems and more with using strategies to address today's issues. Covey (2009) believes that a well-managed entity may be proceeding correctly but, without leadership, may be proceeding in the wrong direction. Leadership must come first to make managing effective. As Govier and Nash (2009) note, if management is efficiency in climbing the ladder, then leadership determines if the ladder is leaning against the correct wall.

A discussion of leadership would not be complete without mention of the emerging role of the clinical nurse leader (CNL). The CNL is a highly skilled master degree–prepared nurse who has completed advanced studies in clinical care with a focus on the improvement of quality outcomes for specific patient populations at the point of care. The CNL coordinates and supervises the care provided by interdisciplinary team members. Like other leadership roles, the CNL role includes development of skills in preceptoring, mentoring, and coaching.

Leadership as an Important Concept for Nurses

Nurses must have leadership to move forward in harmony with changes in society and in health care. Within work settings, nurses as managers are required to ensure that care is delivered in a safe, efficient manner. Nurse leaders are also vital in the workplace to elicit input from others and to formulate a vision for the preferred future.

Leadership is also key for nursing as a profession. The public depends on nurses to advocate for the public's needs and interests. Nurses must step forward into leadership roles in their workplace, in their professional associations and regulatory organizations, and in government and policymaking arenas. Nurses depend on their leaders to set goals for the future and the pace for achieving them. The public depends on nurse leaders to move the health care agenda forward in a patient-focused manner in the interest of the common good.

Leadership as a Primary Determinant of Workplace Satisfaction

Nurse satisfaction within the workplace is an important construct in nursing leadership. Turnover is extremely costly to any work organization in terms of money, expertise, and knowledge, as well as care quality. Thus, being mindful of nurse satisfaction is an economic, as well as a professional, concern.

Canadian researchers provide evidence that leadership practices influence job satisfaction, as well as nurse recruitment and intention to remain in current positions (Cowden, Cummings, & Profetto-McGrath, 2011; Cummings, MacGregor, Davey, et al., 2010). The following leadership practices were found to contribute to higher job satisfaction and greater staff commitment to the organization:
1. Perceived support from leader, manager, and peers
2. Autonomy over practice
3. Recognition for staff contributions
4. Participation in decision making
5. Empowerment to reach full potential
The effective leader needs to be aware of these important work factors that influence followers and find ways to actualize these aspects of work life.

The leader, not the manager, inspires others to work at their highest level. The presence of strong leadership sets the tone for achievement in the work environment. Effective leadership is the basis for an effective workplace, and therefore creating leadership succession is an important consideration. This means that, in addition to supporting current leaders in their roles, new leaders must be encouraged and

developed. According to one Canadian author, nursing lags behind the corporate and other sectors in leadership succession planning (Laframboise, 2011). Succession planning can increase job satisfaction, recruitment, retention, productivity, and quality of service, as it provides leadership stability. Leaders must become "talent scouts," and hire the rising stars of tomorrow and provide them with leadership opportunities; in doing so, they create their own talent pool. Mentoring and networking are essential to leadership succession planning. Succession planning provides the knowledge, skill, attitudes, and competencies nurses need to create vibrant, growing organizations in which many people can lead (Laframboise, 2011). It is an important component of leadership development and a responsibility of nurses at every level of leadership.

EXERCISE 3-2

Health care team members engage in the interactive and interdependent process of leading and following. Follower behaviour nurtures and supports—or deteriorates—leader behaviour. Identify the behaviour you exhibited during your most recent clinical experience. What was supportive of the leader? What did not support the leader?

THE PRACTICE OF LEADERSHIP

Leadership Approaches

How one approaches leadership depends on experience and expectations. Many leadership theories and styles exist. Two of the most popular theory-based approaches are transactional leadership and transformational leadership. (See the Theory Box.)

Transactional Leadership. A transactional leader is the traditional "boss." In a transactional leadership environment, employees understand that a superior makes the decisions, acting within the confines of collective agreements if in place, with little or no input from subordinates. Transactional leadership relies on the power of organizational position and formal authority to reward and punish performance. Followers are fairly secure about what will happen next and how to "play the game" to get where they want to be. A transactional leader uses a *quid pro quo* style to accomplish work (e.g., I'll do *x* in exchange for your doing *y*). Transactional leaders

THEORY BOX

A Comparison of Outcomes in Transactional and Transformational Leadership

TRANSACTIONAL LEADERSHIP	TRANSFORMATIONAL LEADERSHIP
Leader Behaviours	
• Contingent reward (*quid pro quo*)	• Charismatic
• Punitive	• Inspiring and motivating
• Management by exception (active)—monitors performance and takes action to correct	• Intellectually stimulating
• Management by exception (passive)—intervenes only when problems exist	• Individualized consideration
Effect on the Follower	
• Fulfills the contract or gets punished	• Shared vision
• Does the work and gets paid	• Increased self-worth
• Corrects errors in a reactive manner	• Challenging and meaningful work
	• Coaching and mentoring
	• Feeling of being valued
Organizational Outcomes	
• Work is supervised and completed according to the rules	• Increased loyalty
• Deadlines are met	• Increased commitment
• Job satisfaction is limited	• Increased job satisfaction
• Low to stable levels of organizational commitment are achieved	• Increased morale
	• Increased performance

Modified from McGuire, E., & Kennerly, S. M. (2006). Nurse managers as transformational and transactional leaders. *Nursing Economic$, 24*(4), 179–185.

reward employees for high performance and penalize them for poor performance. The leader motivates the self-interest of the employee by offering external rewards that generate conformity with expectations. The status quo is continually reinforced in organizations in which transactional leadership is practised (Weston, 2008).

Transformational Leadership. Transformational leadership is based on an inspiring vision that changes the framework of the organization for employees. Employees are encouraged to transcend their own self-interest. This style of leadership involves communication that connects with employees' ideals in a way that causes emotional engagement. The transformational leader can motivate employees by articulating an inspirational vision; by encouraging novel, innovative thinking; and by providing individualized consideration of each employee, accounting for individual needs and abilities. The result of such leadership is that both leaders and followers have a higher level of motivation and a greater sense of purpose (Rolfe, 2011). Covey (1992) states, "The goal of transformational leadership is to transform people and organizations in a literal

sense, to change them in mind and heart; enlarge vision, insight, and understanding; clarify purposes; make behavior congruent with beliefs, principles, or values; and bring about changes that are permanent, self-perpetuating, and momentum-building" (p. 287).

Kouzes and Posner (2008) identify five key practices in transformational leadership:

1. Challenging the process, which involves questioning the way things have been done in the past and thinking creatively about new solutions to old problems
2. Inspiring a shared vision or bringing everyone together to move toward a goal that all accept as desirable and achievable
3. Enabling others to act, which includes empowering people to believe that their extra effort will have rewards and will make a difference
4. Modelling the way, meaning that the leader must take an active role in the work of change
5. Encouraging the heart by giving attention to those personal things that are important to people, such as saying "thank you" for a job well done and offering praise after a long day

A transformative leader seems particularly suited to the nursing environment.

The literature suggests that transformational leadership produces positive results in the workplace. A systematic review of 23 studies on leadership practices examined the relationship between nurses' perceptions of leadership in the practice environment and nurses' intentions to remain within the organization. Nurses employed in settings where they felt supported by their leaders, valued for their contributions, and empowered to reach their full potential (transformational leadership practices) were generally more satisfied in their jobs and committed to the organization (Cowden et al., 2011). The review also found a positive relationship between transformational leadership practices and staff satisfaction, staff intention to remain in their current positions, and supportive work environments. Another team of researchers reviewed 53 studies on the relationship between leadership style and outcomes for the nursing workforce and work environments. They grouped outcomes into five categories: staff satisfaction with work, role, and pay; staff relationships with work; staff health and well-being; work environment factors; and productivity and effectiveness. Important differences were noted between relational (transformative) and task-focused (transactional) leadership styles and their outcomes for nurses and the work environment. Transformational leadership was found to positively impact nurse satisfaction, recruitment, and retention, and to promote healthy work environments (Cummings et al., 2010).

Clinical leaders who have developed transformational leadership skills have been found to promote effective communication, empowerment, job clarity, continuity of care, and interdisciplinary collaboration among the nursing team (Dierckx de Casterlé, Willemse, Verschueren, et al., 2008). Moreover, a transformational leadership style has been closely associated with followers' well-being and their perceived working conditions—namely influence, involvement, and meaningfulness (Nielsen, Yarker, Brenner, et al., 2008). It is also a key factor in the implementation and sustainability of best practice guidelines (Marchionni & Ritchie, 2008).

Casida and Parker (2011) studied staff nurse perceptions of nurse manager leadership styles and outcomes in a sample of 278 staff nurses and 37 nurse managers. The authors examined whether links existed among the leadership styles (transformational and transactional) of nurse managers and outcomes such as a leader's extra effort, leadership satisfaction, and leadership effectiveness. Results indicated that nurse managers who used a transformational leadership style received higher scores on the variables of leader's extra effort, leadership satisfaction, and leadership effectiveness. Conversely, nurse managers who used a transactional leadership style received lower scores on leader's extra effort, leadership satisfaction, and leadership effectiveness. This study supported the use of a transformational leadership style in achieving leadership effectiveness and leadership satisfaction in acute care hospitals. It also concluded that nurse managers who use a transformational leadership style are likely to reach their leadership goals effectively and satisfactorily, and significantly influence the achievement of organizational strategic goals.

Transformational leadership produces positive outcomes in organizations. It is an effective method for managing a diverse nursing workforce, improving patient outcomes, and inspiring staff to perform beyond expectations. Transformational leadership is needed now more than ever in today's challenging health care environment, and nurses are rising to the challenge, as the following Research Perspective illustrates.

RESEARCH PERSPECTIVE

Resource: Gordon, K., & Melrose, S. (2011). LPN to BN nurses: Introducing a new group of potential health care leaders. *E-Journal of Organizational Learning and Leadership, 9*(1) 121–128.

A qualitative descriptive study applied the Kouzes and Posner's (2008) model of transformational leadership to explore the experiences of ten licensed practical nurses who upgraded their credentials to bachelor of nursing (referred to here as *post LPN to BN nurses*). This longitudinal research project spanned 3 years and involved interview data collected annually, during and after the program of study. Nurses' words were used to illustrate their changing perspectives.

Findings revealed that transformational leadership practices were evident as post LPN to BN nurses transitioned to a new role after graduation. Two key themes illustrated how these nurses changed and grew following their university education. First, post LPN to BN nurses identified a changed awareness of the implications

Continued

RESEARCH PERSPECTIVE—cont'd

of their new role as graduation approached. Second, they developed confidence to begin envisioning themselves as leaders who can make a difference in their profession, and they assumed a new vision of the nursing profession.

Implications for Practice
Transformational, confident, and visionary leaders are needed in today's changing health care environment. This study introduced post LPN to BN graduates as potential health care leaders and provided a glimpse into how these graduates defined their personal values and beliefs differently, embraced the possibility of leadership, and dreamed about a vision for the future of nursing. Educators and nurse leaders need to recognize that post LPN to BN graduates have leadership aspirations and create opportunities for them to model their new way of thinking, guide them toward developing leadership action plans, and encourage them to risk leading initiatives within their organization.

Leadership is the ability to influence people to work toward meeting certain goals. Often this influence requires an ongoing commitment to role-modelling and reinforcing behaviours. The intensity of repeating such influence multiple times can be wearing. In the chaos of health care, nurse leaders face constant change and many challenges. The leader who lasts through these relationships is influential.

Barriers to Leadership

Leadership demands a commitment of effort and time. Many barriers exist to both leading and following. Good leadership and good followership go hand in hand, and both strengthen the mission of the organization. A good leader can accomplish nothing without the presence of a stable and robust team (Rush, 2011).

False Assumptions. Some people have false assumptions about leaders and leadership. For example, some believe that position and title are equivalent to leadership. Having the title of chief executive officer does not

---

EXERCISE 3-3
Define a clinical or management issue that sparks your passion. Assume that you have 6 weeks to make a difference. Create a plan identifying your leadership tasks, the support required from others, and the time frame to move the issue toward resolution. Think about what your message is and how and when you will deliver it. Think about what you would do if no one was responsive to your issue. Think about why the issue may be important for you but not for others.

---

guarantee that a person will be a good leader. Inspired and forward-moving organizations often select executives specifically because of their ability to forge a vision and lead others toward it. Assuming a management role does not automatically confer the title of leader on an individual. Leadership is an earned honour, a privilege, and an action-oriented responsibility. Leaders are those who do the best job of sharing their vision of where the followers want to be and how to get there.

Time Constraints. Leadership requires a time commitment; it does not just happen. The leader must fully comprehend the situation at hand, research options, communicate the vision to others, and continually re-evaluate the situation to ensure that the vision remains relevant and attainable. All of these activities take time. Everyone is busy. Finding time to lead is, therefore, a barrier for many who have inspirational ideas but lack time to develop the skills needed to lead effectively.

LEADERSHIP DEVELOPMENT

Leadership effectiveness depends on mastering the art of persuasion and communication. Success depends on persuading followers to accept a vision by using convincing communication techniques and making it possible for them to achieve their shared goals. Several important leadership tasks will help ensure success (Box 3-2). These are discussed in the following sections.

Select a Mentor

Canadian nurse researchers Earle, Myrick, and Yonge (2011) reported that mentorship, which involves a relationship between a mentor and a mentee, was viewed as the key support that young nurses required to pursue leadership roles. A mentor is someone who models behaviour, offers advice and criticism, and coaches the novice leader or mentee to develop a personal leadership style. A mentor is a knowledgeable and skilled confidante, coach, cheerleader, and teacher who has experience and some success in the leadership realm of

---

BOX 3-2   LEADERSHIP DEVELOPMENT TASKS

1. Select a mentor.	4. Share the rewards.
2. Lead by example.	5. Have a clear vision.
3. Accept responsibility.	6. Be willing to grow.

interest. A respected faculty member, a nurse manager or clinician, or an organizational leader or active member may be a mentor. Mentorship is a two-way street. The mentor must agree to work with the novice leader or mentee and must have some interest in the mentee's future development. A mentor can be close enough geographically to allow both observation and practice of leadership behaviours, as well as timely feedback. A mentor may also be geographically remote and yet well-connected to the mentee. A mentor should provide advice, feedback, and role-modelling. In addition, the mentor has a right to expect assistance with projects, respect, loyalty, and confidentiality. In a mentoring relationship, aspiring leaders soak up knowledge and experience and should expect to return it by serving as a mentor to a young, aspiring leader in the future.

Lead by Example

An effective leader knows that the best way to influence people is to lead by example. Desired behaviour can be modelled. For example, if an organization has a vision of becoming a political player in its province or territory, the leader should be seen engaging in political activities. If the goal is to have improved relationships among the health care team, the leader must exhibit respect and patience with followers. A key skill to develop is the ability to understand that the leader serves the followers. The effective leader does not send members to do a job but, rather, leads them toward a mutual goal as a team.

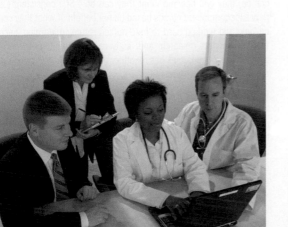

Leading by example helps developing leaders see the mission in action.

Accept Responsibility

The leader is ultimately responsible for the organization or activity. Leaders sometimes react in strange ways when negative outcomes occur, by blaming others or by making excuses for undesirable outcomes. Some refuse to accept any responsibility at all. In accepting responsibility, the leader knows that there is reward in victory and growth in failure. No one plans to fail, but an effective leader sees failures as opportunities to learn and grow so that previous failures are never repeated. This is called *experience*.

Share the Rewards

An effective leader is as eager to share the glory as to receive it. Stepping aside and allowing followers to move forward and share the spotlight of success is a sign of strength (Rush, 2011). The more that respect and trust are shared with others, the more they are returned to the leader. Followers who believe their major task is to make the leader look good will soon tire of the task. Empowerment, the act of sharing power with others, is a dynamic process. In essence, sharing power has a synergistic effect that increases power overall. A team who believes the leader is working to make them look good will form a strong support base for the leader.

Have a Clear Vision

Leaders see beyond where they are and see where they are going. Strong leaders are proactive and futuristic. The effective leader knows why the journey is necessary and takes the time and energy to inspire others to go along. The ability to communicate and promote the vision is a vital part of achieving it. Effective leaders share their vision and empower others to come along to achieve it.

Be Willing to Grow

It is a misconception to think that growth for a person or an organization is automatic. Complacency leads to stagnation. Leaders must continually read about new ideas and approaches, experiment with new concepts, capitalize on a changing world, and seek or create continuing educational opportunities to enhance their abilities to lead. Growth takes risk, planning, investment, and work. Setting goals that complement the vision will help an aspiring leader know where to invest time and energy to grow into the desired role.

Leadership development is a lifetime endeavour. Effective leaders are constantly striving to improve their leadership skills. The good news is that leadership skills can be learned and improved. A commitment to improvement strengthens the leader's ability to lead effectively and raises the bar for followers to achieve. As organizations and health care change, the leader is better able to work effectively with an increasingly diverse workforce. The best leaders bring out the best in their followers, as seen in the following Literature Perspective.

DEVELOPING LEADERS IN THE EMERGING WORKFORCE

Generational differences have always created challenges in the workplace. At the dawn of the twenty-first century, the workplace found an emerging workforce with goals, priorities, and work preferences that were vastly different from those of their Baby Boomer and Generation X parents. Helping each generation understand and tolerate others is often a delicate orchestration of needs and wants, incentives, and motives. Transgenerational leadership must focus on building understanding and acceptance.

LITERATURE PERSPECTIVE

Resource: Holmes, M. (2011). Just say "yes!": Mary Ferguson-Paré and the art of influential leadership. *Nursing Leadership, 24*(1), 23–29. Retrieved from http://www.longwoods.com/content/22330.

With a career that spanned over 40 years, Mary Ferguson-Paré is one of Canada's most widely respected nurse leaders. This article describes her understanding of leadership, a vision that developed over time as she sought to lead individuals, teams, and organizations in the pursuit of excellence in health care. Ferguson-Paré's own voice "takes centre stage" in this descriptive profile of leadership, accompanied by comments from three nurse colleagues who describe the exemplary qualities of leadership that she has personified.

According to colleagues, three commitments have underpinned Ferguson-Paré's leadership: (1) developing nurses, (2) ensuring a quality work life for staff, and (3) developing the highest standard of patient care. All her actions were directed toward these objectives. As a leader in health care, she believes that "you must look after your people so that your people can look after your patients" (Holmes, 2011, p. 25). As a result, she consistently sought input from nurses and listened—really listened—to what nurses told her about their jobs and themselves. This information was then used to create a healthy work environment, thus ensuring a strong platform for nursing leadership.

Ferguson-Paré believes in the importance of focusing on the positive. This realization fundamentally changed her practice. Prior to this realization, when she was looking to make improvements in care, she would identify what staff were doing wrong and then proceed to generate solutions to those errors. Experience taught her that starting from the negative did not work. In the past, strategies for change came from the top down. She learned that creating a "blossoming up" approach, concentrating on the positive and on ideas that came from the actual nursing units, was much more effective.

Ferguson-Paré also developed a new leadership philosophy she calls "just say 'yes'!" This philosophy is intended to prevent people in day-to-day management from "looking at their feet, walking in the same spot and going nowhere!" The point of saying "yes" is to help nurses stay focused on where they want to go rather than on where they currently are. Ferguson-Paré's belief in innovation led staff to come to her with new ideas for implementation. For example, a staff member's proposal to conduct research among practising nurses (little research existed at the unit level) resulted in over 40 teams conducting nursing research at the University Health Network 6 years later.

In addition, a central tenet of Ferguson-Paré's leadership philosophy is empowering people. She believes "if you treat people as they are, they will remain as they are. But if you treat people as they can be, they will become what they can be." She consistently set new expectations for nurses based on her beliefs of what they could become and worked hard to help nurses return to learning, secure funding, conduct research, and apply research findings to patient care. Empowering nurses has resulted in improved satisfaction rates among both patients and staff.

Implications for Practice

Leaders in nursing can increase their leadership effectiveness in practice environments by following the lead of Ferguson-Paré. Nurse leaders can work collaboratively with their staff to empower all nurses to be leaders. According to Ferguson-Paré, nurses can become leaders "first, by thinking about the future they want to move towards as an individual and, next, to clarify and embrace a vision of where they want to travel as a group of capable, courageous caregivers." Ferguson-Paré's leadership philosophy will result in optimal patient-care delivery and the creation of healthy and satisfying work environments for nurses.

The Emerging Workforce: Generations Y and Z

Generation Y (also known as *Nexters* or the *Millennium Generation*), born between 1977 and 1995, share many of the same approaches to work as Generation X but bring their own challenges with no brand loyalty and a blatant disregard for status symbols. They strive to maintain a balance between home and work, and they prefer collaborative approaches to work, with greater autonomy over their practice. They are also technology-savvy and tend to be optimistic and interactive (Wilcox, 2009).

Their younger siblings, Generation Z, born after 1995 are coming of age in 2013. While not a lot is known yet about their approaches to work, they have grown up in a highly sophisticated media and computer environment. They are expected to be even more technology-savvy than their Generation Y siblings. The impact of Generation Z on the workforce bears watching by leaders as this young cohort begins to move into the employment market.

What do these emerging workforce members want in their leaders and work environment? According to a study by Lavoie-Tremblay, Leclerc, Marchionni, et al. (2010), "[G]eneration Y nurses reported that recognition was a key motivator. Their needs are stability, flexible work schedules and shifts, recognition, opportunities for professional development, and adequate supervision" (p. 2). Earle et al. (2011) found that mentorship was a key ingredient the emerging workforce sought in leaders and a necessary requirement in their own pursuit of leadership roles. An Ontario study of the emerging workforce indicated that these young employees want a leader with good people skills who is open to staff participation in decision making and supportive of self-scheduling, continuing education, and career development opportunities for staff (Wilson, Squires, Widger, et al., 2008). They want their leaders to coach and mentor them as well as invest in activities that promote their personal growth and advancement. They are less comfortable in a structured environment, and less likely to agree with their manager's expectations. Rather than managing details of work, nurse managers have to be able to lead this group through coaching and mentoring.

Successfully leading the emerging workforce means the leader must shape a vision and win over the younger workers to follow it. The vision must be one that excites them, because fun and balance are an important part of their lives. A vision that is powerful enough can transform the workplace.

The successful leader must mobilize followers to act. The required actions must provide value to the followers (e.g., learning a new skill or attaining certification). The younger generations are happy to be part of the team as long as they can retain balance in their lives, have information about and input into the decisions that affect them, and see some benefit in the activity. It is the leader's challenge to provide the type of environment in which younger-generation team members want to follow.

The Entrenched Workforce: Baby Boomers and Generation X

Baby Boomers, born after World War II, see work life very differently compared with the emerging workforce. Boomers are more likely to believe in the power of collective action, based on their successes with social movements in their formative years in the 1960s. They tend to mistrust authority and are comfortable with the process of getting to a goal. They find the journey of getting to the goal almost as important as reaching the goal. They are tolerant of, even depend on, meetings and ongoing discussions that the younger generation finds tedious and wasteful.

Generation X (those born between 1965 and 1976) represents the smallest Canadian workforce pool since 1930, with over 4.2 million people, compared with the over 7.8 million Baby Boomers preceding them and the over 7 million Generation Y-ers following them (Statistics Canada, 2008). They have a mindset and work ethic that Baby Boomers who "live to work" do not understand. They are hard workers, but unlike the Baby Boomers, they "work to live," and they do not demonstrate the same loyalty to leaders and institutions as the Boomer generation. Farag, Tullai-McGuinness, and Anthony (2009) reported that they want immediate feedback and gratification for their contributions, expect collaborative decision making, and anticipate mentoring relationships in the job setting while working with effective and knowledgeable leaders. They do not easily follow the regular chain of command and show less concern for the formal organization (Farag et al., 2009). They stay with an employer only as long as there is something that benefits them (Wilcox, 2009), and they change jobs frequently if unhappy with their work environment. They are accustomed to working independently, having grown up as part of the "latch key" generation (so named because often they were left to return home alone while both parents worked) (Keepnews, Brewer, Kovner, et al., 2010).

The preferred leader of the entrenched workforce shares some of the characteristics of the younger generation's preferred leader, such as being motivational, honest, approachable, competent, and knowledgeable. However, Baby Boomers and Generation X-ers expect their leaders to be professional and supportive and have high integrity, a concept not even mentioned by the younger generation, who are not as concerned with the formal organization or the normal chain of command (Farag et al., 2009).

Challenges for the entrenched workforce are sharing leadership with the younger generations, empowering them to lead in their own model, and retaining the younger leaders in leadership ranks. Many younger employees are opting out of traditional work roles to become entrepreneurs. They take their leadership potential with them where there are few older role models for them to follow. A risk for aging Boomers and Gen X-ers is that the best and the brightest potential leaders will lose interest in leading and will opt for personal satisfaction and wealth accumulation rather than leadership and service roles. The values and attitudes of different generations of nurses need to be acknowledged and understood by nurse leaders.

The challenge of generational acceptance is one of many facing twenty-first century leaders. Attention to the needs of both the leader and the followers will create an environment in which everyone thrives.

EXERCISE 3-4

List the names of the people with whom you work most frequently. Determine to which cohort (emerging or entrenched) each belongs. Describe characteristics of the workplace that support each generation's view. (One list may be longer than the other.) What supportive characteristics are absent from the workplace?

SURVIVING AND THRIVING AS A LEADER

The keys to leadership are to believe in the vision and to enjoy the journey. The leader has a responsibility to self, followers, and the organization to stay healthy and enthusiastic for the mission of the group. Surviving and thriving as a leader are based on the rules in Box 3-3. Each rule is discussed in the following sections.

BOX 3-3   THE FIVE RULES OF LEADERS

1. Maintain balance.
2. Generate self-motivation.
3. Build self-confidence.
4. Listen to constituents.
5. Maintain a positive attitude.

The Leader Must Maintain Balance

Time management is essential for an effective leader. Many new leaders, in their zeal to be accessible to their constituents, lose control of their lives. A good strategy for retaining or regaining control is to get control of communication. Good leaders use the simplest and fastest method of communication that makes them accessible but does not tie them down. The keys to success are setting priorities and keeping in control. Planned telephone time and e-mail are excellent ways to keep control of time. Attending to matters as they arise, handling each question or piece of mail once and only one at a time, and focusing on the task at hand without distractions are just some of the time-management strategies used by effective leaders. Saving time, like wasting time, is a learned habit and can therefore be unlearned or relearned. Managing stress and time are further discussed in Chapter 28.

The Leader Must Generate Self-Motivation

Leaders who expect their followers to provide them with motivation, to be grateful for the time spent on staff needs, and to offer lavish praise are in for a painful awakening. Staff in organizations, work situations, and elected constituencies feel they have earned the right to criticize the leader by being followers. As one Canadian nurse leader has noted, "Every word a leader says will be heard, scrutinized and repeated, and will likely become the subject of lunchroom chats—positive or negative, accurate or distorted, and by anyone who listens! Like it or not, everything the leader does and says matters" (Rush, 2011, p. 34). Followers have an opinion about everything. Sometimes the comments are favourable, and sometimes they are not. The reason that self-motivation is so essential is because the leader can expect very little external motivation. Most leaders are risk takers and self-starters who are enthused by and believe in the vision they have created. Enthusiasm leads to an energized base, which is a hallmark of a vibrant, healthy organization.

The Leader Must Work to Build Self-Confidence

An effective leader must have self-confidence. This confidence comes from an acceptance of self, despite imperfections. Self-confidence is a self-perpetuating virtue. Effective leaders perform an honest self-appraisal on a regular basis and work to feel good about the job they are doing. Leaders who are surrounded by people who enhance their leadership characteristics make formidable leaders who have self-confidence in their ability to lead.

The more confident a leader feels, the more likely that success will follow. Success builds self-confidence. Two important factors are related to developing self-confidence. One is avoiding the tendency to become arrogant. The other is maintaining self-confidence despite setbacks.

The Leader Must Listen to His or Her Constituents

Leaders must listen to their constituents and determine whether action is indicated. Active listening requires being attentive to what your team is telling you, both verbally and non-verbally. However, listening does not obligate the leader to any course of action. Clear boundaries must be communicated. A smart leader listens to all sides and makes decisions based on the vision and direction that is best for the group.

The Leader Must Maintain a Positive Attitude

Positive attitude is vital to leadership success. No one wants to follow a pessimist anywhere. People expect the leader to have the answers, to know where the organization is going, and to take the initiative to get the group to its goal. A positive attitude can be a great ally in sharing and maintaining the vision. Attitude is a choice, not a foregone conclusion. The effective leader uses positive thinking and positive messages to create an environment in which followers believe in the organization, the leader, and themselves. The problems and challenges in health care demand that nurses seek and fill leadership positions in a positive and future-oriented manner.

EXERCISE 3-5

Using the five rules for leaders, create a personal description of how you maintain balance, generate self-motivation, build self-confidence, listen to constituents, and maintain a positive attitude.

THE NURSE AS LEADER

Leadership Within the Workplace

Staff Nurse as Leader. Leaders within the workplace are not necessarily those who are entrusted with the role and title of manager. The manager is concerned about budgets, financial performance, staffing, employee evaluations, and employee education and training. All of these activities are paramount concerns of the manager of an operational unit. In contrast, the workplace leader is one who has the ability to envision a preferred future for the quality of the working environment. The leader understands that nurse satisfaction is a central construct of many of the most successful nursing-service delivery systems. A manager may also be an effective leader, and thus others, including staff nurses, can emerge in leadership roles.

Workplace leaders create an environment in which nurses can experience satisfaction and have ideas for increasing the level of workplace satisfaction for nurses on the team. Leaders are those who creatively pose solutions to problems and capitalize on opportunities in the workplace. Furthermore, they support staff nurses who offer solutions to health care issues. Nurses with good ideas for future improvements should volunteer for leadership opportunities through participation on strategic committees such as a nursing council. If the workplace has no formalized mechanism for nurse input into organizational decision making, staff nurses who are leaders should clarify their vision and work to create such mechanisms.

According to the CNA (2009), leadership at the staff nurse level is about the engaged practice of providing evidence-informed exemplary care, advocating for patients, thinking critically, delegating and taking charge appropriately, and pushing the boundaries of practice to new levels. Staff nurses can develop leadership skills in several ways, including employment opportunities (e.g., as clinical nurse leader), professional opportunities (e.g., involvement with provincial nurses associations), and volunteer opportunities (e.g., at a palliative care association). Chapter 29 provides further ideas on how to enhance career development. The CNA supports leadership development at the staff nurse level through conferences, workshops, and the formation of special interest groups. Interested readers can check out the national and provincial or territorial Web sites of their professional association or their college for leadership development opportunities for staff nurses.

The Dorothy Wylie Nursing Leadership Institute is one example of a Canadian health care leadership development program. It offers a unique opportunity for established nurse leaders to partner with emerging leaders (staff nurses), preferably from the same organization, to experience the program together. A mentorship dialogue is essential to the program. Through the institute's program, emergent leaders are identified and a concrete process of leadership development ensues. Staff leaders can subsequently help establish workplaces that are satisfying and rewarding.

Nurse Manager as Leader. Effective management and leadership are a strong combination for success. The nurse in the role of manager ensures that the day-to-day tasks of the workplace are done correctly. Just as the effective manager pays attention to employee selection, hiring, orientation, continuing employee development, and financial accountability, in the role of leader, the manager raises the level of expectations and helps employees reach their highest level of potential excellence. A primary role of the leader is to inspire (Heuston & Wolf, 2011).

Developing with staff nurses a shared vision of the preferred future is a goal of the nurse manager in the role of leader. Staff members tend to resist change that is thrust upon them. When nurses are active participants in change, from its inception, they are more likely to be invested in outcomes.

An essential element of success for the nurse manager as a leader is the inclusion of staff nurses in decision making. This contribution can enhance their organizational commitment and create a sense of pride in successful outcomes. The nurse manager inspires staff by involving them in changing the workplace to make it more satisfying, and, in so doing, also develops personal leadership skills.

Nurse Executive as Leader. A primary goal of the nurse executive is leadership within the workplace. The nurse executive has an outstanding opportunity to shape the future of professional practice by creating opportunities for staff nurses and managers to have optimal input in organizational decision making related to the future. The nurse executive thus helps create a shared vision of the preferred future.

The concept of empowerment is important to the role of leadership for the nurse executive. Empowerment theory suggests that power be shared with others in the organization. Staff nurses may be encouraged to have input into decisions, or they may be given considerable information about how decisions are made. The ability to make or influence changes in the organization is a powerful tool. Nurses must believe that their input and ideas are considered when change occurs. Having input in decisions, having some control over the environment, and receiving feedback about actions taken or not taken, all contribute to a feeling of empowerment and control over one's practice and one's life.

CNA (2009) calls for the coexistence of management and leadership skills as an interdependent skill set. Both management and leadership skills are essential for the nurse executive. The ability to balance the day-to-day operating knowledge with the ability to lead a nursing organization into the future is a winning combination.

Nursing Student as Leader. The goals for leadership at the student level should be kept within a realistic framework. Helping students practise novice leadership skills within the security of an educational program is a reasonable expectation. Novice leadership skills that contribute to future leadership success involve learning how to work in groups, deal with difficult people, resolve conflict, reach consensus on an action, and evaluate actions and outcomes objectively (Figure 3-1). These opportunities foster skills that can lead to some expertise that could transfer to initial practice.

Student development toward true leadership expertise takes place over a long period and should not be expected during the first year or two of nursing school or nursing practice. Boychuck Duchscher (2008), who

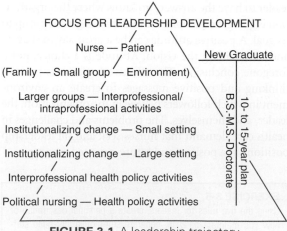

FIGURE 3-1 A leadership trajectory.

has studied the professional role transition of Canadian nursing graduates, concurs that leadership development requires time. Boychuck Duchscher launched Nursing the Future, a pan-Canadian initiative sponsored by provincial governments that offers an annual nursing conference and connects nursing students and new graduates with nursing and health care leaders in their communities through an online support network. Interested readers can visit http://www.nursingthefuture.ca for more information.

Every leader started somewhere. Movement toward an increasingly complex leadership experience allows the new nurse to move from leading and planning with an individual to working with families, groups, or communities and instituting change at different levels. With increasing educational achievement and career experience comes increasing complexity of leadership capabilities.

The Canadian Nursing Students' Association (CNSA) is the national voice of Canadian nursing students. Participation in CNSA provides opportunity to develop and demonstrate leadership and organizational skills and prepares students for future roles within their professional associations or colleges. Through involvement in student associations, nursing students can understand the bigger picture of nursing as a profession.

The best way to begin involvement is to attend a local CNSA chapter meeting and talk with the official and associate delegates. If students are interested in association activities, opportunities exist to serve on committees at the local, regional, or national level or in elected positions on the national board of directors. Examples of leadership development include serving as CNSA representatives on other boards or committees with nurse leaders, such as the executive board of the Canadian Nurses Association or the Canadian Federation of Nurses Unions.

Leadership in Professional Organizations and Unions

A strategic step to becoming a nurse leader is to join a professional organization. In Canada, membership in the CNA shapes career growth and mobility for many nurses. Volunteering for regional committee memberships is a useful way to learn and to grow within the professional association or regulatory college in your province or territory.

Nurses' unions also play a key role in leadership development. In Canada, 80% of nurses are represented by the Canadian Federation of Nurses Unions (CFNU), which is the national voice for nurses in the Canadian Labour Congress. Leadership opportunities are available to union members through attendance at union meetings, participation on committee structures, attendance at educational programs, and by election to leadership positions.

After becoming known at the local level, running for elected office in the district or chapter is a way many leaders within professional associations, colleges, or unions start their leadership careers. Subsequently, leadership efforts at the national level are usually more successful after one has established a record of successful leadership at other levels.

This pathway of leadership involvement—from the student association to the provincial or territorial association, college, or union, and subsequently to the national level—may seem like a linear progression to more global opportunities for leadership in the profession. However, many successful nursing leaders conceptualize the progression as circular rather than linear.

Leadership in the Community

As trusted professionals, volunteers, and opinion leaders, nurses have an opportunity to serve as leaders in their communities. Nurses bring a unique leadership skill set to community activities. The ability to understand complex systems, as well as interpersonal dynamics and communication techniques, constitutes knowledge that is valuable in moulding community opinion and shaping activities that impact community health. From the perspective of the nurse as a community leader, a unique opportunity exists to work with schools, community health boards, city or municipal governments, and other community entities to formulate a vision for improving the health of the community through disease prevention and health promotion. The nurse can be a catalyst for a community to recognize present problems and to develop a plan to reach a preferred future.

Leadership Through Appointed and Elected Office

Nurses are trusted and valuable leaders in elected and appointed offices at the local, provincial or territorial, and federal levels. The numbers of nurses who put their name forward to stand for office at all three levels of government is growing. Currently, three nurses hold national office as members of Parliament in Quebec, Ontario, and British Columbia. Nurses who are elected members of governmental bodies can exert their leadership to shape the vision of the government to help meet the needs of its citizens. Furthermore, many nurses have been called upon to serve on boards, commissions, and agencies that make policy decisions or recommendations to government that have far-reaching health implications for citizens and communities. The CNA and provincial or territorial associations and colleges often play a role in putting forth nominations of members for appointment to such bodies.

The Challenge of Leading

Visionary and authentic leadership is vital to the future success of nursing as an art and a science. Authentic

leaders are those who are true to themselves and their values. They inspire followers by their conviction to act accordingly. They serve as magnets, attracting others and inspiring them to do things they did not believe were possible (Huston, 2008). Professional nursing has been blessed with excellent leaders in the past and will continue to be led by the visionary and authentic nurse leaders of tomorrow.

EXERCISE 3-6

Successful leadership requires leaders and followers. Followers can play an active role in creating a healthy work environment at the unit level to ensure a strong platform for leadership development. As a new graduate, reflect on how you might contribute to a healthy work environment with positive relationships between the leader and the followers. Identify one action you might consider.

💡 A SOLUTION

Consider the following questions:

- *How can Lauren be supported so that she feels heard and knows that her issue is important?*
- *How can the staff involved be approached in a manner that maintains confidentiality?*
- *How can further occurrences of bullying among your staff be prevented?*

Changing behaviour requires changing attitudes. Bullying directed toward newly graduated nurses will not be eliminated unless nurses' attitudes toward students and newly graduated nurses change. It is the responsibility of the nurse manager to deal with this situation professionally while preserving Lauren's confidentiality. It was important for Lauren to know she was heard and that her problem was important. Lauren's feelings of initial excitement were overshadowed by a lack of support and a failure to connect with her colleagues, as well as a sense of isolation resulting from the negative responses she received from her experienced peers. The nurse manager knows that showing Lauren emotional, physical, and educational support in her situation would allow her to feel safe and secure in standing up for herself against her attackers and enable Lauren to feel empowered (Cleary, Hunt, & Horsfall, 2010). This support from the nurse manager is crucial for the success of new graduates like Lauren. To demonstrate support, the nurse manager asked the continuing education nurse to organize staff educational sessions on bullying and specifically teach new graduates strategies to successfully demand respect and ways to confront their abusers. The nurse manager prepared an information package

containing selected articles on confronting and preventing bullying in the workplace and distributed these to new nurses on the unit.

It is important for nurse leaders to identify problems before they occur, to prevent conflicts, to educate and empower staff to work together, to monitor the environment, and to evaluate educational outcomes. To this end, the nurse manager worked with senior management to establish a Violence-Free Task Force whose members were responsible for assisting the continuing education nurse establish and implement a plan to eliminate bullying in the work environment. The nurse manager strategically asked that a new graduate be invited to serve on the task force so that his or her experiential wisdom could be valued and understood and so that he or she could be a point of contact for other new graduates who might be experiencing bullying.

Supporting new graduates like Lauren in the work environment is an ongoing process, as is the process of changing attitudes. Consequently, regular follow-up meetings were scheduled with Lauren to monitor her progress and integration into the nursing unit, reinforce learned strategies for dealing with bullying behaviours, and address any concerns or issues. As a leader, the nurse manager role modelled appropriate workplace relationships in actively promoting zero tolerance of bullying, demonstrated professional behaviour, and supportive transformational leadership practices in dealing with a new graduate who had been a victim of workplace bullying. Violence and incivility in the workplace are discussed in detail in Chapter 25, which offers additional insights to finding solutions to this challenge.

Are these approaches suitable for a nurse manager? Why or why not?

THE EVIDENCE

- More effective leadership promotes effective communication, greater responsibility, empowerment, job clarity, continuity of care, and interdisciplinary collaboration.
- A transformational leadership style is closely associated with followers' working conditions—namely involvement, influence, and meaningfulness.
- A transactional leadership style is weakly associated with a leader's extra effort, leadership satisfaction, and leadership effectiveness, and does not predict leadership outcomes.
- Leaders who use a transformational leadership style are likely to reach their leadership goals effectively and satisfactorily, and significantly influence achievement of organizational strategic goals.
- Transformational leadership is a key factor in the implementation and sustainability of best practice guidelines.
- Emerging workforce members want their leader to coach and mentor them as well as invest in activities that promote their personal growth and advancement. They do not easily follow the regular chain of command and show less concern for the formal organization.

NEED TO KNOW NOW

- Work with others to create a positive environment so that students and others will want to work there.
- Look for leaders, not titles. Communicate with all people you deal with, including patients and their families, by taking generational differences into consideration.
- Leading in the community has great potential to strengthen your skills quickly.
- Leading in professional organizations improves the profession and provides personal connections.
- Succession planning is an important component of leadership development.
- Understand that different generations in the workforce create unique challenges and opportunities for organizations.

CHAPTER CHECKLIST

The role of the nurse leader is to share a vision and provide the means for followers to reach it.

- Excellent leadership in any working environment can improve recruitment and retention efforts and result in satisfied employees.
- Two leadership approaches contrast the leader role:
  - Transactional leaders rely on the power of the organizational position to reward or punish performance to control employees.
  - Transformational leaders ascribe power to interpersonal skills and personal contact in transforming people to make them want to progress.
- Key elements to becoming an effective leader can be learned and practised, as follows:
  - Select an effective and willing mentor.
  - Lead by example through role-modelling.
  - Accept responsibility for undesirable outcomes.
  - Share the rewards with followers.
  - Have a clear vision that followers can support.
  - Be willing to grow and change to meet current needs.
- The emerging workforce (Generations Y and Z) wants a leader who has good people skills and a nurturing attitude. The entrenched workforce (Baby Boomers and Generation X) wants a leader who is tolerant of the process of change and who exhibits high integrity and professionalism.
- To thrive in a leadership position, the nurse must do the following:
  - Maintain balance.
  - Generate self-motivation.
  - Build self-confidence.
  - Listen to constituents.
  - Maintain a positive attitude.

TIPS FOR BECOMING A LEADER

- Take advantage of leadership opportunities.
- Expect to stumble occasionally, but learn from your mistakes and continue.

- Get some help—having a caring mentor is the best way to develop leadership ability.
- Take risks. Leaders forge a vision and bring followers forward.

evolve WEBSITE

Visit the Evolve website for Suggested Readings, Internet Resources, and additional resources related to the content in this chapter: http://evolve.elsevier.com/Canada/Yoder-Wise/leading/.

REFERENCES

Alimo-Metcalfe, B., & Alban-Metcalfe, J. (2008). *Research insight: Engaging leadership: Creating organizations that maximize the potential of their people: Shaping the future.* London, UK: Chartered Institute of Personnel and Development.

Boychuk Duchscher, J. (2008). A process of becoming: The stages of new nursing graduate professional role transition. *Journal of Continuing Education in Nursing, 39*(10), 441–450. doi:10.3928/00220124-20081001-03

Canadian Nurses Association. (2009). *Position statement: Nursing leadership.* Ottawa, ON: Author.

Casida, J., & Parker, J. (2011). Staff nurse perceptions of nurse manager leadership styles and outcomes. *Journal of Nursing Management, 19,* 478–486. doi:10.1111/j.1365-2834.2011. 01252.x

Cleary, M., Hunt, G., & Horsfall, J. (2010). Identifying and addressing bullying in nursing. *Issues in Mental Health Nursing, 31,* 331–335. doi:10.3109/01612840903308531

Covey, S. R. (1992). *Principle-centered leadership.* New York, NY: Simon and Schuster.

Covey, S. R. (2009, February 3). Leadership is a choice, not a position. *Business Standard.* Retrieved from http://www.business-standard.com/article/management/leadership-is-a-choice-not-a-position-stepen-r-covey-109020300076_1.html.

Cowden, T., Cummings, G., & Profetto-McGrath, J. (2011). Leadership practices and staff nurses' intent to stay: A systematic review. *Journal of Nursing Management, 19,* 461–477. doi:10.1111/j.1365-2834.2011.01209.x

Cummings, G. G., MacGregor, T., Davey, M., et al. (2010). Leadership styles and outcome patterns for the nursing workforce and work environment: A systematic review. *International Journal of Nursing Studies, 47,* 363–385. doi:10.1016/j.ijnurstu.2009.08.006

Dierckx de Casterlé, B., Willemse, A., Verschueren, M., et al. (2008). Impact of clinical leadership development on the clinical leader, nursing team and care-giving process: A case study. *Journal of Nursing Management, 16,* 753–763. doi:10.1111/j.1365-2834.2008.00930.x

Earle, V., Myrick, F., & Yonge, O. (2011). Preceptorship in the intergenerational context: An integrative review of literature. *Nurse Education Today, 31,* 82–87. doi:10.1016/j.nedt.2010. 04.002

Farag, A. A., Tullai-McGuinness, S., & Anthony, M. K. (2009). Nurses' perception of their manager's leadership style and unit climate: Are there generational differences? *Journal of Nursing Management, 17,* 26–34. doi:10.1111/j.1365-2834.2008.00964.x

Gordon, K., & Melrose, S. (2011). LPN to BN nurses: Introducing a new group of potential health care leaders. *E-Journal of Organizational Learning and Leadership, 9*(1), 121–128.

Govier, I., & Nash, S. (2009). Examining transformational approaches to effective leadership in healthcare settings. *Nursing Times, 105*(18). Retrieved from http://www.bhs.org.au/sites/default/files/finder/pdf/cnhe/journal%20club/2009/LeadingOpinions Article200909.pdf.

Hader, R. (2011). The truth... and nothing but the truth [Editorial]. *Nursing Management, 42,* 6. doi:10.1097/01.NUMA.0000396493. 28574.cc

Heuston, M. M., & Wolf, G. A. (2011). Transformational leadership skills of successful nurse managers. *Journal of Nursing Administration, 41,* 248–251. doi:10.1097/NNA.0b013e31821c4620

Holmes, M. (2011). Just say "yes!": Mary Ferguson-Paré and the art of influential leadership. *Nursing Leadership, 24*(1), 23–29. Retrieved from http://www.longwoods.com/content/22330.

Huston, C. (2008). Preparing nurse leaders for 2020. *Journal of Nursing Management, 16,* 905–911. doi:10.1111/j.1365-2834.2008.00942.x

Kean, S., Haycock-Stewart, E., Baggaley, S., at al. (2011). Followers and the co-construction of leadership. *Journal of Nursing Management, 19,* 507–516. doi:10.1111/j.1365-2834.2011.01227.x

Keepnews, D. M., Brewer, C. S., Kovner, C. T., et al. (2010). Generational differences among newly licensed registered nurses. *Nursing Outlook, 58,* 155–163. doi:10.1016/j.outlo ok.2009.11.001

Kouzes, J. M., & Posner, B. Z. (2008). *The leadership challenge* (4th ed.). San Francisco, CA: Jossey-Bass.

Laframboise, L. E. (2011). Making the case for succession planning: Who's on deck in your organization? *Nursing Leadership, 24*(2), 68–79. Retrieved from http://www.longwoods.com/publications/nursing-leadership

Lavoie-Tremblay, M., Leclerc, E., Marchionni, C., et al. (2010). The needs and expectations of Generation Y nurses in the workplace. *Journal for Nurses in Staff Development, 26*(1), 2–8.

Marchionni, C., & Ritchie, J. (2008). Organizational factors that support the implementation of a nursing best practice guideline. *Journal of Nursing Management, 16,* 266–274. doi:10.1111/j.1365-2834.2007.00775.x

McGuire, E., & Kennerly, S. M. (2006). Nurse managers as transformational and transactional leaders. *Nursing Economic$, 24*(4), 179–185.

Nielsen, K., Yarker, J., Brenner, S., et al. (2008). The importance of transformational leadership style for the well-being of employees working with older people. *Journal of Advanced Nursing, 63,* 465–475. doi:10.1111/j.1365-2648.2008.04701.x

Rolfe, P. (2011). Transformational leadership theory: What every leader needs to know. *Nurse Leader, 9,* 54–57. doi:10.1016/j.mnl.2011.01.014

Rush, J. (2011). Leading with lustre: Important lessons along the way. *Nursing Leadership, 24*(1), 33–36. Retrieved from http://www.longwoods.com/publications/nursing-leadership.

Senge, P. M. (2006). *The fifth discipline: The art and practice of the learning organization* (Rev. and updated ed.). New York, NY: Doubleday.

Statistics Canada. (2008). *Report on the demographics situation in Canada 2005 and 2006* (Catalogue no. 91-209-x). Ottawa, ON: Author.

Weston, M. J. (2008). Transformational leadership at a national perspective. *Nurse Leader, 6,* 41–45. doi:10.1016/j.mnl.2008.06.001

Wilcox, J. (2009). Challenges of nursing management. In J. Zerwekh & J. C. Claborn (Eds.), *Nursing Today* (6th ed.). St. Louis, MO: Saunders.

Wilson, B., Squires, M., Widger, K., et al. (2008). Job satisfaction among a multigenerational nursing workforce. *Journal of Nursing Management, 16,* 716–723. doi:10.1111/j.1365-2834.2008.00874.x

CHAPTER

4

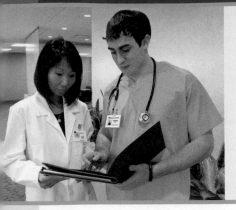

Developing the Role of Manager

Angela L. Stalbaum and Ana M. Valadez
Adapted by Wendy A. Gifford and Nancy Lefebre

This chapter identifies key concepts related to the roles of the nurse manager. It describes the different types of nurse manager roles within the Canadian health care environment. It also presents the basic manager functions, illustrates management principles that are inherent in the role of professional practice, and identifies nurse manager competencies for the nurse manager. Role development is crucial to forming the right questions to ask in a management or clinical situation that will help identify problems and anticipate needs. This chapter provides an overview of the practical skills the nurse manager needs to develop, including the ability to make evidence-informed decisions, manage change, create positive work environments, and manage resources.

OBJECTIVES

- Analyze the roles and functions of a nurse manager within the Canadian health care context.
- Describe the relationship of the nurse manager with others.
- Analyze management of health care settings.
- Understand management resource allocation and distribution.
- Identify the behaviours associated with professionalism in the nurse manager's role.

TERMS TO KNOW

healthy work environment	leader	quality indicators
informatics	manager	role theory
interactional justice	organizational culture	situational leadership

54

? A CHALLENGE

In home health care, staffing presents a unique challenge to front-line nurse managers. Both flexibility and creativity are needed to develop processes related to optimal staffing that ensures client safety while meeting budget expectations. Within senior nurse manager Robert's organization, staff are recruited to work in defined geographical areas and are assigned clients in those specified areas. However, the challenge is that the number of clients to be seen each day varies, depending on the number of hospital discharges and client referrals from community agencies. Unlike hospitals that have a fixed capacity, home health care has no "guaranteed number" of clients. Therefore, nurse managers and staff are required to admit and care for all referred clients, regardless of the pre-existing workload or the number of staff working. Because of the fluctuation in client numbers, it is particularly hard for Robert to determine the number of staff required each day to provide safe and effective nursing care and maintain an acceptable workload. In addition, it is important that changes made to staffing align with the budget while maintaining or improving staff satisfaction. The challenges for Robert are to *not* cut any positions at the point of care and to avoid dramatically increasing the number of clients assigned to each nurse.

What would you do if you were the nurse manager in this situation?

INTRODUCTION

Chapter 1 provided a general overview of leading and managing. This chapter looks at management from different perspectives. Management theory has undergone numerous changes in the past century. In the early 1900s, the theory of scientific management was embraced—a theory based on the idea that there is one best way to accomplish a task. Role theory began with management theory, and although changes in health care delivery no doubt are affecting the roles of nurse managers, role theory remains relevant. Conway's (1978) historic definition, "role theory represents a collection of concepts and a variety of hypothetical formulations that predict how actors will perform in a given role, or under what circumstances certain types of behaviors can be expected" (p. 17), is still appropriate.

Early management theories discounted concern for workers' psychological needs and focused mainly on productivity and efficiency. Between 1930 and 1950, management and leadership research centred on physical and psychological "traits" such as gender, height, appearance, and intelligence, and authoritarianism differentiated leaders from non-leaders (House & Aditya, 1997). Although the search for universal traits of effective leaders has largely been abandoned, the interaction between traits and specific situational demands remains an area of interest in the research (House & Aditya, 1997).

Participative and humanistic management and leadership theories were the dominant perspectives into the 1970s. These perspectives emphasized human relationships, workers' needs, and staff motivation. Situational leadership theories emerged in the late 1970s and early 1980s and continue to be drawn on today. The premise is that no single "best" leadership style exists, but rather that effective leaders and managers adapt their behaviours based on the situation (i.e., the individual, group, and work context) (Hersey, Blanchard, & Johnson, 2008). An example of a situational theory is path goal theory, which contends that the manager will engage in different types of behaviours, depending on the goals of staff and the organization. Effective managers adapt their behaviours based on the individual and group, in addition to the task, job, or goals that need to be accomplished (Hersey et al., 2008).

What is involved in managing? A self-appraisal might lead a potential nurse manager to ask the following questions: Do I have career goals that include gaining experience and education to become a nurse manager? What specific knowledge, skills, and personal qualities do I need to develop to be most effective in practice? Do I have a mentor who can guide me in this direction? Does the organization I currently work for have succession planning? Consider also, what is the role of the nurse manager? Some nurse managers would cite decision making and problem solving as major duties, for which maintaining objectivity is sometimes a challenge. Others would cite collaboration, especially with other professional groups and departments, to enhance quality patient care and outcomes. Truly effective care is the result of efforts by the total health care team. Good collaboration includes honesty, directness, and listening to others' points of view. However, management in nursing is more complex than this.

THE MANAGEMENT ROLE

Management is a generic function that includes similar basic tasks in every discipline and in every society. However, a defining characteristic of all nurse managers is that they must be well-grounded in nursing practice. In Canadian health care organizations, nurse managers work primarily in front-line or executive positions. Front-line nurse managers, often referred to as *managers*, *supervisors*, or *head nurses*, are individuals in a first-level administrative position who manage staff providing direct patient care (Jeans & Rowat, 2005, p. 9). Front-line nurse managers are responsible for managing one or more nursing units or areas; the number of people they supervise directly, or their span of control, sometimes exceeds 100 nursing staff (refer to Chapter 1 for further discussion of *span of control*). Doran, McCutcheon, Evans, et al. (2004) found that the mean span of control for front-line nurse managers in seven Canadian hospitals was 81 staff (ranging from 36 to 258 staff). In contrast, senior nurse managers hold executive positions and are often referred to as *directors*, *administrators*, *vice-presidents*, or *chief nursing officers* (O'Brien-Pallas, Murphy, Laschinger, et al., 2004). Senior nurse managers are typically in charge of nursing and patient care or both and control a large proportion of an organization's operational budget. Due to the large numbers of nurses employed in health care organizations (nurses frequently exceed 50% of all employees), senior nurse managers often have the largest span of control of all health care administrators.

In 1974, Canadian management consultant Peter Drucker identified the following five basic manager functions:

1. Establishes objectives and goals for each area and communicates them to the persons who are responsible for attaining them
2. Organizes and analyzes activities, decisions, and relations needed and divides them into manageable tasks
3. Motivates and communicates with the people responsible for various jobs through teamwork

4. Analyzes, appraises, and interprets performance and communicates the meaning of measurement tools and their results to staff and superiors
5. Develops people, including self

Table 4-1 shows how these basic management functions apply to the nurse manager.

Managers develop initiatives that focus on the individual. Their aim is to enable the person to develop his or her abilities and strengths to the fullest and to achieve excellence. Thus, a manager has a role in helping people develop realistic goals. Goals should be set high enough yet be attainable. Active participation, encouragement, and guidance from the manager and the organization are necessary for the person's developmental efforts

TABLE 4-1	BASIC MANAGER FUNCTIONS AND NURSE MANAGER FUNCTIONS
BASIC MANAGER FUNCTIONS	**NURSE MANAGER FUNCTIONS**
Establishes and communicates goals and objectives	Delineates objectives and goals for assigned area
	Communicates objectives and goals effectively to staff members whose work will help attain goals
Organizes, analyzes, and divides work into tasks	Assesses and evaluates activities on assigned area
	Makes sound decisions about dividing up daily work activities for staff
Motivates and communicates	Role models and emphasizes the importance of being a good team player
	Provides positive reinforcement and recognition
Analyzes, appraises, and interprets performance and measurements	Completes performance appraisals of individual staff members
	Communicates results to staff and management
Develops people, including self	Addresses staff development continuously through mentoring and preceptorships
	Furthers self-development by engaging in reflective practice, attending educational programs, and seeking specialty credentialing

Based on Drucker, P. F. (1974). *Management tasks, responsibilities and practices*. New York: Harper & Row.

to be fully productive. Often, nurse managers who are successful in motivating staff provide a work environment that facilitates goal accomplishment and personal satisfaction.

Leadership is an integral part of a manager's role. The nurse manager must possess the qualities of a good leader: knowledge, integrity, ambition, good judgement, courage, stamina, enthusiasm, communication skills, planning skills, and administrative abilities. While differences between management and leadership roles have long been debated, some overlap exists between management and leadership competencies (see Chapter 1). Moreover, it is widely accepted that managers are in positions of leadership and that leadership is part of the manager's role.

The International Council of Nurses defines *leadership* as "having a vision, or a clear view of what future state to aim for, and then being able to inspire confidence and motivate others so they share the vision and goals, and work together to try to accomplish them" (Shaw, 2007, p. 35). Leaders set a direction, develop a vision, and communicate the new direction to staff. Managers address complexity, whereas leaders address change. Managers address complex issues by planning, budgeting, and setting target goals. They meet their goals by organizing, staffing, controlling, and solving problems. A more detailed comparison of leadership and management roles appears in Chapter 1.

EXERCISE 4-1

In a small group, discuss the services available through hospitals, clinics, hospices. What costs would there be for delivering these services? Hypothesize about what portion of those costs would represent nursing care. How could a manager contribute to the cost-effectiveness of delivering these services?

The literature abounds with the complexities nurse managers face when leading staff. One example is creating a positive work environment that includes multiple generations of nurses: Baby Boomers, Generation X-ers, and Generation Y-ers (*Nexters*, or the *Millennium Generation*) (refer to Chapter 3 for further information on these generations). Carver and Candela (2008) discuss the importance of nurse managers having a strategy to increase job satisfaction, decrease nurse turnover, and increase organizational commitment by considering generational differences.

Managers who know how to relate to the different generations can improve the work environment for nursing. This idea was confirmed in a Canadian study of acute care nurses conducted by Widger, Pye, Wilson, et al. (2007). In that study, data were collected from 8207 registered Ontario nurses and registered practical nurses made up of Baby Boomers, Generations X-ers, and Generation Y-ers. While Baby Boomer nurses showed a high degree of job satisfaction, Generation X and Y nurses did not. The study suggested that if nurse managers want to be more successful in establishing job satisfaction in younger generations, they must consider the following: (1) creating a shared governance structure in which nurses are encouraged to make decisions; (2) providing opportunities for self-scheduling; and (3) providing opportunities for career development as well as supporting education.

The nurse manager is the "environmentalist" of the unit. In other words, the nurse manager is always assessing the context and work environment in which practice occurs, and is responsible for creating and sustaining a healthy work environment for the delivery of safe patient care (a function that requires innovation and adaptability). Healthy work environments are practice settings that maximize the health and well-being of nurses, quality patient outcomes, and organizational and system performance (Registered Nurses' Association of Ontario [RNAO], 2013). Evidence-informed transformational leadership practices help nurse managers create healthy work environments (MacPhee & Bouthilette, 2008). These practices include:

1. Building relationships and trust
2. Creating an empowering work environment
3. Creating an environment that supports knowledge development and integration
4. Leading and sustaining change
5. Balancing competing values and priorities

In today's health care environments—which are often riddled with high ambiguity, uncertainty, and complexity—a manager must be concerned with relationships to be successful in day-to-day operations. Building relationships and trust is foundational to a healthy work environment. A visible and credible front-line nurse manager who builds trust and positive relationships with staff can improve morale and staff motivation while increasing the quality of patient care (Jeans & Rowat, 2005). Respect for the worth of others and fairness are key components of trust (Mishra & Spreitzer, 1998). Canadian researchers have shown that when nurses feel respected, they have higher trust in management, higher job satisfaction, lower emotional exhaustion, and higher ratings of quality of care (Laschinger, 2004).

Through their role, nurse managers aim to help staff develop their abilities and strengths fully to achieve excellence in patient care. Nurse managers who build relationships and trust through their interactions with staff foster work environments that empower staff, increase motivation to succeed, and improve work effectiveness and performance (Laschinger, Wong, McMahon, et al., 1999; McNeese-Smith, 1997; RNAO, 2013).

Management Competencies

What constitutes good management in nursing? What competencies are required for nurse managers? These questions continue to challenge the profession. They are also particularly salient today, as nurse leaders increasingly contribute to the development of the health care system through their influence on practice, policies, and healthy work environments. While the nurse manager's role is important to the integrity of Canadian health care, a number of factors affect the nurse manager's ability to acquire and maintain the necessary skills and competencies. For example, a nurse manager cannot fulfill his or her role without a supportive work environment, clear and reasonable expectations, a reasonable workload, and access to ongoing education programs and mentorship.

According to the nursing literature, the following competencies are important to nurse managers: interpersonal skills, collaboration expertise, analytical thinking, seeing the big picture, resource management, information technology, awareness of the political arena, clinical knowledge, and skills and leadership (Jeans & Rowat, 2005). To understand the competencies required for nurse managers, the Canadian Nurses Association (CNA) commissioned a nation-wide study that included interviews and surveys with 629 senior nurse managers, front-line nurse managers, and staff nurses (Jeans & Rowat, 2005). The top six competencies for nurse managers were as follows: (1) accountability for professional practice, (2) verbal communication, (3) team-building skills, (4) leadership skills, (5) conflict resolution, and (6) knowledge of ethical and legal issues (Jeans & Rowat, 2005).

EVIDENCE-INFORMED DECISION MAKING

Today, the responsibility of nurse managers is twofold: to be active participants in research and to facilitate the use of research both in their own administrative practices and in staff's clinical practice. National policies clearly articulate that nurses must use research evidence in their decision making to ensure high-quality care and positive outcomes for patients (Canadian Nurses Association [CNA], 2010). As part of ongoing quality improvement, nurse managers have a fundamental role to play in helping staff use research evidence in their clinical practice. A literature review has shown that when managers are directly involved in quality and safety improvement initiatives, the success of those initiatives is higher than when managers are not involved (Ovretveit, 2005). Nurse managers can help staff use research evidence in their practice decision making by valuing research, role modelling, providing encouragement, ensuring policies are based on research and are up to date, and monitoring practice and patient outcomes (Davies, Edwards, Ploeg, et al., 2006; Gifford, Davies, Edwards, et al., 2007; Gifford, Davies, Graham, et al., 2013).

Nurse managers can participate in research at their local unit or area level or in large-scale organizational research projects. Through collaboration with nurse researchers and academic institutes, nurse managers are in a strategic position to identify priority gaps in care that could be examined through nursing research. When nurses participate in research, they are more likely to value and subsequently use research findings in their own practice (Tranmer, Lochhaus-Gerlach, & Lam, 2002).

Nurse managers also have a responsibility to use research in their own management decision making. Evidence-informed management reflects the application of empirical research evidence and other forms of evidence in everyday management decision making. Substantial interdisciplinary work is being done in Canada to develop strategies to support evidence-informed management (Canadian Health Services Research Foundation, 2007; Lavis, Robertson,

Woodside, et al., 2003; Lomas, 2000). For evidence-informed management to occur, nurse managers require access to research findings as well as to process and outcome data from their own organization. Health care informatics, the use of technology and information systems to support improvements in patient care and health care administration, is a powerful tool that nurse managers can use to access research related to their own management practice (see "Informatics" later in the chapter).

EXERCISE 4-2

In your current area of work, what type of information system is used? Is there access to research literature? How are the data, information, and evidence used within your clinical area, and who uses them? Are information and evidence used to inform nursing practice, management decision making, or both?

MENTORING

A manager is also concerned about preparing successors. Cherry and Jacob (2008) include the role of mentoring as another role that nurses in leadership or management positions must embrace. Mentoring has been defined as "an intense interpersonal exchange between a senior experienced colleague (mentor) and a less experienced junior colleague (protégé) in which the mentor provides support, direction, and feedback regarding career plans and personal development" (Russell & Adams, 1997, p. 2). Mentoring is an interactive, multi-faceted role that assists staff with setting realistic, attainable goals (Cherry & Jacob, 2008). A meta-analysis of 43 studies on mentoring in diverse settings, including health care, found that individuals who had been mentored had higher career and job satisfaction, had stronger intentions to stay with an organization, and were more likely to be committed to their career compared with individuals who had not been mentored (Allen, Eby, Poteet, et al., 2004).

Mentorship is critical for preparing new leaders and is a key component of career planning and professional development that has a positive impact on job satisfaction and the retention of staff (Cooper & Wheeler, 2010; Cummings, Olson, Hayduk, et al., 2008). Through mentoring, nurse managers can boost staff self-confidence, helping staff gain professional satisfaction when they reach their goals. Nurse managers give clinical guidance to their staff, and they can be instrumental in assisting them with their present work and their career development.

ORGANIZATIONAL CULTURE

In the ever-changing environment of health care, nurse managers need to understand the organizational culture of their work environment and how it supports their unit's mission and goals. Organizational culture can be described as the implicit knowledge or values and beliefs within the organization that reflect the norms and traditions of the organization. Organizational culture is discussed in more detail in Chapter 9. Laschinger (2004) examined nurses' perceptions of respect in a random sample of 500 staff nurses working in Ontario teaching hospitals. Respect is a moral principle that implies valuing another person's dignity and worth, and in organizational theory it is a core value of organizational culture. The instruments used addressed interactional justice (the perceived fairness of the quality of interactions by people who are affected by decisions and subsequent outcomes) and included structural empowerment, respect, work pressures, emotional exhaustion, and work effectiveness. Two hundred and eighty questionnaires were returned, yielding a 52% response rate. The results revealed that the nurses did not consider that their managers shared information about eminent changes in their work environment or showed compassion for the nurses' responses to the changes. The study highlighted the importance of a positive organizational culture and good interpersonal relationships between managers and staff for nurses to feel respected and supported in their work environment.

DAY-TO-DAY MANAGEMENT CHALLENGES

Nurse managers who meet day-to-day management challenges must be able to balance three sources of demand: patient needs, staff needs, and upper management requests. They have to (1) ensure that staff members have opportunities to provide upper management with input regarding changes that affect them, and (2) make unit and staff needs known to upper management. Consumers of health care services today are much better educated and accustomed to providing input into decisions that affect them. Nurse managers must respect patient requests yet maintain care in the broad context of safety and efficiency. Staff members need recognition and independence when carrying out their roles and responsibilities. Nurse managers need to have a sense of when to relinquish control, thus allowing decision making at the point of care.

Additionally, nurse managers must be perceived as credible in the areas they manage. A critical factor in being an excellent nurse manager is understanding how to make decisions that ensure optimal patient outcomes, involve patients and families in the plan of care, and allocate resources in a fair and ethical manner. Sometimes, decisions are made to meet one important patient-care need at the expense of another. That is an important message to convey to staff.

EXERCISE 4-3

Select a nurse manager and a staff nurse follower in one of your clinical areas. Observe them over a certain time (e.g., 2 to 4 hours). Compare the management styles and behaviours they exhibit. Is power shared or centralized? Are interactions positive or negative? What is the nature of their conversations? Is there a link between your observations and the characteristics of managers, leaders, and followers? Review the observed characteristics and behaviours of each nurse: Where were they similar? Where were they different? Describe any times where each nurse demonstrated or used more than one type of characteristic or behaviour.

Workplace Violence

Nurse managers continue to be responsible for ensuring the safety of their staff and patients. Workers in high-risk areas, such as the emergency department, require special attention. For nurse managers, "special attention" translates to their staff receiving adequate on-the-job training to recognize, prevent, and effectively intervene in workplace violence. Such training may include effective techniques relating to crisis intervention and handling highly agitated people who may be carrying a weapon. Four types of violence encountered by nurses in the workplace are worker to worker, patient and family, personal relationship, and criminal intent (RNAO, 2009). From the point of hiring through to a potential disciplinary process, nurse

managers have a responsibility to assess both employees and the workplace to help avert violence and the conditions that lead to it. Senior nurse managers are ultimately responsible for promoting and supporting a workplace free of violence; however, front-line managers must have the knowledge and competencies to prevent, identify, and respond to potential and workplace violence. Refer to Chapter 25 for further information on this topic.

MANAGING HEALTH CARE SETTINGS

Managing health care settings is always challenging for nurse managers, and the current nursing shortage has made the challenge paramount. Nurse managers are key in creating and maintaining a healthy work environment that keeps stress to a minimum so that the staff can achieve optimal work satisfaction. However, to be effective, nurse managers must also be able to reduce their own stress in the work environment. (See the Research Perspective.)

Both in Canada and the United States, professional organizations are speaking out about the need to create work environments that are more conducive to nurses providing safer patient care (Institute of Medicine, 2004; RNAO, 2013). For this to happen, change is required from those in leadership roles, beginning with top-level senior managers and filtering through the hierarchy to front-line unit managers. Five management practices have been found to be effective when instituting change in complex organizations:

1. Managing the change process actively
2. Balancing the tension between efficiency and reliability
3. Creating a learning environment
4. Creating and sustaining trust
5. Involving the workers in the work redesign and the workflow decision making

Staff members often look to the nurse manager to lead them in addressing workplace issues with higher levels of senior management. To do this, the nurse manager must (1) address power sources and define power-based strategies in the work environment, such as organizing other nurse managers with similar concerns; and (2) effectively influence the power holders so that needed change can occur. It is essential for nurse managers to ensure that staff members have an

RESEARCH PERSPECTIVE

Resource: Shirey, M. R., Ebright, P. R., & McDaniel, A. M. (2008). Sleepless in America: Nurse managers cope with stress and complexity. *Journal of Nursing Administration, 38*(3), 125–131. http://dx.doi.org/10.1097/01.NNA.0000310722.35666.73

Through a qualitative, descriptive study, Shirey et al. (2008) looked at what factors contribute to stress in nurse managers. The investigators interviewed five nurse managers ranging in age from 39 to 51 years; their tenure as nurse managers ranged from 5 to 17 years. Interviews with the nurse managers lasted up to 2 hours and produced data that emerged into the following eight common themes:

1. *Nurse manager work:* All the participants saw themselves as "clearing houses" for information affecting the staff. They felt that expectations of them were unrealistic, including "putting out fires" and simultaneously being asked to allow time for strategic planning and innovation.

2. *Sources of stress:* These included such things as demands of the role with not enough resources, leading to unclear role expectations; confusing reporting organizational lines; and a workload that allowed no downtime.

3. *Emotions:* The managers felt that their own emotions took a back seat to the emotions of the staff, and therefore stress was produced when turning "on and off" their own emotional needs.

4. *Value conflicts:* The managers felt that a great source of stress for them was being pushed almost over the line, especially in relation to budgets and what might be best for patients.

5. *Coping strategies:* The managers used two types of coping strategies: emotion-focused, such as anger used with negative situations; and problem-focused for solving specific stress-related problems, such as returning to school.

6. *Social support:* Most of the managers believed that their support came mostly from individuals not connected with their job, such as family, and all of them cited giving more support to staff than they themselves received.

7. *Relationships and communication:* The managers rated building relationships with their staff as a top priority; however, they believed that this category of work was "invisible work" and often sacrificed because of other commitments away from their unit.

8. *Health outcomes:* This theme brought to light how stress affected outcomes such as not being able to sleep, feeling stressed out, being emotionally exhausted, and experiencing physical symptoms of stress such as shortness of breath, palpitations, and tensed muscles.

Although all of the managers loved their jobs, they did feel a work–life imbalance, and although more studies are needed pertaining to stress in nurse managers, this study supports the need that other studies have found—that is, to re-examine and redesign the nurse manager position, which is crucial to their contributions to the overall organization.

Implications for Practice

The findings of the study clearly demonstrate that the stress that nurse managers feel affects not only their physical well-being but also their family life. Several other studies have consistently shown similar results, and the nursing profession needs to address the study findings and develop concrete plans that reduce nurse manager stress. Nurse managers are not expendable, and nursing needs to re-examine and develop mechanisms that reduce the stress in these essential management leaders.

opportunity to provide feedback to senior management and simultaneously advocate for staff needs. In their interviews of 24 nurse leaders, Antrobus and Kitson (1999) found that effective nurse leaders act as both interpreters and translators for the macro issues of senior organizational decision makers and the micro issues of practice. For example, front-line managers translate staff issues (such as workload) into language and priorities that are understood by senior management (such as costs and patient safety). They also interpret senior management decisions and then translate them into language and actions that are meaningful to staff (such as staffing and scheduling). Through this process, effective nurse managers position issues and concerns in ways that are meaningful

to the audience they are targeting, be it front-line staff, senior managers, or organizational decision makers. Refer to Chapter 18 for an in-depth discussion on leading change.

Staff members also look to the nurse manager to lead them in ethical, value-based management. The nurse manager's commitment to the mission and vision of the organization must be demonstrated in everyday behaviour, not merely recited on special occasions. This ongoing commitment lends stability in a time of constant change. In other words, although the strategies and approaches to address an issue may change, the core values remain the same, and the actions and decisions of the nurse manager must reflect the mission and vision of the organization. Therefore, the nurse manager must understand how the work of the unit supports the mission, values, and goals of the organization. Without this understanding, which is almost palpable, staff nurses may be skeptical about the nurse manager's commitment to both the organization and them. Nurse managers must translate their commitment so that staff know they are valued in accomplishing the work of the unit that furthers the mission of the organization. One way of demonstrating that employees are valued is through recognition. Recognizing staff's efforts is part of effective management practices (Yukl, 2006). Employees who have exceeded expectations in meeting the needs of the patient, department, or institution deserve recognition. Recognition may occur in many forms, for example, personal memos or "Bravo Cards" that acknowledge communication, performance, personal leadership, respect, teamwork, or staff's efforts to implement best practices.

EXERCISE 4-4

The senior nurse manager for the local public health department has just undergone a tremendous challenge because of an influenza outbreak in the vicinity. Many staff members, despite their own family needs, assisted victims with their needs, which ranged from crisis care to adequate follow-up of chronic disorders. The senior nurse manager wants to establish a recognition program for the staff members who gave endless hours to their community. How would you approach establishing this recognition program? What resources would you need, and where would you go to seek the needed resources? How would you want to be recognized in a similar situation?

MANAGING RESOURCES

Many of the concepts inherent in managing resources are addressed in depth elsewhere in this book, but the key point is that the nurse manager must manage resources and integrate these efforts with others. The practice settings of tomorrow will no doubt continue to include in-hospital care; however, numerous innovative practice models operating from a community-based framework are emerging. Predictors of positive outcomes for quality patient care include (1) all-care settings where patients receive comprehensive interprofessional care; (2) precise outcome-oriented quality-assurance processes, such as critical pathways;

and (3) concerted efforts to control spiralling health care costs by ensuring the provision of effective evidence-informed health care. Other practice models, differentiated practice, shared governance, and restructured work environments make use of all levels of health care personnel.

The nurse manager is responsible for managing all resources designated to the unit of care. This includes all personnel, health care providers and others, under the nurse manager's span of control (see also Chapter 9). Delegation and interdisciplinary collaboration are essential to the nurse manager's role and are covered in Chapter 26. The wise nurse manager quickly determines that a unit must function economically and, in so doing, realizes that many opportunities exist to reshape how nursing is delivered. Sare and Ogilvie (2010) have envisioned nursing in the twenty-first century based on a business paradigm with the goal of empowering the profession. They suggested combining existing nursing theories with business theories to depict the nurse as a change agent in health care. For Sare and Ogilvie, nurses must know and be able to apply fundamental business practices to take a stronger position within their organizations. Why are business theories important to the role of the nurse manager? The answer is simple yet very germane: because many of the tenets of business theories such as management, leadership, personnel, and systems are inherent in the role of the nurse manager.

Budget and personnel have always been considered critical resources. However, as technology improves, informatics must be integrated with budget and personnel as a critical resource element. Basing practice on research findings (evidence-informed care), networking with other nurse managers, sharing concerns and difficulties, and being willing to step outside of tradition can assist future nurse managers in decisions about resource use.

INFORMATICS

Informatics in health care is constantly changing and growing. Much technology and many systems are available to health care organizations to assist in improvements. Electronic medical records give quick and ready access to current and retrospective clinical patient data. Electronic patient classification systems allow managers to better measure the acuity of nursing areas, as well as assist in budget planning and the need for resources. New technologies such as Smart Beds are patient beds being used in some hospital settings; they have computers that do things such as weigh patients, help prevent pneumonia and bed sores, and replace the manual process of documenting patients' vital statistics. Smart Beds have the capacity to collect information for nurses, thus creating real time for nurses to think critically about what to do regarding the data.

The accessibility and use of the Internet facilitates the education of staff, patients, and their families. Nurse managers must stay abreast of, and in touch with, changing technologies in health care and be ready to advocate and defend the need for them to make improvements. In addition, managers must role model early adoption of new technology to demonstrate its value to staff. Older generations of nurses (e.g., Baby Boomers) may not have had the same exposure to electronic informatics systems as Generation X-ers and Generation Y-ers, and therefore may have more difficulty adapting to new electronic technologies (for more on technology in nursing, see Chapter 12).

BUDGETS

Budgetary allocations, whether they are related to the number of dollars available to manage a unit or related to full-time equivalent employee formulas, may be the direct responsibility of nurse managers. For highly centralized organizations, only senior managers at the executive level decide on budgetary allocations. Within less hierarchical organizations with "flat" organizational structures and decentralized management decision-making responsibilities, front-line nurse managers with responsibilities for patient care manage fiscal resources for their designated unit. Nurse managers require business and financial skills to prepare and justify detailed budgets that reflect the short-term and long-term needs of their unit.

Perhaps the most important aspect of a budget is the provision for a mechanism that allows nurse managers to have some budgetary control, such as decision making at the point of service, which does not require previous hierarchical approval.

> **EXERCISE 4-5**
> While in your clinical placement, examine the information system used by that health care setting. What type of information system is used? Are both paper (hard copy) and computer sources used? What can you assume about the budget, based on the physical appearance of the setting? Does any equipment appear dated? How do the employees (and perhaps volunteers) function? Do they seem motivated? Ask two or three to tell you, in a sentence or two, the purpose (vision and mission) of the organization. Can you readily identify the nurse manager? What does the nurse manager do to manage the three critical resources of personnel, finances, and technological access?

QUALITY INDICATORS

The nurse manager is consistently concerned with the quality of care that is being delivered on his or her unit. Using data to identify nursing's contribution to quality care is an important part of the nurse manager's role and requires reliable and valid nursing-sensitive indicators and outcomes. In the late 1970s, data sets such as the Universal Minimum Health Data Set and the Discharge Abstract Database (DAD) were developed, but they did not include information specific to nursing care, thereby rendering nurses' contribution to patient care and outcomes invisible (Doran, Mildon, & Clarke, 2011). To address this information gap, initiatives have been undertaken in Canada and around the world to develop nursing minimum data sets (NMDSs). For example, the American Nurses Association (ANA) developed the National Database of Nursing Quality Indicators (NDNQI) (www.nursingquality.org). The NDNQI measures are specifically concerned with patient safety and aspects of quality of care that may be affected by changes in the delivery of care. The quality indicators (measurable elements of quality that specify the focus of evaluation and documentation) address staff mix and nursing hours for acute care settings, as well as other care components. The NDNQI project is designed to assist health care organizations identify links between nursing care and patient outcomes. Participating organizations collect and adhere to certain core measures concerned with quality and outcomes of care. Hospitals are compared with other hospitals across the United States in these measurements. Examples of the core measures are practices associated with acute myocardial infarctions, care for the patient with congestive heart failure, and care associated with the treatment of pneumonia.

Work is currently underway to advance NMDSs and develop core measures of nursing-sensitive indicators for a national nursing report card (for more information, visit http://nhsru.com/publications/toward-a-national-report-card-in-nursing-a-knowledge-synthesis). Nursing-sensitive indicators are a set of generic outcomes relevant for adult populations in acute care, home care, long-term care, and complex continuing care settings and include, for example, pain, nausea, dyspnea, fatigue, pressure ulcers, and falls (Doran et al., 2011). Databases of nursing-sensitive indicators in Canada include the Health Outcomes for Better Information and Care project in Ontario (HOBIC) and Canada-HOBIC (C-HOBIC), which involves Saskatchewan and Manitoba (http://c-hobic.cna-aiic.ca/about/default_e.aspx).

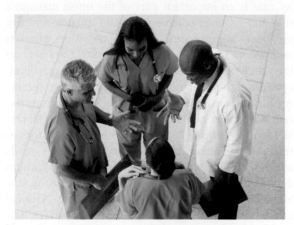

Nurse managers are constantly concerned with the quality of care that is being delivered on their unit.

PROFESSIONALISM

Nurse managers must set examples of professionalism, which include academic preparation, roles and competencies, and increasing autonomy. Nursing is a self-regulating profession in Canada, which means that provincial and territorial governments delegate to the nursing profession the power to regulate itself in the interest of the public. To this end, the CNA developed the *Code of Ethics for Registered Nurses* (CNA, 2008), which articulates the specific values and ethical responsibilities expected of registered nurses in Canada. The code of ethics serves as a framework through which

nurse managers can understand nursing's accountability to those who receive care and advocate for quality work environments that enable the provision of safe, compassionate, and ethical care (CNA, 2008). Professional nursing within an ethical framework also involves endeavouring to address broad aspects of social justice that are associated with health and well-being. For example, a nurse manager's professional philosophy should include patient rights. The primary values within the code of ethics that support patient rights include preserving dignity, promoting and respecting informed decision making, and maintaining privacy and confidentiality (CNA, 2008).

EXERCISE 4-6

Mr. Jafri, a patient who had foot surgery 3 days ago, has asked Daniel, a young nurse on a surgical orthopedic unit, several times during his 12-hour day shift for some medication for pain. Daniel's assessment of Mr. Jafri leads him to believe that he is not having that much pain. Although the patient does have an oral medication order for pain, Daniel independently decides to administer a placebo by subcutaneous injection and documents his medication intervention. Mr. Jafri does not receive any relief from this subcutaneous medication. When the 12-hour night nurse relieves Daniel, Daniel gives the nurse a report of his intervention concerning Mr. Jafri's pain. The following morning, the night nurse reports Daniel's medication intervention to you, the nurse manager. You will have to address Daniel's behaviour. What will you do? What resources will you use to handle Daniel's behaviour? How will you demonstrate professionalism?

Professionalism is all-encompassing; the way a manager interacts with personnel, other disciplines, patients, and families reflects a professional philosophy. Professional nurses are ethically and legally accountable for the standards of practice and nursing actions delegated to others. Conveying high standards, holding others accountable, and shaping the future of nursing for a group of health care providers are inherent behaviours in the role of a nurse manager.

Nurse managers are the closest link to direct care staff. They set the tone, create the work environment, and manage while providing professional role-modelling to develop future managers and leaders. (See the Theory Box for two approaches to motivating employees.) They influence staff members' decisions to stay or leave. Nurse managers are critical to the success of any health care setting.

THEORY BOX

Theory X/Theory Y

THEORY/CONTRIBUTOR	KEY IDEA	APPLICATION TO PRACTICE
McGregor (1960)	**Theory X:** Authoritarian • People do not like to work. • People need to have the threat of punishment. • People want to be told what to do.	This style might be useful when quick action or critical decisions must be made in which everyone must perform in the same way. In general, it is ineffective with professionals and creates workplace issues. However, in situations such as violence, this strategy may be necessary.
	Theory Y: Participative • Work is natural, and people like to work. • People use self-control. • People accept responsibility. • People like to solve problems.	This style might be useful when sufficient time is available or when the group must agree to a plan. In general, this approach is effective in health care and helps reinforce the concept of team. It is especially effective when a group is dealing with a quality initiative.

Data from McGregor, D. (1960). *The human side of enterprise.* New York, NY: McGraw-Hill.

A SOLUTION

As senior nurse manager, Robert looked at the current processes and developed a plan to allow for maximum flexibility of nursing staff, maintain patient quality care and continuity, and promote staff satisfaction. His solution was to create a staffing model that allowed flexibility in the staffing of geographical areas and self-scheduling, while maintaining an adequate mix of both full-time and part-time staff.

The geographically based approach allowed nurse managers to assign nurses to specific areas and use a "group practice" or team model approach to patient care. Through group practice, nurses became familiar with a distinct physical area and built their knowledge of locations and resources that reduced travel time between patients. Having flexibility in the staffing of geographical areas meant that the nurse managers could assign nurses outside their prescribed geographical areas or receive staff into prescribed geographical areas as the demand for services increased or decreased in different areas. However, this approach was only possible because nurses and nurse managers from different regions worked together as a team, collaborating and accepting accountability to meet the care needs of the population.

The foundation of this model is nurse self-scheduling and using all nurses to their full scopes of practice. Self-scheduling allowed nurses to select their work hours to accommodate patient needs, while allowing a balance between work and home. This provided greater job satisfaction while ensuring adequate numbers of licensed nursing staff each day. The use of the "right" number of full-time and part-time staff also allowed for greater flexibility; when patient numbers went up, staff could be increased, and when patient numbers went down, staff could work outside their geographical area, take time off, or share a reduced workload with other staff. The model was further complemented by using a mix of nurses to their full scopes of practice; nurses with differing competencies were able to manage their own caseload or share appropriate patients with other nurses as needed. These changes allowed for the full use of all nursing staff, improved job satisfaction, and an appreciation of staff for the skills and knowledge each group in the care team brings. Since implementing the new staffing model, staff nurses and nurse managers have reported increased job satisfaction, greater stability and continuity in their workload, and a better work–life balance.

Would this be a suitable approach for you? Why or why not? What might you do differently?

THE EVIDENCE

Hall, Doran, and Pink (2008) conducted a quasi-experimental study in Ontario to understand how interventions designed to improve nursing work environments impact patient and nurse outcomes. The study involved 16 nurse managers, 1137 patients, and 296 observations by registered nurses. Data were collected preintervention and 3 and 6 months postintervention. Interventions included enhancing documentation, improving linen supply, increasing availability of stock medications, and improving communication related to patient transfers and basic equipment needs for staff. The most significant finding was an increase in how nursing staff felt about the quality of their work life. After participation in the intervention, nurses reported higher perceptions of their work and work environment. Patients' perceptions of the quality of care also increased significantly as a result of the change interventions. Study results made it apparent that nurse managers can positively influence nursing staff's perceptions of nurses' work environments. In addition, positively impacting nursing staff increases patients' perceptions of quality of care.

NEED TO KNOW NOW

- Understand and respect the individual needs of the different generations of nurses currently working together in health care settings.
- Engage in a unit-based, shared-governance council inclusive of staff, allowing for empowerment.
- Provide professional development opportunities and support for furthering education.
- Encourage, support, and model the use of evidence-informed practice.
- Participate in the rewarding and recognition of nursing staff.

CHAPTER CHECKLIST

The role of the nurse manager is multi-faceted and complex. Integrating clinical concerns with management functions, synthesizing leadership abilities with management requirements, and addressing human concerns while maintaining efficiency are the challenges facing the nurse manager. Thus, the nurse manager's role is to ensure effective operation of a defined area, contribute to the overall mission of the organization, and create an environment that supports quality of care for patients.
- The five basic functions of a manager are as follows:
  - Establishes and communicates goals and objectives
  - Organizes, analyzes, and divides work into tasks
  - Motivates and communicates
  - Analyzes, appraises, and interprets performance and measurements
  - Develops people, including self
- A nurse manager is responsible for the following:
  - Relationships with those above themselves, peers, and staff for whom they are accountable
  - Professionalism
  - Management of resources

TIPS FOR IMPLEMENTING THE ROLE OF NURSE MANAGER

- Aspects of the role of the nurse manager include being a leader as well as a follower. To be effective in the role, the nurse manager must be dedicated to the following:
  - A management philosophy that values people
- A commitment to patient-focused quality of care outcomes that include both evidence-informed processes and patient health outcomes
- The desire for ongoing learning about health care change and its effect on the nurse manager's role and functions

Evolve WEBSITE

Visit the Evolve website for Suggested Readings, Internet Resources, and additional resources related to the content in this chapter: http://evolve.elsevier.com/Canada/Yoder-Wise/leading/.

REFERENCES

Allen, T. D., Eby, L. T., Poteet, M. L., et al. (2004). Career benefits associated with mentoring for protégés: A metaanalysis. *Journal of Applied Psychology, 89*, 127–136. doi:10.1037/0021-9010.89.1.127

Antrobus, S., & Kitson, A. (1999). Nursing leadership: Influencing and shaping health policy and nursing practice. *Journal of Advanced Nursing, 29*, 746–753. doi:10.1046/j.1365-2648.1999.00945.x

Canadian Health Services Research Foundation. (2007). *Is research working for you? A self-assessment tool and discussion guide for health services management and policy organizations.* Ottawa, ON: Author.

Canadian Nurses Association. (2008). *Code of ethics for registered nurses (2008 centennial edition).* Toronto, ON: Author. http://www.cna-aiic.ca/cna/documents/pdf/publications/Code_of_Ethics_2008_e.pdf.

Canadian Nurses Association. (2010). Evidence-informed decision making and nursing practice: CNA position statement. http://www.cna-aiic.ca/CNA/documents/pdf/publications/PS113_Evidence_informed_2010_e.pdf.

Carver, L., & Candela, L. (2008). Attaining organizational commitment across different generations of nurses. *Journal of Nursing Management, 16*(8), 984–991. doi:10.1111/j.1365-2834.2008.00911.x

Cherry, B., & Jacob, S. R. (2008). *Contemporary nursing, issues, trends and management.* St. Louis, MO: Mosby.

Conway, M. E. (1978). Theoretical approaches to the study of roles. In M. E. Hardy & M. E. Conway (Eds.), *Role theory: Perspectives for health professionals* (pp. 17–28). New York, NY: Appleton-Century-Crofts.

Cooper, M., & Wheeler, M. M. (2010). Building successful mentoring relationships. *Canadian Nurse, 106*(7), 34–35.

Cummings, G. G., Olson, K., Hayduk, L., et al. (2008). The relationship between nursing leadership and nurses' job satisfaction in Canadian oncology work environments. *Journal of Nursing Management, 16*(5), 508–518. doi:10.1111/j.1365-2834.2008.00897.x

Davies, B., Edwards, N., Ploeg, J., et al. (2006). *Determinants of the sustained use of research evidence in nursing: Final report.* Ottawa, ON: Canadian Health Services Research Foundation.

Doran, D., McCutcheon, A. S., Evans, M. G., et al. (2004). *Impact of the manager's span of control on leadership and performance.* Ottawa, ON: Canadian Health Services Research Foundation.

Doran, D., Mildon, B., & Clarke, S. (2011). Towards a national report card in nursing: A knowledge synthesis. *Nursing Leadership, 24*, 38–57. doi:10.12927/cjnl.2011.22464

Drucker, P. F. (1974). *Management tasks, responsibilities and practices.* New York, NY: Harper & Row.

Gifford, W. A., Davies, B., Edwards, N., et al. (2007). Managerial leadership for nurses' use of research evidence: An integrative review of the literature. *Worldviews on Evidence-Based Nursing, 4*, 126–145. doi:10.1111/j.1741-6787.2007.00095.x

Gifford, W. A., Davies, B. L., Graham, I. D., et al. (2013). Developing leadership capacity for guideline use: A pilot cluster randomized control trial. *Worldviews on Evidence-Based Nursing, 10*(1), 51–65. doi:10.1111/j.1741-6787.2012.00254.x

Hall, L. M., Doran, D., & Pink, L. (2008). Outcomes of interventions to improve hospital nursing work environments. *Journal of Nursing Administration, 38*(1), 40–46. doi:10.1097/01.NNA.0000295631.72721.17

Hersey, P., Blanchard, K. H., & Johnson, D. E. (2008). *Management of organizational behavior: Leading human resources* (9th ed.). Upper Saddle River, NJ: Pearson Prentice Hall.

House, R. J., & Aditya, R. N. (1997). The social scientific study of leadership: Quo vadis? *Journal of Management, 23*, 409–473. doi:10.1177/014920639702300306

Institute of Medicine (IOM). (2004). *Keeping patients safe: Transforming the work environment of nurses.* Washington, DC: The National Academy Press.

Jeans, M. E., & Rowat, K. M. (2005). *Competencies required of nurse managers.* Ottawa, ON: Canadian Nurses Association.

Laschinger, H. K. (2004). Hospital nurses' perception of respect and organizational justice. *Journal of Nursing Administration, 34*(7–8), 354–363.

Laschinger, H. K., Wong, C., McMahon, L., et al. (1999). Leader behavior impact on staff nurse empowerment, job tension, and work effectiveness. *Journal of Nursing Administration, 29*, 28–39. doi:10.1097/00005110-199905000-00005

Lavis, J., Robertson, D., Woodside, J., et al. (2003). How can research organizations more effectively transfer research knowledge to decision makers? *Milbank Q, 81*, 221–248. doi:10.1111/1468-0009.t01-1-00052

Lomas, J. (2000). Using "linkage and exchange" to move research into policy at a Canadian foundation. *Health Affairs, 19*, 236–240. doi:10.1377/hlthaff.19.3.236

MacPhee, M., & Bouthilette, F. (2008). Developing leadership in nurse managers: The British Columbia Nursing Leadership Institute. *Nursing Leadership, 21*, 64–75. doi:10.12927/cjnl.2008.20061

McGregor, D. (1960). *The human side of enterprise.* New York, NY: McGraw-Hill.

McNeese-Smith, D. K. (1997). The influence of manager behavior on nurses' job satisfaction, productivity, and commitment. *Journal of Nursing Administration., 27*, 47–55.

Mishra, A., & Spreitzer, G. (1998). Explaining how survivors respond to downsizing: The roles of trust, empowerment, justice and work redesign. *Academy of Management Review, 23*, 567–588. doi:10.5465/AMR.1998.926627

O'Brien-Pallas, L., Murphy, G. T., Laschinger, H., et al. (2004). *Survey of employers: Health care organizations' senior nurse managers.* Ottawa, ON: The Nursing Sector Study Corporation.

Ovretveit, J. (2005). Leading improvement. *Journal of Health Organization and Management, 19*, 413–430. doi:10.1108/14777260510629661

Registered Nurses' Association of Ontario. (2009). *Preventing and managing violence in the workplace.* Toronto, ON: Author.

Registered Nurses' Association of Ontario. (2013). *Developing and sustaining nursing leadership.* Toronto, ON: Author.

Russell, J. E. A., & Adams, D. M. (1997). The changing nature of mentoring in organizations: An introduction to the special issue on mentoring in organizations. *Journal of Vocational Behavior, 51*, 1–14.

Sare, M. V., & Ogilvie, L. A. (2010). *Strategic planning for nurses: Change management in health care*. Boston, MA: Jones and Bartlett Publishers.

Shaw, S. (2007). *International Council of Nurses: Nursing leadership*. Oxford, UK: Blackwell.

Shirey, M. R., Ebright, P. R., & McDaniel, A. M. (2008). Sleepless in America: Nurse managers cope with stress and complexity. *Journal of Nursing Administration, 38*(3), 125–131. doi:10.1097/01.NNA.0000310722.35666.73

Tranmer, J. E., Lochhaus-Gerlach, J., & Lam, M. (2002). The effect of staff nurse participation in a clinical nursing research project on attitude towards, access to, support of and use of research in the acute care setting. *Canadian Journal of Nursing Leadership*, 15, 18–26. doi:10.12927/cjnl.2002.19137

Widger, K., Pye, C., Wilson, B., et al. (2007). Generational differences in acute care nurses. *Nursing Leadership*, 20(1), 49–61. doi:10.12927/cjnl.2007.18785

Yukl, G. A. (2006). *Leadership in organizations* (6th ed.). Upper Saddle River, NJ: Pearson Prentice Hall.

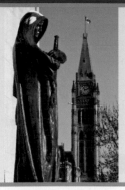

Legal Issues

Lyle G. Grant

Legal issues have become a growing concern for nurses as nursing practices continue to expand in scope and involve higher degrees of expertise, autonomy, and accountability. Nursing practice is legally defined as distinct from and independent of other health care practices, and this distinction has changed traditional views of nursing liability. Laws related to nursing actions cover areas such as the governance of nursing, individual rights, autonomy, privacy, consent, substitution decision making, record maintenance, freedom of information, and labour relations. Laws can add not only certainty but also complexity to nursing practice. A basic understanding of the laws that apply to nursing actions and patients forms part of the skills and knowledge nurses need to meet most provincial or territorial nursing regulations and applicable codes of ethics. Nurse leaders need increased working knowledge in a number of key legal areas to properly supervise staff and manage liability risk. This chapter provides an introduction to legal issues important to nurses in Canada. The law is constantly changing and must be viewed in light of individual situations, so it is not possible within a single chapter to include all areas of law that may be relevant to nursing practice or to outline the law completely in the areas identified. The purpose of this chapter is to create awareness of select areas of law affecting nursing leadership as a starting point for continued learning.

OBJECTIVES

- Identify the sources of Canadian law.
- Identify key legal differences in nursing practices and nursing regulation.
- Identify key areas of liability of concern to nurses.
- Understand key areas where positive duties to act exist around reporting, risk management, and public protection.
- Understand how various legal matters—including negligence, malpractice, privacy, confidentiality, reporting statutes, employment law, and insurance—affect leading and managing roles in nursing.
- Describe the purposes and components of documentation and record keeping.
- Identify areas of law relevant to information and health record management, including leader responsibilities.
- Describe how institutional policies, procedures, and protocols integrate patient care and legal responsibility.
- Understand the role of nurse leaders in developing institutional policies, procedures, and protocols that address legal issues.

TERMS TO KNOW

battery	liability	privacy
circle of care	licensure	regulatory body
collective agreements	malpractice	risk management
common law	natural law	scope of practice
confidentiality	negligence	statute
foreseeability	nursing practice act	tort
informed consent	personal liability	vicarious liability

❓ A CHALLENGE

Jessica is a nurse on a hospice and palliative care unit located next to a small suburban hospital. Jessica is one of two nurses who have worked a 12-hour-day shift and are due to be relieved by the next shift at 1930 hours. However, one of the nurses on the next shift has called in sick at the last minute and Jessica's manager asks her to stay on to work until a replacement nurse is located. This is Jessica's fourth shift in four days, so she is feeling weary. After 3 hours, Jessica advises her manager that she is so tired that she feels unsafe to practise any longer and needs replacing now. The manager advises that she has been unsuccessful in obtaining a replacement nurse despite best efforts and asks Jessica to stay for the balance of the night shift.

She confirms that Jessica may take an extended break commencing in 1 hour; this will allow her to sleep for 6 hours on the unit, but also leave her available to assist the other nurse in an urgent situation so that patient safety is maintained. Jessica advises that she does not feel competent to stay any longer, and the manager reminds her that she has a legal obligation not to abandon her patients, so unfortunately she must stay for the sake of patient safety.

What would you do if you were Jessica? What legal issues may affect resolution of this situation?

SOURCES OF LAW

The laws applicable to nurses and nurse managers in Canada originate from multiple sources. Primarily, laws have *legislative* and *common law* sources. Legislation refers to law (commonly regarded as "written law") that is constructed and modified by a legislative body. In Canada, the two primary sources of legislation are provincial legislative bodies (e.g., legislative assemblies, provincial parliaments, and Lieutenant Governors) and federal Parliament, which consists of the House of Commons, the Senate, and the Governor General. Legislation can be found in the various *acts* or statutes of Canada and its provinces and territories accompanied by associated regulations. Legislation is relatively easy to locate.

A hallmark of Canada's democratic system is that law making ultimately rests in legislative bodies, which is referred to as the *supremacy of Parliament*. Parliament can ultimately take responsibility for making, amending, and repealing all laws. Canada also operates under a federal system of government that divides these legislative powers exclusively between national and provincial governments. This division of powers is outlined in the *Constitution Act* (1867) of Canada and creates an important background to understanding some of the political contexts of the Canadian health care system and its system of public funding and regulation. For instance, most matters of health care and hospitals fall under provincial jurisdiction. However, under the *Canada Health Act* (1985) federal authorities have used spending powers to gain participation of provinces and territories in medicare, effectively influencing the provision of provincial health care services by attaching terms and conditions to the transfer of federal funds to provinces. Medicare, our publicly funded national health insurance program, is a fundamental and valued part of making health care available to all Canadians without financial barrier. The federal government, by controlling large portions of the monies necessary to fund medicare, indirectly exercises substantial influence over health care delivery and policy in Canada (Downie, Caulfield, & Flood, 2011).

Common laws are those laws that have been derived from the system of courts that operate in Canada and are commonly referred to as "judge made." Common laws are located by a review of relevant case law and the decisions of courts; they are not collected in any one place. Canada's common law system is derived from the English common law system. The system is structured with courts that have different levels of authority. Moreover, the decisions of higher courts govern lower courts and courts at the same level are governed by consistency in subsequent rulings on similar matters. Quebec has a slightly different legal system than the rest of Canada, and most of its provincial laws are limited to and contained within a single written civil code based on the French civil code. Quebec does not have a set of common laws like the rest of Canada, and court decisions related to Quebec provincial laws are often restricted to how courts interpret the civil code.

Canadian law is also influenced by expert opinions and scholarly consensus on how to interpret laws, customary practice, and natural laws. **Natural laws** are those *higher* laws that apply to all human beings and thus should override human-made laws. They include matters such as the right to defend oneself from harm as well as concepts of natural justice, such as the right to be heard. International laws that have been ratified in Canada may also be binding on Canadians. Finally, various activities in the health care system are governed by private laws. Private laws are those laws administered between persons and include agreements that the courts will enforce as law; contracts are an example of this type of law. Contracts or agreements that are not otherwise illegal in their intent, with a few exceptions, are generally enforceable in Canadian courts, giving them the full effect of law. Contracts play an important part in health care service delivery and employment arrangements. While much of contract law is common law, some types of contracts, such as insurance and employment contracts, have been given special attention by legislators over time and are subject to specific statutes. More recently, health care issues involving Aboriginal populations in Canada have drawn on international laws and rely heavily on private laws and fiduciary and treaty obligations of the federal state.

Federal statutes related to nursing include criminal laws and laws related to human rights, social welfare, copyright, patents, medications, interprovincial matters, health care funding, and Aboriginal people. Provincial and territorial laws vary in form and name between provinces and territories, but they all address the regulation of unions, health care

providers, employment, insurance, health insurance systems, hospitals, privacy, consent, mental illness, human rights, and information. Laws at all levels and of all types are subject to change over time due to their interpretation by the courts and as amended or repealed by parliaments. Legislation is an important instrument for implementing government policy, and it shapes and influences the political and policy environments of health care.

THE REGULATION OF HEALTH CARE WORKERS

In Canada, health care and its workforce are highly regulated, but these regulations differ significantly across provinces and territories. Commonly, health care workers who must be licensed to practise are referred to as "regulated" and health care workers who do not require a licence are referred to as "unregulated." Regulated health care workers include nurses, pharmacists, and occupational therapists. They conduct reserved health care–related actions authorized by licensing. Unregulated health care workers include care aides and certain therapists or counsellors. However, simply distinguishing regulated from nonregulated workers oversimplifies the regulatory realities of health care workers in Canada and the transitions underway in regulatory frameworks governing professional health care workers and their authorized practices.

The regulation of who may provide designated health care services may involve licensure, certification, or registration. Traditionally, **licensure** effectively granted a monopoly to a group of qualified individuals to perform regulated activities and to identify as a member of that group through use of a designation or credential. Nursing is an example of an occupation where licensure is necessary before designated nursing actions can be performed; registered nurse (RN) is one type of licensed nursing designation. Licensing bodies are often referred to as *colleges*, *associations*, or *professional regulatory bodies*. *Certification* was typically viewed as less restrictive than licensure, but certifying bodies may limit the use of a reserved title (that may include the word *certified*) to recognize members as having met certain predetermined qualifications (Epps, 2011, p. 82). For example, in Nova Scotia, use of the title "massage therapist" is restricted to those who have met certain educational requirements to join the Massage

Therapists Association of Nova Scotia. *Registration* is the least restrictive regulation governing health care occupations and may simply require individuals to register with a designated employer to obtain membership (Epps, 2011, p. 83). Registration also offers the least regulatory protection to the public. These terms continue to evolve in their use and meaning.

Under evolving regulator schema in provinces such as British Columbia, Alberta, and Ontario, health profession regulation is being re-conceptualized to accommodate changing scopes of practice and practice realities. While a full description of these new regulatory frameworks is beyond the scope of this chapter, umbrella legislation governing all health care providers provides for the making of regulations that authorize or license acts reserved to specific health care providers. An act associated with professional practices may simultaneously be authorized to those holding different professional designations. For example, an authorized nursing act, like injecting a substance subcutaneously, may be part of registered nurse, practical nurse, and psychiatric nursing scopes of practice. Additionally, advanced nursing practice acts can be authorized to those who are "certified" to conduct these acts. These new regulatory frameworks blur the traditional distinctions among designated professional practices (monopolies) and are examples of changes to certification and licensing.

The actions and duties that nurses can legally perform as set out in legislation (including its regulations) and complemented by standards, guidelines, and policy positions of provincial or territorial nursing regulatory bodies define scope of practice (Canadian Nurses Assocation, 2007, p. 13). The ability for licensed practical nurses, registered nurses, registered psychiatric nurses, registered practical nurses, and nurse practitioners to use nursing titles and to conduct designated procedures, processes, and actions is generally set out in nursing practice acts or legislation that creates regulatory authorities or regulatory bodies. For example, registered nurses in British Columbia must be registered with the College of Registered Nurses of British Columbia, a regulatory body created under the province's *Health Professions Act* (1996), to be able to practise; other provinces have similar bodies and acts. These legislative acts and their associated regulations create a form of self-regulating profession: they control who can be licensed, the types of actions that are regulated, reserved, or authorized to nurses, and scope of practice; set out educational and examination requirements for registration and continuing competency requirements; and establish governing bodies and processes for monitoring professional conduct and acting on misconduct. Within nursing, various designations help distinguish scope of practice and expected competencies. Advanced nursing practices or specialized nursing actions that exceed the basic scope of practice may also need to be authorized through special certification. Additionally, nurses limit their own individual actions based on their assessment of personal skills, experience, and competencies. Professional regulations, defined scopes of practice, and individual competencies are important to determining legal authority and responsibilities for nursing actions performed by individuals. They are the primary mechanisms for protecting the public from incompetent or unethical actions. Moreover, when a health care worker is regulated through licensing, professional sanctions accompany other available legal actions to protect the public from harm.

IMPLICATIONS AND LIABILITY

Liability and professional sanctions may arise from wrongful, inappropriate, or unethical actions. The law also imposes a special duty on health care workers to protect individuals who are considered vulnerable, such as older adults, those who are incapacitated, and children. A law is a form of public policy that represents a collective set of values and beliefs important to maintaining a peaceful society. Liability and deterrence for wrongful actions are mechanisms to ensure compliance. The consequences faced by nurses who perform wrongful actions fall into four basic categories: criminal liability, civil liability, professional sanctions, and employment ramifications.

Criminal Liability

Criminal liability is largely codified in the *Criminal Code* (1985) of Canada, but some quasi-criminal sanctions and penalties may exist in other federal or provincial or territorial legislation. Criminal actions have a higher standard of proof than do actions involving other liability, and criminal sanctions generally have jail time as a penalty option. In criminal law, people are presumed to be innocent until proven guilty beyond reasonable doubt. Criminal prosecution also requires proof of the criminal act (*actus reas*) and criminal intent (*mens rea*). A conscious, rational person is seen to intend the natural consequences of his or her acts, but *mens rea* prevents criminal liability for those who may be mentally ill, insane, or completely unaware of their actions because of some mental impediment. The following acts are subject to criminal investigation and potential prosecution: certain forms of negligence, assault, and nuisance; actions that result in the spread of communicable diseases; drug-related matters; and actions that intentionally, wantonly, or recklessly bring about death.

Civil Liability

Civil liability is an important mechanism in ensuring quality health care services (Epps, 2011, p. 80), and it generally arises when a civil wrong (such as a tort or breach of contract) is committed. Civil law allows an injured person to bring a lawsuit to claim for damages, commonly referred to as *being sued*. Damages are generally reduced to a monetary payment for a wrongful act as compensation to an injured party where some legal duty was breached. The nature of such liability can arise from legislation or common law. Traditionally, the largest source of civil liability has been negligence and malpractice. Nurses have rarely been held personally liable to pay damages because their actions were often seen as being directed by others; they were poorly paid and lacked substantive resources on which to collect any judgement for damages; or their employer was seen as "vicariously liable" because of the employer–employee relationship. Common law liability is generally found in a branch of law called *tort law*. A **tort** is a civil wrong or injury, not related to a contract, for which a court will provide a remedy (usually monetary damages). The standard of proof in civil liability cases is based on a balance of probabilities rather than the stricter "beyond a reasonable doubt" burden of proof required in criminal law; for example, liability may be found where it was judged *more probable than not* that an action caused the damage. Civil liability claims typically require a person (the plaintiff) to bring a legal action against another (the defendant). Different from criminal prosecutions (which are brought by the state), civil liability cases can be initiated by a person or a business.

Professional Sanctions

Professional sanctions are imposed by regulatory bodies and arise from a delegation of regulatory authority from provinces or territories to self-regulate their members. These professional bodies assume responsibility for administrative and profession-specific decisions, such as setting minimum education requirements, setting clinical standards, and addressing ethical, investigative, and disciplinary matters (Epps, 2011, p. 82). Most health professions in Canada are regulated in this manner. Disciplining members is the primary mechanism by which professional bodies enforce their standards, and enforcement is an important part of protecting the general public. Professional sanctions and disciplinary actions generally arise from three unacceptable behaviours: (1) misconduct, (2) incompetence, and (3) conduct unbecoming a member of the profession (Downie et al., 2011, p. 91). *Misconduct* is unacceptable behaviour within the scope of the profession's practice; *incompetence* is a failure to meet minimum generally accepted standards; and *conduct unbecoming a member of the profession* is behaviour outside a profession's practice that may bring the profession into disrepute (Epps, 2011, p. 91). Professional sanctions may include loss of licence or any one or a combination of reprimand, censure, fine, remediation requirements, further education, or practice restrictions. Professional sanctions do not restrict other legal actions and remedies.

To protect the public interest, professional regulatory bodies have powers of inquiry into member registrant practices and conduct that can be initiated by the regulatory body or that may be required upon receipt of a complaint from a member of the public. Nurses should be aware of the mechanisms and procedures that may be undertaken by their respective regulatory bodies in response to a public complaint or inquiry. The powers of a regulatory body may also extend to investigation, inspection of records, search and seizure (with a court order), sanction, and the ability to charge back the costs of these actions to the registrant if wrongdoing is found. Inquiries contested by a registrant or those of a particularly serious nature may advance to a disciplinary hearing open to the public. These approaches are consistent with principles of transparency and a public mandate to act in the public's best interest.

Regulatory bodies must follow administrative law procedures in adjudicating wrongdoing and imposing professional sanctions on their members. Professional sanctions have potentially serious consequences for people's careers and lives, and the more serious the consequence proposed, the more important administrative law becomes to the process. Administrative legal principles will help determine that regulatory bodies act within their legal authority, demonstrate principles of fairness in dealing with complaints and disciplinary matters, and apply principles of natural and administrative justice. Regulatory bodies must also act without bias and discrimination. A disciplinary hearing, usually conducted by a disciplinary committee, is the most serious practice review mechanism available to regulatory bodies. A nurse who is responding to a disciplinary hearing may be represented by legal counsel, and some jurisdictions permit representation by a union representative or other agent. Additionally, a nurse undergoing disciplinary proceedings will have an opportunity to present evidence, make submissions, cross-examine witnesses, and receive written reasons for decisions within a reasonable period of time. Nurses do not always have legal representation during investigative and sanctioning proceedings and, arguably, principles of natural justice would require that options for legal representation be made available to nurses at these times. Decisions of regulatory body disciplinary proceedings may be appealed to the superior court in the province or territory of the proceeding.

EXERCISE 5-1

Locate and review literature that both supports and refutes the self-regulation of professions as good public policy. Consider the ultimate aims and objectives of regulating health professions and how self-regulation may contribute to or confound achievement of these objectives.

Employment Ramifications

Employment ramifications may be imposed directly by an employer or may flow indirectly from sanctions imposed by a professional body. Failure to meet employment obligations permit an employer to take various forms of action. Common law, labour law, and employment law regulate the employer–employee relationship and the remedies that employers may take. Collective agreements associated with unionized workplaces are special types of agreements that outline collectively negotiated terms of employment between employers and employees and often have detailed processes for discipline that must be followed. Collective agreements are discussed in detail later in this chapter, and as part of collective bargaining, discussed in Chapter 20. Depending on the employment breach, direct consequences may be punitive in nature and include loss of employment, reprimand, increased monitoring, and additional conditions of continued employment. By contrast, the consequences may be more supportive in an effort to remediate unacceptable practices and include increased mentorship, education, and support for change. Indirect consequences generally arise from licensing or practice restrictions imposed by professional bodies that affect the registrant's ability to meet employment requirements and expectations. For example, employment may be difficult to maintain if the limitations placed on a licence are strict.

LEADERSHIP PERSPECTIVES

Entire books are devoted to laws relevant to nursing, and even they do not fully encompass the legal issues that nurse leaders may face. What follows is a brief outline of key areas of legal concern for nurse leaders. Nurses have a responsibility to undertake further inquiry and learn about the full range of legal issues related to their practice areas and responsibilities.

Duty to Report

Some recent nursing regulations impose new statutory duties on nurses to report other nurses or health care providers to their registration bodies where concern exists that a professional is dangerous to the public or demonstrates sexual misconduct. Of concern here is an individual health care provider's fitness to practise and the protection of the public. As well, medical practitioners who treat another health care provider who has been admitted to a psychiatric hospital or a drug or alcohol addiction treatment facility may be required to report this to the relevant regulatory body and may also need to include information about the person's condition, treatment, prognosis, and fitness to practise. The British Columbia *Health Professions Act* (1996) is an example of legislation that imposes reporting duties on health care providers across the province. Statutes similar to the British Columbia *Health Professions Act* create relatively new legal requirements to report the inappropriate conduct of another health care provider when he or she is potentially dangerous to the public. Failure to report where a requirement exists may invite inquiry into one's own practice. In British Columbia, the statutory duty to report extends to all health care professions, but this statutory duty does not exist in all provinces and territories; however, nurses may also be ethically bound or required under standards of practice to make such reports even without statutory requirements.

Provinces and territories may have statutes that require reporting of certain events of abuse witnessed by nurses in the course of duty. The aim is to protect people in care from abuse whether they be in residential care, psychiatric treatment facilities, nursing homes, or hospitals (see, e.g., Alberta's *Protection for Persons in Care Act*, 2009). Statutes may require that individuals and managers report abuse and alleged abusers to external agencies that may include the police. Other examples of reporting obligations are considered in the section below, Protective and Reporting Laws. Nurses may be affected by a variety of laws that require reporting, and many statutes provide whistle-blower provisions to protect those who report from reprisals or retaliatory actions by employers or others as a result of the reporting. The intent is to advance the protection of the public and those who take action to safeguard it.

Insurance

Insurance law is an area often neglected in the discussion of laws relevant to nursing. The damages for personal injuries related to health care can be large, and nurses may be found personally liable for these amounts. Insurance offers a form of indemnity for these losses, effectively paying the economic losses on behalf of the nurse if the damages arose from a risk covered under a policy of the insurance (an *insured risk*). Insurance is a form of managing an individual's financial risk. It is based on many people paying premiums into a pool of funds that can be used to pay out individual liability claims; the effect is to pool or spread risk so that individuals are protected from large, contingent, economic burdens. The system is sustained as long as the premiums collected exceed payouts; the size of the pool and the relative risk will determine the stability of the premiums over time. The medicare system in Canada was a grassroots form of insurance that started in Saskatchewan, applying the notion of pooled risk, and is now a much larger, specialized, public insurance system.

Most registered nurses in Canada, except those in British Columbia and Quebec, are covered under the Canadian Nurses Protective Society insurance policy (see http://www.cnps.ca). British Columbia and Quebec nurses have separate insurance underwriters for their registrants' coverage. In Ontario, alternative insurance options may be available, as is sometimes the case with advanced practice nurses, including nurse practitioners. Registered psychiatric nurses and licensed or registered practical nurses should look to their respective registration organizations to confirm insurance coverage. By example, the Canadian Nurses Protective Society policy premium is sometimes collected as a part of nurse registration fees in their respective province or territory of registration, but this type of automatic insurance inclusion is not the case for all nurses, and sometimes membership in another provincial nurses' association or other insurance options must be explored. The College of Nurses of Ontario, which governs the registration of all nurses in the province, does not include the provision of personal liability protection insurance as part of its registration fee, but as of March 31, 2014, required all registrants to have this insurance in place by other means (College of Nurses of Ontario, 2013). Typically, this type of insurance covers the civil liability of individual nurses, including legal expenses for the defence of alleged breaches of statutes, as well as criminal proceedings. However, it does not cover expenses related to professional disciplinary proceedings. The amount of liability covered under an insurance policy is limited, and nurses will want to make sure that additional and optional insurance is separately purchased and maintained where individual work circumstances have increased liability risk. For example, advanced practice roles may increase individual nurse exposure to liability that may exceed the basic limits contained in the policy. Coverage in all nursing circumstances should not be assumed. Nurses who work independently or outside the country may not be covered under the insurance policies provided through provincial or territorial nurse registration bodies or associations. Nurses should check with their insurer to determine the amount and nature of their coverage. Nurse registration organizations generally cover nurse practitioners under separate policies of insurance that carry higher limits. However, nurse practitioner practices vary widely in Canada, so nurses are advised to confirm adequate coverage that reflects the liability risks associated with their individual practices.

Insurance law is a special type of contract law. The insurance contract or policy may vary depending on the type of risk being insured and the person or entity being insured. Insurance-specific statutes impose many legal requirements on the terms and conditions of these contracts. For individual nurses, it is important to understand the nature and type of insurance in place, the risks insured (i.e., what elements of their practice are insured under what circumstances), and the obligations owed to the insurer when a potential insurance claim arises. Nurses who breach elements of an insurance contract may find themselves with limited or no insurance coverage.

Under insurance law, the insurer and the insured (the individual nurse) have a very special type of trust relation. The insured is said to have a relation of *uberrima fides* with the insurer, which roughly translates to a position of "utmost good faith." So the duties owed by an insured to the insurer exceed the normal laws of trust to a position of ultimate trust that include abundant good faith, absolute and perfect candour, openness, and honesty. If an insured person violates this trust, for example, by lying to the insurer, then the insurance policy may be voided by law. Other duties include that the insured nurse notify the insurer as soon as he or she is aware of a potential claim against the insurance policy, and certainly as soon as any legal action is commenced against him or her; the insurer requires full information and involvement from the outset to best manage its risk position.

Employers, particularly public health authorities, also typically carry professional liability insurance that protects employees, including nurses, from civil liability when acting within their scope of employment. Additionally, the legal notion of **vicarious liability** creates indirect liability of the employer for the actions of an employee acting within his or her scope of employment, thus protecting nurses and nurse managers from **personal liability** (a person's responsibility at law for his or her own actions). Vicarious liability reflects common law principles that recognize

employment arrangements are founded on generating economic gains for employers, so they must therefore bear the risk of employees who act within their scope of employment. Institutional policies and procedures are important determinants and indicators of what falls within the scope of an individual's employment. An employee who exceeds his or her scope of employment may expect to be personally liable for any liability that arises.

Documentation Requirements

The requirement of accurate, readable, and timely charting and record keeping has multiple legal sources. Institutional policies and procedures provide the first point of guidance for nurses, but additional documentation may be required to meet practice standards, practice expectations, and changes in patient condition. The timeliness of charting is critical to patient care and well-being. Medical charts are part of interdisciplinary communications that must be up-to-date to ensure proper patient care and to avoid potential legal liability. Charting alerts everyone to potential changes and developments in patient condition. These records also serve to protect nurses from ill-founded accusations of negligence or other improper conduct (Peppin, 2011, p. 173). Nursing notes entries are required with minimum frequency as dictated by patient condition, as necessary for quality care, and as directed by institutional policies and procedures. Taken routinely and contemporaneously, nursing notes are generally admitted by courts during legal proceedings as establishing the truth of the events recorded, unless others can prove them inaccurate. As with all health records, entries should be clear, factual, precise, made as close to the timing of an event as possible, permanent, and dated. Additionally, the maker of the notation should be clearly indicated with the appropriate nursing or professional designation (e.g., RN, RPN, LPN). Single lines drawn through deletions help ensure that no attempt was made to hide a portion of the record, but merely to correct the record of clerical error. Corrections made at the time of entry should clearly indicate the change and be initialled by the original entry maker. All attempts should be made to avoid alteration after the record is made and to avoid interlineations or markings that suggest alterations. Clear explanations for necessary changes or additions made late are necessary. Legal proceedings involving medical incidents do not often surface for four or more years after the event. Memories of the necessary details of the medical events that are the subject of the proceedings will have faded, so clarity of charting notations is important to reconstructing events and refreshing memories.

PRIVACY AND CONFIDENTIALITY

Canadians take their privacy seriously, and various remedies are available to Canadians if they believe their privacy and confidentiality have been compromised by health care workers. **Privacy** may be defined as "the right of the individual to determine when, how, and to what extent he or she will release personal information" (*R. v. Duarte*, 1990) and **confidentiality** relates to holding in private any information provided and protecting the exchange of information with an obligation to prevent release of information to those who are unauthorized (Gibson, 2011, p. 254). Confidentiality may encompass holding private information related to individuals and other entities, such as organizations. Nurses are likely to encounter legal issues with privacy and confidentiality frequently in the workplace and may find themselves under personal scrutiny for actions performed or neglected regarding patient information. Important changes to legal issues regarding privacy and confidentiality protection continue.

Legal duties to protect the confidentiality of patient information likely arise from common law principles rooted in the Hippocratic oath taken by physicians (Gibson, 2011, p. 254); health care practitioners act like trustees of personal information obtained from patients. With these trust-like relationships come a host of fiduciary duties around acting in the best interest of patients and protecting the confidentiality of information. Ethical duties also exist to preserve confidentiality, often incorporated in related codes of ethics, as do professional obligations under various health care provider regulations. The common law duties respecting confidentiality have been modified by various statutory provisions. The legal landscape of this legislation is complicated by at least two factors: first, the division of legislative powers between provinces and territories and the federal government and the fact that information often flows across provincial borders; and second, the enactment by some provinces of general privacy and information protection acts only,

while others have also included health-information-specific acts. The nature of information handled by health care institutions and nurse managers may therefore fall under consideration of between one and three specific privacy and information acts. For example, in Ontario employment data on a nurse working at a hospital is not considered health information and is covered under the *Freedom of Information and Protection of Privacy Act (FIPPA)* (1990), but if that nurse were admitted or treated as a patient at the hospital, all health information related to that employee would be covered under the *Personal Health Information Protection Act, 2004 (PHIPA)* (2004). It is necessary for nurse managers to understand under which acts information is governed in order to discharge the appropriate legal obligations and duties respecting the treatment of that information.

Health information legislation aims "to provide for protection of personal health information being collected, used, stored, or disclosed by an entity other than the individual who is the information source" (Gibson, 2011, p. 269). A list of some major information protection statutes in force in Canadian jurisdictions is outlined in Table 5-1. These statutes address the custody, access, disclosure, and use of health information obtained by health care practitioners and the institutions for which they work, including the companies that process, store, or handle the data on their behalf. Those who access health data are often referred to as *custodians* of health information in the legislation. A careful read of some of the definitions of who is a custodian of information and what information is deemed personal health information may surprise some. For example, Ontario legislation includes the expected cadre of health care providers as "information custodians" but excludes faith healers, traditional Aboriginal healers, and midwives.

The general duty of custodians and trustees of personal health information is to protect the information from disclosure except where such disclosure is authorized by the information provider. There are, however, exceptions. Generally, information may be shared with the patient's "circle of care," unless the patient has specifically instructed the trustee of the information not to make such a disclosure. A **circle of care** may be specifically defined by the relevant legislation but is generally understood as referring to the individuals and institutions directly connected to an individual's health care

TABLE 5-1	SELECT STATUTES RELATING TO PRIVACY, CONFIDENTIALITY, AND INFORMATION ACCESS IN HEALTH CARE	
JURISDICTION	**NAME OF ACT**	**COMMON ACRONYM**
Canada	*Personal Information Protection and Electronic Document Act*, SC 2000, c. 5	PIPEDA
	Privacy Act, RSC 1985, c. P-21	
	Access to Information Act, RSC 1985, c. A-1	
Alberta	*Personal Information Protection Act*, SA 2003, c. P-6.5	PIPA
	Health Information Act, RSA 2000, c. H-5	HIA
	Freedom of Information and Protection of Privacy Act, RSA 2000, c. F-25	FOIP
British Columbia	*Personal Information Protection Act*, SBC 2003, c. 63	PIPA
	Freedom of Information and Protection of Privacy Act, RSBC 1996, c. 165	FOIPPA
	Privacy Act, RSBC 1996, c. 373	
Manitoba	*The Personal Health Information Act*, SM 1997, c. 51, CCSM, c. P33.5	PHIA
	The Privacy Act, RSM 1987, c. P125, CCSM, c. P125	FIPPA
	The Freedom of Information and Protection of Privacy Act, SM 1997, c. 50, CCSM, c. F175	
Ontario	*Personal Health Information Protection Act*, 2004, SO 2004, c. 3, Sch. A	PHIPA
	Freedom of Information and Protection of Privacy Act, RSO 1990, c. F.31	FIPPA
New Brunswick	*Personal Health Information Privacy and Access Act*, SNB 2009, c. P-7.05	PHIPAA
	Right to Information and Protection of Privacy Act, SNB 2009, c. R-10.6	
Newfoundland and Labrador	*Personal Health Information Act*, SNL 2008, c. P-7.01	PHIA
	Access to Information and Protection of Privacy Act, SNL 2002, c. A-1.1	ATIPPA
Northwest Territories	*Access to Information and Protection of Privacy Act*, SNWT 1994, c. 20	
Nova Scotia	*Freedom of Information and Protection of Privacy Act*, SNS 1993, c. 5	FOIPOP
	Hospitals Act, RSNS 1989, c. 208	
Nunavut	*Access to Information and Protection of Privacy Act*, SNWT (Nu) 1994, c. 20, as duplicated for Nunavut by s. 29 of the *Nunavut Act*, SC 1993, c. 28	ATIPP
Prince Edward Island	*Freedom of Information and Protection of Privacy Act*, RSPEI 1988, c. F-15.01	FOIPP
Quebec	*An Act Respecting the Protection of Personal Information in the Private Sector*, RSQ 1993, c. P-39-1	
Saskatchewan	*Health Information Protection Act*, SS 1999, c. H0.021	*HIPA*
	Freedom of Information and Protection of Privacy Act, SS 1990-91, c. F-22.01	*FOIP*
Yukon	*Access to Information and Protection of Privacy Act*, RSY 2002, c. 1	

(Kosseim & Brady, 2008, para. 96). The consequences of mismanaging health data or disclosing personal information can be serious and include fines and civil liability.

Incident reports contain information that may be legally significant—even though that information is not focused on individual care. Incident reports typically collect information on adverse events, near misses, or incidents that potentially place patients or staff at risk. Usually, these reports are not referred to in patient health records to prevent them from becoming part of the patient record. Incident reports and the related procedures and follow-ups are important to continuous quality improvement, staff development, and patient and staff safety. These documents would likely fall outside of most health-information-specific protection acts, although they may contain references to individual patients. Procedures around documenting incident reports often strip patient-identifying information from the data at some stage, but procedures for completing these forms, the type of information they should contain, and how the data are handled require clear institutional policy and procedures to minimize unwanted legal use of this information.

Privacy can also relate to the more physical aspects of patient care; for example, intimate aspects of nursing care that, if made public, might cause a patient embarrassment and distress. Nurses are ethically bound to preserve dignity in patients, which helps reduce the incidence of embarrassment and distress. Callous or inappropriate actions of nurses who fail to protect the dignity and privacy of patients may bring on disciplinary action and legal liability. Such actions have been cast as a type of invasion of privacy tort, but Ontario courts have raised doubt on the success of such a legal advance, while British Columbia, Manitoba, Saskatchewan, and Newfoundland and Labrador have privacy acts that authorize the courts to award damages for invasion of privacy (Peppin, 2011, p. 179). The circumstances would likely have to involve a gross violation of privacy to warrant legal action from a practical perspective, but legal actions for violation of privacy may be sustainable despite any pragmatic outcome to the injured person.

Privacy laws in Canada remain a bit of a patchwork. Generally, these personal information laws provide for the protection of personal health information and impose obligations and responsibilities on health care institutions and their employees. Privacy laws have made the collection, storage, exchange, and disclosure of personal health information more regulated and, accordingly, more complex. Health care employers need clearly developed policies and procedures that follow privacy laws within their jurisdiction to help staff manage these complex laws and guard against liability. Nurses are well advised to review the personal information protection acts that apply in their jurisdiction of practice, and fully regard themselves as trustees of patient information with all the legal standards required of those standing in positions of trust. The standards to which nurses are held in protecting the personal information of patients are high.

Electronic Records

In the information age, the storage of electronic information has raised new privacy concerns. Access to information by those unauthorized to view and use it is of greatest concern. The portability of computer and storage devices makes data more easily stolen. Information systems that transmit data over the airwaves give rise to security concerns about who may be able to intercept this information flow. Information systems designed to track hospital supplies and equipment in real time to support health care and provide timely services to patients can raise privacy concerns. When tracking devices are attached to patients, it may be tantamount to tracking an

individual (Information Privacy Commission of Ontario and Hewlett-Packard [Canada] Co., 2008).

As Canada contemplates and attempts a move to electronic health records that are portable across provinces and territories and health care professions, issues of data protection remain unanswered and topical. The *USA Patriot Act* (2001) provides a salient example of how individual health data may unintentionally be accessible to state authorities in the United States if the data are stored or transmitted through the United States. Canadian health authorities have been careful to ensure that data storage, transmission, and processing remain in Canada. Structuring a balanced policy approach that is universal enough to make electronic health records portable across Canada and across health disciplines is challenging and has been slow moving (Ries, 2006).

Confidentiality

Nurses have access to large amounts of personal and confidential information regarding patients and families. Canadian society has typically valued the privacy of the individual, and this view is reflected in many Canadian laws. Disclosure of confidential information, particularly in health care settings, can have significant, sometimes life-changing consequences to individuals and their families. The increasing use of electronic storage of this confidential information and the vulnerability of technologies raises concerns about how to best protect confidential information in health care settings. Laws relating to the legal responsibilities of users of confidential personal information continue to undergo significant changes, and negative consequences befall those who might breach these laws. Part of confidentiality is not accessing patient information that you do not have need to access as part of your usual nursing duties. Institutions should develop and implement policies and procedures for who may access what patient information, lockouts, and monitoring mechanisms to help protect patient confidentiality.

PROTECTIVE AND REPORTING LAWS

In certain circumstances, it may be deemed in the public interest for privacy and confidentiality not to be protected, such as when health care providers need to report information to other public authorities. Earlier you were introduced to one special protective law in Alberta that aims to protect those in care facilities from abuse: the *Protection for Persons in Care Act* (2009).

It is an example of a protective law that places a positive duty, or burden, on nurses and nurse managers to act to protect an identified subgroup of the Canadian population. All provinces and territories have acts that make reporting mandatory when an individual reasonably suspects a child is subject to inadequate care (neglect) or any physical or sexual abuse. Some provinces have extended this requirement to include those individuals who, due to physical or mental disability, are incapable of protecting themselves from such abuse, regardless of age. Reporting in these cases does not require consent to disclose, and the disclosure may contain information that would otherwise be confidential.

Other miscellaneous laws impose duties to report. For example, in the interests of public health protection and promotion, all provinces and territories have public health acts that require health care providers to report patients with communicable diseases such as hepatitis and tuberculosis to public health authorities. Several Canadian jurisdictions have also added duty to report gunshot or stab wounds to local police authorities (see, e.g., Alberta's *Gunshot and Stab Wound Mandatory Disclosure Act*, 2009). More generally, disclosure may be made without the consent of the information provider or patient in situations where a patient is at risk of doing serious bodily harm to self or others, and disclosure can help eliminate this risk (e.g., see *Personal Health Information Protection Act*, 2004). Duty to report laws create legal obligations for health care workers to report the actions of others to protect individuals viewed as vulnerable or the general public.

LABOUR AND EMPLOYMENT

Within any facility, employment and labour laws can be complex. Some employees will be covered under collective agreements and some will not. Employees in different occupational categories may be covered under different collective agreements. As a result, health care providers need to know the common laws respecting their employment situation, statutory laws that outline minimum standards of employment, and employment-specific collective agreements and related legislation. Specialists in human resources departments at large organizations can be particularly helpful to nurse managers in sorting through the array of employment and labour laws relevant to their workplace.

Basic employment law is found in common law and includes a duty for employees to follow legitimate employer commands related to their work. These commands may take the form of a manager's direct request and are also contained within institutional rules, policies, and procedures. Common law also provides for reasonable notice for termination of employment, unless it is for just cause. Failure to provide adequate notice is commonly the subject of wrongful dismissal lawsuits claiming money in lieu of such notice. Determining the nature of appropriate notice is not always straightforward and depends on a number of factors, including the nature of the work, seniority, and the ability to find similar work at similar compensation. Common laws are modified by employment standards legislation. Employment standards legislation provides details on minimum wage requirements, prohibition regarding the employment of minors, pay periods, when overtime is to be calculated, maternity and parental leave, minimum notice periods for termination, and vacation entitlements.

A substantial portion of the health care workforce is unionized. Specific labour relations legislation both permits and protects employee ability to create unions and negotiated collective agreements that displace employment standards legislative provisions. **Collective agreements** are a special type of employer–employee contract, and the labour relations acts under which they are governed provide for certification of unions, basic contents of collective agreements, guidelines for negotiations, and procedures for arbitration where differences arise (Morris & Clarke, 2011, p. 311). Collective agreements maintain a right of management with the employer, but often contain various procedural, grievance, and appeal procedures in dealing with employee issues. Collective agreements cover a wide range of employment situations including wages, benefit entitlement, job protection, graduated procedures for terminating an employ for cause, duty to accommodate employees with disability, employment leaves, and procedures in matters affecting employment status or disciplinary actions including employee rights to union representation. Nurse managers must be knowledgeable and skilled in dealing with the provisions of collective agreements within their workplace.

Related to employment laws, and often augmented by collective agreements, health care institutions have duties to staff and patients around issues of safety and ability to practise. Duties extend to ensuring that staffing is sufficient to permit patient safety and safe clinical practice, that staff is provided with adequate orientation to the work environment, that policies and procedures are in place to provide a safe workplace, and that adequate equipment, tools, supplies, and systems exist to maintain safety. Employers must also adequately train, instruct, and supervise employees, which includes instruction in and training on the proper use of equipment and devices so that employees remain safe (Morris & Clarke, 2011, p. 335). Health care facilities, for example, have some of the highest rates of violence toward nurses, and employers have a duty to reduce risk to employees. Occupational health and safety legislation gives employees the right to refuse to work where that work, including the operation of equipment, machines, or devices, poses a danger to themselves or others. However, this right is not absolute. Health care workers do not have the right to refuse work where the perceived danger is within their usual or inherent scope of work. So, for example, nurses may not refuse to treat someone with a contagious disease, as this is within the normal and expected scope of nursing work. Additionally, health care workers cannot refuse to work where refusal would directly endanger the life, health, or safety of another person.

Other miscellaneous laws affect managers' interaction with employees and employment-related matters. Examples include reporting and record-keeping requirements under employment standards acts, the *Employment Insurance Act* (1996), and Canada's *Pension Act* (1985). Leaders must also take care in providing accurate and fair employee work-related references. For example, negative reference letters may attract liability under defamation laws, and failing to provide a reference that can assist an employee in locating new employment when he or she has been dismissed can increase damages for wrongful dismissal. Centralizing the provision of references within human resources departments or with select managers helps manage the legal risks. Finally, human rights legislation and the *Canadian Charter of Rights and Freedoms* (1982) outline many of the provisions that prohibit discrimination in the workplace based on national origin or ethnicity, race, religion, age, colour, gender, sexual orientation, or mental or physical disability. Workplaces are well advised to develop policies

and procedures that guide managers and reflect the current state of law in these areas.

Mental Health Laws

Mental health acts create special legal considerations in dealing with individuals undergoing treatment for mental health illness. All provinces and territories have legislation that specifically addresses this subgroup of patients. Significantly, these statutes provide for involuntary detention of patients and define when consent for medical treatment is and is not necessary. These acts also contain special provisions for the protection of the rights of involuntary patients. Nurses are often at the front line of ensuring that patients have been afforded the correct legal protections and rights under the mental health acts. Moreover, nurse managers are often designated with particular statutory responsibilities under the mental health acts. Familiarity with the provisions of these acts and how to discharge one's legal and professional obligations to patients in care is not always as straightforward as one might believe. As an example, differences in statutory provisions exist between provinces and territories regarding whether involuntary patients can be forced to take antipsychotic medications believed to benefit their condition. Professional and ethical duties to advocate on behalf of the patient may at times seem to contradict the provision of mental health acts. It is fundamental to understand that even involuntary patients under mental health acts have all the rights and privileges of other patients and Canadians, except where specifically limited by legislation. This may mean, for example, that an involuntary patient cannot refuse to take antipsychotic medication, but may have the right to refuse to take a prescribed multivitamin or validly withhold consent to surgery not considered emergency surgery. Interpretation of laws that restrict individual freedoms and rights will favour the least limiting approach.

DRUG LAWS

Access to and the use of drugs is heavily regulated by law and institutional procedures and includes the regulation of those who may prescribe and dispense medications to patients. Nurses must understand their legal capacity to handle, administer, and dispense various drugs and drug types, and legal requirements for accountability and documentation to avoid legal difficulties. Criminal and civil liability may result if drug laws are contravened.

CONSENT TO TREATMENT

Canadian law supports the fundamental right for patients to be free of unwanted medical treatment (Robertson, 2008) and contact by another person of their body (Peppin, 2011, p. 153). For example, a patient has the right to provide or withhold consent to medical treatment. Common law creates a legal duty for practitioners to disclose relevant information about treatments to patients so that they can provide informed consent, having fully understood and weighed the risks of accepting or rejecting the proposed treatments (*Hollis v. Dow Corning Corp.*, 1995). Failure to obtain informed consent before performing an act on a patient, or where an act exceeds the consent given, results in what is termed a *battery* in tort law. Battery takes place when someone intentionally touches another without consent (Peppin, 2011, p. 155). Two important points should be remembered: first, intent to touch is generally inferred by the physical act, regardless of the good intention of the person touching; and second, a person who has legal capacity to grant consent maintains the right to refuse treatment no matter how unreasonable it may seem to others.

Consent laws have been modified by statutory provisions that vary between provinces and territories. Nurses should be aware of the consent laws in the jurisdiction of their practice to avoid legal entanglements. Importantly, legislation dealing with matters of informed consent specifically address when someone has the legal capacity to grant consent, who may make substitute decisions when an individual is unable to make decisions on his or her own, and what legal process is available for obtaining consent. Comprehensive consent acts have been implemented in British Columbia, Ontario, Prince Edward Island, and Yukon (e.g., see Yukon's *Adult Protection and Decision-Making Act*, 2003). Issues of consent are also considered under statutes that deal with those without legal capacity to make these decisions; for example, statutes that address adult guardianship, mental illness, substitute decision making, health care directives, powers of attorney, and care facility legislation. It is beyond the scope of this chapter to provide a complete listing of the statutes involved in considering consent or the details of these statutes. The basic information necessary for informed choice as part of valid consent is outlined in Box 5-1 and must be considered in the circumstances of individual patients and procedures. Mental incapacity, temporary or otherwise, is the most common reason why a patient may be legally incapable of providing informed consent. The known wishes of a patient and any consents given prior to a loss of this capacity are important starting points in determining whether a medical or nursing procedure has been authorized by a patient.

MALPRACTICE

Malpractice, in strict legal terms, encompasses a number of professional wrongdoings and liability (Irvine, Osborne, & Shariff, 2013), but it is commonly understood as a type of medical or nursing negligence. Negligence that has caused suffering or injury may be legally actionable as a claim for damages (and reduced to a claim for money) as a result. Malpractice is a type of tort that has been established in common law and requires an injured person to prove, on balance of probabilities, that (1) he or she was owed a duty of care, (2) the duty of care was not met or was breached,

---

BOX 5-1   INFORMATION REQUIRED FOR INFORMED CONSENT

- An explanation and patient understanding of the proposed treatment or procedure to be performed, the expected results, and the health condition it addresses
- An invitation to ask questions and receive understandable answers about the treatment or procedure and risks
- Disclosure of the material risks (those probable, unusual, serious, or likely to influence an individual patient's consent)—elective procedures may require disclosure that is more thorough

- The benefits likely to result because of the treatment or procedure
- Options to the proposed course of action, including absence of treatment
- Name of the person(s) performing the treatment or procedure
- Statement that the patient may withdraw his or her consent at any time

Peppin, P. (2011). Informed consent. In J. G. Downie, T. A. Caulfield, & C. M. Flood (Eds.), *Canadian health law and policy* (4th ed., pp. 153–194). Markham, ON: LexisNexis Canada.

(3) there was reasonable foreseeability, (4) injury or damages were suffered because of the breach, and (5) the damages or injury would not have occurred but for the negligence (Dickens, 2011, p. 117). *Reasonably foreseeable* (which is called **foreseeability**) means that injuries and damages resulting from some action or failure to act are not simply accidents or errors in judgement (Dickens, 2011; Irvine et al., 2013). Table 5-2 presents an example of the six elements that must be presented in a successful malpractice suit.

Duty of Care and Standards of Practice

The standards of care owed by health care providers to patients are largely derived from the standards of practice of the respective professions. For example, in nursing in all provinces and territories, standards of practice are the primary measure of what a reasonably prudent nurse would do in similar circumstances and timing (College of Registered Nurses of British Columbia, 2011). See the following Literature Perspective for an example of how standards of practice affect nurses, patients, and health care agencies. Management

decisions that create work overloads, designate tasks to improperly trained or equipped personnel, fail to adequately orient staff to work environments, or fail to provide adequate resources to allow professionals to meet expected standards of care may shift liability to managers or institutions (Dickens, 2011, pp. 129–130). Hospitals, for example, may also be negligent and owe their patients and communities duties to "(1) select and maintain competent, adequate staff, (2) provide proper instruction and supervision to staff, (3) provide and maintain proper and adequate equipment and facilities to staff, and (4) establish systems necessary for the safe operation of the hospital" (Dickens, 2011, p. 147).

LITERATURE PERSPECTIVE

Resource: Beal, G., Chan, A., Chapman, S., et al. (2007). Consumer input into standards revision: Changing practice. *Journal of Psychiatric and Mental Health Nursing, 14,* 13–20. http://dx.doi.org/10.1111/j.1365-2850.2007.01034.x

Focus groups were conducted with consumers of mental health services in acute care and community settings to gather their input on mental health services. That information was then used to inform quality improvement in and amendments to the *Canadian Standards for Psychiatric-Mental Health Nursing.* Recognizing the public mandate of nursing, the standards of practice document sets out specific expectations of nurses, articulates minimum standards of clinical practice, and communicates information on the nature of psychiatric nursing practice and expected competencies. Inviting consumers to participate in informing the standards of practice offered new opportunities for reflection on personal nursing practice and nursing leadership while acknowledging accountability to those whom nursing serves. Knowing the consumer and building strong therapeutic relationships within relational and reflective nursing practices were critical to consumers. Focus on behaviour, control, and management failed to support strong therapeutic relationships. The complexity of therapeutic relationships requires ongoing learning. Nurse leaders are obliged to seek opportunities for appropriate, non-performance-based, clinical supervision that fosters learning and development of nurses to match desired competencies and standards.

Implications for Practice
Nurse leaders have an obligation to develop and implement standards, policy, procedures, and work environments that support practice—relevant, core competencies in nursing. Standards of practice are important sources of knowledge and reflect the standards and competencies on which the public can rely. The patient or consumer is central to standards of practice. Thus, inviting patients or consumers to inform the development of nursing standards is essential to promoting positive patient outcomes and meeting the public mandate of nursing.

TABLE 5-2	ELEMENTS OF MALPRACTICE
ELEMENTS	**EXAMPLES**
Duty owed the patient	Duty to regularly monitor a patient's condition at a frequency suited to the acuity and anticipated stability of the patient
Breach of the duty owed	Failure to regularly monitor the blood pressure of a patient 1 hour post-surgery or to communicate change in patient status to the primary health care provider
Foreseeability	Blood pressure changes following surgery are an indication of adverse post-surgical events that require intervention to reduce endangerment to life and limb
Causation	Failure to provide adequate monitoring of a patient or adequate patient education
Injury or damages	Fractured hip and head concussion after a patient fall leading to loss of employment income for additional recovery time, future medical and nursing care needs and costs

RISK MANAGEMENT

Portions of risk management fall under the practice of most nurse managers. Risk management is the systematic identification, assessment, and prioritization of risks and the development and implementation of strategies to reduce adverse events and liability associated with these risks. Chapter 21 provides additional information on risk management. Risk management not only reduces losses but also enhances quality outcomes in health care delivery.

Institutional Liability and Insurance

Policy and procedures help improve the safety of staff and patient care and also help limit institutional liability and personal liability in managers. Contributing to the development and implementation of well-developed policy and procedures is an important management function.

Managers have a duty to their employer to manage exposure to liability risks where assessment of this risk is possible and insurance coverage may be adversely affected without proper management actions. Where the potential for liability exists, it is incumbent on managers to notify the institution's insurance company. Larger health care institutions often have a risk manager, a legal officer, or an institutional lawyer to whom a manager can turn for advice and guidance about potential legal risks. However, the task of recognizing and appropriately documenting the events that lead to or potentially lead to a liability risk often rests with managers.

Workers' compensation programs exist in all provinces and territories and are a form of employment-based, mandatory insurance that managers must know about. These programs offer compensation and rehabilitation support to employees injured at the workplace. Failure to comply with policies, procedures, and workplace orders originating from workers' compensation boards can result in various forms of liability.

Occupational health and safety legislation and associated regulations address general workplace safety issues as well as the use of hazardous materials, radiation, and chemicals. Additionally, this legislation addresses issues such as workplace violence and harassment and imposes obligations on employers for the development of policies, procedures, safety programs, reporting, and documentation (see, e.g., Part III of Ontario's *Occupational Health and Safe Act*, 1990).

Health Records

Record keeping is generally part of the professional standards of regulated health care professions, but it is also part of the tasks of health care workers who are unregulated. Moreover, health care institutions may be regulated by specific legislative acts to collect and maintain certain types of records on patients. For example, in British Columbia the *Continuing Care Act* (1996) requires that records be maintained on patients receiving continuing care in areas such as home oxygen supply, home support, meal programs, adult day care services, and continuing care respite services. Special records, such as narcotic control documentation, may also be necessary, and failure to follow legal requirements for such records can result in prosecution. Good quality health records are important not only in meeting legal requirements but also in providing quality health care to patients. From a nurse leader's perspective, record keeping must meet professional standards, fulfill legal requirements, benefit patients, and help establish or protect legal claims and legal defences. In terms of general guidelines, records must correctly identify the patient and be accurate, intelligible, made in ink or an indelible medium that does not lend itself to invisible correction after the event (Dickens, 2011, p. 150), complete, made routinely and contemporaneously, and dated with a clear indication (signature or initial) of who made each entry. Institutional policies and procedures should capture the necessary elements of record keeping to help avoid legal liability.

Access to Health Records

Relatively recent case law from the Supreme Court of Canada has helped clarify ownership and access issues surrounding patient health records. It is important to keep in mind that this case law may be specifically modified by health record legislation in individual provinces and territories. However, most jurisdictions in Canada have closely followed the court's direction on the issue. As a general rule, the patient does not own the actual health record housed by the health care institution, physician's office, or record keeper. Although ownership rests with the maker and holder of the record, patients ordinarily have the legal right to access the record, subject to some limitations (*McInerney v. MacDonald*, 1992). Patients may not be entitled to immediately access their record or see portions of it while they are in active treatment in the hospital, where a physician believes that it is not in their best interests or where disclosure may put a third party at risk. Additionally, patients may require supervision, interpretative assistance, and professional explanation of their records to avoid harmful misinterpretation. Hospitals should develop and maintain clear policies and protocols regarding patient access to their own health records and patient ability to photocopy them (*McInerney v. MacDonald*, 1992). Under many health information privacy acts, patient requests to access their health records must be tracked by an information officer if the records are kept by a custodian under the relevant legislation. This makes it that more important that procedures and policies are in place and known by all staff. Staff also need to be fully cognizant of who may ultimately view health records when contemplating making entries into them. In a changed era of patient–health care provider relationships, the law makes health care providers and institutions trustees of personal health information; this trusteeship recognizes that liberal access to one's own health record is part of a "philosophy of openness and candour better suited to cultivating mutual trust between patients and their healthcare providers" (Irvine et al., 2013, p. 262).

Patient Safety

In recent years, the emphasis on patient safety and quality care has grown. Creating and maintaining environments that promote patient safety means fostering and developing cultures of safety that move from finding individual blame to looking at how systems can contribute to safety. Fears of liability and cultures of blame associated with revealing adverse events have hampered movement to improved cultures of safety that serve to benefit patients. New legislation in Canada (see, e.g., Manitoba's *Apology Act*, 2007) that prevents apology letters to patients for adverse events being entered into evidence in courts to substantiate wrongdoing and legal liability is one step signalling a movement away from a culture of blame and liability to one that looks for a systematic approach to enhancing patient safety (Robertson, 2008). Moving to cultures of safety that incorporate blamelessness and understanding encourages the reporting of errors and harm to patients so that environments of safety can develop and additional education and training can be offered to avoid harmful recurrence.

Canadian courts have been reluctant to hold hospitals vicariously liable for physician negligence where the physician is not an employee of the hospital (*Yepremian v. Scarborough General Hospital*, 1980). However, hospitals are liable for actions of their employees under laws of vicarious liability. Such legal responsibility is intended, in part, to operate as a deterrent of poor practices so that health care facilities might conscientiously address systematic approaches to reducing risk (*John Doe v. Bennett*, 2004) and thus increase patient safety. Managers must remain attentive to addressing quality of care and patient safety systematically to avoid institutional liability.

Contract Law

Managers may have authority to enter into contracts on behalf of the institutions and employers for which they work. Some basic understanding of contract law will assist them in making sure that contracts can be properly enforced and that liability is not inadvertently created.

DISTINGUISHING LAW AND ETHICS

While laws should be rooted in ethical and moral principles, laws and ethics differ and may offer different or contradictory solutions to individual situations. As a result, there is value in considering legal and ethical issues separately in health care decision making. In this chapter, legal issues particular to nursing leadership were highlighted. The next chapter addresses ethical issues.

A SOLUTION

The issues raised in A Challenge are not unusual and provide the opportunity for staff and management to address important issues around safe practice and patient safety. It is important to consider professional standards and the duty to withdraw from practice when it is unsafe or a nurse feels unfit. Nurses cannot abandon patients under their standards of practice, but they can provide their employer with sufficient notice of the need for rest or for replacement when their practice is becoming unsafe. With adequate notice of need for relief to maintain safe practice, responsibility shifts to employers to find replacement staff. Although not ideal, this might mean drawing on staff from other areas of the hospital who lack specialized qualifications, but who can perform general nursing duties under the direction of the regular palliative care nurse to enhance patient safety. If the issues are ongoing, unions and nursing regulatory bodies may offer assistance.

Nurses leave themselves and their institutions open to liability if errors or omissions occur from working while fatigued or on excessive overtime. Consider the elements of malpractice in these circumstances. Employers and nurses have a duty to maintain safe work environments for the protection of staff and patients and this should include planning for these contingencies, particularly if recurrent. Guidelines and agreement on what is reasonable notice to find replacement staff at the end of a shift and what communication is needed to clarify expectations between staff and management facilitate necessary policy development and ultimately enhance patient care and safety. Knowing her legal obligations as a nurse and owning her own fitness to practise makes Jessica a leader.

If you were in a similar situation, how might you approach your manager with this information?

THE EVIDENCE

Nurses should be aware of the unique privacy issues associated with electronic medical records (EMRs). In one of its *InfoLaw* information sheets for nurses, the Canadian Nurses Protective Society (2009) addressed unique issues of access, accuracy, theft, and disposal of electronic records. With the growing presence of and reliance on electronic records in health care, these issues are highly relevant to practising nurses.

Inappropriate access—that is, accessing a patient's personal information for which you have no legitimate use in the performance of your duties and care of your current patients—may be subject to sanctions. For example, a clerk in a plastic surgeon's office was charged and fined $10 000 for accessing the medical records of an individual who was not a patient of the surgeon but known to the clerk. Development and enforcement of clear policies, strong password protections, and audit trails and periodic audit procedures should form part of an organization's plan to guard against improper access to EMRs.

In another case, a patient who had requested a copy of his own medical record was inadvertently provided with information on other patients because the data were not appropriately separated, a situation that arose from the inclusion of multiple patients' data in one file or on one DVD. Clear policies to prevent data mixing, provide ongoing education, and establish careful checks for patient information should be in place before use or disclosure of that information.

Theft of electronic devices containing protected patient information is a problem that seems to appear regularly in media reports. Risk management procedures should include strong password protection and encryption of storage media if personal health information is stored on portable devices. Additionally, risk management issues arise in the transfer of data when governments and health care providers see a value to patients in making their EMRs widely available to health care professions at multiple service points within the patients' circles of care. Similarly, wireless communications and transfers of data, while they enable improvements to patient care through use of portable devices at the bedside or at patients' homes, raise new data security issues.

The disposal of electronic records is also problematic. For example, data deleted on an electronic device may not actually be erased from the storage device, but marked as available for overwriting. Policies and practices must address how data can be wiped from storage devices and how storage devices can be destroyed or rendered inoperable in ways that do not allow data retrieval of any residual information. It is equally important to understand that personal information may automatically be stored on devices containing memory or storage capacities, such as fax machines, photocopiers, and personal data devices; this type of storage requires management to avoid inadvertent disclosure. To protect patient information from inappropriate disclosure, nurses must be aware of privacy protection laws, where confidential data exists, and policies and procedures for data access and destruction, audits, and due care.

NEED TO KNOW NOW

- Understand the legal ramifications of the nurse manager role, especially in terms of federal, provincial, and territorial laws. Query legal staff and privacy officers at your employer, administration, and the nursing regulatory agencies and associations as needed.
- Understand where liability for your own actions may occur; particularly, understand your personal obligations toward protecting patient privacy and confidentiality, your duty to practise in accordance with nursing standards as a reasonably prudent nurse acting within your scope of practice, and personal practice competencies.
- Consult with your regulatory or professional association if you have questions about insurance issues that protect you against personal liability for errors and omissions occurring in the course of your professional practice. Know what activities may not be covered by your insurance policy, such as independent practice and volunteer board work.

- Consult your union for assistance in navigating legal issues and legal questions you may have related to your employment. (The majority of nursing workplace environments are unionized.)
- Your regulatory body or nursing association may offer assistance with assessing and avoiding legal issues with your professional practice.
- Understand the laws in your province or territory that address informed consent and substitute decision making to help inform and keep your practice patient-centred and respectful of the wishes of your patient.
- Keep records accurately, precisely, and in a timely fashion as warranted by patient condition; focus on facts and be accountable for your entries.
- Expect laws affecting your practice to change and accept responsibility for keeping up to date with the changes that affect your practice.
- If legal and ethical issues are contradictory, legal aspects are enacted first.

CHAPTER CHECKLIST

This chapter explores multiple legal issues as they pertain to managing, leading, and following in nursing.

Legal areas that all nurses must understand include the following:

- The source of law (federal, provincial, territorial, and common law)
- The regulatory and licensing structures that relate to those working in health care
- Sources of legal liability and practice implications:
  - Criminal liability
  - Civil liability, including malpractice, duty of care, and practice standards
  - Professional sanctions
  - Employment ramifications
- Privacy, confidentiality, and access to information laws that vary across provinces and territories and are generally outlined in statute law

- Laws that govern duty to report and protective laws that are aimed at protecting individuals viewed as vulnerable or at discouraging crime
- Leadership includes knowing what laws affect your practice and keeping abreast of changes to these laws. Some important changes are occurring around the following:
  - Duty to report
  - Insurance
  - Documentation and the importance of protecting privacy and confidentiality
  - The impact of electronic record keeping and related laws

Managers must have enhanced understanding of the following:

- Labour and employment laws
- Duty of care owed by employers to others
- Patient rights and patient decision making

CHAPTER CHECKLIST—cont'd

- While management may require enhanced knowledge, all nurse managers have a part to play in risk management, including individual roles in addressing the following:
  - Institutional liability and insurance
  - Health records maintenance by those not governed by professional standards

- Access to health records
- Patient safety and quality of care
- Contracts

Law and ethics, while related, are distinguishable and may yield different answers to issues arising in nursing practice.

evolve WEBSITE

Visit the Evolve website for Suggested Readings, Internet Resources, and additional resources related to the content in this chapter: http://evolve.elsevier.com/Canada/Yoder-Wise/leading/.

TIPS FOR INCORPORATING LEARNING ABOUT LEGAL ISSUES IN PRACTICE SETTINGS

- Locate and read the relevant scope of practice documents and nursing standards of practice within your jurisdiction.
- Apply legal principles in all health care settings.
- Legal issues can be complex and may not always have simple answers. Know when you are faced with a complex legal issue and seek additional expert opinion before acting.

- Continue to look for ways to influence policy and procedures in your work area that support expert practice, promote patient safety, and assist in risk management and quality improvement.
- Locate and read your local policies on patient information protection and disclosure.

REFERENCES

Statutes

Adult Protection and Decision-Making Act, SY 2003, c. 21, Sch. A (Yukon).
Apology Act, SM 2007, c. 25, CCSM c. A98 (Manitoba).
Canada Health Act, RSC 1985, c. C-6 (Canada).
Canadian Charter of Rights and Freedoms, Part I of the Constitution Act, 1982, being Schedule B to the Canada Act 1982, (UK), 1982, c. 11.
Constitution Act, 1867 (U.K.), 30 & 31 Vict, c. 3.
Continuing Care Act, RSBC 1996, c. 70 (British Columbia).
Criminal Code, RSC 1985, c. C-46 (Canada).
Employment Insurance Act, SC 1996, c. 23 (Canada).
Freedom of Information and Protection of Privacy Act, RSO 1990, c. F-31 (Ontario).
Gunshot and Stab Wound Mandatory Disclosure Act, SA 2009, c. G-12 (Alberta).
Health Professions Act, RSBC 1996, c. 183 (British Columbia).
Occupational Health and Safety Act, RSO 1990, c. O.1 (Ontario).
Pension Act, RSC 1985, c. P-6 (Canada).

Personal Health Information Protection Act, 2004, SO 2004, c. 3, Sch. A (Ontario).
Protection for Persons in Care Act, SA 2009, c. P-29.1 (Alberta).
USA Patriot Act of 2001, 115 USC Stat. 272 (2001).

Case Law

Hollis v. Dow Corning Corp. [1995] SDJ 104, [1995] SCR 634 at paras. 24–25.
John Doe v. Bennett, 2004 SCC 17, [2004] 1 SCR 436.
McInerney v. MacDonald [1992] 12 CCLT (2d) 224 (SCC).
R. v. Duarte, [1990] 1 SCR 30.
Yepremian v. Scarborough General Hospital (1980), 28 OR (2d) 494, 110 DLR (3d) 513 (Court of Appeal).

Texts

Beal, G., Chan, A., Chapman, S., et al. (2007). Consumer input into standards revision: Changing practice. *Journal of Psychiatric and Mental Health Nursing, 14,* 13–20. doi:10.1111/j.1365-2850.2007.01034.x

Canadian Nurses Assocation. (2007). *Framework for the practice of registered nurses in Canada.* Ottawa, ON: Author. Retrieved from http://www.cna-nurses.ca/CNA/practice/scope/default_e.aspx.

Canadian Nurses Protective Society. (2009, December). Privacy and electronic medical records. *InfoLaws, 18*(1). Retrieved from http://www.cnps.ca/index.php?page=140.

College of Nurses of Ontario. (2013). *College of Nurses of Ontario by-laws.* Toronto, ON: Author. Retrieved from http://www.cno.org/Global/docs/general/46005_bylaws.pdf.

College of Registered Nurses of British Columbia. (2011). *Legal issues for registered nurses.* Vancouver, BC: Author. Retrieved from https://www.crnbc.ca/Standards/Lists/StandardResources/422LegalIssuesforRNs.pdf.

Dickens, B. (2011). Medical negligence. In J. G. Downie, T. A. Caulfield, & C. M. Flood (Eds.), *Canadian health law and policy* (4th ed., pp. 115–151). Markham, ON: LexisNexis Canada.

Downie, J. G., Caulfield, T. A., & Flood, C. M. (Eds.). (2011). *Canadian health law and policy* (4th ed.). Markham, ON: LexisNexis Canada.

Epps, T. (2011). Regulation of health care professionals. In J. G. Downie, T. A. Caulfield, & C. M. Flood (Eds.), *Canadian health law and policy* (4th ed., pp. 75–114). Markham, ON: LexisNexis Canada.

Gibson, E. (2011). Health information: Confidentiality and access. In J. G. Downie, T. A. Caulfield, & C. M. Flood (Eds.), *Canadian health law and policy* (4th ed., pp. 253–294). Markham, ON: LexisNexis Canada.

Information Privacy Commission of Ontario and Hewlett-Packard (Canada) Co. (2008). *RFID and privacy: Guidance for health-care providers.* Toronto, ON: Authors. Retrieved from http://www.longwoods.com/articles/images/rfid-healthcare.pdf.

Irvine, J. C., Osborne, P. H., & Shariff, M. (2013). *Canadian medical law: An introduction for physicians, nurses, and other health care professionals* (4th ed.). Scarborough, ON: Thomson Carswell.

Kosseim, P., & Brady, M. (2008). Policy by procrastination: Secondary use of electronic health records for health research purposes. *McGill Journal of Law & Health, 2*(1), 5–46.

Morris, J. J., & Clarke, C.D. (2011). *Law for Canadian health care administrators* (2nd ed.). Markham, ON: Butterworths.

Peppin, P. (2011). Informed consent. In J. G. Downie, T. A. Caulfield, & C. M. Flood (Eds.), *Canadian health law and policy* (4th ed., pp. 153–194). Markham, ON: LexisNexis Canada.

Ries, N. M. (2006). Patient privacy in a wired (and wireless) world: Approaches to consent in the context of electronic health records. *Alberta Law Review, 43*(3), 681–712.

Robertson, G. B. (2008). A view of the future: Emerging developments in health care liability. *Health Law Journal* (Special edition), 1–12.

Ethical Issues

Sandra A. Pike-MacDonald

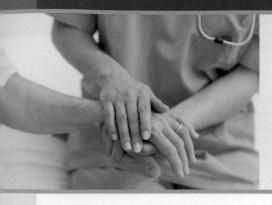

This chapter highlights and explains ethical issues as they relate to nurse managers, leaders, and staff nurses. Relational ethics, principles of bioethics, and codes of ethics are discussed. Nursing has been described as a "moral activity, a moral act, and even an ethical force in society" (Raya, 1990, p. 506), which means that nurses are expected to act ethically. This chapter also examines how ethical decision making can be applied to everyday clinical practice.

OBJECTIVES

- Define *ethics*.
- Discuss the principles of relational ethics.
- Analyze the bioethical principles of autonomy, justice, beneficence, and nonmaleficence.
- Apply nursing codes of ethics from a nurse manager's perspective.
- Explore ethical violations, dilemmas, and distress.
- Discuss how law, morality, and professional accountabilities can influence nurses' managerial and clinical decision making.
- Apply a framework to prevent and resolve ethical conflicts.
- Understand the ethical obligations of nurse managers and leaders.
- Analyze the role of clinical ethics committees.
- Understand the nurse manager's responsibility to develop policy using an ethical decision making framework.

TERMS TO KNOW

autonomy	ethical (or moral) distress	nonmaleficence
beneficence	ethical violation	relational ethics
bioethics	ethics	social justice
confidentiality	justice	
ethical dilemma	moral uncertainty	

? A CHALLENGE

Mirella is the nurse manager working on a paediatric oncology out-patient clinic in a large tertiary care hospital. The nurses are currently caring for a five-year-old patient, Adam, who was recently diagnosed with a brain tumour. He has been receiving radiation therapy for the past eight months and today is receiving his last treatment. One of the nurses has approached Mirella to ask for her help to deal with an ethical issue that the nurses have been discussing since yesterday. Adam's haemoglobin is very low, and he is experiencing symptoms of weakness, dizziness, and shortness of breath. The need for a blood transfusion has been thoroughly discussed with all members of the health care team and Adam's

parents. However, Adam's parents are Jehovah's Witnesses and have expressed their religious belief that Adam is not to receive any blood or blood products. Thus, although the parents understand the situation, they refuse to allow the blood transfusion. The nurses are very upset with the parents' decision because they think Adam will be negatively affected if he does not receive the blood transfusion.

How would you deal with this situation if you were Mirella? What ethical principles could guide your actions?

INTRODUCTION

Nurses and nurse managers are held to a high level of ethical accountability and are expected to act as an ethical force in society, especially when making decisions regarding patient care. To be viewed as ethical, nursing management decisions and actions are guided by three elements: ethical principles, professional accountabilities, and the law (Figure 6-1). Each of these elements interconnects to influence the development of the nurse's moral self, which in turn influences the nurse's decisions and actions. Ethical decision making and ethical practice can be challenging for nurses in today's health care environment. Rising patient acuity, staff shortages, heavy workloads, recruitment and retention issues, and ever-expanding treatment options all place extraordinary ethical demands on nurses (Bjarnason, 2011; Pavlish, Brown-Saltsman, Hersh, et al., 2011). Nurse managers and leaders must maintain an ethical perspective when

making managerial decisions to ensure that patients and nursing staff are *cared for* and *cared about* in a manner that reflects mutual respect as well as valuing (Woods, 2012). This chapter provides an introduction to the ethical theories and principles that nurse managers, nurse leaders, and staff nurses must consider when making decisions in a clinical setting. Relational ethics and the principles of bioethics are also explored, especially as they relate to the nurse manager's role.

THE RELATIONAL CONTEXT OF ETHICS

Ethics is a division of moral philosophy that involves the moral practices, beliefs, and standards of individuals or groups (Toren & Wagner, 2010). It includes consideration of whether thoughts and actions are "right" or "wrong." *Ethics* and *morality* are often considered to have the same meaning. However, *ethics* is a branch of philosophy that deals with what is right and wrong, whereas *morality* is the code of conduct advanced and accepted by a society, a group, or an individual (Merriam Webster, n.d.; Stanford Encyclopedia of Philosophy, 2011). Morality can be reflected in personal, cultural, and professional values, and it is based on ideas about right and wrong. Ethics can be divided into three branches: (1) meta-ethics, (2) normative ethics, and (3) applied ethics. *Meta-ethics* explores the broader theory and meaning of morality, and the foundation and scope of moral values, words, and practice (Stanford Encyclopedia of Philosophy, 2007). *Normative ethics* is concerned with the standards most people use to guide their behaviours (e.g., murder is wrong), and how they are determined (Encyclopedia Britannica, n.d.). Finally,

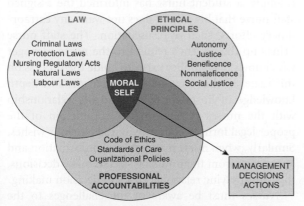

FIGURE 6-1 The interface of law and morality.

applied ethics relates ethical principles to real-life moral issues, such as how to provide nursing care and how to conduct research on human subjects. A division of philosophical thought within applied ethics is *bioethics*, which focuses on questions about science and human life often in the context of health care and incorporates the principles of autonomy, justice, beneficence, and nonmaleficence (Risjord, 2014). Understanding the study of ethics can help nurse managers and leaders develop the strategies they need to engage in ethical decision making and ethical nursing practice.

Ethics in health care recognizes the importance of human relationships in ethical decision making. A key area of ethical nursing practice is the therapeutic relationship between the nurse and the patient (Beckett, Gilbertson, & Greenwood, 2007). Whether this relationship involves direct one-on-one care provided by a staff nurse or indirect care provided by a nurse manager or leader, it is central to nursing care. The relationships that develop between nurses and individuals, groups, and communities form the relational context of ethical practice. Although each relationship is unique and includes different individual experiences, thoughts, and actions, all can be grounded in the core elements of relational ethics.

RELATIONAL ETHICS

Relational ethics involves asking not only *What should I do?* but also *What should I do for others?* In an effort to answer these questions, relational ethics focuses on ethical action that takes place in relationships. The core elements of relational ethics are engaged interactions, mutual respect, embodied knowledge, uncertainty and vulnerability, and interdependent environment (Austin, Goble, & Kelecevic, 2009; Kunyk & Austin, 2012; Shaw, 2011). According to a relational ethics approach, nurses must consider those who will be influenced by their thoughts and actions (Falk-Rafael & Betker, 2012) (Box 6-1).

A relational ethics approach to nursing includes engaged interactions that promote the interpersonal aspects of relationships (Leung & Esplen, 2010; Olmstead, Scott, & Austin, 2010). In nursing practice, engaged interactions are not confined to the nurse–patient relationship; they also occur between nurses and the health care team, nurse managers and staff, and nurse managers and the health care team (Wright & Brajtman, 2011). These engaged interactions with individuals and

BOX 6-1	CORE ELEMENTS OF RELATIONAL ETHICS

- Engaged interactions
- Mutual respect
- Embodied knowledge
- Uncertainty and vulnerability
- Interdependent environment

Based on Austin, W., Goble, E., & Kelecevic, J. (2009). The ethics of forensic psychiatry: Moving beyond principles to a relational ethics approach. *Journal of Forensic Psychiatry & Psychology, 20*(6), 835–850. http://dx.doi.org/10.1080/14789940903174147; Kunyk, D., & Austin, W. (2012). Nursing under the influence: A relational ethics perspective. *Nursing Ethics, 19*(3), 380–389. http://dx.doi.org/10.1177/0969733011406767; Shaw, E. (2011). Relational ethics and moral imagination in contemporary systemic practice. *Australian & New Zealand Journal of Family Therapy, 32*(1), 1–14. http://dx.doi.org/10.1375/anft.32.1.1

groups can help form the basis for ethical decision making for nurse managers, nurse leaders, and staff nurses.

Another important principle of relational ethics is mutual respect. Mutual respect is inherent in the relationships that are developed between nurses and patients, families, the health care team, and nurse managers. For example, nurse managers show mutual respect for students, nurses, and the health care team by facilitating interprofessional team meetings to discuss and plan patient care. Team meetings provide an opportunity to value everyone's contributions and demonstrate mutual respect, which is a critical aspect of effective teamwork. Relationships that are based on mutual respect can provide guidance for nurse managers to take ethical actions.

When nurse managers base their decisions on embodied knowledge, they are also applying the principles of relational ethics to their actions. Embodied knowledge can include research, policies, and the information obtained through the nurse manager's relationships with staff and the health care team. For example, a student nurse has informed the assigned staff nurse that his patient does not want any extraordinary efforts, such as resuscitation. The staff nurse brings up the patient's request to the nurse manager who knows that a policy exists to guide the process on this issue. In this way, the nurse manager's in-depth knowledge of hospital policies and her relationship with the nurses resulted in the completion of the proper legal form to comply with the patient's wishes. Similarly, when nurse managers seek information and knowledge from their nursing staff to make decisions, they are applying relational ethics to decision making.

Nurses must be aware of the challenges to the integrity of the nurse–patient relationship and the uncertainty inherent in decisions about patient care. It is the nurse's and the health care team's responsibility to assess the vulnerability of the patient and to evaluate any harm or susceptibility for harm to the patient. Nurses have an ethical obligation to be aware of the vulnerable status of their patients and adjust care accordingly to prevent harm; for example, by ensuring that consent for surgery is given prior to administering a relaxant pre-op medication to the patient.

Nurse managers must also be aware of the challenges to the integrity of nurse manager–staff relationships. It is the nurse manager's responsibility to evaluate any harm or susceptibility for harm to staff and adjust the work environment accordingly. Nurse managers have an ethical obligation to be aware of any safety issues in the workplace and intervene to correct those issues.

According to a relational ethics approach, the workplace is considered to be an interdependent environment that extends beyond the individual nurse manager and staff relationships to include relationships that connect the staff to the health care system, the community, and the world (an idea embodied in the International Council of Nurses Code of Ethics for Nurses [2012]). In an interdependent environment, nurse managers, nurse leaders, and staff nurses recognize individuals' social and political nature. A relational ethics approach suggests that individuals often apply their personal values within their social worlds (Kenny, Sherwin, & Baylis, 2010). This concept implies that nurse managers should involve different nurses and roles in matters of health policy and create an environment where nurses and the health care team are encouraged to apply their personal values to the development of policy and standards of care. For example, when developing new policies and protocols for the care of post–cardiac arrest patients receiving therapeutic hypothermia treatment, the nurse manager must involve the direct care nurses and members of the health care team in the development of those policies and protocols to ensure they accurately reflect the needs of patients. When developing or revising health policies, nurses must consider that within a relational ethics approach, individuals are considered to be social, independent beings who bring a unique perspective to policy development.

Applying the principles of relational ethics to practice and managerial decisions related to patient care can help nurse managers think about the fundamental question *What should I do for others?* In an effort to answer that this question, the relational ethics perspective focuses on the nurse–patient relationship and the relationships that develop within the health care team as important elements in the development and maintenance of a moral self. A relational ethics perspective can help nurse leaders realize that relationships are critical in the development and maintenance of the nurse managers' and leaders' roles and actions. A relational ethics approach helps nurse managers and leaders reflect on how they ought to act and think, and to consider the relationships they have with their staff, patients, families, communities, and groups in an effort to provide ethically sound nursing care and make ethical decisions in the clinical setting. Box 6-2 shows how the core elements of relational ethics can be applied to nursing leadership.

THE PRINCIPLES OF BIOETHICS

Bioethics (also referred to as *biomedical ethics*) is a division of applied ethics rooted in biological research and medicine and increasingly concerned with questions related to health care. Its major principles are autonomy, justice, beneficence, and nonmaleficence. Bioethics applies to real-life situations, such as ensuring informed consent and making ethical managerial decisions. How each of the principles of bioethics applies to nurse managers and leaders is discussed next.

Autonomy

Autonomy is derived from the Greek words *autos* ("self") and *nomos* ("rule"), which means to self-rule. Autonomy is the freedom and the right to choose what will happen to one's own person. Applying the principle of autonomy to nursing practice means that nurses focus on the patient's specific needs, opinions, and preferences for care, while balancing the preferences for care of the health care team (Risjord, 2014). When nurses apply the principle of autonomy to guide their ethical practice and decision making, they recognize the right of patients to be involved in decisions about their own lives to the extent they are able. Helping people be involved in making decisions about their own lives is a basic principle of informed consent. Informed consent requires that a patient be competent to make decisions about his or her care; it can only be obtained from a competent patient who at a minimum is orientated to

BOX 6-2   THE CORE ELEMENTS OF RELATIONAL ETHICS APPLIED TO NURSING LEADERSHIP

CORE ELEMENTS	NURSE LEADER'S ROLE	NURSE LEADER'S ACTIONS
Engaged interactions	Communicator Counsellor Teacher Decision maker	Attends team meetings Fosters nurse–patient relationship Provides education for patients and staff Is a member of hospital ethics committee
Mutual respect	Negotiator Team builder Patient advocate	Participates in patient rounds Facilitates interprofessional team meetings Participates in discussions with family about care
Embodied knowledge	Researcher Coordinator of care Professional development supporter Policy and procedure administrator Expert clinician	Participates in research Understands patient-care needs Attends conferences Is a member of policy and procedure committee Reads appropriate literature
Uncertainty and vulnerability	Advocate Consultant Risk manager	Develops policy and procedures Is a member of ethics committee Advocates for quality care
Interdependent environment	Team leader Advocate for social justice	Applies code of ethics to practice Actively participates in professional associations Actively participates in policy development

time, person, and place. (Elements of informed consent are also considered in Chapter 5.)

EXERCISE 6-1

Nurse Susan is completing the preoperative checklist for Mr. Wright prior to a transurethral resection of the prostate (TURP). During their discussions, Mr. Wright says, "I hope the cut doesn't take too long to heal." Recognizing Mr. Wright's lack of knowledge related to the surgery, Nurse Susan brings her concerns to Nurse Manager Khan, stating that Mr. Wright does not have enough information about the surgical procedure. How could Nurse Susan and Nurse Manager Khan use the core elements of relational ethics to help them decide on a course of action?

When nurse managers apply the principle of autonomy to guide their ethical practice and managerial decision making, they recognize the importance of involving their staff in decisions that affect their work lives. Applying the principle of autonomy suggests that nurse managers are aware of their responsibility to consider staff's needs. For example, a nurse manager who is preparing the budget for the next two years asks her staff to participate in developing a list of priority items to be purchased for their unit. By doing so, the nurse manager involves staff in decisions that affect them directly. On occasion, however, it is the sole responsibility of the nurse manager to make decisions (e.g., in times of crisis). The nurse manager can still seek input from staff and promote respect for staff autonomy, but must make the final decision alone. Good followership suggests that staff provide needed input to inform important decisions. Managers who respect autonomy respect their staff as individuals who have individual goals and aspirations; for example, a manager respects and supports a staff nurse's right to request a leave of absence from work to return to school and complete her degree even though it means the unit will now be short one staff.

One criticism of the principle of autonomy is that it can lead to a focus on the rights or needs of one individual at the expense of the rights or needs of others (including entire groups). However, a relational approach to autonomy recognizes that respecting the autonomy of one individual should not come at the expense of the autonomy of others and acknowledges that individuals have different social, political, and economic backgrounds. For example, one staff nurse believes that she should make decisions autonomously about patients under her care without consulting with other health care team members. However, aspects of patient care depend on the availability of other health care team members to provide specialized care such as physiotherapy. The nurse should consider how her autonomy for patient-care decisions should not supersede other health care team members' autonomy to make decisions about patient care. The perceived rights of one have infringed on the rights of many. As such, autonomy is respect not only for the individual but for others. A relational approach to autonomy suggests that autonomy is best promoted through social change rather than through protecting an individual's freedom of choice (Kenny, Sherwin, & Baylis, 2010).

Justice

Justice refers to the principle that everyone should be treated equally and fairly; for example, all patients should be provided with quality care. Moral justice guides the actions of nurses by promoting the principle that those who are poor, sick, and vulnerable must be given more help than those who have adequate resources, are healthy, and can defend their rights on their own. In the health care setting, patients are often vulnerable, and once they enter the health care system, nurses become their advocates, or their "voice," to ensure they receive the best care possible. It is not enough that nurses support the principle of justice; they must actually engage in those good and right actions that show justice is being done. For example, if a nurse observes an unsafe practice, he or she must report it rather than ignore it. The principle of justice also suggests that benefits and burdens should be distributed in a just manner in society (a concept known as *distributive justice*).

Nurse managers who apply the principle of justice in their nursing practice and managerial decision making ensure that staffing and workload are fairly distributed among the nursing staff. It is not enough to recognize that one nurse has a heavier workload than another; the nurse manager must change that workload to ensure equal distribution of the work (although equality is not, of itself, always fair and just). Performance appraisals by nurse managers ought to be guided by the principle of justice. For example, if one nurse is disciplined for being late, then all nurses who are late should be disciplined in the same way. Or, if one nurse is rewarded with time off for attending an education session, then all nurses who attended the same education session should also be given the same time off. In this way, when managers are guided by the bioethical principle of justice, everyone should be treated equally and fairly.

The Canadian Nurses Association (CNA) proposes the principle of social justice, and considers it an organizational priority that has a role to play in CNA's national and international work (Canadian Nurses Association, 2006, p. 5). Social justice refers to the fair distribution of society's benefits, responsibilities, and consequences for all. It focuses on the position of one social group in relation to others and encourages nurses to explore the root causes of disparities and what can be done to eliminate them (Myllykoski, 2011; Peter, 2011; Woods, 2012). Social justice principles are in keeping with a relational approach to ethics because the focus extends beyond individuals to include social groups who may be affected by practices and policies that have the potential to create inequalities. Nurse managers often have to make tough decisions about the allocation of scarce health care resources, and using the principle of social justice can help them make a case for allocating resources to certain patient populations. For example, cardiac rehabilitation units and cardiac post-surgical units are competing for more nursing resources to meet what they see as elevated and specialized care requirements. A nurse manager may suggest a compromise from both units to balance nursing allocation or advocate for increases to both units based on the social justice principle that each patient population is equally deserving of care and neither should be disparaged or have enhanced benefit to the exclusion of the other.

Beneficence

Nurses are bound by a professional, legal, and ethical duty to provide quality, safe care. The principle of beneficence states that the actions one takes should "do good." This principle is reflected in the provision of quality care based on competent, compassionate practice. Nurses must be educated in accredited nursing education programs and then maintain their competence through active practice and continuing professional education. Nurse managers must support staff nurses in their pursuit of continuing competency as well as maintain their own competency in practice and management.

Nonmaleficence

The principle of nonmaleficence states that the actions one takes should "do no harm." This principle is reflected in practice, administration, education, and research. Nurses in practice must be competent as well as be aware of any safety concerns for patients and anticipate any risks of treatment. Nurse managers must consider patient safety, but they must also consider staff safety and recognize their responsibility to establish safe, quality professional practice environments for their staff. Nurse managers must help establish standards of practice and develop policies that promote a safe work environment with systems for professional appraisal and professional development.

CODE OF ETHICS FOR NURSES

Nurses have access to several key documents that can guide their ethical conduct in practice, including codes of ethics for licensed practical nurses (LPNs) (called *registered practical nurses* in Ontario), registered psychiatric nurses (RPNs), and registered nurses (RNs). The Canadian Nurses Association (CNA), the International Council of Nurses (ICN), and provincial or territorial regulatory colleges for the three nursing groups have all developed or adopted codes of ethics, which can be applied to guide the ethical conduct of nurses, nurse managers, and nurse leaders. While these codes of ethics may contain differences, many of the principles are essentially the same as those identified in the CNA and the ICN code of ethics (International Council of Nurses, 2012). It is recommended that all nurses seek out their specific provincial regulatory code of ethics when exploring guidelines for practice.

The CNA *Code of Ethics for Registered Nurses* describes the ethical values that guide registered nurses' actions (CNA, 2008). The CNA code states that nurses are ethically committed to persons with health care needs and to those receiving nursing care. The code outlines seven primary values that serve as bases for the relationships that nurses have with their patients, students, colleagues, and other members of the health care team, which are, for example, similar to those identified in the code of ethics for LPNs of British Columbia (College of Licensed Practical Nurses of BC, 2004) and the code of ethics for LPNs of Newfoundland and Labrador (College of Licensed Practical Nurses of Newfoundland and Labrador, 2011). Those values include a responsibility to provide safe, compassionate, competent, and ethical care and to

intervene to address unsafe, noncompassionate, unethical, or incompetent practice or unsafe working conditions (Box 6-3). These seven primary values can also be applied as guidelines for the nurse manager's conduct. For example, nurse managers are morally obligated to ensure that nursing staff are providing safe, competent, and ethical nursing care. To meet this obligation, nurse managers may need to organize education sessions for nursing staff on ethics, and they may need to intervene if nursing staff are unsafe or incompetent.

BOX 6-3   PRIMARY NURSING VALUES: CNA CODE OF ETHICS FOR REGISTERED NURSES

1. Provide safe, compassionate, competent, and ethical care.
2. Promote health and well-being.
3. Promote and respect informed decision making.
4. Preserve dignity.
5. Maintain privacy and confidentiality.
6. Promote justice.
7. Be accountable.

Canadian Nurses Association [CNA]. (2008). Code of Ethics for Registered Nurses (2008 Centennial Edition). Toronto, ON: Author. © Canadian Nurses Association. Reprinted with permission. Further reproduction prohibited.

The CNA code of ethics stresses the importance of nurses maintaining their competency while adhering to the values of the code. Nurses are expected to care for patients while collaborating with the team to plan that care. Nurses respect the wishes of their patients and share information to help patients make informed decisions. Nurses must also intervene to preserve the dignity of patients and never judge, discriminate, label, demean, stigmatize, or humiliate patients. Finally, nurses must be accountable for their practices, whether nurses work in direct care, education, administration, or research. Nurses are expected to adhere to the principles of the CNA code of ethics.

The ICN code of ethics states that nurses have a moral obligation "to promote health, to prevent illness, to restore health, and to alleviate suffering" (International Council of Nurses, 2012, p. 1). In light of this moral obligation, the ICN has identified four principal elements that outline the standards of ethical conduct that guide nurses' actions: (1) nurses and people; (2) nurses and practice; (3) nurses and the profession; and (4) nurses and co-workers. Each of these principal elements can be applied by practising nurses, nurse managers, educators, and researchers. Box 6-4 demonstrates

BOX 6-4   ELEMENTS OF THE ICN CODE OF ETHICS APPLIED TO THE NURSE MANAGER'S ROLE

ELEMENT	NURSE MANAGER'S ROLE
People	Provide leadership that respects patient and staff rights and is sensitive to the values, customs, and beliefs of all people.
	Provide education for staff on ethical principles to guide practice.
	Ensure staff have adequate information to advocate for the patient's right to choose or refuse treatment.
	Maintain the confidentiality of staff information (e.g., professional appraisals)
Practice	Establish a working environment that promotes quality care.
	Establish a system for the professional appraisal of staff.
	Establish systems of the professional development of staff.
	Monitor and promote the personal health of staff.
Profession	Set standards and policies to guide ethical practice.
	Foster the use of research and evidence for practice.
	Promote participation in federal, provincial, territorial, and international nursing associations.
Co-workers	Create awareness of the benefits of interprofessional team collaboration.
	Support common professional ethical values and behaviours among staff.
	Prevent unsafe practices and work environments.

EXERCISE 6-2

Adrian is a nurse manager on a busy surgery floor, and it has been brought to his attention that it is common practice for the nurses working on the night shift to take 1 hour for their break and sleep in the visitors' lounge. Adrian is currently planning a unit meeting with all of the nursing staff, and he is trying to decide if he will discuss this matter at the meeting. Which of the elements of the CNA code of ethics or the ICN code of ethics could Adrian apply to help make an ethical decision about this problem?

how the ICN code of ethics can be applied specifically to the nurse manager's role.

THE INTERDEPENDENT ENVIRONMENT OF NURSING

Within a relational ethics approach to ethics, nurse managers and leaders must consider the interdependent environment that goes beyond the individual nurse to include connections to the community and globally. Recall that three factors can have an influence on nurses' managerial and clinical decision making: laws, ethical principles, and professional accountabilities (see Figure 6-1, page 91). A relational ethics approach promotes the idea that the workplace is an interdependent environment that fosters relationships that connect nurses to their patients, one another, members of the health care team, local and international professional organizations, the community, and globally.

Many laws affect nursing actions and decision making, including nursing regulation acts, common laws, natural laws, and labour laws. Some of these laws are discussed in Chapter 5. Laws are generally rooted in ethical and moral principles, but laws and morality can differ and even contradict one another. Laws are grounded in ethical values and principles, and many of today's laws have been influenced by ethical values that have been in existence for thousands of years, such as "thou shall not kill" and "do not steal." As society's ethical values change, so do laws. It can be argued that the first early laws of society developed as a result of ethical inquiry into wrongful acts. Murder is one of the clearer examples of how society's ethical values have affected the development of laws that punish wrongful acts. However, there is a continuing interface between law and ethics, whereby changing community standards and ethics begin to affect a change in laws. For example, once considered unethical, patients and their families are encouraged to clearly outline their wishes regarding end-of-life decisions (e.g., no extraordinary measures), thus upholding the ethical principle of autonomy that protects a patient's right to make decisions about his or her own care (e.g., informed consent). In 2013, the Parliament of Quebec tabled Bill 52, which reflects community standards and ethical principles on ensuring that end-of-life patients are provided with care that is respectful of their dignity and autonomy, including guidelines on terminal palliative sedation and medical aid in dying (Quebec National Assembly, 2013).

The interface of law and morality can also impact the professional accountabilities of nurses. Just as society's ethical values influence the law, so too laws and ethical values influence the professional accountabilities of nurses and nurse managers. For example, laws exist to ensure that patients provide informed consent, so those laws and the bioethical principle of autonomy work in concert to influence the nurse–patient relationship.

Another example of how the law and ethical principles can impact professional accountabilities is confidentiality. Confidentiality can be viewed as both an ethical and a legal concept. It includes an ethical obligation for nurses to uphold the privacy and security of privately held personal information and a legal obligation under common law to protect personal information divulged to health care providers and not release that information without the patient's explicit permission (Cornock, 2011). An organization-wide policy on privacy and confidentiality is based on laws such as the *Personal Health Information Protection Act, 2004* and the ethical principle of autonomy. Both legal and ethical implications must be considered in policy development. Based on the legal requirements of the statutory law (the Act), such a policy would have to provide guidance on how to access, disclose, and handle patient information (Box 6-5). Nurses must consider the interface of law and ethics when establishing professional standards and policies to guide actions in the clinical setting. Confidentiality is discussed in further detail in Chapter 5.

BOX 6-5   EXAMPLE OF A PRIVACY AND CONFIDENTIALITY POLICY

Values
Wellness Hospital is dedicated to protecting the privacy and confidentiality of personal health information. We are legally and ethically obligated to keep all information collected within our services confidential, including how we collect, use, access, maintain, and destroy personal information.

Principles
All personal health information collected at Wellness Hospital is to be held in the strictest confidence and only collected, used, or disclosed for reasons of patient care or education. Collecting, sharing, discussing, and disposing of information must be in accordance with relevant legislation, professional standards, and codes of ethics. Information to be kept confidential includes but is not limited to patients' personal health information or personal information and any financial information.

DEFINING ETHICAL PROBLEMS FOR NURSE MANAGERS

Nurse managers and leaders are faced with a variety of ethical issues and concerns that sometimes can be difficult to define, and staff nurses often turn to their managers for help with ethical concerns (Zuzelo, 2007). Being able to define the type of ethical concern being experienced can help nurses discuss it further with colleagues. The CNA code of ethics suggests several terms that nurses can apply when they must define ethical issues and concerns, including *moral uncertainty*, *ethical violations*, *ethical dilemmas*, and *ethical distress*.

At the simplest level, an ethical experience is a situation that creates a sense of moral uncertainty: "when a nurse feels indecision or a lack of clarity or is unable to even know what the moral problem is, while at the same time feeling uneasy or uncomfortable" (Canadian Nurses Association, 2008, p. 6). The situation makes the nurse feel uncomfortable, but she or he is uncertain about the ethical nature of the issue, such as when a patient complains that he didn't know he was going to have an HIV test. Situations that provoke moral uncertainty may be resolved by discussing the problem with the patient, colleagues, and the health care team members.

📖 LITERATURE PERSPECTIVE

Resource: Zuzelo, P. R. (2007). Exploring the moral distress of registered nurses. *Nursing Ethics, 14*(3), 344–359.

As the author notes, nurses are confronted every day with practice issues that can evoke moral distress. This research-based article describes the causes of RNs' moral distress and the frequency of morally distressing events in practice. The Moral Distress Scale was administered to 100 direct care RNs working in a variety of settings, including medical–surgical, maternal–child, and critical care. RNs identified that the two most morally distressing events in their practice were related to working with "unsafe" levels of nursing staff and working with physicians who were not as competent as the patient care required. Comments from the RNs indicated that they resented it when physicians were reluctant to address death and dying issues with patients and their families. Another very frequent distressing event for RNs was carrying out orders for unnecessary treatments and tests. RNs also identified that their nurse managers and supervisors were their most important supports when dealing with ethical issues.

Implications for Practice

Nurses practising in different settings and with different patient groups (including neonates, adults, and older people) all experience moral distress. One example of a morally distressing event often reported by nurses in practice includes unsafe levels of staffing. Nurses rely on their nurse managers to provide advice on ethical issues. Therefore, making nurse managers aware of specific ethical issues may be an important first step in enhancing the ethical reasoning and moral assertiveness of nurses in practice. Nurse managers can also implement other strategies to address the moral distress of RNs, such as ethics rounds, improving access to ethics consultations, and increasing involvement of RNs on ethics committees.

Ethical violations "involve actions or failures to act that breach fundamental duties to the persons receiving care or to colleagues and other health care providers" (Canadian Nurses Association, 2008, p. 7). Ethical violations reflect a nurse's neglect of moral obligations and a breach of duty (e.g., when a nurse discusses patient information in the cafeteria). **Ethical dilemmas** or questions "arise when there are equally compelling reasons for and against two or more possible courses of action, and when choosing one course of action means that something else is relinquished or let go" (Canadian Nurses Association, 2008, p. 6). With ethical dilemmas, reasons exist for and against a particular course of action, but only one option can be selected (e.g., when deciding to continue treatment for a patient who is likely to die). Finally, **ethical (or moral) distress** "arises in situations where nurses know or believe they know the right thing to do, but for various reasons (including fear or circumstances beyond their control) do not or cannot take the right action or prevent a particular harm" (Canadian Nurses Association, 2008, p. 6). Ethical distress occurs when the nurse knows the right thing to do, but he or she cannot act on that insight. Ethical distress can often provoke feelings of guilt, concern, or distaste; for example, a family wants their mother resuscitated, but the mother signed a "do not resuscitate order." Ethical distress can result from unresolved or repeated ethical uncertainty or ethical violations. Repeated, unresolved ethical distress can result in work dissatisfaction and may cause nurses to leave the workplace (Chiarella & McInnes, 2008).

It is important for nurse managers to focus on the resources that are needed to resolve the ethical issues and concerns experienced by nursing staff. Managers must examine organizational barriers that may prevent resolving ethical problems. An excessive workload, unsafe levels of staffing, or a lack of clear policies can contribute to unresolved ethical dilemmas and ethical distress (Gaudine, LeFort, Lamb, et al., 2011). Managers must ensure that nurses are safe, competent, and ethical practitioners who provide compassionate care. This goal can be partly achieved through a written annual performance appraisal and regular coaching when necessary. Nurse managers should also develop a system for rewarding "good behaviour" with praise; for example, praise can be documented in a performance appraisal, given verbally, or written in a letter for the nurse's file.

Nurse managers must help ensure that nurses have an understanding of the ethical principles that guide practice and decision making. Nurse managers must support the continued professional development of nursing staff in understanding how ethics applies to practice. Organizing educational workshops to discuss ethical principles for practice (e.g., the CNA code of ethics) or educating staff on the role of the hospital ethics committee are examples of activities that can help promote the discussion and resolution of ethical dilemmas and ethical distress in practice. Finally, nurse managers must be ethical role models for staff and support staff in making ethical decisions every day in their practice. Occasionally, when ethical concerns cannot be resolved at the nurse manager level, they must be referred to and discussed with the hospital or clinical ethics committee.

ETHICS COMMITTEES

Most health care organizations in Canada have ethics committees or consultants with expertise in dealing with bioethical issues. The primary role of an ethics committee is to create a forum for the discussion of ethical issues or problems and to generate feasible solutions to those issues or problems (Cesta, 2011a, 2011b). Ethics committees are multidisciplinary by nature, and members can include a health care ethicist, legal experts, nurses, managers, physicians, clergy, social workers, pharmacists, and dieticians (Gaudine, Lamb, LeFort, et al., 2011). The committees provide structure and guidance for clinical ethical decision making and fulfill a patient advocacy role. Ethics committees are often involved in conflict resolution and, in some cases, the ethical review of research proposals

(Larkin & Schotsmans, 2008). Ethics committees are interactional and usually make decisions by consensus.

Nurse managers can promote the use of ethics committees by ensuring that staff understand the roles and functions of such committees. Nurse managers can do so by educating staff on the mandate of their organization's ethics committee and on the ethical consultation process. Most ethics committees require a written request for consultation. It is a nurse manager's responsibility to consult with the ethics committee to help make ethical decisions in the clinical setting and to also support the staff if they decide to consult the committee. Information about how to consult the ethics committee is critical information for staff, if the committee is to be used effectively.

EXERCISE 6-3

Consulting with an ethics committee usually requires a written submission of the ethical issues to be considered by the committee. Think about an ethical issue that would require consultation with the hospital ethics committee, for example, a do not resuscitate or refusal of treatment. Complete the "Request for Ethics Committee Consultation" form found on the accompanying Evolve site under Additional Resources for this text, and recommend the best course of action to address the issue. Discuss the ethical issue and the proposed solution with a fellow student. Did he or she agree with your recommended action?

Request for Ethics Committee Consultation

Contact Name: _____
Date: _____
Unit: _____
Description of Concerns:
   Patient
   Family
   Health Care Team
Summary of Ethical Issue:
Recommended Action:
   Patient
   Family
   Health Care Team

A MODEL FOR ETHICAL DECISION MAKING FOR NURSE MANAGERS AND LEADERS

Nursing codes of ethics emphasize that it is important for nurses to engage in ethical reflection and discussion. Time for ethical reflection is necessary when there is a need to clarify or determine how a particular ethical value impacts the professional accountabilities of the nurse and nurse manager. A variety of ethical decision making models can help nurses reflect on and apply ethical values to decision making. In general, ethical decision making models follow similar steps (Box 6-6). Effective nurse managers are prepared to facilitate these steps and promote ethical reflection.

One of the first steps in making ethical decisions is to *clarify the need* for the decision and its urgency; for example, the need to decide whether to remove a patient from a ventilator is different from the need to implement the do-not-resuscitate order of an acutely ill patient. Timelines for making the decision at hand must be established and agreed upon by all involved, including the patient, family, and the health care team. When clarifying the need for the decision, it is also important to collect all of the available information that will be used to make the decision (e.g., diagnostic tests). Once a need to make a decision has been established, it is important to *identify all of those involved* and directly affected by the decision and *arrange a meeting* with them to discuss the issue.

Discussing ethical issues such as removing a patient from a ventilator can be a very difficult process for everyone involved. The health care team usually includes the patient and family, nurses, physicians, clergy, social workers, and other health care providers, but when an ethical issue arises, the team may be expanded to include a patient representative and a health care ethicist. Once the meeting has been arranged, it is appropriate for the group to *select a*

BOX 6-6   STEPS IN ETHICAL DECISION MAKING

1. Clarify the need.
2. Identify all involved.
3. Arrange a meeting.
4. Select a facilitator or chair.
5. Identify areas of agreement.
6. Identify areas of disagreement.
7. Offer resources.
8. Seek outside advice if necessary.
9. Make a decision.
10. Implement the decision.

facilitator or chair who is not directly involved in the decision and can be impartial (e.g., a nurse manager from another unit). The key to a productive meeting is to ensure that an open discussion and a safe environment exists in which all can comfortably express personal views.

The facilitator should establish key areas for discussion, including *areas of agreement* and *areas of disagreement* between members of the group. The roles and responsibilities of each member of the group should be established and clarified (e.g., patient representative, staff nurse, the unit's nurse manager). All members must be given the opportunity to express their views and be heard. If a decision cannot be made together with the patient, family, and health care team, *outside advice may be necessary* (such as from the clinical ethics committee). Ideally, everyone should agree and understand the implications of the decision that is being made. Consensus may be difficult to achieve, so the group must decide on who will *make the final decision* (e.g., the patient) and how to *implement the decision*. The ethical decision making process can help the group reflect on the ethical values that may have an impact on the decision.

EXERCISE 6-4

You are the nurse manager of a busy intensive care unit (ICU), and the team has approached you to help them make a decision about the care of a comatose patient. Three successive electroencephalograms (EEGs) have revealed that the patient is "brain dead," and his wife has given permission to remove all life support. The patient's daughter, however, refuses to agree with the decision, and she is preventing the team from carrying out the wife's wishes. This morning, the wife has informed the team that she no longer wants to remove life support. Using the process outlined, explain the steps you would take to help the health care team and the family make an ethical decision.

CONCLUSION

Ethical principles, moral thought, the law, and professional accountabilities guide both nurses' and nurse managers' decisions and actions. This chapter provides an introduction to the ethical theories and principles important to nurse managers and leaders making decisions in clinical settings. Guidelines for ethical conduct were presented and applied to the nurse manager's role, and a framework for ethical decision making was outlined to help managers and decision makers engage in ethical reflection when decisions involving ethical issues are required in practice.

A SOLUTION

Mirella held a team meeting with the nurses involved in Adam's care. Together, they explored not only the ethical principle of autonomy in relation to Adam's parents' ethical and legal right to make decisions about their child's care but also the ethical, legal, and professional obligations of the nurses to ensure that the parents were informed of the risks and benefits of those decisions. Using the principles of relational ethics helped the nurses recognize that although Adam was in a vulnerable situation, they had fulfilled their obligations by ensuring the parents understood the risks associated with the situation. Mirella discussed the importance of maintaining the therapeutic relationship the nurses had already established with Adam and his family, so that they could continue to provide safe, compassionate care for Adam. Mirella also stressed the importance of listening to Adam and his parents, and of continuing to seek their input in future decisions about his care. Finally, Mirella discussed the process for consulting other members of the health care team and the hospital ethics committee if the nurses continued to feel ethical distress about this situation.

Would this be a suitable approach for you? Why or why not?

THE EVIDENCE

Nurse managers are often involved with ethical decision making in clinical practice and are confronted with the need to choose the ethically right solution for patients, staff, and the nursing profession. Toren and Wagner (2010) suggested that by using an ethical decision making model, nurse managers can maintain patients' and nurses' rights and still fulfill their obligation to the organization and the nursing profession. They propose an ethical decision making model that has several steps, including defining the ethical issue or problem, clarifying the personal and professional ethical principles involved, initiating a discussion with all parties, and identifying and choosing an action. They recommend open discussions with everyone involved and basing decisions on the ICN code of ethics. The nurse manager's responsibility is to care for both patients and staff in a fair manner, but they are also responsible for caring about the nursing profession, whose goal is to give the best care possible. An ethical decision making model can help nurse managers fulfill their obligations and effectively resolve ethical dilemmas in clinical practice settings.

NEED TO KNOW NOW

- Know the principles of bioethics that guide nursing practice and administration.
- Understand how the principles of relational ethics can be applied to nursing practice, leadership, and management.
- Use the CNA and ICN codes of ethics to guide your ethical conduct, and understand how those principles can be applied to the work of a staff nurse, nurse manager, or nurse leader.

- Understand that laws and professional accountabilities may impact your ethical nursing practice, leadership, and management.
- Develop a general process for making ethical decisions in your institution.
- Know your institution's policies and procedures regarding ethical decision making in practice.
- Know how to consult with your organization's ethics committee.

CHAPTER CHECKLIST

This chapter focused on ethical issues as they relate to the role of nurse managers and leaders. In particular, relational ethics was discussed with a focus on its core elements: engaged interactions, mutual respect, embodied knowledge, uncertainty and vulnerability, and interdependent environment. Nurses must consider the relationships they have with those who will be influenced by their thoughts and actions. The major principles of bioethics were also presented: autonomy, justice, beneficence, and nonmaleficence. An understanding of these ethical principles can help nurse managers and leaders develop the strategies they need to engage in ethical decision making and practice. Nurse managers experience a variety of ethical issues on a daily basis. Therefore, it is important for managers and leaders to be aware of the strategies to deal with these issues, including the role of hospital ethics committees and how to establish a clear process for ethical decision making.

The following key concepts apply to ethical decision making in everyday clinical practice:

- Nurse managers' decisions and actions are guided by ethical principles, professional accountabilities, and the law.
- Ethics involves moral practices, beliefs, and standards of individuals or groups.
- Principles of relational ethics include engaged interactions, mutual respect, embodied knowledge, uncertainty and vulnerability, and interdependent environment.
- The major principles of bioethics are autonomy, justice, beneficence, and nonmaleficence.
- Ethical problems can be defined as ethical violations, ethical dilemmas, or ethical distress.
- Ethics committees can provide a framework to prevent and resolve ethical conflicts in practice.
- The steps in ethical decision making are clarify the need, identify all involved, arrange a meeting, select a facilitator or chair, identify areas of agreement, identify areas of disagreement, offer resources, seek outside advice if necessary, make a decision, and implement the decision.

TIPS FOR DECISION MAKING AND PROBLEM SOLVING

- Reflect on the ethical principles to guide your practice and decisions.
- Seek guidance from CNA and ICN codes of ethics.
- Talk with colleagues and the health care team about ethical issues or concerns.

- Research journal articles and the relevant sections of textbooks to increase your knowledge base of ethical issues in practice.
- Consult with the hospital ethics committee when necessary.

Evolve WEBSITE

Visit the Evolve website for Suggested Readings, Internet Resources, and additional resources related to the content in this chapter: http://evolve.elsevier.com/Canada/Yoder-Wise/leading/.

REFERENCES

Statutes

Personal Health Information Protection Act, 2004. SO 2004, c. 3, Sch. A. Retrieved from http://www.e-laws.gov.on.ca/html/statutes/english/elaws_statutes_04p03_e.htm#BK65.

Texts

Austin, W., Goble, E., & Kelecevic, J. (2009). The ethics of forensic psychiatry: Moving beyond principles to a relational ethics approach. *Journal of Forensic Psychiatry & Psychology, 20*(6), 835–850. doi:10.1080/14789940903174147

Beckett, A., Gilbertson, S., & Greenwood, S. (2007). Doing the right thing: Nursing students, relational practice, and moral agency. *Journal of Nursing Education, 46*(1), 28–32.

Bjarnason, D. (2011). Moral leadership in nursing. *Journal of Radiology Nursing, 30*(1), 18–24. doi:10.1016/j.jradnu.2011.01.002

Canadian Nurses Association. (2006). Social justice: A means to an end, an end in itself. *Canadian Nurse, 102*(6), 18–20.

Canadian Nurses Association. (2008). *Code of ethics for registered nurses (2008 centennial edition).* Toronto, ON: Author. http://www.cna-aiic.ca/cna/documents/pdf/publications/Code_of_Ethics_2008_e.pdf.

Cesta, T. (2011a). Every day, the case management department faces multiple dilemmas over ethics. *Hospital Case Management, 19*(8), 118–119.

Cesta, T. (2011b). Solution: Committees on organizational ethics. *Hospital Case Management, 19*(8), 119–121.

Chiarella, M., & McInnes, E. (2008). Legality, morality and reality: The role of the nurse in maintaining standards of care. *Australian Journal of Advanced Nursing, 26*(1), 77–83.

College of Licensed Practical Nurses of BC. (2004). *CLPNBC code of ethics for LPNs: Companion guide.* Burnaby, BC: Author.

College of Licensed Practical Nurses of Newfoundland and Labrador. (2011). *Standards of practice and code of ethics for Licensed Practical Nurses of Newfoundland & Labrador.* St. John's, NL: Author.

Cornock, M. (2011). Confidentiality: The legal issues. *Nursing Children & Young People, 23*(7), 18–19. doi:10.7748/ncyp2011.09.23.7.18.c8682

Encyclopedia Britannica. (n.d.). Normative ethics. Retrieved from http://www.britannica.com/EBchecked/topic/418412/normative-ethics.

Falk-Rafael, A., & Betker, C. (2012). Relational ethics in public health nursing practice. *International Journal for Human Caring, 16*(3), 63.

Gaudine, A., Lamb, M., LeFort, S., et al. (2011). Barriers and facilitators to consulting hospital clinical ethics committees. *Nursing Ethics, 18*(6), 767–780. doi:10.1177/0969733011403808

Gaudine, A., LeFort, S., Lamb, M., et al. (2011). Ethical conflicts with hospitals: The perspective of nurses and physicians. *Nursing Ethics, 18*(6), 756–766. doi:10.1177/0969733011401121

International Council of Nurses. (2012). The ICN code of ethics for nurses. Geneva, Switzerland: Author.

Kenny, N., Sherwin, S., & Baylis, F. (2010). Re-visioning public health ethics: A relational perspective. *Canadian Journal of Public Health, 101*(1), 9–11.

Kunyk, D., & Austin, W. (2012). Nursing under the influence: A relational ethics perspective. *Nursing Ethics, 19*(3), 380–389. doi:10.1177/0969733011406767

Larkin, P., & Schotsmans, P. (2008). A relational ethical dialogue with research ethics committees. *Nursing Ethics, 15*(2), 234–242. doi:10.1177/0969733007086021

Leung, D., & Esplen, M. (2010). Alleviating existential distress of cancer patients: Can relational ethics guide clinicians? *European Journal of Cancer Care, 19*(1), 30–38. doi:10.1111/j.1365-2354.2008.00969.x

Merriam-Webster. (n.d.) Ethic. Retrieved from http://www.merriam-webster.com/dictionary/ethic/.

Myllykoski, H. (2011). Social justice: Who cares? *Alberta RN, 67*(4), 28–29.

Olmstead, D., Scott, S., & Austin, W. (2010). Unresolved pain in children: A relational ethics perspective. *Nursing Ethics, 17*(6), 695–704. doi:10.1177/0969733010378932

Pavlish, C., Brown-Saltzman, K., Hersh, M., et al. (2011). Nursing priorities, actions, and regrets for ethical situations in clinical practice. *Journal of Nursing Scholarship, 43*(4), 385–395. doi:10.1111/j.1547-5069.2011.01422.x

Peter, E. (2011). Fostering social justice: The possibilities of a socially connected model of moral agency. *Canadian Journal of Nursing Research, 43*(2), 11–17.

Quebec National Assembly. (2013). Bill 52: An act respecting end-of-life care. Retrieved from http://www.assnat.qc.ca/en/travaux-parlementaires/projets-loi/projet-loi-52-40-1.html.

Raya, A. (1990). Can knowledge be promoted and values ignored? Implications for nursing education. *Journal of Advanced Nursing, 15*(5), 504–509. doi:10.1111/j.1365-2648.1990.tb01848.x

Risjord, M. (2014). Nursing and human freedom. *Nursing Philosophy, 15*(1), 35–45. doi:10.1111/nup.12026

Shaw, E. (2011). Relational ethics and moral imagination in contemporary systemic practice. *Australian & New Zealand Journal of Family Therapy, 32*(1), 1–14. doi:10.1375/anft.32.1.1

Stanford Encyclopedia of Philosophy. (2007). Metaethics. Retrieved from http://plato.stanford.edu/entries/metaethics/.

Stanford Encyclopedia of Philosophy. (2011). The definition of morality. Retrieved from http://plato.stanford.edu/entries/morality-definition/.

Toren, O., & Wagner, N. (2010). Applying an ethical decision-making tool to a nurse management dilemma. *Nursing Ethics, 17*(3), 393–402. doi:10.1177/0969733009355106

Woods, M. (2012). Exploring the relevance of social justice within a relational nursing ethic. *Nursing Philosophy, 13*(1), 56–65. doi:10.1111/j.1466-769X.2011.00525.x

Wright, D., & Brajtman, S. (2011). Relational and embodied knowing: Nursing ethics within the interprofessional team. *Nursing Ethics, 18*(1), 20–30. doi:10.1177/0969733010386165

Zuzelo, P. R. (2007). Exploring the moral distress of registered nurses. *Nursing Ethics, 14*(3), 344–359. doi:10.1177/0969733007075870

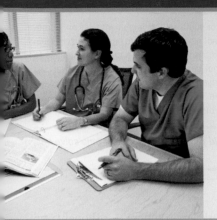

Making Decisions and Solving Problems

Ena L. Howse

This chapter presents an overview of problem solving and decision making. It examines the intellectual processes involved in problem solving and decision making, including rational thinking, critical thinking, creative thinking, and intuition, as well as individual and group decision biases. It also explores problem-solving and decision-making approaches, group decision-making strategies, and a variety of decision-making support tools.

OBJECTIVES

- Distinguish between the terms *problem* and *decision*, and understand the relationship between problem solving and decision making.
- Identify the intellectual processes involved in problem solving and decision making within the health care context.
- Describe how the scientific method, critical thinking, nursing process, creative thinking, and intuitive thinking relate to decision making.
- Explain the effect of decision biases, fallacies, and personal attributes on the quality of decisions.
- Understand how problem-solving skills apply to nursing practice.
- Compare three models of decision making: the rational decision-making model, the bounded rationality model, and the Clinical Judgement Model.
- Describe the group decision-making process and understand its importance for interdisciplinary health care teams.

TERMS TO KNOW

availability bias	group invulnerability	optimizing decision
confirmation bias	group polarization	problem solving
creative decision making	groupthink	prudence trap
critical thinking	heuristics	satisficing decision
decision bias	hindsight bias	six thinking hats
decision making	intuition	SWOT analysis
fallacies	nominal group technique	team dynamics

? A CHALLENGE

Shyanne, a recently hired nurse at a youth walk-in clinic, was thrilled about being hired for her first full-time job. As team leader of the Youth Engagement program, she would be working with a staff of three experienced mental health workers to develop and deliver workshops on health and wellness, social interaction, and leadership skills. Shyanne had worked at the clinic during the summer for the past two years and was comfortable with her co-workers and supervisor. She was eager to start planning workshops that would help her young patients develop the tools they need to solve their problems, become more confident, and learn basic life skills. Her co-workers were supportive and very interested in

Shyanne's new ideas for youth skill development. Her only problem was that she was not getting through to her supervisor, Rhea. Although Rhea was responsive to Shyanne's ideas and seemed to accept them, she did not share her enthusiasm about advancing the plan. Rhea's response to Shyanne's request to move forward was "let's wait and see." Shyanne was discouraged at first, but the more Rhea stalled, the more frustrated Shyanne became.

What advice would you give to Shyanne to help solve her problem?

INTRODUCTION

Problem solving and decision making are essential skills for nurse managers, nurse leaders, and staff nurses. According to Mintzberg (1973), managers have three key roles: interpersonal contact, information processing, and decision making. Problem-solving skills are universal and can be applied in any situation. Numerous technological, social, political, and economic changes have dramatically increased the need for problem solving in health care and nursing. Increased patient acuity, shorter hospital stays, a shortage of health care providers, an increase in technology use, greater emphasis on quality and patient safety, the diversity of patient populations, and the continuing shift from inpatient to community care are a few of the changes that require nurses to be able to problem solve effectively and make sound decisions. More emphasis is now placed on involving patients and work teams in decision making and problem solving. The complexities and problems that result from rapid changes strain the abilities of nurses to process large quantities of information, understand the interrelationships among elements in the organization, and keep pace with new developments. Keeping pace requires a good knowledge of traditional and contemporary approaches to problem solving and decision making.

PROBLEM SOLVING AND DECISION MAKING

The Difference Between a Problem and a Decision

Effective problem-solving and decision-making skills are essential for dealing with ambiguity and

uncertainty in work environments. Although problem-solving and decision-making skills are accepted core functions of nursing, many nurses are often too busy to apply these skills in a purposeful way. However, by using problem-solving and decision-making skills on a regular basis, nurses will be able to perceive difficult clinical issues as intellectual challenges that develop their critical-thinking skills and good judgement. Sound knowledge of the core concepts and skills related to problem solving and decision making begins with a good understanding of associated terminology, processes, and models.

A *problem* is a recognized difference between current and desired conditions or a gap between "what is" and "what should be" with an accompanying perception that something should be done to resolve it. Some problems demand immediate attention, while others can be resolved over time. A *decision* is a choice between alternative courses of action or interventions that are selected for implementation.

The Relationship Between Problem Solving and Decision Making

Although often thought of as the same process, decision theorists distinguish between problem solving and decision making. **Problem solving** is a comprehensive, sequential, cognitive process used to solve a problem by reducing the difference between current and desired conditions. A review of the literature on problem solving and decision making shows a difference of opinion about these concepts, which may partly explain the variety of models that exist. Some see the problem-solving process as an integrated process, with decision making dispersed throughout (Huitt, 1992). Others argue that the two concepts are interchangeable. Certain scholars question the value of defining a structured problem-solving or decision-making process because structured and purposeful processes do not appear to reflect what people actually do when they solve problems or make decisions (Tanner, 2006). Others see problem solving as a comprehensive, overarching process with decision making as "a process within a process," taking place at a distinct point or step in the problem-solving process and as a recurring activity (Kepner & Tregoe, 1965). This perspective is presented in this chapter. Figure 7-1 helps illustrate where decision making occurs within the problem-solving process. Regardless of the theoretical perspective, the two elements essential to solving any problem are problem analysis and decision making. Problem analysis includes identifying, clarifying, and verifying a problem, while decision making focuses on developing cognitive strategies to solve a problem.

Decision making is "a process that chooses a preferred option or a course of actions from among a set of alternatives on the basis of given criteria or strategies" (Wang & Ruhe, 2007, p. 73). Decision making in risky situations involves estimating the probability of success of alternatives, given the complexity, level of risk, and the certainty of outcome of each alternative (Riabacke, 2006). Decision making is most often associated with the rational decision-making model (Lunenburg, 2010), which will be discussed later in the chapter. Decision-making skills are also applicable to nursing practice. For example, the College

of Nurses of Ontario (2011) has developed a "three-factor framework" to help nurses make effective decisions regarding which category of nurse (registered nurse or registered practical nurse) matches patient needs.

INTELLECTUAL PROCESSING IN PROBLEM SOLVING AND DECISION MAKING

Intellectual processes are mental operations that enable one to acquire new knowledge, apply that knowledge in both familiar and unique situations, and control the mental processing that is required for knowledge acquisition and use. These processes are reflected in the problem-solving and decision-making models that are presented below. Mental operations, such as conceptualizing and synthesizing, can be applied in a sequential critical-thinking process to generate new knowledge or solve problems.

Scientific Method

The scientific method is a rational and logical approach to problem solving that is widely used and has proven to be effective over time. It is the foundation for many models of decision making. It is a familiar process that reflects the cognitive behaviours that occur in a predictable order when conducting experiments or solving problems. The six steps in the scientific method are (1) identify and clarify a problem, (2) determine the problem's significance and relevance, (3) gather data about the problem and its causes, (4) generate hypotheses and choose alternatives to solve the problem, (5) test selected alternatives, and (6) plan, implement, and evaluate the effects of the selected alternatives.

Critical Thinking

Effective problem solving and decision making are based on an individual's ability to think critically. Although *critical thinking* has been defined in numerous ways, Scriven and Paul (2007) describe critical thinking as "the intellectually disciplined process of actively and skillfully conceptualizing, applying, analyzing, synthesizing, and/or evaluating information gathered from, or generated by, observation, experience, reflection, reasoning, or communication, as a guide to belief and action" (para. 1). Glaser (1941) asserted that critical thinking is based on critical

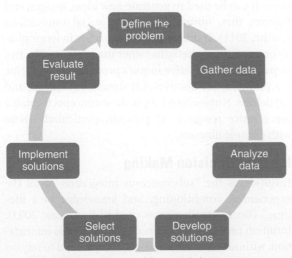

FIGURE 7-1 The problem-solving process.

inquiry (logic and argumentation). Based on this view, critical thinking is associated with a thoughtful and orderly approach to considering problems, knowledge of methods of logical inquiry and reasoning skills, and the ability to apply them. In practice, critical thinking involves recognizing problems and finding ways to solve them by gathering pertinent information, appraising evidence, and evaluating arguments. It requires an examination and testing of beliefs, assumptions, and relationships among propositions in light of evidence to reach valid conclusions. Glaser's view of critical thinking is particularly valuable for ethical decisions and other complex problems.

Problem-Solving Process

The problem-solving process is based on the scientific method. Various models are described in the literature, but most include essential cognitive components. The traditional seven-step problem-solving process is cyclic: steps in the process are repeated to solve a problem (Figure 7-1). Feedback from failed attempts to solve a problem is used to reactivate the problem-solving process, using different alternatives.

Decision-Making Process

The decision-making process is an integral component of the problem-solving process and is mainly associated with making choices among alternatives for action. Two commonly used models of decision making are the rational decision-making model and the bounded rationality model. These models will be compared later in this chapter. The rational decision-making model consists of five steps that are similar to the problem-solving process: (1) define a problem or opportunity, (2) set goals (outcomes) and identify evaluation criteria, (3) identify alternatives for each outcome, (4) evaluate alternatives for each outcome, and (5) choose the preferred alternative.

Nursing Process

The five-step, systematic nursing process is also based on the scientific method and is tailored to the field of nursing. The steps in the process are (1) assessment, (2) diagnosis, (3) planning, (4) implementation, and (5) evaluation. The steps are sequential, interactive, and cyclic. The nursing process is goal directed and guides nurses in problem solving for health conditions.

Decision making is particularly evident in the diagnosis and planning steps.

Ethical Decision Making

The steps in ethical decision making are similar to those in the rational decision-making model. However, ethical principles and arguments are applied in the intellectual-reasoning process to determine alternatives or options for action. These principles are highly relevant for health care problems. Ethical issues are fully discussed in Chapter 6.

Creative Decision Making

Creative decision making, which is associated with lateral or divergent thinking, is described as the generation of new and imaginative ideas that are critical for problem solving (Fulcher, 2009). Divergent thinking is needed in problem solving to overcome the tendency to see problems in a conventional way; it involves inducing decision makers to see the problem in a variety of new contexts. Creative decision making is a combination of divergent thinking and rational decision making. The decision-making process involves the use of brainstorming and other techniques, such as "mind tools," to generate different and novel ideas.

Appreciative inquiry is a creative approach to problem solving. It "seeks out the best of 'what is' to help ignite the collective imagination of 'what might be.' The aim is to generate new knowledge that expands the 'realm of the possible' and helps people envision a collectively desired future" (Kaminski, 2012). Like other logical models, appreciative inquiry follows sequential steps. It can be used to generate new ideas, images, and theories that, ultimately, lead to social innovations (Bushe, 2011). It differs from approaches in its emphasis on examining strengths rather than deficits. The five steps in the appreciative inquiry process are: (1) define the problem, (2) discover, (3) dream, (4) design, and (5) deliver. Nurses could apply these concepts to enable the creative resources of patients, particularly those with chronic illnesses.

Intuitive Decision Making

Intuition is the "subconscious integration of all the experiences, conditioning, and knowledge of a lifetime" (Bruce Henderson as cited in Bonabeau, 2003). Intuition provides instantaneous access to this information, without conscious thought. People tend to rely on intuition primarily when in stressful situations where information is limited and the problems are unclear. In such instances, people respond to cues in the situation and draw from stored information (tacit knowledge that is hard to describe) in the subconscious to make rapid decisions instead of taking an incremental, analytical approach such as that found in the rational decision-making model. Rational thinking and intuitive thinking are complementary, and successful decision making is a balance between the two approaches. The role of intuition in nursing has been supported by Benner and Tanner (1987). It is most commonly used in the decision making of expert practitioners. In nursing, "gut feeling" responses are associated with intuition, and themes that emerge from intuition are referred to as "knowing or understanding" (Smith, 2007, p. 16). Intuition can be enhanced through decision-making strategies such as brainstorming and group discussions (Smith, 2007). Nurses must always be vigilant that their intuition does not lead to the identification or imposition of suboptimal decisions.

Putting It All Together

Figure 7-2 illustrates the relationships among the foregoing intellectual processes. The scientific method is at the core of rational, systematic models of critical thinking, problem solving, and the nursing process. Creative decision making and intuitive decision-making processes are not regarded as rational-thinking approaches. Although both include sequential steps,

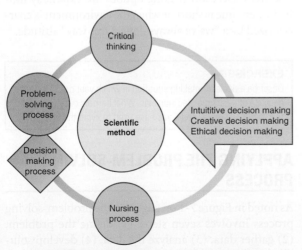

FIGURE 7-2 Intellectual processing models.

the intellectual processes differ. Creativity and intuition feed rational-thinking processes and, therefore, can be seen as complementary thinking processes. Similarly, ethical decision making is a systematic, values-oriented approach to reasoning that complements the scientific method.

FACTORS THAT AFFECT THE QUALITY OF DECISIONS

Individual Decision Biases

Many factors, such as past experiences, personal attributes, and cognitive biases, interfere with the quality of a decision (Henriksen & Dayton, 2006). Often, people tend to make decisions based on **heuristics**, which are educated guesses or "rules of thumb." Heuristics are based on experience and general knowledge about how things work, as opposed to specific information about the situation at hand. Mostly they are helpful, especially when time is not available to collect and assess relevant information. However, they can lead to **decision bias**, or error in judgement, when relevant information is omitted. A number of individual decision biases have implications for nurses and other health care providers. **Confirmation bias** is the tendency for people to seek information that reaffirms past experience and to discount information that contradicts past judgements. This bias might lead to an incorrect hiring decision if only past negative experiences are used to judge a job candidate. **Availability bias** is the tendency for people to base their judgement on a preceding and memorable event that is readily recalled rather than complete information on the present situation. **Hindsight bias** is the tendency for people to overestimate their ability to predict an event after the fact, which the phrase "I knew it all along" suggests. Hindsight bias interferes with people's ability to learn from the past because it leads them to be overconfident in their predictive skills, which can interfere with their ability to make good judgements. **Prudence trap** is the tendency for people to be too cautious and avoid risks that may be justified. Nurse managers and leaders need to be alert to individual decision biases and address how to avoid them in staff meetings and with individual nurses.

Group Decision Biases

Decision biases can also affect the group decision-making process and its outcomes. **Groupthink**, the most common group decision bias, is a phenomenon in which group members are so concerned with avoiding conflict and supporting their leader and other members that important facts, concerns, and differing views are not raised that might indicate an alternative decision. Recall how being a good follower may require you to raise important overlooked facts and concerns. Failure to bring up options, explore conflict, or challenge the status quo results in ineffective group functioning and decision outcomes. Group polarization is the tendency for groups to make decisions that are more extreme (risky or conservative) than the privately held beliefs of individual group members. When groups polarize toward one extreme or the other, their decisions could lead to negative outcomes, such as financial loss or failed projects. The reasons for such radical shifts in decisions vary. One explanation is that groups are more confident than individuals because of strength in numbers and a sense that responsibility for the decision is shared. Group invulnerability is the perception of group members that the group cannot be wrong, which can lead the group to make overly optimistic or overly risky decisions. Nurse managers and leaders need to monitor group processes for group decision biases to maintain the quality of group decisions.

Fallacies

Fallacies are beliefs that appear to be correct but are found to be false when examined by logical reasoning rules. Logical reasoning uses syllogisms to make valid arguments. A *syllogism* is "a formal argument consisting of a major and a minor premise and a conclusion" ("Syllogism," n.d.). The major premise states a general rule, followed by a minor premise, which includes statements of fact about a person, thing, or group. The conclusion connects the premises, sequentially, into a general principle. The premises, when true, support the conclusion. For example, "All humans have brains; Dan is human and, therefore, Dan has a brain" is a syllogism, and the conclusion is true. "All humans have brains; Bugsy has a brain and, therefore, Bugsy is human" has some logical pattern, but it contains a fallacy because Bugsy is a dog.

Fallacious arguments can result in wrong decisions and actions. Numerous types of fallacies exist, but a complete discussion of these fallacies is beyond the scope of this chapter. However, examples help demonstrate the importance of recognizing fallacies. The *gambler's fallacy* is a common fallacy related to probabilities.

With a fair coin, the probability of getting heads or tails on a single toss is ½ (one in two). If we have tossed 20 heads in a row, we might believe that the chance of the next coin toss being tails has increased. However, each coin toss has the same probability, regardless of the previous toss, so an equal chance (i.e., 50-50) remains that the next toss will be tails. Another common fallacy is the *hasty generalization*, which is a broad claim based on assumptions and insufficient facts. A *post hoc error* occurs when it is quickly and incorrectly assumed that an event was caused by the one that preceded it. Time constraints, interruptions, heavy workloads, and other factors interfere with logical reasoning and effective decision making. Awareness of fallacies is the first step in learning how to avoid them.

Personal Attributes

Certain personality factors, such as self-esteem and self-confidence, affect whether one is willing to take risks in solving problems or making decisions. Keynes (2008) stated that individuals may be influenced by social pressures. For example, one may be inclined to make decisions to satisfy people to whom they are accountable and from whom they feel social pressure.

Personal internal and external factors can influence how a decision-making situation is perceived. Internal factors include variables such as the decision maker's physical and emotional state, personal philosophy, biases, values, interests, experience, knowledge, attitudes, and risk-seeking or risk-avoiding behaviours. External factors include environmental conditions, time, and resources. Decision-making options are externally limited when time is short or when the environment is characterized by a "we've always done it this way" attitude.

> **EXERCISE 7-1**
> Describe a decision-making situation in which your decision failed because of a personal decision bias. What barriers did you encounter? What strategies could you have used to avoid the error?

APPLYING THE PROBLEM-SOLVING PROCESS

As noted in Figure 7-1 on page 107, the problem-solving process involves seven steps: (1) define the problem, (2) gather data, (3) analyze the data, (4) develop solutions, (5) select solutions, (6) implement the solutions, and (7) evaluate the result. People adopt different approaches to problem solving and decision making, ranging from intuition to in-depth logical processing. The approach used often depends on the circumstances and the individual's level of problem-solving expertise. The nursing process is the most commonly used formal problem-solving process in nursing. In the problem-solving example that follows, a generic seven-step model of problem solving, which incorporates the nursing process, illustrates how the steps in the process apply to nursing practice. The problem-solving steps that rely heavily on decision-making processes are indicated.

Problem Solving in Nursing Practice

Step 1: Define the Problem. Problem analysis begins with an investigation of the presenting problem. Patients who enter the health care system often have a number of interrelated problems. On admission, a complete intake history and patient assessment is conducted to identify and clarify any problems. Identifying a problem entails collecting preliminary data from as many sources as possible to describe fully the patient's problem or problems. The most common cause for failure to resolve a problem is the improper identification of the problem; therefore, problem recognition and identification are considered the most vital steps. The quality of the patient outcome depends on accurate identification of the problem, which is likely to recur if the true underlying causes are not targeted.

Step 2: Gather Data. Once the preliminary investigation is completed and the problem is identified, nurses can focus on in-depth data collection to resolve the issue using relevant and evidence-based resources. The data gathered should consist of objective (facts) and subjective (feelings) information. Facts that are gathered should be valid, accurate, relevant to the issue, and timely. Data collection is influenced by many factors, including the amount and accuracy of available information, the values, attitudes, and experiences of those involved, and time. Sufficient time should be allowed for the collection and organization of data. Data collection tools, such as the five *W*'s—who, what, when, where, why—can be used to improve the quality of information. A list of questions could include the following:

- Who is affected by the problem? Who is responsible for addressing the problem?
- What is the nature of the problem?

- When did the problem start?
- Where did the problem originate?
- Why did the problem occur?

Step 3: Analyze the Data. Data should be carefully analyzed to explore the full extent of the problem, root causes, and contributing factors. Nurses can refer to clinical reasoning guides and a compendium of nursing diagnoses for this purpose. This analysis should lead to a nursing diagnosis and potential solutions to the problem.

Step 4: Develop Solutions (Decision Making). Patient outcomes are linked to nursing diagnoses. By linking outcomes to nursing diagnoses, nurses can discover which solution would be most appropriate for a patient. Not all possible solutions can be applied, but it is important to consider the advantages and disadvantages of each, based on a set of priorities. One source of outcomes is evidence-informed best practices that have been formulated for clinical use through decision analyses, such as systematic reviews (see Khan, 2010). Systematic reviews involve extensive research analyses of previous problems to identify, select, and validate best practices. Valid findings are incorporated into books, compendiums of best practice, and professional journals. Nurses use their professional judgement to determine the outcomes that might have the most value for the patient.

Step 5: Select Solutions (Decision Making). After possible patient outcomes have been generated, decisions are made about which alternatives are most appropriate. This involves a deliberate process of determining the alternatives to meet each outcome, establishing priorities among alternatives, and choosing the most appropriate patient outcome for implementation. An outcome for a patient in pain after surgery might be "to achieve a level of pain that the patient can reasonably tolerate." Alternatives for pain control might be assessed, using general knowledge or decision rules about how to assess pain and the appropriate interventions for each level of pain.

If the investigation indicates that no action should be taken because the problem is beyond the nurse leader's control or the problem is likely to resolve itself spontaneously, a *purposeful inaction* or a "do nothing" approach might be taken (Burrow, Kleindl, & Everard, 2007). For example, in certain instances, a nurse manager may decide to leave things as they are by being indifferent. This indifference could be focused on a particular issue or a chronic pattern of problems. If the response is to a chronic pattern, the nurse leader's behaviour might be construed as a lack of caring, which could have a negative effect on staff and patients. It is important for nurse leaders to communicate the underlying reasons for purposeful inaction.

Step 6: Implement the Solutions. Implementing a plan of action to solve a problem requires attention to details. If the plan introduces an innovation, the adjustment to it may create problems. If the intervention does not address root causes, it may be ineffective. Any deviations in the patient's condition or unexpected responses should be monitored and decisions should be made to adapt the care plan. The implementation phase should include a contingency plan to deal with negative consequences if they arise.

Step 7: Evaluate the Result. An evaluation of patient outcomes reflects the quality of problem analysis, decision making, and interventions. Feedback that is obtained from the health care team and the patient is assessed and used to revise or continue with the plan. Considerable time and energy are usually spent on identifying the problem or issue, generating possible solutions, selecting the best solution, and implementing the solution. In the past, evaluation and follow-up were often neglected. Today, health care organizations have to meet stringent quality control standards. It is important to delegate responsibility for evaluation and monitoring of outcomes early in the problem-solving process. Typically, health care teams assume this responsibility and continuously monitor practices to identify areas for improvement. Deviations from quality control standards usually occur to maintain high quality of care. This topic is addressed in Chapter 21.

EXERCISE 7-2

Find a case description of a patient's condition in a journal. Use a five *W*'s approach (described in Step 1 of "Problem Solving in Nursing Practice") to generate questions for gathering data from the case. What information did you obtain in response to your questions? What gaps did you identify in the case description?

DECISION-MAKING MODELS

For health care providers, decision making in health care settings has become increasingly challenging. As a

result, the trend in health care has been to adopt well-established business models of decision making and decision support tools. A decision-making model is a guide to decision making for individuals or groups. The rational decision-making model, the bounded rationality model, and the Clinical Judgement Model are common approaches to decision making. These models will be explored in this section, together with decision support tools that complement them.

Rational Decision-Making Model

The rational decision-making model (sometimes called the *rational choice model*) originated in the field of economics and has been adopted by many other fields, including nursing and management. The model holds that patterns of human behaviour in society reflect choices that people make as they try to maximize their benefits and minimize their costs (Green, 2002). As a result, people will compare different options and courses of action. Rational decision making involves choosing a rational action, based on individuals' preferences. Three assumptions are made about individuals' preferences: (1) all actions can be ranked according to preference, (2) all actions can be compared with other actions, and (3) alternatives are independent. These assumptions explain the structure and content of the rational decision-making model. In applying this model, goals are set first, and then the criteria are stated and weighted according to importance. Finally, alternatives are generated and compared to determine which best satisfies the criteria (Box 7-1). Although this model appears to be reliable, it is not always easy to use to make good decisions (Korte, 2003; Lunenburg, 2010).

BOX 7-1   A SIX-STEP RATIONAL MODEL FOR DECISION MAKING

1. Define the problem and identify goals to solve them.
2. Identify decision criteria that must be met to achieve each goal.
3. Weight (rank) the criteria according to level of importance.
4. Generate alternatives or courses of action to solve the problem.
5. Rate each alternative in its ability to satisfy each criteria.
6. Evaluate each alternative against the weighted criteria to determine the alternative with the highest total score, which is the optimal choice.

Typically, most people use less stringent models to ill-defined problems and uncertain situations. Although these models appear to be prescriptive, they are usually not applied deliberately or in logical order. Experienced decision makers tend to be flexible in their approach to decision making moving back and forth through the steps or applying several steps simultaneously.

A Rational Decision-Making Tool. Decision tools help visualize options under consideration and allow the comparison of options using common criteria. Criteria, which are determined by the decision makers, may include time required, ethical or legal considerations, equipment needs, and cost. The relative advantages and disadvantages should be listed for each option. For example, the nurse manager of a hospital education department is assessing whether it is better to retain the services of an outside consultant to coordinate an advanced cardiac life support (ACLS) course in the hospital, pay the per-person fees to send the staff to another hospital for training, or train staff as ACLS instructors who can then provide training in-house. The type of information this nurse manager might compile includes a breakdown of the costs for the three options, equipment needs, the benefits of each option, the number of nurses who need the course, and future training needs.

The weighted decision matrix, illustrated in Figure 7-3, is commonly used to calculate preferred alternatives when using the rational decision-making model (Borysowich, 2006). The matrix uses the following steps:

1. Identify a desired outcome.
2. Enter criteria that can fulfill the desired outcome in the left column.

3. In column 2, rank each criterion (e.g., 0–5 scale, with 5 being most important) in order of importance.
4. Generate different options that might meet all of the criteria and enter them in the second row from the top.
5. In the rows, rank (e.g., 0–5 scale) each criterion on how well the alternative meets that criterion (e.g., satisfaction level).
6. Multiply the weight for each criterion by its rating for each alternative and enter the result in the score columns (weight × rating = score).
7. Total the scores for each alternative. The highest score indicates the preferred option.

EXERCISE 7-3

Use the weighted decision matrix to select a job offer from three options in three different cities. Discuss the value of this decision-making tool for job selection.

Bounded Rationality Model

The bounded rationality approach to decision making succeeded the rational decision-making model. The bounded rationality model was proposed by Nobel Prize–winner Herbert Simon, who observed that the rational (choice) decision-making model did not fit with observations of behavioural psychologists (Jones, 1999). He argued that people were constrained or "bounded" by personal and environmental factors that limited their abilities to make rational decisions. Limits on important factors such as knowledge, capacity to process information, expertise, resources, and unfavourable or uncertain environment conditions prevent people from making optimal decisions. In fact, in such cases, people are most likely to make a **satisficing decision**, which means that the option is acceptable but not necessarily the best option, when an **optimizing decision** is not feasible. An *optimizing decision* is the act of selecting the ideal solution or option to achieve goals. An example of a satisficing approach is the tendency of a decision maker to rely on heuristics (defined earlier) to select the solution that minimally meets the objective or standard for a decision. It allows for quick decisions and may be most appropriate when time is an issue. To illustrate, a nurse practitioner may rely on a reliable, short questionnaire to decide whether to place a patient with chest pain on an observation

Outcome:		ALTERNATIVES (Options)					
ACLS Instruction		Consultant		Send off site		Train trainer	
Criteria	Weight	Rating	Score	Rating	Score	Rating	Score
Time	4	2	8	5	20	3	12
Workload issues	3	3	9	3	9	1	3
Cost	2	3	6	3	6	2	4
Total			23		35		19
Preferred option					35*		

FIGURE 7-3 Weighted decision matrix on how to train nurses in ACLS. *ACLS,* advanced cardiac life support.

unit or on a low-intensity medical unit upon admission. The trend toward standardizing decision making by modelling and testing such heuristics can improve decision making in the health care environment. Some decisions are based on firmly established criteria in health care, such as traditions, values, doctrines, culture, and the policies of the organization. Every leader or manager has to comply with organizational mandates. Best practice guidelines are an example of standard guidelines for decision making. Nurses must have advanced decision-making skills, however, to make independent judgements on problems that are not readily solved through clinical guidelines.

Tools for Making Bounded Rationality Decisions. The tools commonly associated with practical (bounded rationality) decisions in health care are heuristics, medical algorithms, and portable digital instruments. The tools used to make bounded rationality decisions should match the situation. They should be easy to use, practical, and not require in-depth analyses because of time constraints. They should be able to capture essential data that will be sufficient, rather than optimum. The fishbone diagram used in quality improvement programs to identify problems quickly is a good example of a tool that is effective in unstructured work environments.

The fishbone diagram, also known as a *cause-and-effect diagram*, is a useful model for categorizing the possible causes of a problem (Six Sigma, 2011), and many versions are available on the Internet. This tool displays, in increasing detail, all of the possible causes related to a problem to try to discover its root causes. It encourages problem solvers to focus on the content of the problem and not be sidetracked by personal interests, issues, or the agendas of team members. It also collects a snapshot of the collective knowledge of the team and helps build consensus around the problem. The "effect" is generally the problem statement, such as decreased morale. The major categories of "causes" are the main bones, and these are usually supported by smaller bones, which represent issues that contribute to the main causes. In creating a fishbone diagram, the problem or issue is inserted at the "head" of the fish. Bones of the fish are labelled by category.

The major categories can be the four *M*s (methods, machines [equipment], manpower [people],

and materials), the four *P*s (place, procedure, people, and policies), or the four *S*s (surroundings, suppliers, systems, and skills). One particular set of categories may be more relevant to a particular problem. Applying the four *P*s category to nursing, *place* could be the location or facilities for holding wellness clinics, *procedures* could include communication problems or lack of protocols, *people* could include inadequate staffing or staff mix and knowledge or skills deficits, and *policies* could include rules or guidelines that relate to activities such as training programs and equipment.

An example of a fishbone diagram based on the four *M*s appears in Figure 7-4.

EXERCISE 7-4

Use a fishbone diagram and the four *P*s category to identify all the factors (causes) that might explain low attendance at smoking cessation classes that you are conducting for a group of public service utility workers on Fridays at 17:00. List as many issues or root causes as possible. Discuss your diagram with a classmate. Brainstorm together for additional causes to determine the most important causes of low attendance. Give some examples of actions that you could take for each cause to increase attendance at your classes.

Clinical Judgement Model

The Clinical Judgement Model described by Tanner (2006) in the Literature Perspective on page 116 emphasizes the role of intuition in decision making by nurses, particularly expert nurses (Tanner, 2006, p. 204). This model is systematic and similar in its sequence of steps to other models, although the thinking processes involved differ. Tanner identified four decision-making phases: (1) *noticing*: responding to cues based on knowledge and experience, (2) *interpreting*: reasoning and sense making, (3) *responding*: deciding on the best options, and (4) *reflecting*: examining one's own actions, patient responses, and subsequent learning. It is an intuitive, rather than a prescriptive model. Nurses use clinical reasoning to reach judgements about the most appropriate interventions. Clinical reasoning occurs in transitions and during reappraisal as situations unfold. Intuition is used when problems are complex, the decision maker has the expertise for solving similar complex problems, subtle changes are difficult to detect, information is unclear or confusing, factors in the external environment are challenging,

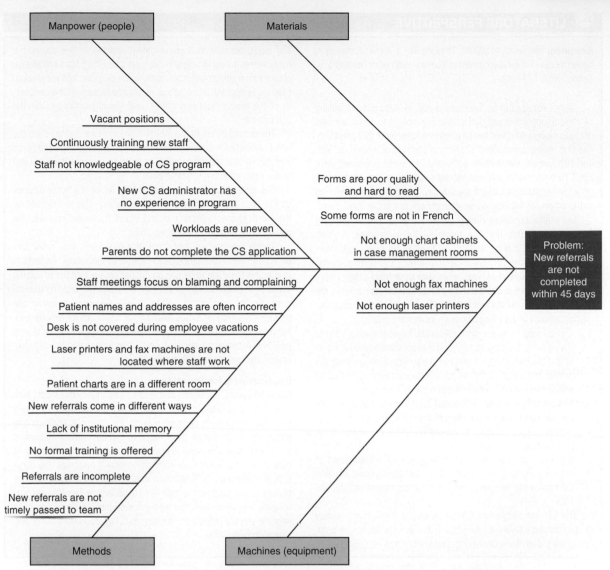

FIGURE 7-4 Fishbone diagram showing root causes of referral problems. *CS*, Children Services.

and changes in the patient's condition are occurring rapidly.

Clinical Judgement Support Tool for Students. Clinical journalling is prescribed for students who use the Clinical Judgement Model. This established teaching tool can be used to assess students' knowledge, skills, and affective development. By regularly recording their thoughts in a journal, students can capture data that can be interpreted for specified reasons, such as comprehension, skill development, and cognitive reflection on the meanings and implications

of experiences. Tanner's (2006) Clinical Judgement Model can be used to guide retrospective reflection on decision making.

GROUP DECISION MAKING

Like individual decision making, group decision making involves identifying a problem, determining alternative solutions, evaluating alternatives, and selecting a solution. For unpredictable problems, satisficing or intuition may apply. In groups, decision making is

LITERATURE PERSPECTIVE

Resource: Tanner, C. A. (2006). Thinking like a nurse: A research-based model of clinical judgment in nursing. *Journal of Nursing Education, 45*(6), 204–211.

Tanner engaged in an extensive review of 200 studies focusing on clinical judgement and clinical decision making to derive a model of clinical judgement that can be used as a framework for instruction. The first review summarized 120 articles and was published in 1998. The 2006 article reviewed an additional 71 studies published since 1998. Based on an analysis of the entire set of articles, Tanner proposed five conclusions, which are listed below. The reader is referred to the article for detailed explanation of each of the five conclusions.

The author considers clinical judgement as a "problem-solving activity." She notes that the terms *clinical judgement*, *problem solving*, *decision making*, and *critical thinking* are often used interchangeably. For the purpose of aiding in the development of the model, Tanner defined *clinical judgement* as actions taken based on the assessment of the patient's needs. Clinical reasoning is the process by which nurses make their judgements (e.g., the decision-making process of selecting the most appropriate option):

1. Clinical judgments are more influenced by what nurses bring to the situation than the objective data about the situation at hand.
2. Sound clinical judgment rests to some degree on knowing the patient and his or her typical pattern of responses, as well as an engagement with the patient and his or her concerns.
3. Clinical judgments are influenced by the context in which the situation occurs and the culture of the nursing care unit.
4. Nurses use a variety of reasoning patterns alone or in combination.
5. Reflection on practice is often triggered by a breakdown in clinical judgment and is critical for the development of clinical knowledge and improvement in clinical reasoning. (Tanner, 2006, p. 204)

The Clinical Judgement Model developed through the review of the literature involves four phases that are similar to the problem-solving and decision-making steps described in this chapter.

The model starts with a phase called *noticing*. In this phase, the nurse comes to expect certain responses resulting from knowledge gleaned from similar patient situations, experiences, and knowledge. External factors influence nurses in this phase such as the complexity of the environment and values, and typical practices within the unit culture.

The second phase of the model is *interpreting*, during which the nurse understands the situation that requires a response. The nurse employs various reasoning patterns to make sense of the issue and to derive an appropriate action plan.

The third phase is *responding*, during which the nurse decides on the best option for handling the situation. This is followed by the fourth phase, *reflecting*, during which the nurse assesses the patient's responses to the actions taken.

Tanner emphasized that "reflection-in-action" and "reflection-on-action" are major processes required in the model. Reflection-in-action is real-time reflection on the patient's responses to nursing action with modifications to the plan based on the ongoing assessment. On the other hand, reflection-on-action is a review of the experience, which promotes learning for future similar experiences. Nurse educators and leader or managers can employ this model with new and experienced nurses to aid in understanding thought processes involved in decision making.

Implications for Practice

Nurse educators, managers, and leaders can employ this model with new and experienced nurses to aid in understanding the thought processes involved in decision making. For example, students and practising nurses can be encouraged to maintain reflective journals to record observations and impressions from clinical experiences. In clinical post-conferences or staff development meetings, the nurse educator, manager, or leader can engage staff in applying the five phases Tanner proposed to their lived experiences. The ultimate goal of analyzing their decisions and decision-making processes is to improve clinical judgement, problem-solving, decision-making, and critical-thinking skills.

done through collaboration among group members who share common goals and are mutually supportive. Groups tend to make better decisions than individuals because of accumulated expertise and resources, and because members are likely to commit to alternatives that they develop. In deciding to use the group process for decision making, it is important to consider group composition. Homogeneous groups may be more compatible; however, highly cohesive groups may be ineffective in decision making if they succumb to group biases, such as group polarization or groupthink. Heterogeneous groups, such as interprofessional teams, may be more successful in problem solving because divergent thinking is useful in creating best decisions.

Work groups and work teams are interdependent collections of individuals who share common goals and specific outcomes for their organizations, with work teams typically having more formal status than work groups (Nielsen, 2012). In health care, loosely organized work groups and teams are transitioning from multidisciplinary to interdisciplinary teams (see Chapter 26). This change in how care is delivered requires leadership training to help members from different disciplines function as a unit. With a growing emphasis on quality care and workplace safety, it is expected that interdisciplinary teams will become more involved in clinical decision making. In health care, an interdisciplinary team is "a structured entity with a common goal and a common decision-making process . . . [and] is based on an integration of the knowledge and expertise of each professional, so that solutions to complex problems can be proposed . . . in an open-minded way" (D'Amour, Ferrada-Videla, San Martin Rodriguez, et al., 2005, p. 120). Generally, interdisciplinary teams have authority and accountability for planning, decision making, and implementing goals. Increasingly, management decisions are being assigned to these types of teams when problems are complex, information is needed from many sources, a quality decision is required, and commitment to the decision is necessary for implementation of the decision.

Leadership and Team Development for Decision Making

Teams share decision making in order to meet their goals and are successful when members have the necessary decision-making and group-interaction skills to perform as a team. Shared decision making involves important elements of leadership and followership. Understanding and appreciating professional roles and responsibilities, and communicating effectively are among the most valued group member competencies in shared decision making (Suter, Arndt, Arthur, et al., 2009).

Kozlowski and Ilgen (2006) identified key cognitive and behavioural processes that enable group members to achieve their goals. These are coordination, cooperation, and communication; group member competencies; regulations; and group performance dynamics. The group leader is the most important facilitator of these processes. The Research Perspective supports the importance of leadership in shared decision making. Morgeson, DeRue, and Karam (2010) identified the specific leadership support needs of team members from a meta-analysis of studies on team leadership. They developed a taxonomy of these needs, which includes leadership functions for team building (transition phase) and team performance (action phase). Team building needs include competent, motivated

RESEARCH PERSPECTIVE

Resource: MacPhee, M. Wardrop, A. & Campbell, C. (2010). Transforming work place relationships through shared decision making. Journal of Nursing Management, 18, 1016–1026.

The shared decision-making model is a professional practice model that promotes nurses' control over and accountability for decisions that affect themselves and their patients. It is facilitated by access to information, resources, supports, and informal or formal lines of power. The authors examined the effect of shared decision making between nurses and nurse leaders around workload issues. Specifically, they examined the relationships within project teams (members and front-line leaders) and the relationships between project teams and mid-level leaders.

Four nurse-led project teams participated in the study to learn how to work together in a new nursing workload project. The study used participatory action research as its methodological approach. Participatory action research is a dynamic, collaborative process for helping people address social issues influencing their lives. The approach involves cycles of planning, acting, and reflecting, giving people the opportunity to bring about change and social improvement. Data were collected through observation, field notes, interviews, and focus groups. The participant observers also acted as facilitators of the project to enable nurses to gradually assume control over practice.

Shared decision making led to a number of successful outcomes, including team pride, the team's ability to engage in discussions with the nurse leader about work issues, and team involvement in shared decision making. Conflict and communication issues surfaced related to history, power dynamics, hierarchical differences, and roles and responsibilities. The study concluded that leadership has a critical role in transforming workplace relationships through shared decision making. It also confirmed the importance of leadership competencies related to communication, team building, conflict resolution, and change management.

Implications for Practice
This study provides nurse managers and leaders with insight into the complexity of team building, which occurs simultaneously with changing team members' roles and relationships. In reflecting on the process, the authors commented on the importance of strategic planning for future programs and the need for nurse managers and leaders to have strong team-building, communication, and conflict-resolution skills. Conflict is inevitable in group development, particularly in the early stages of development. Differences in goals, values, attitudes, role expectations, role changes, communication barriers, and historical issues all contribute to team conflict. In this study, conflict took place in the early stage of group development. It would be interesting to compare these observations with those at a later stage of group development.

members; clear goals and expectations; training; help with sense making; and feedback. Leadership functions needed for team performance are team monitoring; management of team boundaries; assistance with tasks; help with solving problems; resources; encouragement for self-management; and support for the social climate. This taxonomy focuses on followers in a group or team and the leadership support that they need, regardless of source, to help them fulfill goals such as effective group decision making.

Team Development. In most organizations, team leaders are responsible for team development and team performance. As coaches, team leaders are expected to provide guidance and direction to individuals to help them fulfill their roles. They take responsibility for their own development and serve as models to their followers. Leadership is discussed further in Chapters 1, 3, 18, and 19. The competencies described here include some of the important learning needs identified by team members and leaders.

Coordination, Cooperation, and Communication. Coordination involves synchronizing tasks among other health care providers and agencies to deliver patient care in different health agencies. In health care, work is streamlined in an orderly way to ensure completion of tasks on schedule and to reduce the incidence of omissions and errors. However, the coordination of services in health care is challenging when patients require multiple services from different agencies and health care providers (Khan, 2010). Effective nurse managers and leaders build efficient teams that can integrate and organize work as well as liaise with networks outside the team's boundaries to ensure continuity of care. Computer technology and standardized protocols and guidelines can enhance coordination and delivery of services. These support tools also facilitate decision making at different points in the care continuum. Students are involved in work coordination across departments and agencies, which gives them many opportunities to study and promote coordination.

Cooperation is the voluntary effort on the part of individuals to work with others to achieve common goals in a noncompetitive manner. When people cooperate willingly, more positive work outcomes can be expected. Cooperation in teams involves sharing goals, information, expertise, and resources for task completion. Effective nurse managers and leaders

promote cooperation between individuals and teams by setting clear goals, delegating tasks appropriately, monitoring workflow, and providing assistance for resolving conflicts that are related to joint task performance and decision making.

Effective communication is vital for group decision making. Poor communication, which can cause conflict and misunderstandings, can reduce team effectiveness. In health care teams, communication problems have been associated with hierarchical differences among team members, differences in expertise, the complexity of care, rapid decision making, role conflict, blocked upward communication, and interpersonal power issues (Suter et al., 2009). These factors present challenges for group function, group decision making, and patient care, which means that training in communication and decision-making skills is essential for nurse managers and leaders.

Team Competencies. Competencies are task-related knowledge, skills, and attitudes that reflect a task and can be measured. It is difficult to measure competencies for the team as a whole, but individual team members are accountable for their own task performance. Team building requires clear goals and expectations, task training, and feedback on performance. Decision making is a challenging task in interdisciplinary teams and one that is not easily managed. Advances in training resources, such as virtual team-building programs, can be used to promote effective decision making and team building and assist nurse managers and leaders to gain these requisite competencies for team building. Other resources, including professional programs, can enhance skill development in leaders. Feedback provided by leaders to team members on their performance is important for motivation and continuous learning.

Team Performance Dynamics. Team dynamics is defined as the way team members interact and react to changing circumstances. Positive team dynamics are conducive to shared decision making (Morgeson et al., 2010).

Persistent problems, such as group polarization, groupthink, conflicts of interest, and different perspectives can lead to team dysfunction. Conflicts within the team may be related to task, relationships, or behaviours. For example, disagreements can arise about team decision-making tasks (Jehn,

Greer, Levine, et al., 2008). Research has shown that moderate amounts of conflict may be helpful for motivating team members, but, in general, conflict can interfere with work satisfaction, cognitive processes, and the willingness of group members to work together. By carefully monitoring the team's progress, team leaders can detect and address conflict before it escalates. Conflict resolution strategies are discussed in Chapter 23.

A competency-based training program for effective team dynamics can be used by nurse managers and leaders to set standards for behaviour. The following competencies can help foster positive team performance dynamics:

- Establish ground rules for the team climate (ethical behaviour, work ethic, trust, shared decision making).
- Work with team members to set strategic goals for the team.
- Promote effective team communication (listening, encouraging participation, negotiating).
- Manage dysfunctional conflict in the team (conflict resolution strategies).
- Manage dysfunctional communication in the team (jargon, interruptions).
- Provide coaching for tasks and give constructive feedback.
- Use decision tools to help solve complex problems.
- Engage team members in reflection on team performance.

Team Decision Support Tools

Making decisions in a team can be challenging, particularly in interdisciplinary teams. Professional differences and independent focus of practice can make it difficult for team members to cross boundaries and negotiate to reach consensus on patient-care outcomes. Collaborative decision tools can help minimize some of these barriers and assist the team in reaching a consensus to resolve issues.

Electronic Meetings. Electronic meetings allow numerous team members in different geographical locations to interact with one another to instantly access information, consult with experts, generate new ideas, make presentations, conduct research, and complete work efficiently. Electronic meetings are beneficial for collaborative teams who are focused on task coordination and task completion. However, electronic meetings may not have the same positive effects in situations where social interaction among team members is low, trust among team members has not been established, and language and cultural barriers exist. Compared with face-to-face groups, electronic meeting groups may suffer from information overload, little social bonding, negative behaviours because of anonymity, and less input from all members. These deficits could have a negative effect on the quality of decision making.

Brainstorming. Brainstorming is a useful technique for stimulating the creative, spontaneous, and free-flowing thoughts of individuals and teams. It is important for generating novel ideas and focusing attention on specific issues. To ensure that creativity is not stifled, participants are asked to state whatever comes to mind when responding to questions. Responses should not be censored or ridiculed. Many ideas can be generated quickly and at minimal cost through brainstorming. The quantity of responses is not as important as the quality, which is achieved through a process of categorizing and evaluating content at the end of a brainstorming session. This method is useful for teams who get stalled in the problem analysis phase of decision making or when generating alternatives for interventions to solve problems. It also helps relieve tensions among members who are locked into a particular position that others are unable to accept. However, brainstorming does have some disadvantages that limit its success. For example, it is difficult to sort content into useful categories for analysis, some people are intimidated by sharing ideas that pop into their heads, and facilitators may not have the needed skills for the task. The introduction of electronic brainstorming has transformed this process. Content can be captured anonymously so that inhibited members can participate, and people's ideas are instantly visible and can be sorted into manageable categories for analysis. Some disadvantages of electronic brainstorming limit its appeal, such as cost, limited accessibility, information overload, and difficulties with evaluating data.

Six Thinking Hats. Six thinking hats is a powerful decision-making tool that can be used by groups to look at problems laterally from six different perspectives (De Bono, 2009). The hats have different colours, and each represents a different style of parallel thinking or role that a wearer assumes in a group. As participants switch from one hat to another, they are able to examine and reconsider their own style of thinking and how it affects their decision making. The six thinking hats are as follows:

- *Black hat:* negative, critical
- *Blue hat:* rational, decisive
- *Green hat:* creative, innovative
- *Red hat:* intuitive, emotional
- *Yellow hat:* positive, optimistic
- *White hat:* objective, factual

This decision tool is highly rated for critical thinking, communication, collaboration, and creativity. It has a positive effect on group dynamics when everyone has a chance to participate and can be objective in their approach to decision making.

Nominal Group Technique. The **nominal group technique** involves asking individual group members to respond to questions posed by a moderator and then asking participants to evaluate and prioritize the ideas of all group members ("Gaining Consensus," 2006). This technique is efficient and useful for controlling negative group behaviours (such as discussion domination by a few members) and increasing the participation of all group members in the problem-solving process.

In the nominal group technique, the process begins by presenting a problem. Participants are given a period of approximately 10 minutes of silence to generate and record their ideas on how to address the problem. Then, all ideas are shared with the group, using a chalkboard, flip chart, or computer screen. After the ideas have been shared, the group discusses the ideas for clarity and evaluates the merits of each idea. Next, each member silently and independently ranks each idea. The solution chosen is the one that receives the highest ranking by the majority of participants.

This technique is most useful when in-depth thinking from a variety of perspectives about options and strategies is needed to reach a quality decision. However, some members may feel that the process involved is too formal and may not like the restricted social interaction during decision making.

SWOT Analysis. **SWOT analysis** is a study of an organization's internal strengths and weaknesses, as well as its external opportunities and threats (Pearce, 2007). It is commonly used in strategic planning or marketing efforts but can also be used by individuals and groups in decision making. During a SWOT analysis, team members list the *S*trengths, *W*eaknesses, *O*pportunities, and *T*hreats related to the situation under consideration. Table 7-1 shows how SWOT analysis can be used to facilitate a nursing decision to transfer a nurse who has worked in a medical–surgical unit for 5 years to a critical care unit (CCU). SWOT analysis is an efficient tool for scanning the internal and external environments of an organization so that it can minimize and correct its weakness and threats, and to build on strengths and opportunities. However, the knowledge gained about the state of the internal and external environment may be too costly to change or impossible to change. The cost of equipment and supplies may escalate internally, and external policies and mandated programs may increase costs.

EXERCISE 7-5

SWOT analysis is a practical tool for decision making. Use the example in Table 7-1 to conduct a SWOT analysis of a hospital discharge plan for a patient to decide if the plan is appropriate.

EXERCISE 7-6

Use the Research Perspective on page 117 to generate options for managing group conflict in the shared decision-making program between nurses and nurse leaders around workload issues. Which decision-making tool would be most helpful to guide the selection of a best option? Explain your answer.

CONCLUSION

Problem-solving and decision-making skills are essential for nurse managers and leaders. However, health care problems are often complex and difficult to solve. Decision-making models and tools are helpful but can be limited by flaws in decision making, interpersonal conflict, and unpredictable conditions such as crises. Continuous skill building will improve the ability of nurse managers and leaders to think critically and solve complex problems.

TABLE 7-1   SWOT ANALYSIS

INTERNAL	
STRENGTHS	**WEAKNESSES**
• Familiar with the health care system • Clinically competent and has received favourable performance appraisals • Good communication skills; well liked by her peers • Recently completed 12-lead electrocardiogram (ECG) interpretation class	• Has not attended the critical care class • Has had a prior unresolved conflict with one of the surgeons who frequently admits to the critical care unit (CCU) • Is uncertain whether she wants to work full-time, 12-hour shifts
EXTERNAL	
OPPORTUNITIES	**THREATS**
• Anticipated staff openings in the CCU in the next several months • Critical care course will be offered in 1 month • Advanced cardiac life support (ACLS) course offered four times a year • A friend who works in CCU has offered to mentor her	• Possible bed closures in another CCU may result in staff transfers, thus eliminating open positions • Another medical–surgical nurse is also interested in transferring

A SOLUTION

Shyanne's supervisor, Rhea, seems to have made a conscious decision to avoid implementing the project, which has confused and frustrated Shyanne. Rhea's passive, but not indifferent, response makes it difficult for Shyanne, a new employee, to confront the issue. Shyanne should first determine if a problem exists, by searching for cues. Talking with a trusted co-worker might confirm her perception that Rhea is avoiding the decision to go forward with the project. Shyanne could invite her co-worker to brainstorm with her to generate reasons for Rhea's passive behaviour. Shyanne might conclude that Rhea may not want to invest in the project if the outcomes are uncertain or that Rhea may feel that the current youth skill development programs are working well. This exercise should help Shyanne take a more objective view of the problem and increase her confidence in approaching her supervisor. Shyanne could also use the problem-solving process to generate alternatives that she could discuss with her supervisor.

Would this be a suitable approach for you? Why or why not?

THE EVIDENCE

Penz and Bassendowski (2006) examined barriers to evidence-based nursing in clinical practice. They observed that while nurse educators and clinical nurse educators have a mandate to model and facilitate evidence-based practice, barriers in clinical settings make it difficult for nurses to apply their evidence-based knowledge and skills. The current emphasis on evidence-based practice comes from concerns within medicine about deficits in the quality of medical practice. Defined by Sackett et al. (1996) as "the conscientious, explicit, and judicious use of current best evidence in making decisions about the care of individual patients" (p. 71), evidence-based practice has become a requirement in many health care disciplines. Different definitions of evidence-based nursing practice exist, but most definitions address the importance of basing practice decisions on recent research that is validated through nurses' knowledge and systematic reviews. Other elements, such as nurse's intuition and sound judgement, are associated with definitions of evidence-based nursing practice. Some of the barriers to evidence-based practice in the current study were lack of time; insufficient access to libraries near clinical settings, current research journals and the Internet; inadequate research knowledge and learning opportunities; and unsupportive clinical cultures. Based on previous

THE EVIDENCE—cont'd

research, the authors emphasized the importance of helping nursing students develop critical-thinking skills and independent thinking to guide systematic investigations. Developing intellectual curiosity is necessary to help students explore beyond the traditional approaches to practice. In practice settings, clinical educators should know how to search for and evaluate evidence. The authors recommended journal clubs to facilitate analysis of emerging research, critical inquiry, and increased accessibility to research evidence.

The authors drew on accumulated research to emphasize the value of clinical educators as change agents for evidence-based practice to mitigate some of the barriers to implementation of evidence-based practice. Clinical educators can be role models for practitioners and set the tone for change in the clinical setting. Using their sound foundation in evidence-based research, they can establish orientation programs that promote evidence-based practice and ensure that valid practices are incorporated into policies, procedures, and practice guidelines. An evidence-based nursing approach will improve patient outcomes and decision making by clinical nurses.

NEED TO KNOW NOW

- Know how to distinguish a problem from its symptoms.
- Know how to use diagnostic tools to gather and analyze data about problems.
- Know how to use decision-making models to guide the decision-making process and determine best alternatives for action.
- Understand the importance of evidence-informed literature for nursing practice.
- Understand the importance of creativity, intuition, and shared decision making.
- Understand the importance of effective problem solving and decision making for health care providers.

CHAPTER CHECKLIST

The ability to make good decisions and encourage effective decision making in others is a hallmark of nursing leadership and management. A nurse manager or leader is in a good position to facilitate effective decision making by individuals and groups. Doing so requires good communication, conflict resolution, and mediation skills; knowledge of group dynamics; and the ability to foster an environment conducive to effective problem solving, decision making, and creative thinking.

- Problem solving is a comprehensive, sequential, cognitive process used to solve a problem by reducing the difference between current and desired conditions.
- Decision making is a phase of problem solving, which includes a reasoning process to analyze proposed alternatives (options) for action to determine the most appropriate choice.

- The scientific method is a rational, logical, and widely used problem-solving approach. It is the foundation for many models of decision making.
- Creativity and intuition feed rational-thinking processes and, therefore, can be seen as complementary thinking processes.
- Decision bias, or error in judgement, is a concern when relevant information is omitted. Groupthink is an example of a group decision bias.
- Decision-making styles and personal factors, such as self-esteem and self-confidence, influence decision making.
- Decision-making tools support decision making, especially in groups.
- The situation and circumstances should dictate the leadership style used by a nurse manager or leader to solve problems and make decisions.

TIPS FOR DECISION MAKING AND PROBLEM SOLVING

- Be conscious of personal influence on problem situations and decision-making processes; use safeguards against known biases.
- Research journal articles and relevant sections of textbooks to increase your knowledge base.

- Examine new approaches to problem resolution through experimentation, and calculate the risk to self and others.
- Become skilled in using decision-enabling tools.

℮volve WEBSITE

Visit the Evolve website for Suggested Readings, Internet Resources, and additional resources related to the content in this chapter: http://evolve.elsevier.com/Canada/Yoder-Wise/leading/.

REFERENCES

Benner, P., & Tanner, C. (1987). Clinical judgment: How expert nurses use intuition. *American Journal of Nursing, 1*, 23–31.

Bonabeau, E. (2003). Don't trust your gut. *Harvard Business Review, 81*(5), 116–123.

Borysowich, C. (2006). Constructing a weighted matrix. Retrieved from http://it.toolbox.com.

Burrow, J. L., Kleindl, B., & Everard, K. E. (2007). *Business principles and management*, 12th ed. Mason, OH: Thomson South-Western.

Bushe, G. R. (2011) Appreciative inquiry: Theory and critique. In D. Boje, B. Burnes, & J. Hassard (Eds.), *The Routledge Companion to Organizational Change* (pp. 87–103). Oxford, UK: Routledge.

College of Nurses of Ontario. (2011). RN and RPN practice: The client, the nurse and the environment. Toronto, ON: Author. Retrieved from http://www.cno.org/learn-about-standards-guidelines/standards-and-guidelines/.

D'Amour, D., Ferrada-Videla, M., San Martin Rodriguez, L., et al. (2005). The conceptual basis for interprofessional collaboration: Core concepts and theoretical frameworks [Review]. *Journal of Interprofessional Care, 19*(Suppl. 1), 116–131. doi:10.1080/13561820500082529

De Bono, E. (2009). *Six thinking hats*. London, UK: Penguin.

Fulcher, E. (2009). *Foundations of cognitive psychology*. n.p.: GEFT Consultancy Services. Retrieved from http://www.eamonfulcher.com.

Gaining consensus. (2006, November). Evaluation Briefs, Centers for Disease Control and Prevention. Retrieved from http://www.cdc.gov/healthyyouth/evaluation/pdf/brief7.pdf.

Glaser, E. M. (1941). *An experiment in the development of critical thinking*. New York, NY: Teachers College, Columbia University.

Green, S. L. (2002). Rational choice theory revisited: An overview. Waco, TX: Baylor University.

Henriksen, K., & Dayton, E. (2006). Organizational silence and hidden threats to patient safety. *Health Services Research, 41*(4, Pt2), 1539–1554.

Huitt, W. (1992). Problem solving and decision making: Consideration of individual differences using the Myers-Briggs Type Indicator. *Journal of Psychological Type, 24*, 33–44. Retrieved from http://www.edpsycinteractive.org/papers/prbsmbti.htm.

Jehn, K.A., Greer, L.L., Levine, S., et al. (2008). The effects of conflict types, dimensions, and emergent states on group outcomes. *Group Decision and Negotiation, 17*, 465–495. Retrieved from http://www.academia.edu/2094806.

Jones, B. D. (1999). Bounded rationality. *Annual Review of Political Science, 2*, 297–321.

Kaminski, J. (2012). Theory applied to informatics—Appreciative inquiry. *Canadian Journal of Nursing Informatics, 7*(1). Retrieved from http://cjni.net/journal/?p=1968.

Kepner, C. H., & Tregoe, B. B. (1965). The rational manager: A systematic approach to problem solving and decision-making. New York, NY: McGraw-Hill.

Keynes, M. (2008). Making good decisions: Part 1. *Nursing Management, 14*(9), 32–34.

Khan, E. (2010). Team-based care interventions involving nurses and primary care or community pharmacists improve hypertension control. *Evidence Based Nursing, 13*, 47–48. doi:101136/2bn1036

Korte, R. F. (2003). Biases in decision making and implications for human resource development. *Advances in Developing Human Resources, 5*(4), 440–457. doi:10.1177/1523422303257287

Kozlowski, S, W, J, & Ilgen, D. R. (2006). Enhancing the effectiveness of work groups and teams. *Psychological Science in the Public Interest, 7*(3), 78–124. doi:10.1111/j.1529-1006.2006.00030.x

Lunenburg, F. C. (2010). The decision-making process. *National Forum of Educational Administration and Supervision, 4*(1), 27, 1–12. Retrieved from http://nationalforum.com/Electronic%20Journal%20Volumes/Lunenburg,%20Fred%20C.%20The%20Decision%20Making%20Process%20NFEASJ%20V27%20N4%202010.pdf.

MacPhee, M., Wardrop, A., & Campbell, C. (2010). Transforming work place relationships through shared decision making. *Journal of Nursing Management, 18*, 1016–1026.

Mintzberg, H. (1973). *The nature of managerial work*. New York, NY: Harper & Row.

Morgeson, F. P., DeRue, D. S., & Karam, E. P. (2010). Leadership in teams: A functional approach to understanding leadership structures and processes. *Journal of Management, 36*(1), 5–39. doi:10.1177/0149206309347376

Nielsen, T. M. (2012). The evolving nature of work teams: Changing to meet the requirements of the future. In C. Wankel (Ed.), *21st century management: A reference handbook* (pp. 3–14). Thousand Oaks, CA: Sage. Retrieved from http://www.sagepub.com/northouse6e/study/materials/reference/reference12.1.pdf.

Pearce, C. (2007). Ten steps to carrying out a SWOT analysis. *Nursing Management, 14*(2), 25.

Penz, K. L., & Bassendowski, S. L. (2006). Evidence-based nursing in clinical practice: Implications for nurse educators. *The Journal of Continuing Education in Nursing, 37*(6), 250–254.

Riabacke, A. (2006). Leader or managerial decision making under risk and uncertainty. IAENG *International Journal of Computer Science, 32*(4). Retrieved from http://www.iaeng.org/IJCS/issues _v32/issue_4/IJCS_32_4_12.pdf.

Sackett, D. L., Rosenberg, W. M. C., Gray, J. A. M., et al. (1996). Evidence-based practice: What it is and what it isn't. *BMJ, 312*(13), 71–72.

Scriven, M., & Paul, R. (2007). Defining critical thinking. Retrieved from http://www.criticalthinking.org/aboutCT/definingCT.cfm.

Six Sigma. (2011, February 19). What is a fishbone diagram or fishbone analysis? Retrieved from http://sixsigmatutorial.com/f ishbone-analysis.

Smith, A. J. (2007). Embracing intuition in nursing practice. *Alabama Nurse, 34*(3), 16–17.

Suter, E., Arndt, J., Arthur, N., et al. (2009). Role understanding and effective communication as core competencies for collaborative practice. *Journal of Interprofessional Care, 23*(1), 41–51. doi:10.1080/13561820802338579

Syllogism. (n.d.). In *Merriam-Webster's online dictionary*. Retrieved from http://www.merriam-webster.com/dictionary/syllogism.

Tanner, C. A. (2006). Thinking like a nurse: A research-based model of clinical judgment in nursing. *Journal of Nursing Education, 45*(6), 204–211. Retrieved from http://www.ncbi.nlm.nih.gov/pubmed/16780008.

Wang, Y., & Ruhe, G. (2007). The cognitive process of decision making. *International Journal of Cognitive Informatics and Natural Intelligence, 1*(2), 73–85. Retrieved from http://www.uc algary.ca/icic/files/icic/67-IJCINI-1205-DecisionMaking.pdf.

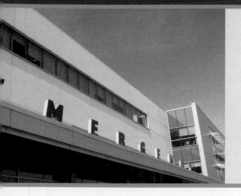

Health Care Organizations

Ena L. Howse and Lyle G. Grant

Nurses need to understand the basic framework and operations of the Canadian health care system as the context for their health care organization and their own work. This chapter presents the key elements of the Canadian health care system—such as its funding structure and the organization of health care services—that affect the provision of health care services. It also considers health care organizations within their dynamic context and the primary forces that influence how they operate. Finally, this chapter explores the health human resources that sustain health care, including the education, type of practice, and scope of practice associated with key health care provider roles.

OBJECTIVES

- Describe the Canadian health care system and the five criteria established by the *Canada Health Act* for federal government financial support of health care in the provinces and territories.
- Describe the current challenges faced by the Canadian health care system.
- Identify the roles and responsibilities of the federal, provincial, and territorial governments in funding, organizing, and delivering health care services.
- Describe the types and classifications of health care services.
- Analyze health care organizations from an open-systems perspective, and describe the influence of external forces.
- Identify the education, type of practice, and scope of practice associated with key health care provider roles.

TERMS TO KNOW

accreditation	open-systems theory	primary health care (PHC)
health care system	primary care	social determinants of health

Alex, the emergency department (ED) nurse manager, anxiously watched the patient census rise in the already crowded ED. The trauma room, all patient cubicles, and the holding room for patients awaiting transfer to inpatient units were filled. Patient overflow was in the hallways, service rooms, and the waiting room. This situation was not unusual; the ED admitted over 300 patients daily. Occasionally, overcrowding meant that the hospital had to declare gridlock and patients would be rerouted to other hospitals. Alex would have to alert administration because he expected more patients to arrive. He knew from experience that overcrowding was a cyclical problem and that his options were limited, but he was obligated to follow hospital policy to reduce wait times in the ED. In his role as nurse manager, Alex was familiar with the routine responses to overcrowding: he would ask for volunteers to work an extra shift and consult with the triage nurse, ED physicians, laboratory staff, and diagnostic imaging staff to see whether their workflow could be accelerated. The ED team generally worked to full capacity and was highly efficient; however, it was never easy to discharge patients from the holding room, which meant that fewer beds were available for incoming patients.

What would you do if you were Alex to help discharge patients from the holding room?

INTRODUCTION

Health care is one of the largest and most complex industrial and service sectors in Canada. Services are delivered by a multitude of health care organizations that differ in size, type, structure, and internal complexity. While each organization is different, all share common features: a collection of people oriented toward achieving established health care goals; work that is divided into specialized functions; and work that is coordinated to maintain the stability and continuity of the organization over time (Johns & Saks, 2001). Understanding these features makes it possible to study the nature of the health care organization, identify its components, and determine how tasks and responsibilities are divided for efficiency and coordinated to achieve common goals. It is also important to know how health care organizations are affected by internal forces such as input from health care providers, nurse managers, patients, and others who have a stake in the organization. Together, these forces help explain why health care organizations fail or remain stable and productive.

The Canadian health care system has been undergoing reform to improve performance and patient outcomes for a number of years. A 2000 First Ministers' conference focused on developing an action plan for health system renewal, and the First Ministers agreed to work in partnership with health care providers and citizens to reform the health care system. Three years later, they passed the *2003 First Ministers' Accord on Health Care Renewal* and in 2004 presented *A 10-Year Plan to Strengthen Health Care* (Health Canada, 2011).

As part of the renewal efforts, the Health Council of Canada was established to monitor the progress and health outcomes of these accords (Health Council of Canada, 2011). Included in the ten-year plan were recommendations to decrease wait times; increase funds for home care, Aboriginal health, and the supply of health care providers; introduce electronic health records; and develop primary care. Since 2004, all provinces and territories have made changes to improve health care.

However, recent reports show that the health care system continues to face significant challenges (Health Council of Canada, 2014). Health care costs continue to rise, and the current state of the global economy suggests that funding health care at its present level will be difficult in the future. Public demands for better quality of care and access to care are still major concerns. Moreover, as the population ages, the demand will increase. The success of reform efforts requires capable nurse managers and leaders who understand how their health care organization functions and how to influence others in increasing organizational effectiveness within the context of not only the organization but also the Canadian health care system.

THE CANADIAN HEALTH CARE SYSTEM

A health care system is "the sum total of all the organizations, institutions and resources whose primary purpose is to improve health" (World Health Organization [WHO], 2005). According to the World Bank (2007), a health care system has four key functions: (1) stewardship or governance, (2) financing, (3) human and physical resources, and (4) organization and management of service delivery. Canada's health care system can be viewed as an interlocking set (system) of ten provincial and three territorial health insurance plans that share common features and standards of coverage (Health Canada, 2011). In practice, the federal and provincial/territorial governments typically collaborate to establish health care principles, finance health care, and address the organization and delivery of health care services despite their distinct jurisdictions, reflecting the key functions that are associated with health care systems. However, provinces and territories have primary responsibility for the organization and delivery of health care services.

The *Canada Health Act* establishes the criteria for federal government financial support of a national health care insurance plan that aims to ensure Canadians have reasonable access to medically necessary hospital and physician services without direct personal cost. Federal funding is transferred to the provinces and territories so that they can provide these basic services, assuming that the provinces and territories meet specific criteria and conditions. As such, the *Canada Health Act* defines the central tenets of basic and universal medicare available to Canadians.

To qualify for federal health care funding, provinces and territories must meet the following five criteria:

1. Public administration (provincial and territorial health insurance plans must be administered on a not-for-profit basis by public authorities that are accountable to the governments);
2. Comprehensive (provincial and territorial health insurance plans must cover all insured health care services, which include physician services, hospital care, and medically required dental procedures performed in a hospital);

3. Universality (all residents of a province or territory must have access to public health care insurance and insured health care services on uniform terms and conditions);
4. Portability (provinces and territories must cover insured health care services provided to their citizens when temporarily absent from their province or from Canada, and services must be uninterrupted when citizens move from one province or territory to another); and
5. Accessibility (insured persons must have reasonable and uniform access to insured health care services, free of financial or other barriers). Contributions by patients through user charges or extra billing are prohibited (Health Canada, 2013).

HEALTH CARE SERVICES FUNDING

Federal Funding

The federal government fulfills its fiscal responsibility to the provinces and territories mainly through transfer payments. Table 8-1 shows the amount of transfer and equalization payments made from 2007 to 2012. The amount of individual transfer payments for health care services is determined by a formula that is based on the financial capacity of each jurisdiction to deliver services. Equalization payments are distributed to those provinces and territories that do not have sufficient capacity to provide necessary services. Additional federal health care allocations, such as funding to reduce wait times, are made at the discretion of the federal government. For example, federal funding has been expanded to include funding for the renewal of primary health care services. In the 2003 First Ministers' accord, the federal government committed to allocating $16 billion for health renewal initiatives in

TABLE 8-1	FEDERAL SUPPORT TO PROVINCES AND TERRITORIES: MAJOR TRANSFERS, 2010–2015				
	2010–2011	2011–2012	2012–2013	2013–2014	2014–2015
	(IN $ MILLIONS)				
Canada Health Transfer	25 672	26 952	28 569	30 283	32 114
Canada Social Transfer	11 179	11 514	11 859	12 215	12 582
Equalization Payments	14 372	14 659	15 423	16 105	16 669

Adapted from Department of Finance Canada. (2014). Federal support to province and territories. Retrieved April 11, 2014 from http://www.fin.gc.ca/fedprov/mtp-eng.asp. Reproduced with the permission of the Minister of Finance Canada, 2014.

the areas of primary health care, home care, and catastrophic drug coverage (Health Canada, 2003).

In addition, the federal government directly funds services to groups such as First Nations and Inuit, military personnel, prisoners in federal penitentiaries, and recent immigrants (Butler & Tiedemann, 2013). It also has criminal law powers to protect Canadians through control of possible hazards from products or matters such as food and drugs, controlled substances, medical devices, industrial and consumer products, cosmetics, tobacco, radiation-emitting devices, and pest control products (Butler & Tiedemann, 2013).

Provincial and Territorial Funding

Health care spending represents the largest single budget item for provincial and territorial governments and is, therefore, a constant concern (Canadian Institute for Health Information [CIHI], 2013b). Figure 8-1 shows how provinces and territories compare in their health care spending. All governments make efforts to contain

How do the provinces and territories compare?

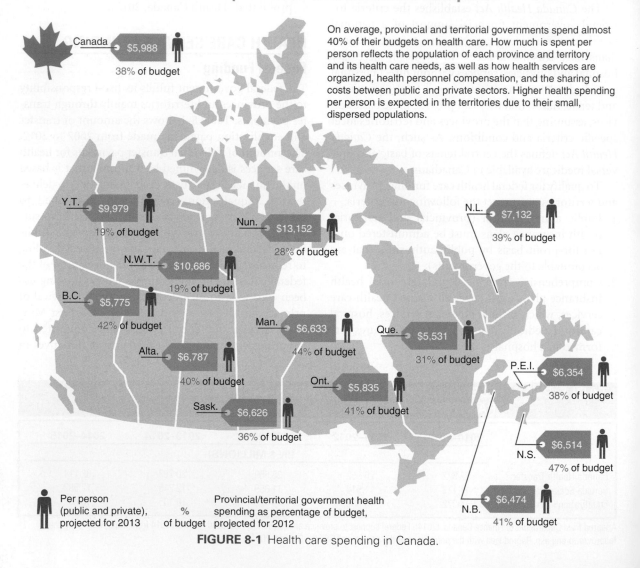

On average, provincial and territorial governments spend almost 40% of their budgets on health care. How much is spent per person reflects the population of each province and territory and its health care needs, as well as how health services are organized, health personnel compensation, and the sharing of costs between public and private sectors. Higher health spending per person is expected in the territories due to their small, dispersed populations.

Canada $5,988   38% of budget

Y.T. $9,979   19% of budget
Nun. $13,152   28% of budget
N.L. $7,132   39% of budget
N.W.T. $10,686   19% of budget
B.C. $5,775   42% of budget
Man. $6,633   44% of budget
Que. $5,531   31% of budget
P.E.I. $6,354   38% of budget
Alta. $6,787   40% of budget
Ont. $5,835   41% of budget
Sask. $6,626   36% of budget
N.S. $6,514   47% of budget
N.B. $6,474   41% of budget

Per person (public and private), projected for 2013
% of budget
Provincial/territorial government health spending as percentage of budget, projected for 2012

FIGURE 8-1 Health care spending in Canada.

health care costs while maintaining quality care. Health care spending in Canada in 2011 was $200.1 billion and was expected to reach $211.2 billion by 2013 (an average of $5988 per capita), or 11.2% of Canada's gross domestic product (GDP) (CIHI, 2013c, p. 11). A comparison of health care spending (in US dollars) in Organisation for Economic Co-operation and Development (OECD) countries appears in Table 8-2.

The high and rising costs of health care are important constraints on the ability of Canadian health care organizations to deliver safe and effective health care. Federal transfer payments only account for about 20% of provincial/territorial health budgets. To carry out their health care responsibilities within the mandate of the *Canada Health Act*, the provinces and territories make up the remaining health budget with revenues from taxation (Health Canada, 2013). The majority of health care funding (about 70%) comes from federal and provincial tax revenues, and the remaining funding is paid out-of-pocket (15%), by private health insurance (13%), and by social insurance funds (1%) (Marchildon, 2013).

Each provincial and territorial government has its own public health insurance plan. The plan's funds are used to deliver a broad range of services, such as those in large tertiary/quaternary care health science centres; small, community primary care hospitals; drug benefits; laboratory/imaging and other diagnostic services; and services of health care providers. Most plans also provide coverage for medications for people over 65 years of age and for people requiring social assistance.

An increase in private funding in the Canadian health care system has raised concerns that private funding will compromise the public health care system. The growth rates of private health expenditures were expected to be 3.4% in 2012 and 2.9% in 2013. In 2013, private health expenditures were forecast to reach $63 billion (CIHI, 2013c). In comparison, the growth rates of public health expenditures were expected to be 2.7% in 2012 and 2.5% in 2013, which indicates a slowing rate of growth in public health spending (CIHI, 2013c). Private funding primarily comprises out-of-pocket payments and private health insurance payments. Other industrialized countries also have a mix of public–private health funding (Table 8-2). The *Canada Health Act* does not specifically prohibit private funding, but some provinces prevent private insurance plans from covering services that are identified in the *Canada Health Act* as medically necessary.

ORGANIZING THE DELIVERY OF CARE

As well as allocating funds to meet health care needs, the provinces and territories are responsible for hospital care and the primary care provided by physicians, nurses, physiotherapists, and allied professionals (Health Canada, 2011). The health care system consists of many connected services and health care providers, including hospitals, ambulatory clinics, and community health programs such as home care, mental health care services, and public health organizations. It also includes many support services, such as diagnostic services, regulatory bodies, and professional associations. All services and health care providers are interconnected and interacting parts of a complex, unpredictable, and

TABLE 8-2	HEALTH CARE SPENDING IN OECD COUNTRIES RANKED BY GDP, 2011			
COUNTRY	**PER CAPITA ($US)**	**% OF GDP**	**% PUBLIC SPENDING**	**% PRIVATE SPENDING**
United States	8508	17.7	48	52
Netherlands	5099	11.9	86	14
France	4118	11.6	77	23
Germany	4495	11.3	77	23
Canada	**4522**	**11.2**	**70**	**30**
Switzerland	5643	11.0	65	35
Denmark	4448	10.9	85	15
United Kingdom	3405	9.4	83	17
Australia	3800	8.9	68	32
OECD Average	**3410**	**9.3**	**73**	**27**

Adapted from Canadian Institute for Health Information. (2013c). *National health expenditure trends 1975 to 2013.* Ottawa, ON: Author. Retrieved from https://secure.cihi.ca/free_products/NHEXTrendsReport_EN.pdf.

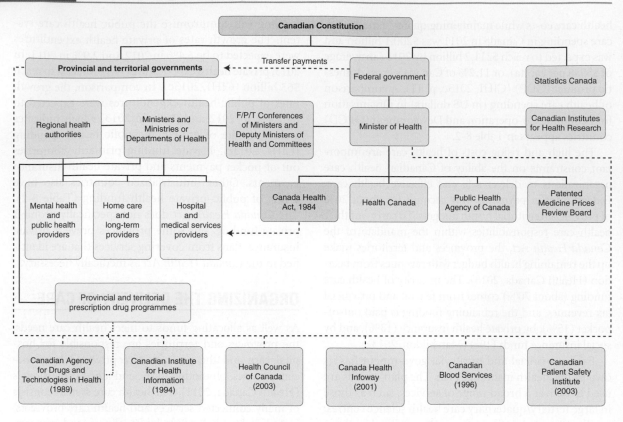

Note: Solid lines represent direct relationships of accountability while dotted lines indicate more indirect or arm's length relationships.

FIGURE 8-2 Organization of the Canadian health care system. *F*, federal; *P*, provincial; *T*, territorial.

dynamic health care system. Figure 8-2 illustrates how the health care system is organized in Canada. In such a complex system, management and leadership skills are needed to motivate people, coordinate work, and produce quality outcomes. Governments accomplish these and other objectives by sharing responsibility with regulatory bodies, such as Regional Health Authorities (RHAs) that oversee health care delivery, and self-regulatory authorities called "colleges" or "orders" that regulate health care provider groups.

APPROACHES TO DELIVERING CARE

Regional Health Administration

The equitable and efficient allocation of health care resources dominates public discussion in many Western countries. In the late 1980s, most provincial health ministries created regional branches based on geographical boundaries called *health regions* and made them responsible for the local delivery and administration of health care services. Health regions offer some localized control over health care services delivery. Health ministries also determined that delegating provincial responsibilities for service delivery to regional bodies would be useful to containing costs and improving efficiencies in health care delivery, while being responsive to local needs. Provinces have revised the size and structures of health regions over time, and these regions may have different names from one province to another. For example, in many provinces, health regions are called *Regional Health Authorities*, but Ontario has a system of *Local Health Integration Networks (LHINs)* that plan, integrate, and fund health care services. Health regions are responsible for governing, planning, prioritizing, budgeting, and allocating funds to health agencies, and delivering and managing health care services within predetermined regional areas (Morris & Clarke, 2011). The regional health administration system is consistent with population health and wellness approaches to health care and reflects the primary care goals of reducing exclusion and social disparities, organizing health care services around people's needs, integrating health into all sectors, pursuing collaborative models of policy dialogue, and increasing stakeholder participation (World Health Organization, 2014a).

Typically, health regions are governed by a board made up of local health care providers and community stakeholders. In Ontario, LHINs have slightly less authority for decision making than do other health region organizations in other provinces.

Over time, the challenges in organizing and funding the delivery of health services have motivated some provinces to reduce the number of health regions and contemplate and trial other cost-saving initiatives. The costs of health care are high and continue to escalate. Efforts to reduce health care services to regions may be divisive if they are perceived to distribute funds unfairly or inequitably among similar regions within a province. Drawing similarities across health regions is also considerably complex because of the vast geographical areas and the diversity of populations. Knowledge and skill will be needed to reconcile these issues and gain the trust of health care organizations to lead effectively.

Public–Private Partnership

Public–private partnerships (P3s) began gaining acceptance at the change of this century. They represent a new form of collaboration between private, for-profit industry and public, not-for-profit organizations. These partnerships now seem to have a permanency in how health care delivery is funded and provided. Governments, which are pressed to control the costs of delivering health services, have turned to private industry to share the risks of large investments in infrastructures necessary for service delivery and to seek their expertise in finding economic efficiencies. P3s have been used to develop and support new technologies that support operational aspects of health care delivery, to provide diagnostic services with in-house and centralized laboratories and specialized

professionals, to deliver publicly funded "nonhospital" surgeries, to expand retail business ventures, and to provide services not covered by public funding, including services to foreign patients (Morris & Clarke, 2011). P3s have become the most popular means of funding large capital projects, such as new hospitals or hospital expansions. Usual arrangements include the industry partner building the structure and then the hospital renting back the space at an agreed rate over the useful life of the asset (usually decades). Proponents of using P3s for large capital projects suggest that this arrangement shifts some of the burden of capital costs to the private sector, creates shared risks related to building delays and cost over-runs, and harnesses the efficiencies private enterprise can bring to a public-sector undertaking. Detractors suggest that cost savings are overestimated, that the capital costs associated with nongovernment borrowing result in higher costs of borrowing, and that the long-term costs to government unnecessarily include the costs of ensuring that the private industry partner generates a profit.

Initiatives that contract out services that were previously provided within health care organizations are also examples of P3s. Increasingly laundry, food, parking, security, and housekeeping services are being contracted out to private, for-profit enterprises. The long-term impact and costs of these service delivery changes are not fully known, but the rationale for adopting these approaches includes cost containment, increased standardization, and the shifting of financial risks from public- to private-sector partners. Detractors are concerned that P3s provide lower standards of service than public-sector health care services, which they suggest will negatively affect overall health care goals. Recently, Canadians have begun to take issue with the rising costs of parking at hospitals because of P3 arrangements. These parking costs are often hardest on families visiting relatives or attending tertiary or quaternary services on a regular basis, compounding other financial challenges facing these families (CBC News, 2013).

Effective leaders broadly assess the advantages and disadvantages of P3s on health care delivery in the short and long term, as well as the impact on those most affected by P3 arrangements. Based on this assessment, effective leaders advocate for decisions that most closely align with the overarching health goals in Canadian health care delivery, including patient-centredness and primary health care goals.

TYPES AND CLASSIFICATIONS OF HEALTH CARE SERVICES

Health care delivery can be classified in various ways. Conceptual divisions that consider the sequencing and classification of health care services offer an understanding of the roles of different organizations, the way in which they relate to one another, and the overall provision of health care services. In Canada, health care services are classified based on the sequence in which they are delivered: (1) primary health care services (what happens first), (2) secondary health care services (what happens next), and (3) additional (supplementary) health care services (Health Canada, 2011). These health care services can be further classified based on types of care: (1) public health services/ prevention services, (2) community care services, and (3) hospital care services. Community care services are further divided into residential care, community mental health and addiction services, and home care services. Hospital care services are further divided into primary, secondary, tertiary, and quaternary health care. Table 8-3 presents the basic framework of health care services and service classifications in Canada. The distinction between types of services is not always clear-cut, especially from the patients' or users' perspective, but the framework presented in Table 8-3 can serve as a guide to health care delivery in Canada.

Basic Framework of Services

Primary Health Care Services. Terminology related to primary health care can be confusing. In Health Canada documents, as in Table 8-3, *primary health care services* are generally the first point of contact for individuals with the system; at this point of care, health care providers also help coordinate health care services and ensure continuity of care for patients across the system (Health Canada, 2011). However, this terminology has not been universally adopted. *Primary health care* and *primary care* are often used interchangeably, but they are distinct concepts. Primary care is the first point of entry in the Canadian health care system and deals with the majority of health issues. Primary care comprises the assessment, diagnosis, and treatment of an individual by a general practitioner or family physician, nurse practitioner, or other authorized health care provider; it is considered part of the larger concept of primary health care. According to the World

Health Organization (WHO, 1978), primary health care (PHC) is a community-based health care service philosophy that is focused on illness prevention, health promotion, treatment, rehabilitation, and identification of people at risk. Through access to resources and education, people are empowered to be responsible, self-reliant, and participate in their health care. Health care services are provided by teams of health care providers (e.g., physicians, nurses, midwives, other practitioners, community members) close to where people live and work. Practical, affordable, scientifically sound methods and technologies are encouraged to maintain quality care and manage costs (Canadian Nurses Association [CNA], 2005). Primary health care is a comprehensive systems approach focused on preventing illness and promoting health (CNA, 2005). It is also the level at which individuals, families, and communities enter the health care system to access services, thus primary care is considered an aspect of primary health care. Box 8-1 on page 134 outlines the key articles of WHO's Declaration of Alma-Ata that underpin primary health care in Canada.

Health care organizations may provide primary health care that includes routine care, care for urgent but minor health problems, mental health care, psychosocial services, nutritional counselling, and other services (Health Canada, 2014). In Canada, health policymakers continue to consider that primary health care principles hold the most promise for creating the best health care system and the healthiest population in the world (Health Canada, 2014). A key feature of primary health care reform has been a shift from single provider practices, such as solo physician practices, to teams of providers who are responsible for providing patients with comprehensive care (Health Canada, 2014). The success of these teams depends on many factors, including the ability of health care providers to sustain collaboration. Nurse managers and leaders play a key role in developing interprofessional teams by modelling leadership skills, being effective communicators and negotiators, and using conflict-resolution behaviours (see also Chapter 26).

Secondary Health Care Services. Secondary health care services take place after the initial patient contact with primary health care services. For example, a patient may be referred for specialized care to a hospital or other facility. Secondary health care services can also be provided in the home, community

TABLE 8-3 TYPES AND CLASSIFICATIONS OF HEALTH CARE SERVICES

TYPE	DESCRIPTION
Basic Framework of Services	
Primary health care services	• First-contact services for routine problems and emergencies • Provision of coordination of patients' health care services to ensure continuity of care and ease of access across the health care system • Holistic approach to health promotion and disease prevention
Secondary health care services	• Referrals to specialized care in hospitals, long-term care, or in the community • Services that may be provided in the home, community, or institution (mostly long-term care facilities)
Additional health care services	• Prescription drugs, dental care, vision care, and other therapies not usually covered by public health insurance • Sometimes part of first-contact services, sometimes part of secondary services
Service Classifications	
Public Health Services/ Prevention Services	• Service to individuals and communities to promote health, prevent disease, and control infectious diseases
Community Care Services	
Continuing care and rehabilitation	• Complex continuing care (CCC) and rehabilitation services care for ill, medically complex, and disabled patients • Services that are sometimes attached to or within close proximity of hospital services
Residential care	• Care provided in residential settings (e.g., long-term care, supportive housing, and retirement homes)
Community mental health and addiction services	• Care provided in nonacute care institutions, community settings, and group homes to promote health, support recovery from mental illness, and provide programs and resources
Home care services	• Care delivered in community settings, including private homes to people needing health care supports to remain independent and community dwelling • Sometimes used temporarily to aid patients with acute and chronic conditions recovering at home • Mental health services often have a component of home care services for those living in private homes • Palliative care services or end-of-life health services that are provided at home
Hospital Care Services (Primary, Secondary, Tertiary, Quaternary Care)	• Primary care: generally offered by a general practitioner, family physician, or nurse practitioner outside of hospital • Secondary care: the starting point of hospital inpatient care, it is treatment by specialists to whom a patient has been referred by a primary care provider or been admitted through urgent care services located at the hospital (typically community hospitals) • Tertiary care (or tertiary hospital). Highly specialized services (e.g., academic teaching hospital) • Quaternary care: centres for treatment of extremely rare medical conditions (generally part of a large, tertiary care hospital)
Ambulatory care	• Care provided to outpatients, ranging from primary care to urgent care in clinics or emergency departments • Care provided by hospitals for special health care needs that cannot easily be offered through home care services; patients do not stay at the hospital overnight
Emergency care	• Treatment of urgent to life-threatening problems
Acute care	• Treatment for a disease or severe episode of illness or surgery for a short period of time
Specialized services	• Treatment for trauma, specified injuries, joint replacements, organ replacements • The classification often used to help monitor service provision goals

Based on Canadian Institute for Health Information. (2014). Information about health care. Retrieved from http://www.cihi.ca/CIHI-ext-portal/internet/EN/Theme/types+of+care/cihi000002; Health Canada. (2011). Canada's health care system. Retrieved from http://www.hc-sc.gc.ca/hcs-sss/pubs/system-regime/2011-hcs-sss/index-eng.php.

BOX 8-1   KEY ARTICLES RESPECTING PRIMARY HEALTH CARE FROM THE DECLARATION OF ALMA-ATA

Declaration:

VI

Primary health care is essential health care based on practical, scientifically sound and socially acceptable methods and technology made universally accessible to individuals and families in the community through their full participation and at a cost that the community and country can afford to maintain at every stage of their development in the spirit of self-reliance and self-determination. It forms an integral part both of the country's health system, of which it is the central function and main focus, and of the overall social and economic development of the community. It is the first level of contact of individuals, the family and community with the national health system bringing health care as close as possible to where people live and work, and constitutes the first element of a continuing health care process.

VII

Primary health care:

1. reflects and evolves from the economic conditions and sociocultural and political characteristics of the country and its communities and is based on the application of the relevant results of social, biomedical and health care services research and public health experience;
2. addresses the main health problems in the community, providing promotive, preventive, curative and rehabilitative services accordingly;
3. includes at least: education concerning prevailing health problems and the methods of preventing and controlling them; promotion of food supply and proper nutrition; an adequate supply of safe water and basic sanitation; maternal and child health care, including family planning; immunization against the major

infectious diseases; prevention and control of locally endemic diseases; appropriate treatment of common diseases and injuries; and provision of essential drugs;
4. involves, in addition to the health sector, all related sectors and aspects of national and community development, in particular agriculture, animal husbandry, food, industry, education, housing, public works, communications and other sectors; and demands the coordinated efforts of all those sectors;
5. requires and promotes maximum community and individual self-reliance and participation in the planning, organization, operation and control of primary health care, making fullest use of local, national and other available resources; and to this end develops through appropriate education the ability of communities to participate;
6. should be sustained by integrated, functional and mutually supportive referral systems, leading to the progressive improvement of comprehensive health care for all, and giving priority to those most in need;
7. relies, at local and referral levels, on health workers, including physicians, nurses, midwives, auxiliaries and community workers as applicable, as well as traditional practitioners as needed, suitably trained socially and technically to work as a health team and to respond to the expressed health needs of the community.

VIII

All governments should formulate national policies, strategies and plans of action to launch and sustain primary health care as part of a comprehensive national health system and in coordination with other sectors. To this end, it will be necessary to exercise political will, to mobilize the country's resources and to use available external resources rationally.

World Health Organization. (1978). Declaration of Alma-Ata. International Conference on Primary Health Care, Alma-Ata, USSR, 6–12. Retrieved from http://www.who.int/publications/almaata_declaration_en.pdf.

(e.g., community clinics), or long-term care or chronic care facility. Referrals to this type of care can be made by primary health care providers, community-based health organizations, families, and patients themselves (Health Canada, 2011). The "secondary" in *secondary health care services* refers only to the timing and referral of these services after primary health care services have occurred.

Additional Health Care Services. Additional health care services are not usually covered by public health insurance. For example, prescription medications (with some exceptions), dental care, vision care, and acupuncture therapies are not usually covered by public health insurance. Typically, supplemental health

insurance (available from some employers) or private purchases are used to cover such costs. Moreover, the escalating costs of drugs has led a number of governments to decide to subsidize catastrophic drug coverage and engage in deliberations with pharmaceutical corporations on cost control.

Service Classifications

Public Health Services/Prevention Services. The primary goal of the Public Health Agency of Canada is to strengthen Canada's capacity to protect and improve the health of Canadians and to help reduce pressures on the health care system (Public Health Agency of Canada, 2013). While predominantly funded by the federal government in the past, the costs and responsibilities for public health services are now shared among all levels of government. In Ontario, for example, much of the funding for public health comes from provincial and municipal governments. The public health system encourages good health in Canadians by helping prevent injuries and chronic diseases, promoting a healthy lifestyle, and preventing the spread of infectious diseases. Public health nurses and community nurses take on a wide range of educational and support roles in the community, manage communicable diseases in the community, and are among the first responders to public health crises.

Community Care Services. Community care services include a large range of services delivered in private homes, long-term residential care settings, retirement communities, and community clinics, excluding those services related to public health and prevention services. Community care services include continuing care and rehabilitation services for individuals with medically complex conditions or disabilities.

Long-term residential care includes the care provided in nursing homes, personal care facilities, private homes, and assisted-living arrangements. Many long-term residential care facilities are privately owned, although most receive public funding for certain care services. For example, provincial and territorial plans usually cover the costs of the medical services provided in long-term care facilities, while individuals remain responsible for their room and board costs (in some cases, individuals receive subsidies for room and board) (Health Canada, 2011). The operation of long-term care facilities is governed by provincial or territorial legislation.

Community care services are delivered by independently practising health care providers, professional groups, multidisciplinary teams, and public and private agencies. Home services coordinators or nurses might provide professional at-home care and support to clients who need acute and chronic health care services. Home service coordinators also manage long-term care placements. Most community care services case managers are nurses, but other health care providers, such as physiotherapists and occupational therapists, can assume this role in the community. Mental health services are provided in the community by case managers, independently practising health care providers, or multidisciplinary teams that include physicians, psychiatrists, nurses, psychologists, social workers, recreational and occupational therapists, and other support staff. Clinics and special programs for addictions are available throughout Canada.

Hospital Care Services. Hospitals play a major role in the delivery of health care. "Hospital services" are outlined in the *Canada Health Act* and include (1) standard or public ward accommodation and meals, (2) nursing service, (3) diagnostic procedures such as blood tests and X-rays, (4) the administration of medications, and (5) the use of operating rooms, case rooms, and anaesthetic facilities. Hospitals that are described as private, not-for-profit entities receive public funds for their services. Some hospitals are governed by boards that make decisions about the hospital's operations and its priorities, but increasingly this decision-making responsibility is being delegated to Regional Health Authorities. Provincial and territorial governments have authority over the amount of public money that will be allocated to a hospital, the services that it provides, and penalties for hospitals that fail to operate within their budget. Hospitals are represented by professional associations that lobby on behalf of their constituents in the best interests of their organizations and influence government health care policy.

Hospital care ranges from ambulatory to highly specialized services. Community hospitals typically provide general and comprehensive care that does not require specialists or advanced diagnostic and treatment facilities. Tertiary hospitals provide acute and complex care, such as consultation, diagnostics, intensive care, and emergency care to patients who are referred to them. In larger centres, tertiary hospitals may form networks. Hospital stays are usually short, but treatment may be transferred to home care. Highly specialized care (quaternary care) is provided in tertiary care hospitals or specialized centres for rare or experimental procedures.

EXERCISE 8-1

Visit the Ministry of Health Web sites for two provinces and/or territories and compare their home care services. What similarities and differences exist between the jurisdictions' home care services? How does home care service coverage differ for palliative care patients versus patients who are not deemed palliative? What differences in services exist between the two jurisdictions? What home care services are typically available to those with severe and persistent mental illness, and how do these differ between the two jurisdictions?

A THEORETICAL PERSPECTIVE

Systems Theory

Managing within dynamic and unpredictable health care organizations can be a challenge for nurse managers and leaders. By viewing the operational processes of health care organizations from a systems theory perspective, nurse managers and leaders are in a better position to find productive and innovative responses to forces within and outside their organizations. A systems theory perspective attempts to explain productivity in terms of a unifying whole as opposed to a series of unrelated parts (Thompson, 1967). Systems can be either closed (self-contained) or open (interacting with both internal and external forces).

Open-systems theory views organizations as dynamic, interactive systems that are strongly influenced by internal and external forces (W. R. Scott, 2002). The system is open, as opposed to closed, because it constantly interacts with and adapts to both internal forces and external forces. The characteristics of open-systems organizations, such as health care organizations, are outlined in Box 8-2.

Simply defined, a *system* is a group of interacting, interdependent elements that form a complex whole (W. R. Scott, 2002). A biological system is often used as a model for understanding the relevance of open-systems theory to social organizations. A biological system consists of separate but interdependent parts (e.g., organs) that function together to achieve common purposes. Inputs (e.g., food) are received from the external environment and processed to produce outputs (e.g., nutrients and waste products). The system seeks internal balance, or homeostasis. Adjustments to achieve internal balance are made through the input–cycle and feedback mechanisms (Liebler & McConnell, 2012).

An open-systems model is useful for a holistic assessment of a health care organization and its external environment. Knowledge of the impact of external forces can be used to guide efforts to identify and adapt to change by modifying or developing strategies (processes) for survival. Health care managers who are guided by an open-systems approach to practice proactively scan internal and external forces to assess and respond to organizational changes. They are aware of how work units (components) interrelate and how work should be coordinated among them. They understand how the system is affected by external forces, such as funding changes or sociocultural changes, which will help them recognize changes and respond to them accordingly. They also understand the importance of feedback in monitoring and improving the system. As a result, they seek timely performance feedback (such as statistics on mortality and morbidity), accreditation reports that show adherence to or deviation from national health performance standards, benchmarking data that identify successful practices of comparable organizations, environmental safety audits, and staff performance evaluations. The Theory Box below lists the basic components of an open-systems model. A representation of an open-systems model for a health care organization appears in Figure 8-3.

BOX 8-2	CHARACTERISTICS OF OPEN-SYSTEMS ORGANIZATIONS

- Organizations are dynamic and continuously interact with their external environment.
- The internal environment consists of independent, interactive components.
- A change in any single component can affect others.
- Inputs are acquired from the external environment and processed into products or services to be released as outputs.
- As a synergistic unit, a system can produce greater effects than the sum of the effects achieved by its independent components.
- Feedback on performance influences the subsequent selection of inputs.
- A system will change, adapt, and develop to survive, or it will deteriorate.

⬤ THEORY BOX

Basic Open-Systems Model Components

Inputs → Processes → Outputs ← Feedback

Inputs: people, materials, equipment, funds, information, policies, infrastructure

Processes: communication, decision making, collaboration, coordination

Outputs: quality care, patient safety, patient satisfaction, wellness

Feedback: performance standards achievement, budget variances, errors, infection rate changes (positive and negative outcomes, and areas for improvement)

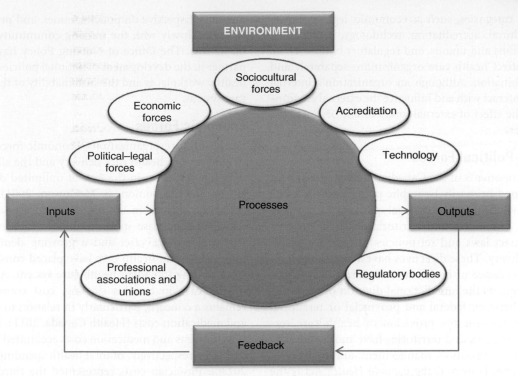

FIGURE 8-3 An open-systems model of a health care organization.

Chaos Theory

Chaos theory can extend open-systems theory or augment understandings of organizations in their contexts by relaxing assumptions of linear, cause-and-effect predictable relations to include random or unpredictable events as affecting organizations. Health care is not always as predictable and orderly as systems theorists would have us believe. In contrast to the somewhat orderly universe described in systems theory, in which an organization can be viewed in terms of a linear, cause-and-effect model, chaos theory sees the universe as filled with unpredictable and random events (Hawking, 1998). According to the proponents of chaos theory, organizations must be self-organizing and adapt readily to change in order to survive. Organizations, therefore, must accept that change is inevitable and unrelenting. When one embraces the tenets of chaos theory, one gives up on any attempt to create a permanent organizational structure. Using creativity and flexibility, successful managers will be those who can tolerate ambiguity, take risks, and experiment with new ideas that respond to each day's unique situation or environment.

INTERNAL FORCES INFLUENCING HEALTH CARE ORGANIZATIONS

The internal forces influencing health care organizations are numerous, and many are discussed in other chapters of this text so are not repeated here. For example, organizational structures are discussed in Chapter 9, technology in Chapter 12, costs and budgets in Chapter 13, care delivery strategies in Chapter 14, and staffing and scheduling in Chapter 15. People, materials, equipment, funds, information, policies, and infrastructure that support the operations of organizations may all be viewed as inputs to the internal processes of organizations, and the diversity of these inputs and those involved mean managing them can be complex.

EXTERNAL FORCES INFLUENCING HEALTH CARE ORGANIZATIONS

Organizations are strongly influenced by many changes, events, and conditions in their surrounding environments. These external forces are typically grouped into distinct categories, such as economic, legal–political, sociocultural, accreditation, technology, professional associations and unions, and regulatory bodies. These forces affect health care organizations separately and in combination. Although an organization's internal forces interact with and influence the external environment, the effect of external forces on the organization is greater.

Legal–Political Forces

The components of the Canadian health care system are shaped primarily by public policy and therefore are heavily influenced by legal–political forces. The federal, provincial, and territorial levels of government enact laws and set policies to regulate health care delivery. These directives have a major effect on the governance of health care organizations. Chapter 5 presents the jurisdictional division of responsibilities between federal and provincial or territorial governments for the provision of health care services. Provinces and territories have most authority over the organization, management, and delivery of health care. However, the *Canada Health Act* is the most influential legislation in health care. As mentioned earlier, the Act established five criteria that the provinces and territories must meet in order to receive federal funds for health care. These criteria encourage the provinces and territories to support and adhere to the principles of the *Canada Health Act*. Health Canada, a federal department, is responsible for administering provisions of the *Canada Health Act* and has either total or partial responsibility for other health-related acts, such as the *Controlled Drugs and Substances Act*, *Department of Health Act*, *Financial Administration Act*, and *Quarantine Act*. These Canadian statutes can be accessed at http://laws-lois.justice.gc.ca/eng/acts/.

Health Canada has a Strategic Policy Branch that plays a key role in health policy, communications, and consultations. It includes the Health Care Policy Directorate and the Office of Nursing Policy. The Health Care Policy Directorate is responsible for improving the access, quality, and integration of health care services to better meet the health needs of Canadians wherever they live or whatever their financial circumstances. This oversight ensures that the *Canada Health Act* will be implemented as it was intended. The Office of Nursing Policy advises Health Canada on the nursing perspective on policies, issues, and programs. It works closely with the nursing community to fulfill its role. The Office of Nursing Policy has been a partner in the development of national policies such as healthy workplaces and the sustainability of the health care system.

Economic Forces

For health care organizations, economic forces relate to efficiency in health care delivery and the allocation of scarce resources in the face of unlimited demands (R. D. Scott, Solomon, & McGowan, 2001). Scarce resources, increasing costs, a variable economy, an anticipated increase in the number of older adults who will require care, and a growing demand for improvement in health care have placed considerable strain on the Canadian health care system. Although the increase in costs is slowing, cost containment remains a concern, particularly in relation to hospital and medication costs (Health Canada, 2011). In 2011, hospital costs and medication costs accounted for 30% and 16%, respectively, of total health spending (CIHI, 2013c). Physician costs represented the third-largest cost at 15% of total health spending and also had the highest percentage growth among the top-three cost categories (3.6% compared with a 2.6% and 2.4% growth for hospital and medication costs, respectively) (CIHI, 2013c).

Hospitals have long been associated with high costs and inefficient management. Overlapping effort, wasted resources, and poor patient outcomes are areas of concern. Work inefficiency has been linked to poor quality of care and high costs. Integrated health care systems (Health Canada, 2011) and interprofessional clinical teams (Reeves, MacMillan, & van Soeren, 2010) are viewed as solutions to rationalizing health care costs and improving patient outcomes in hospitals. Strengthening primary health care is a proposed solution for controlling costs while improving access to community-based care. By focusing on chronic disease prevention and health promotion, the goal is to reduce chronic diseases, assist people to better manage their health, and avoid hospitalization for conditions that can be managed through community-based care.

The chronic shortage of nurses across Canada is a concern to governments and health care employers because it restricts productivity and future economic prospects (Knox, 2010). From an economic perspective, health care delivery is heavily dependent on health human resources, and efficiencies in services delivery can be achieved through unrestricted access to human resources. Access to the total pool of available nurses in Canada can be blocked by barriers to mobility that can be associated with differing professional regulatory requirements and regulations across provinces and territories. In 2012, the First Ministers issued the *Agreement on Internal Trade*, an intergovernmental trade agreement among the provinces and territories to encourage professional labour mobility (Internal Trade Secretariat, 2012). Dating back to 2006, Alberta, British Columbia, and Saskatchewan adopted the mutual recognition principle in their *Trade, Investment and Labour Mobility Agreement* (2006) that makes nurse mobility nearly seamless between these provinces. Nurses in these three provinces have unrestricted access to seek work. Provincial and territorial governments are also increasing efforts to foster the mobility of internationally qualified health care providers.

Sociocultural Forces

Sociocultural forces—such as customs, values, beliefs, education, level of income, and patterns of behaviour—influence lifestyle and well-being. Attitudes toward health and patterns of accessing health care may be shaped by these factors. For example, compared with affluent people, those of lower socioeconomic status are more likely to have poor health and to require more care. In 2005, WHO identified the social determinants of health, which are the conditions in which people are born, live, and work; these conditions are shaped by economics, social policies, and politics. According to WHO (2014b), "the social determinants of health are mostly responsible for health inequities." The social determinants of health are listed in Box 8-3. In 2009, the Canadian Nurses Association (CNA) published a position paper confirming the integral role of nurses in acting on the social determinants of health. Those social determinants of health subject to modification involve macro economies and broad social agendas of governments. Part of the role of nurses is to influence these agendas through advocacy and political action. Nurse managers and leaders also need to consider how the social determinants of health affect

---

BOX 8-3 SOCIAL DETERMINANTS OF HEALTH

Income and social status
Social support networks
Education and literacy
Employment/working conditions
Social environments
Physical environments
Personal health practices and coping skills
Healthy child development
Biology and genetic endowment
Health services
Gender
Culture

the patient population in their health care organizations to best facilitate organizational planning and operations.

Accreditation

Many health care organizations participate in accreditation, which is "a process of assessing health services against standards, to identify what is being done well and what needs to be improved" (Accreditation Canada, 2013). The accreditation process is ongoing and involves the periodic evaluation of the extent to which the organization is meeting the set standards. Accreditation evaluations by external reviewers (surveyors) often require accredited hospitals and other accredited health care organizations to implement changes. Thus, for organizations seeking to maintain accreditation, the need to achieve the minimum standards set for accreditation effectively becomes an external force for change. Chapter 21 provides more details on accreditation.

ISO international standards (http://www.iso.org) may also apply to select ancillary and supply organizations in the health care sector.

Technology

In the health care field, technological advances can influence the ability of health care providers to improve clinical practice and communication (Anvari, 2007). They are also essential to improving quality of life and life expectancy (see also Chapter 12).

Consider the advances made in joint replacements, diagnostic imaging, and coronary procedures as examples. Some might argue that these innovations are not cost effective and that their costs will likely increase in the future due to the demands of a large, aging population. Less expensive and effective innovations may reduce costs in the short term, but as the population of older adults grows, the high demand for these innovations will increase and so too will their costs.

Information technology, now regarded as an essential investment for health care delivery, has the capacity to improve the efficiency of work processes in health care organizations. Electronic health records, for example, can improve the accuracy of information and accelerate the flow of a patient's information to all those who are directly involved in the patient's care (Gagnon, Ouiment, Godin, et al., 2010). Manual errors, such as the duplication of tests and errors in recording can be reduced. Ordering and dispensing medications can be streamlined and controlled. Tracking systems can be used for storage and retrieval of information that can be recalled for treatment and research purposes. Videoconferencing networks, such as the Ontario Telestroke Program, facilitate emergency neurological consultations and provide timely access for patients in areas that do not have access to specialists.

The new Canadian Classification of Health Interventions (CCI) database represents a significant advance in data on health care procedures (CIHI, 2009). The database classifies a range of interventions more precisely than in the past, which makes it more responsive to user needs. It is the new national standard for classifying diagnostic, therapeutic, support, and surgical interventions for all health care provider groups. The frequency of interventions can be tracked over time through the CCI. The new database also includes codes for nursing that were not included previously, making it possible to link positive nursing-specific actions to patient outcomes (Albanese, Evans, Schantz, et al., 2010). However, if a code does not exist for an intervention that is not easily defined (e.g., emotional support), that intervention will not be added to the database, even though it contributes to patient outcomes.

In Canada, the drive to implement electronic health records (EHR) and other health information technology as widely as possible has been strong. The implementation of EHRs requires skilled leadership and management to negotiate best uses. Canada Health Infoway was established in 2001 as a not-for-profit organization funded by the federal government to work with health care organizations and others to foster and "accelerate the development, adoption and effective use of digital health innovations across Canada . . . [to] help deliver better quality and access to care and more efficient delivery of health services for patients and clinicians" (Canada Health Infoway, 2014, p. 1). Early stages of development will require training and vigilance in developing this technological system.

> **EXERCISE 8-2**
> Identify sociocultural patient-care needs that you have observed in health care organizations. Give examples to show what you would do to address these needs.

Professional Associations and Unions

Professional associations are not-for-profit, voluntary organizations that act in the interests of their members and their patients (see Chapters 5 and 20). They promote the advancement of the discipline by facilitating continuing education and research; mentoring in career development; advocating on issues relevant to the discipline; promoting interaction among members through conferences and networking; and providing access to personal or career-related benefits. Unions are not-for-profit organizations that have significant influence on the organization of health human resources (the labour force) in health care. Those employed in a position covered by a collective agreement are normally required to join the union and contribute financially to union operations through the payment of union fees. Like professional associations, union organizations also support advancement of the nursing discipline, continuing education, research, mentorship, advocacy, healthy work environments, advocacy, and networking. In Canadian health care organizations, professional associations and unions have a major influence on policymaking, organizational structures, work, and professional practices that affect health care organizations.

Influence on Policy. Many health care provider associations and unions lobby governments on behalf of their disciplines and members. National organizations, such as the Canadian Medical Association and the Canadian Nurses Association, lobby governments to influence policy development or changes to advance the interests of patients, the community, and their profession. Each province and territory has its own professional health associations and regulatory bodies that may lobby parliamentary committees for changes in policy or new policy directions to improve the status of a group or deal with its issues (Chapter 2 provides a complete list of nursing regulatory bodies). The Canadian Nurses Association is a federation of provincial and territorial nursing associations and, therefore, represents a national voice when seeking to influence policymakers. Similarly, unions from across the provinces and territories often have associated national federations to bring a national voice to important issues. They use a variety of media to gain support for a proposal, including press releases, position papers, campaigns, radio or television interviews, and posters. Access to politicians and government officials can be helpful to influence change. Nurses have successfully influenced policies on entry to practice, scope of practice, work environments, and health promotion initiatives. Large organizations have the ability, time, and resources to be successful in lobbying, but some issues require sustained lobbying effort over years to achieve results.

Influence on Organizational Structures. Both Canadian professional nursing associations and union organizations have drawn attention to the structure and health of work environments and limitations of care delivery models, all of which have been sources of concern for the past two decades. Over this period, many studies were conducted highlighting heavy workloads, excessive overtime, inflexible scheduling, safety hazards, poor management, and few opportunities for leadership and professional development (Shamian & El-Jardali, 2007). However, despite the support of available research study data and the efforts of many to change work environments, these issues persist and continue to require the consideration of effective leaders. Managers and leaders can draw on research to support their efforts to make changes in their organizations. See the Research Perspective for an example of a study on empowering work environments.

🔍 RESEARCH PERSPECTIVE

Resource: Greco, P., Laschinger, H. K., & Wong, C. (2006). Leader empowering behaviours, staff nurse empowerment and work engagement/burnout. *Nursing Leadership, 19*(4), 41–56.

The authors suggest that the nurse leader's empowering behaviours can be pivotal in the way nurses react to their work environment. The objective of this survey of 322 staff nurses in acute care hospitals was to test a model examining the relationship between nurse leaders' empowerment behaviours, perceptions of staff empowerment, and areas of work life and work engagement using Kanter's (1979) theory of structural power in organizations. The authors' findings showed that staff nurses perceived their leaders' behaviours to be somewhat empowering and their work environment to be moderately empowering. In all, 53% of staff nurses reported severe levels of burnout. The staff nurses reported that leader-empowering behaviour had an indirect effect on their emotional exhaustion (burnout) through structural empowerment and overall fit in the six areas of work life studied. These findings indicate that the leader's empowering behaviours can enhance the compatibility between a nurse and his or her job and may prevent burnout.

Implications for Practice
The authors suggested that when leaders develop organizational structures that empower nurses to deliver optimal care, they promote a greater sense of fit between nurses' expectations of work life quality and organizational goals and processes. This greater sense of fit can create a stronger work engagement and lower burnout. Reforms in health care delivery may lead to greater empowerment of nurses.

Influence on Practice and Research. The influence of professional associations and unions on practice and research is significant, although often indirect. For example, since 1999 the Registered Nurses' Association of Ontario (RNAO) has established over 50 best practice guidelines; 10 of these best practice guidelines pertain to healthy workplaces (http://rnao.ca/bpg/guidelines). Specialty practice groups facilitate professional development of their members by preparing them for certification and helping them gain research skills. Members are encouraged to share their practices and research at conferences and professional gatherings. Some groups provide scholarships for graduate work. The Canadian Federation of Nurses Unions lobbies governments to improve the working conditions of nurses.

Many nonprofessional specialty organizations influence health care organizations. Not-for-profit volunteer groups run by members of the community and supported by health care providers manage organizations such as the Canadian Diabetes Association and the Heart and Stroke Foundation of Canada. These organizations raise funds to support research, education, personal care, and disease control. They also lobby governments.

EXERCISE 8-3

Visit the Web site of the nurses' association or college that licenses nurses in your province or territory. Examine the processes for licensing nurses and monitoring nursing care. What processes are in place to ensure the public's safety? What regulatory processes are in place to support the interests of the public?

Regulatory Bodies

Health care organizations are regulated and monitored by external organizations. Chapter 5 also presents some of the regulations that affect health care organizations. Most health care organizations are legally accountable to federal and provincial or territorial ministries of health and are mandated to protect the health and safety of the patients and the communities they serve. In addition, individuals who belong to professional groups, such as nurses, are accountable to the professional regulatory organizations that license and monitor them. As the number of policy-driven interventions increases in response to changing circumstances, organizations will have to become more involved with government agencies to plan, implement, and evaluate projects.

Managing regulatory changes can be challenging. As new regulations are applied to policies and practices in response to health care concerns, people often experience information overload, a steep learning curve, and, in some instances, a resistance to change. The demands on individuals will likely increase as the integration of health care providers and organizations increases.

The following examples illustrate how regulatory changes impact health care organizations.

The recent emphasis on patient safety and quality care emerged from an international concern about troubling data on medication errors, drug-resistant infections within hospitals, and other negative indicators. Canada, together with a number of other industrialized countries, instituted programs and measures to change practices within health care organizations.

In Canada, two agencies were established to guide improvements in education, system innovation, communication, regulatory affairs, and research that influence improved safety practices: the Canadian Patient Safety Institute (CPSI; http://www.patientsafetyinstitute.ca) and the Institute for Safe Medication Practices (ISMP; http://www.ismp-canada.org). ISMP, CIHI, and Health Canada developed the Canadian Root Cause Analysis Framework for health care organizations to analyze contributing factors that led to a critical incident or close-call medication error. Consistent with other countries, health care organizations responded by implementing health promotion programs, such as an intensive handwashing campaign to control the spread of infection. Cooperation and adherence with policy was encouraged, and work was monitored closely to ensure good results.

In 2010, Ontario passed the *Excellent Care for All Act* to strengthen quality care, safety, and accountability in all Ontario health care organizations. The Act requires that health care providers set up quality committees to guide and report on specific quality initiatives, prepare quality improvement plans, make results of interventions available to the public, conduct patient satisfaction surveys, and develop ways to improve public relations. The Act mandated a more rigorous approach to quality control, called quality improvement (QI). QI achieves quality through an "incremental change" to solving persistent and elusive problems in the workplace. Incremental change is believed to be effective because small, well-developed changes that build on previous successes tend to be more effective and last longer than radical change (Dunphy, 2008). Health care organizations responded by implementing QI principles to set goals and guide work performance. They also instituted QI teams, trained people to use QI, and implemented QI programs. QI is discussed in more detail in Chapter 21.

HEALTH HUMAN RESOURCES

The large workforce that sustains health care delivery in Canada comprises many health care providers, including regulated and unregulated health care providers. The focus in this chapter is on the regulated nursing workforce. Regulated nurses comprise the largest proportion of health care providers in Canada (CIHI, 2013a). Between 2008 and 2012, Canada's regulated nursing workforce grew by 7%, outpacing both the growth in the Canadian labour force and the general population (CIHI, 2013d). In 2010, there were 1040 regulated nurses per 100 000 population compared with 237 physicians, 59 dentists, and 89 pharmacists per 100 000 population (CIHI, 2013a). Most health care providers work in hospitals, including 57% of the regulated nurses in Canada (CIHI, 2013d). In 2012, there were 365 422 regulated nurses in Canada, with registered nurses representing 74%, practical nurses 24%, and psychiatric nurses 2% of all regulated nurses (CIHI, 2013d). Between 2008 and 2012, the practical nurse workforce grew by more than 18%, registered nurses by 4%, and psychiatric nurses by less than 5% (CIHI, 2013d). A 15-year percentage growth rate report on 16 health care provider groups (1997 to 2011) ranked the top three growth areas as social workers (163%), dental hygienists (102%), and occupational therapists (102%); it ranked the bottom three growth areas as medical laboratory technologists (15%), registered nurses (18%), and dentists (28%) (growth rates of practical nurses and psychiatric nurses were not reported because of data variations) (CIHI, 2013a). Each health care provider group and professional designation has specific educational requirements and is associated with a type and scope of practice based on regulation. These factors influence decisions made by managers and leaders about the availability of nurses and the mix of skills required in various organizations (see Chapter 14).

Education

Most professional disciplines require a minimum of four years of undergraduate education to enter practice (CIHI, 2013a). Registered nurses require a baccalaureate degree (except in Quebec) to enter practice, and practical nurses and psychiatric nurses require a diploma to enter practice. National exams are required for all regulated nurses entering practice in Canada. Master's degrees in nursing can generally be completed in two years, and a doctor of philosophy (PhD) in nursing can generally be completed in four to six years. A master's degree for entry to practice as a nurse practitioner is not required in every province or territory, but it is required in most. The number of nurse practitioners grew by 96% between 2008 and 2012 and reached a total of 3286 (CIHI, 2013d). Chapter 29 discusses educational options in professional nursing practice.

Type of Practice

Health care in Canada has traditionally focused on episodic and responsive primary care delivery models, with a focus on hospitals (Health Canada, 2011). However, with changing demographics and focus on finding sustainable solutions to maintaining a top-rated health care system shifts to more distributed, community-based care, health promotion and prevention are modifying the emphasis on types of health care provider practices (Health Canada, 2011). Nurses practise in most areas of health care, at different levels of care, as generalists and specialists, and along the full continuum of care. Most nurses are employed by organizations, but nurse practitioners and some specialty nurses may maintain independent practices. Funding cuts in the past decade have influenced the ratio of regulated nursing staff to unregulated staff assisting in the delivery of nursing services, which has raised concerns among nurses about the quality of care and safety of the work environment in which they work. Staff shortages, heavy workloads, and work delivery models are among the contributing factors to workplace problems (O'Brien-Pallas, Murphy, Laschinger, et al., 2005).

Scope of Practice

Expanding the scope of practice for nurses is expected to alleviate the costs of delivering care, improve access to care, and increase work efficiency. In Canada, unregulated health care providers have been assigned some traditional nurse tasks, such as administering routine medication and obtaining routine vital signs. Additionally, the roles and responsibilities of licensed practical nurses have expanded to help meet the needs of nursing staff and cost management. Efforts continue within health care organizations to best match or rationalize qualifications and competencies to essential health provision tasks. New roles, such as physician's assistant, navigator in case management, and program manager have also been introduced. Several provinces and territories have expanded the scope of practice for a number of health care providers; for example, in some jurisdictions, nurse practitioners are authorized to set broken bones, dentists can write prescriptions, pharmacists can write refills for medications, and physiotherapists can order X-rays and treat injuries. Fricke (2005) provided a rationale for extending physiotherapy into a primary care role as first contact or consultant for musculoskeletal conditions. A study of the effectiveness of geriatric advanced practice nurses in rural, underserviced areas showed that these practitioners were not only effective in providing essential health care services to older adults but also could be expected to make major contributions to changing gerontology practice (Higuchi, Hagen, Brown, et al., 2006). Leaders will have roles in both influencing and responding to changing landscapes around scope of practice in health care providers.

EXERCISE 8-4

Ask a public health nurse and a community nurse who provide direct patient care about their roles. How do their roles differ?

CONCLUSION

Knowledge of the contexts in which health care organizations operate is important to understanding the potential effects of various forces on organizational goal achievement. External forces such as legal–political, economic, sociocultural, accreditation, technology, professional associations and unions, and regulatory bodies will continue to shape health care delivery in Canada. The key principles of the *Canada Health Act*, continued emphasis on advancing reform in primary health care goals, and emphasis on patient safety, cost economies, and quality improvement remain paramount. A systems theory perspective offers a holistic approach to understanding health care organizations and the internal and external forces that influence them. Nurses represent a significant portion of the health human resources necessary for health care organizations to reach their goals, and all nurses—whether leaders or followers—benefit from an increased understanding of the context in which health care organizations operate. With this knowledge, nurses can better understand organizational structures, planning, operations, and responses to change as organizations attempt to achieve their goals. Savvy nurse managers and leaders assess the internal and external forces that influence their health care organization when planning and before acting.

💡 A SOLUTION

Alex found that many patients remained in the emergency department after their medical issues were resolved because of emotional or mental health issues. Therefore, he contacted the Mental Health Assessment Group to get their help in prioritizing these patients' management and discharge. He also found that a number of patients were waiting for nursing, physiotherapy, and other support staff services to coordinate plans for discharge. Alex also alerted administration about the need for a more rapid patient assessment and management plan. Often patients await consultation from physicians who are otherwise occupied with other patients. Alex raised the problematic emergency department overcrowding issue with the physicians and asked for their help in accelerating patient discharge.

Would these solutions work for you? Why or why not?

▌ THE EVIDENCE

A study by Edwards, Davies, Ploeg, et al. (2007) set out to describe the impact of implementing six nursing Best Practice Guidelines (BPGs) on nurses' familiarity with patient referral resources and referral practices.

Although referring patients to community care services is important for optimum continuity of care, referrals between hospital and community sectors are often problematic. A pre- and post-study design was used. For each BPG topic, referral resources were identified. Information about these resources was presented at education sessions for nurses. Pre- and post-questionnaires were completed by a random sample of 257 nurses at 7 hospitals, 2 home visiting nursing services, and 1 public health unit. Average response rates for pre- and post-implementation questionnaires were 71% and 54%, respectively. Chart audits were completed for three BPGs ($n = 421$ pre- and 332 post-implementation). Post-hospital discharge patient interviews were conducted for four BPGs ($n = 152$ pre- and 124 post-implementation). Statistically significant increases occurred in nurses' familiarity with resources for all BPGs, and they self-reported referrals to specific services for three guidelines. Higher rates of referrals were observed for services that were part of the organization where the nurses worked. There was almost a complete lack of referrals to Internet sources. No significant differences between pre- and post-implementation referral rates were observed in the chart documentation or in patients' reports of referrals. Implementing nursing BPGs, which

included recommendations on patient referrals, produced mixed results. Nurses' familiarity with referral resources does not necessarily change their referral practices. Nurses can play a vital role in initiating and supporting appropriate patient referrals. BPGs should include specific recommendations on effective referral processes, and this information should be tailored to the community setting where implementation occurs.

NEED TO KNOW NOW

- Understand that the Canadian health care system faces ongoing challenges.
- Know the role of federal and provincial or territorial governments in funding, organizing, and delivering care.
- Know the role of Regional Health Authorities and public–private partnerships.
- Be able to describe the types and classifications of health care services.

- View the health care organization as an open system. Be aware of both the internal forces and external forces (legal–political, economic, sociocultural, technology, accreditation, professional associations, regulatory bodies) that influence a health care organization.
- Identify the trends and impact of health human resources on health care organizations.

CHAPTER CHECKLIST

- The health care organization, related governmental structures, and funding arrangements that support Canadian health care services are key to understanding heath care organizations in their contexts.
- According to the *Canada Health Act*, to qualify for federal health care funding, provinces and territories must meet five criteria:
  - Public administration
  - Comprehensiveness
  - Universal coverage
  - Portability
  - Accessible
- Canadian health care is funded through federal taxation and provincial or territorial taxation, with most revenue coming from income taxes and consumption taxes.
- Contemporary health care organizations have adopted a more flexible, responsive, team-oriented approach to management, consistent with the principles of open-systems theory.
- As part of health care reform, most provincial health ministries have delegated the responsibility for the delivery and administration of health services to Regional Health Authorities.

- Health care services in Canada can be divided into a framework based on the sequence of access: primary care services, secondary care services, to additional health care services:
  - Primary health care services are first-contact services for routine problems and emergencies. They are also the point of referral and coordination of patient care through the continuum of care. Primary care and primary health care are distinct. *Primary care* is the first point of contact with a general practitioner, and *primary health care* is a community-based health care service philosophy that is focused on illness prevention, health promotion, treatment, rehabilitation, and identification of people at risk.
  - Secondary health care services take place after the initial patient contact with primary health care services. The primary care practitioner refers the patient to specialized care that may be provided in a hospital, home, community, or long-term care or chronic care facility.
  - Additional health care services are those services (e.g., prescription medications [with some

exceptions], dental care, and vision care) not usually covered by public health insurance.
- Health care services can also be classified by type of service:
  - Public health services/prevention services
  - Community care services
    - Continuing care and rehabilitation
    - Residential care
    - Community mental health and addiction services
    - Home care services
  - Hospital care services (primary, secondary, tertiary, quaternary)
    - Ambulatory care
    - Emergency care
    - Acute care
    - Specialized services
- An organization survives by acquiring inputs from its external environment and interacts with other components to process them into products or services to be released to the external environment as outputs.

- Open-systems theory is a conventional way of viewing the health care organization that allows examination of the organization as a dynamic, interactive system.
- Health care organizations are affected by internal and external forces, an understanding of which helps with leading and managing organizations.
- Legal–political, economic, sociocultural, accreditation, technology, professional associations and unions, and regulatory bodies are broad categories of external forces that influence health care organizations.
- Health human resources represent a mix of regulated and unregulated health care providers. Nurse shortages, the educational requirements of nurses, and type and scope of practice affect health care organization performance.
- Public insurance covers the following hospital services: standard or public ward accommodation and meals; nursing service; diagnostic procedures such as blood tests and X-rays; the administration of medications; and the use of operating rooms, case rooms, and anaesthetic facilities.

TIPS FOR NURSE MANAGERS AND LEADERS

- Understand the contexts and large organizational frameworks in which health care organizations work to better understand the influences that act upon health care organizations and are critical to effective organizational leadership and management.
- Understand that nurses represent a significant portion of the health human resources necessary for health care organizations to reach their goals. All nurses, whether leaders or followers, benefit from an increased understanding of the contexts in which health care organizations operate.

- Gain knowledge of the external forces that affect health care organizations to be able to systematically assess the external environment for threats and opportunities.
- Understand why primary health care principles hold the most promise for creating the best health care system. The social determinants of health are important indicators for primary nursing practice.
- Research new health care delivery models, such as integrated primary care, to continually acquire new knowledge and skills in leadership for managing integrated teams.

evolve WEBSITE

Visit the Evolve website for Suggested Readings, Internet Resources, and additional resources related to the content in this chapter: http://evolve.elsevier.com/Canada/Yoder-Wise/leading/.

REFERENCES

Statutes

Canada Health Act, RSC 1985, c. C-6 (Canada).
Excellent Care for All, SO 2010, **c. 14 (Ontario)**.

Texts

Accreditation Canada. (2013). Accreditation basics. Retrieved from http://www.accreditation.ca/accreditation-basics.

Albanese, M. P., Evans, D. A., Schantz, C. A., et al. (2010). Engaging in clinical nurses in quality and performance improvement activities. *Nursing Administration Quarterly, 34*(3), 226–245.

Anvari, M. (2007). Impact of information technology on human resources in healthcare. *Healthcare Quarterly, 10*(4), 84–88.

Butler, M., & Teidemann, M. (2013). *The federal role in health and health care (in brief)*. Ottawa, ON: Library of Parliament.

Canada Health Infoway. (2014). 2014–2015 Summary corporate plan: Improving health care through innovation. Retrieved from https://www.infoway-inforoute.ca/index.php.

Canadian Institute for Health Information. (2009). Canadian classification of health interventions, Vol. 3—Tabular list. Retrieved from http://www.cihi.ca.

Canadian Institute for Health Information. (2013a). *Canada's health care providers, 1997–2011—A reference guide*. Ottawa, ON: Author. Retrieved from https://secure.cihi.ca/estore/productFamily.htm?pf=PFC2161&lang=en&media=0.

Canadian Institute for Health Information. (2013b). Health spending in Canada. Retrieved from http://www.cihi.ca/CIHI-ext-portal/internet/en/document/spending+and+health+workforce/spending/release_29oct13_infogra1pg.

Canadian Institute for Health Information. (2013c). *National health expenditure trends 1975 to 2013*. Ottawa, ON: Author. Retrieved from https://secure.cihi.ca/free_products/NHEXTrendsReport_EN.pdf.

Canadian Institute for Health Information. (2013d). *Regulated nurses, 2012—Summary report*. Ottawa, ON: Author. Retrieved from https://secure.cihi.ca/estore/productFamily.htm?locale=en&pf=PFC2385.

Canadian Institute for Health Information. (2014). Information about health care. Retrieved from http://www.cihi.ca/CIHI-ext-portal/internet/EN/Theme/types+of+care/cihi000002.

Canadian Nurses Association. (2005). *Primary health care: A summary of the issues*. Ottawa, ON: Author. Retrieved from http://www.cna-aiic.ca/sitecore%20modules/web/~/media/cna/page%20content/pdf%20fr/2013/09/05/19/03/bg7_primary_health_care_e.pdf#search=%22primary health care a summary%22.

Canadian Nurses Association. (2009) Position statement: Determinants of health. Retrieved from http://yrna.ca/wp-content/uploads/CNA-Determinants-of-Health-2009.pdf.

CBC News. (2013, March 28). Hospital parking rates a "tax" on sick Canadians. Retrieved from http://www.cbc.ca/news/canada/hospital-parking-rates-a-tax-on-sick-canadians-1.1346722.

Department of Finance Canada. (2014). Federal support to provinces and territories. Retrieved from http://www.fin.gc.ca/fedprov/mtp-eng.asp.

Dunphy, D. (2008). Sustainable organizations. In T. Cummings (Ed.), *Organizational Development* (pp. 216–219). Newbury Park, CA: Sage.

Edwards, N., Davies, B., Ploeg, J., et al. (2007). Implementing nursing best practice guidelines: Impact on patient referrals. *BMC Nursing, 6*(4). doi:10.1186/1472-6955-6-4

Fricke, M. (2005). *Physiotherapy and primary health care: Evolving opportunities*. Winnipeg, MB: Manitoba Branch of the Canadian Physiotherapy Association, the College of Physiotherapists of Manitoba and the Department of Physical Therapy, School of Medical Rehabilitation, University of Manitoba.

Gagnon, M. P., Ouiment, M., Godin, G., et al. (2010). Multi-level analysis of electronic health record adoption by health care providers: A study protocol. *Implementation Science, 5*, 30. doi:10.1186/1748-5908-5-30

Greco, P., Laschinger, H. K., & Wong, C. (2006). Leader empowering behaviours, staff nurse empowerment and work engagement/burnout. *Nursing Leadership, 19*(4), 41–56.

Hawking, S. (1998). *A brief history of time*. London, UK: Bantam Press.

Health Canada. (2003). 2003 First Ministers' accord on health care renewal. Retrieved from http://www.hc-sc.gc.ca/hcs-sss/delivery-prestation/fptcollab/2003accord/fs-if_2-eng.php.

Health Canada. (2011). Canada's health care system. Retrieved from http://www.hc-sc.gc.ca/hcs-sss/pubs/system-regime/2011-hcs-sss/index-eng.php.

Health Canada. (2013). *Canada Health Act annual report 2012–2013*. Ottawa, ON: Author.

Health Canada. (2014). About primary health care. Retrieved from http://www.hc-sc.gc.ca/hcs-sss/prim/about-apropos-eng.php.

Health Council of Canada. (2011). Progress report 2011: Health care renewal in Canada. Retrieved from http://healthcouncilcanada.ca/rpt_det.php?id=165.

Health Council of Canada. (2014). *Progress timeline 2003–2013: Highlights of health care reform*. Toronto, ON: Author. Retrieved from http://www.healthcouncilcanada.ca/rpt_det.php?id=481.

Higuchi, K. A., Hagen, B., Brown S., et al. (2006). A new role for advanced practice nurses in Canada: Bridging the gap in health services for rural older adults. *Journal of Gerontology Nurses, 32*(7), 49–55.

Internal Trade Secretariat. (2012). *Agreement on internal trade (consolidated version)*. Winnipeg, MB. Retrieved from http://www.ait-aci.ca/en/ait/ait_en.pdf.

Johns, G., & Saks, A. M. (2001). Organizational behaviour. Toronto, ON: Pearson Education.

Kanter, R. M. (1979). Power failure in management circuits. *Harvard Business Review, 57*, 65–75.

Knox, R. (2010). Who can work where? Reducing barriers to labour mobility in Canada: Backgrounder, CD Howe Institute. Retrieved from http://www.cdhowe.org/pdf/backgrounder_131.pdf.

Liebler, J. G., & McConnell, C. R. (2012). *Management principles for health professionals*. Mississauga, ON: Jones & Bartlett Learning.

Marchildon, G. P. (2013). Canada: Health system review. *Health Systems in Transition, 15*(1), 1–179. Retrieved from http://www.euro.who.int/__data/assets/pdf_file/0011/181955/e96759.pdf.

Morris, J. J., & Clarke, C. D. (2011). *Law for Canadian health care administrators* (2nd ed.). Markham, ON: Butterworths.

O'Brien-Pallas, L., Murphy, G. T., Laschinger, H., et al. (2005). *Canadian survey of nurses from three occupational groups.* Ottawa, ON: The Nursing Sector Study Corporation.

Public Health Agency of Canada. (2011). What determines health? Retrieved from http://www.phac-aspc.gc.ca/ph-sp/determinants/index-eng.php.

Public Health Agency of Canada. (2013). Background. Retrieved from http://www.phac-aspc.gc.ca/about_apropos/back-cont-eng.php.

Reeves, S., Macmillan, K., & van Soeren, M. (2010). Leadership of interprofessional health and social care teams: A socio-historical analysis. *Journal of Nursing Management, 18*(3), 258–264. doi:10.1111/j.1365-2834.2010.01077.x

Scott, R. D. II, Solomon, S. L., & McGowan, J. E. Jr. (2001). Applying economic principles to health care [Special issue]. *Emerging Infectious Diseases, 7*(2), 282–285.

Scott, W. R. (2002). *Organizations: Rational, natural, and open systems.* Upper Saddle River, NJ: Prentice Hall.

Shamian, J., & El-Jardali, F. (2007). Healthy workplaces for health workers in Canada: Knowledge transfer and uptake in policy and practice. *Healthcare Papers, 7,* 6–25.

Thompson, J. D. (1967). *Organization in action.* New York, NY: McGraw-Hill.

Trade, Investment and Labour Mobility Agreement. (2006). *Trade, Investment and Labour Mobility Agreement.* Retrieved from http://www.tilma.ca/the_agreement.asp.

World Bank. (2007). Strategy for HNP results—Healthy development: Annex L. Retrieved from http://siteresources.worldbank.org.

World Health Organization. (1978). Declaration of Alma-Ata. International Conference on Primary Health Care, Alma-Ata, USSR, 6–12. Retrieved from http://www.who.int/publications/almaata_declaration_en.pdf.

World Health Organization. (2005). What is a health system. Retrieved from http://www.who.int/features/qa/28/en/.

World Health Organization. (2014a). Primary health care. Retrieved from http://www.who.int/topics/primary_health_care/en/.

World Health Organization. (2014b). What are social determinants of health? Retrieved from http://www.who.int/social_determinants/sdh_definition/en/.

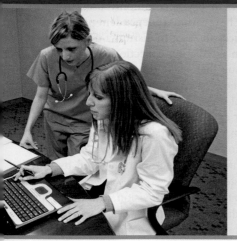

Understanding and Designing Organizational Structures

Mary E. Mancini
Adapted by Carol A. Wong

This chapter explains key concepts related to organizational structures and provides information on designing effective structures. This information can be used to help new managers function in an organization and to design structures that support work processes. An underlying theme is designing organizational structures that will respond to the continuous changes taking place in the health care environment.

OBJECTIVES

- Analyze the relationships among mission, vision, and philosophy statements and organizational structure.
- Analyze factors that influence the design of an organizational structure.
- Compare and contrast the major types of organizational structures.
- Evaluate the forces that are necessitating reengineering of organizational systems.

TERMS TO KNOW

bureaucracy	organization	service-line structure
chain of command	organizational chart	shared governance
flat organizational structure	organizational culture	span of control
functional structure	organizational structure	staff function
hierarchy	organizational theory	system
hybrid organizational structure	philosophy	systems theory
line function	redesign	vision
matrix structure	re-engineering	
mission	restructuring	

❓ A CHALLENGE

A new hospital was created by the merger of two former small community hospitals. This new organization has experienced two different leadership structures since the merger over 5 years ago. These two leadership structures contributed to at least two sets of sometimes conflicting operating policies that direct care. As a result, the standard of care was also driven by two different sets of policies. After Nurse Laurie's appointment as director of Patient Care Programs, she was responsible for leading implementation of a new organizational plan. However, implementation of the plan was hindered because several of the nurse manager and supervisor positions were vacant. Sometimes no nurse manager was available to clarify which practice should be followed or to recognize any major clinical conflicts that could lead to significant patient-care problems.

What might you do if you were Laurie?

INTRODUCTION

People have always organized themselves into groups. The term **organization** has multiple meanings. It can refer to a business structure designed to support specific business goals and processes, or it can refer to a group of individuals working together to achieve a common purpose. Regardless of how the term is used, learning to determine how an organization accomplishes its work, how to operate productively within an organization, and how to influence organizational processes is essential to a successful professional nursing practice.

Organizational theory (sometimes called *organizational studies*) is the systematic analysis of how organizations and their component parts act and interact. Organizational theory is based largely on the systematic investigation of the effectiveness of specific organizational designs in achieving their purpose. Organizational theory development is a process of creating knowledge to understand the effect of identified factors, such as (1) organizational culture; (2) organizational technology, which is defined as all the work being carried out; and (3) organizational structure or organizational development. A purpose of such work is to determine how organizational effectiveness might be predicted or controlled through the design of the organizational structure.

Specific organizational theories provide insight into areas such as effective organizational structures,

motivation of employees, decision making, and leadership. **Systems theory** is commonly used in health care to analyze how various independent parts interact to form a unified whole or to disrupt a unified whole. A **system** is an interacting collection of components or parts that together make up an integrated whole. The basic tenet of systems theory is that the individual components of any system interact with each other and with their environment. To be effective, professional nurses need to understand the specific part—role and function—they play within a system and how they interact, influence, and are influenced by other parts of the system.

An organization's mission, vision, and philosophy form the foundation for its structure and performance as well as the development of the professional practice models it uses. An organization's **mission**, or reason for the organization's existence, influences the design of the structure (e.g., to meet the health care needs of a designated population, to provide supportive and stabilizing care to an acute care population, or to prepare patients for a peaceful death). The **vision** is the articulated goals to which the organization aspires. A vision statement conveys an inspirational view of how the organization wishes to be described at some future time. It suggests how far to strive in all endeavours. Another key factor influencing structure is the organization's **philosophy**. A philosophy expresses the values and beliefs that members of the organization hold about the nature of their work, about the people to whom they provide service, and about themselves and others providing the services.

EXERCISE 9-1

Consider how you might use the information in the Introduction (1) to analyze an organization that you are considering joining to determine whether it fits your professional development plans, (2) to assess the functioning of an organization of which you are already a member, or (3) to make a plan to reengineer the structure or philosophy to better accomplish the mission of an organization you are considering joining or of which you are already a member.

MISSION

The mission statement is a formal written document that identifies the organization's unique purpose; its core values; the patients served; and the types of programs or services offered, such as education, supportive nursing care, rehabilitation, acute care, and home care (Williams, Smythe, Hadjistavropoulos, et al., 2005). The mission enacts the vision of the organization.

The mission statement sets the stage by defining the services to be offered, which, in turn, identify the kinds of technologies and human resources to be employed. The mission statement of health care systems typically refers to the larger community the organizations serve as well as the specific patient populations to whom they provide care. In Canada, health regions, also called *Regional Health Authorities (RHAs)*, are a governance model used by most provincial governments to administer and/or deliver health care to its citizens. Mission statements are generally developed for each RHA, and individual hospitals and other health care agencies that link to that RHA may or may not have their own mission statements. The Saskatoon Health Region in Saskatchewan has vision, mission, and values statements: its vision is "healthiest people, healthiest communities and exceptional service"; its mission is "to improve health through excellence and innovation . . ."; and its values include respect and

compassion, which are core to its vision (Saskatoon Health Region, 2014). Hospitals' or RHAs' missions are primarily health and treatment oriented; long-term care facilities' missions are primarily oriented toward maintenance, social support, and quality of life; and the missions of nursing centres are oriented toward promoting optimal health status for a defined group of people. The definition of services to be provided and its implications for technologies and human resources greatly influence the design of the **organizational structure** (how work is divided within an organization). Hospitals or health care organizations may also have vision, mission, and values statements specific to particular clinical services or professional departments such as nursing. An example of a mission statement for nursing at University Health Network (UHN), a large urban hospital, appears in Box 9-1.

Nursing, as a profession providing a service within a health care organization, often formulates its own mission statement that describes its contributions to achieve the organization's mission. One of the purposes of the nursing profession is to provide nursing

---

BOX 9-1 VISION, MISSION, STRATEGIC PRIORITIES/GOALS, AND PRACTICE PHILOSOPHY FOR NURSING AT UNIVERSITY HEALTH NETWORK

Nursing Vision
- Global Leaders in Nursing—New Knowledge and Innovation in Patient-Centred Care

Nursing Mission
- We provide competent, compassionate, collaborative care to patients and their families through a commitment in patient care, education, and research.

Nursing's Strategic Priorities/Goals
- Developing innovative nursing recruitment and retention strategies
- Creating a dynamic, high-quality practice environment
- Fostering high staff and patient satisfaction
- Offering leadership development; learning opportunities and professional development
- Creating a spirit of inquiry
- Giving voice to nurses at all levels

Practice—Patient-Centred Care
Patient-centred care at UHN [University Health Network] is about identifying and respecting the patient's perspective about what matters most to them and then tailoring the care we provide to enhance their experience in our care. At UHN, patients are a part of the team

and help to lead the team with what matters most to them and their family.

Patient-centred care incorporates other related efforts in pain management, patient education, health care provider-to-provider communication, patient safety, and cultural diversity. UHN policies, processes, systems, and physical environments are also being designed to support patient-centred care.

At University Health Network, each of us has a role to play—and the power to lead from where we stand to make a difference in the experience that patients and families have at UHN. Sometimes, it might be as simple as stopping to provide directions to family members. While at the bedside, it will mean taking the time to ask patients about their priorities, hopes, and dreams and to listen intently when asking about their questions, concerns, fears or anxieties about their care. To embrace our responsibility to respond compassionately to vulnerable persons, patient-centred care also requires practitioners and leaders to engage in guided self-reflection. This practice helps staff personally connect with the patient-centred care values of respect, dignity, and person as leader so their daily practice is continually directed by these values and so UHN leaders can have the courage to lead for patient-centred care.

Richards, J. (2014a). About nursing; Richards, J. (2014b). *Practice Patient-centred care.* UHN Nursing.

care to patients. The statement usually defines nursing and may be based on theories that ground the model of nursing used to guide nursing care delivery. Nursing's mission statement tells why nursing exists within the context of the organization. It is written so that others within the organization can know and understand nursing's role in achieving the employer's mission. The mission should be the guiding framework for decision making. It should be known and understood by other health care providers, by patients and their families, and by the community. It indicates the relationships among nurses and patients, employer personnel, the community, and health and illness. This statement provides direction for the evolving statement of values and beliefs or philosophy and the organizational structure. It should be reviewed for accuracy and updated routinely by professional nurses providing care.

VISION

Vision statements are future-oriented, purposeful statements designed to identify the desired future of an organization. They serve to unify all subsequent statements toward the view of the future and to convey the core message of the mission statement. Typically, vision statements are brief, consisting of only one or two phrases or sentences. An example of a vision statement for nursing appears in Box 9-1.

PHILOSOPHY

A philosophy is a written statement that articulates the values and beliefs held about the nature of the work required to accomplish the mission and the nature and rights of both the people being served and those providing the service. It states the nurse managers' and practitioners' vision of what they believe nursing management and practice are and sets the stage for developing goals to make that vision a reality. For example, the mission statement may incorporate the provision of individualized care as an organizational purpose. The philosophy statement would then support this purpose through an expression of a belief in the responsibility of nursing staff to act as patient advocates and to provide quality care according to the wishes of the patient, family, and significant others. Box 9-1 includes a statement of philosophy about the

practice of patient-centred care by nurses and other care team members of the UHN.

Philosophies are evolutionary in that they are shaped both by the social environment and by the stage of development of professionals delivering the service. Nursing staff reflect the values of their time. The values acquired through education are reflected in the nursing philosophy. Technology developments can also help shape philosophy. For example, information systems can provide people with data that allow them greater control over their work; workers are consequently able to make more decisions and take action that is more autonomous. Philosophies require updating to reflect the extension of rights brought about by such changes.

Many health care organizations focus primarily on short and succinct descriptions of their core values, which are the foundation for their mission and goals, rather than extended descriptions of philosophy. A review of Canadian hospital mission statements by Williams et al. (2005) found that values predominated other types of content and that the primary values included commitment to patient care, respect and esteem for staff, teamwork, commitment to community, education and research, trust, caring, and compassion.

EXERCISE 9-2

1. Take a few minutes to develop a personal philosophy statement based on your own vision values, and beliefs for your nursing practice.
2. Obtain a copy of the vision and philosophy statement for nursing at an organization you are familiar with or one you could see as your future employer. How do the vision, values, and beliefs in these documents compare with your own philosophy about nursing practice? Is there a fit or a mismatch for you?
3. Search the Web sites of your local regional health authority and/or health care agencies such as hospitals, nursing homes, or public health units and examine how they have described their missions, visions, values, and beliefs (or philosophy) for the services they provide. What commonalities and differences can you identify by employer?

ORGANIZATIONAL CULTURE

An organization's mission, vision, and philosophy shape and reflect organizational culture. Organizational culture is the implicit knowledge or values and beliefs within the organization that reflect the norms and traditions of the organization. It is exemplified by rituals and customary forms of practice, such as dress policy, the celebration of promotions, and professional performance. Examples of norms that reflect organizational culture are the characteristics of the people who are recognized as heroes by the organization and the behaviours—either positive or negative—that are accepted or tolerated within the organization.

In organizations, culture is demonstrated in two ways that can be either mutually reinforcing or conflict producing. Organizational culture is typically expressed in a formal manner via mission, vision, and philosophy statements; job descriptions; and policies and procedures. Beyond formal documents and verbal descriptions given by administrators and managers, organizational culture is also represented in the day-to-day experience of staff and patients. To many, it is the lived experience that reflects the true organizational culture. Do the decisions that are made within the organization consistently demonstrate that the organization values its patients and keeps their needs at the forefront? Are the employees treated with trust and respect, or are the words used in recruitment ads simply empty promises with little evidence to back them up? When there is a lack of congruity between the expressed organizational culture and the experienced organizational culture, confusion, frustration, and poor morale often result (Casida, 2008; Melnick, Ulaszek, Lin, et al., 2009).

Organizational culture can be effective and promote success and positive outcomes, or it can be ineffective and result in disharmony, dissatisfaction, and poor outcomes for patients, staff, and the organization. A number of workplace variables are influenced by organizational culture (Chen, 2008). A recent study by Laschinger, Finegan, and Wilk (2009) demonstrated the positive influence of two key aspects of organizational culture—collective perceptions of unit leadership and workplace empowerment—on individual nurses' organizational commitment in acute care hospitals. Workplace empowerment at the unit level can be construed as an aspect of unit or organizational culture. Similarly, culture may include the values and norms that influence how supportive the unit or workplace is as a learning environment for students or new staff members during orientation. The manner and degree to which students and/or orientees are respected, welcomed, and supported by members of the unit or organization may be determined by the culture (Henderson, Cooke, Creedy, et al., 2012). In addition, a culture that encourages seeking new ways of improving practice and promotes professional development of members also improves care outcomes.

When seeking employment or advancement, nurses need to assess the organization's culture and develop a clear understanding of existing expectations as well as the formal and informal communication patterns. Various techniques and tools can help nurses perform a cultural assessment of an organization, such as the Denison Organizational Culture Survey described by Casida (2008) and Hatch's three-perspective approach used in the systematic review of organizational culture research in nursing by Scott-Findlay and Estabrooks (2006). With a solid understanding of organizational culture, nurses will be better able to be effective change agents and help transform the organizations in which they work. The Research Perspective presents a qualitative study that explored the organizational attributes that best support the work of Canadian public health nurses. One of the major attributes was the local organizational culture (Meagher-Stewart, Underwood, MacDonald, et al., 2010).

RESEARCH PERSPECTIVE

Resource: Meagher-Stewart, D., Underwood, J., MacDonald, M., et al. (2010). Health policy: Organizational attributes that assure optimal utilization of public health nurses. *Public Health Nursing, 27*(5), 433–441. http://dx.doi.org/10.1111/j.1525-1446.2010.00876.x

This Canada-wide project included an investigation of the salient organizational attributes necessary to promote optimal use of public health nurses (PHNs). Considerable knowledge exists about work environment conditions that best support acute care nursing practice, but less is known about the organizational conditions that support public health nursing. As part of a pan-Canadian research program examining community nursing workforce capacity, this project used focus group methodology to identify the organizational attributes that best support PHNs to work effectively. Qualitative data were collected from 156 participants in 23 focus groups in 6 geographically diverse regions of Canada over a 6-month period in 2007–8. The focus groups included 12 groups of 85 front-line PHNs (from urban or rural/remote settings) and 11 groups of 71 policymakers or managers involved with public health nursing practice (from urban or rural/remote settings). Values and effective leadership were identified as key organizational attributes at all levels of the public health system. Three subthemes of

Continued

🔍 **RESEARCH PERSPECTIVE—cont'd**

attributes relevant to organizational culture were as follows: (1) a shared vision—participants stressed that effective organizations maintained a clear vision, mission, and goals for public health; (2) a culture of creativity and responsiveness to community needs at both the front-line and management levels; and (3) effective leadership, which participants identified as showing respect, trust, and support for PHNs working to their optimal capacity.

Implications for Practice
Findings from this study highlight the relevance of organizational culture and leadership to optimizing nursing outcomes in Canadian public health. The range of practice settings (rural/remote and urban) represented in the study increased the potential for application to other public health settings. Moreover, the consistency of findings across positions highlighted the importance of shared responsibility for creating organizational culture and vision. The need for effective and positive leadership at all levels is key to facilitating optimal work environments and practice outcomes.

FACTORS INFLUENCING ORGANIZATIONAL DEVELOPMENT

To be most effective, organizational structures must reflect the organization's mission, vision, philosophy, goals, and objectives. Organizational structure defines how work is organized, where decisions are made, and the authority and responsibility of workers. It provides a map for communication and outlines decision-making paths. As organizations change through restructuring (including mergers of hospitals, government mandates, and specific losses or additions of care programs), it is essential that structure changes to accomplish revised missions.

Probably the best theory to explain today's nursing organizational development is chaos (complexity, nonlinear, quantum) theory (see also Chapter 8). In essence, chaos theory suggests that lives—and organizations—are really web-like. Pulling on one small segment rearranges the web, a new pattern emerges, and yet the whole remains. This theory, applied to nursing organizations, suggests that differences logically exist between and among various organizations and that the constant environmental forces continue to affect the structure, its functioning, and the services. Brafman and Beckstrom (2008), in their aptly named book *The Starfish and the Spider*, identified how organizations differ and yet are successful. Spider organizations are built like a spider,

and when the head is destroyed, the spider dies. The starfish, on the other hand, can lose an appendage, and it just grows another one. In fact, a starfish, when cut in half, creates two starfish. Organizations that are controlled in a heavily centralized way can diminish quickly without the strong, central figure. Organizations that are self-generating quickly share leadership as needed and often continue to thrive. The important point for any organization is to find what is known as the "sweet spot," the point of balance between centralization and decentralization.

The issues in health care delivery, with their concomitant changes such as increases or decreases in government funding with new regulations and the development of networks for delivery of health care, have profound effects on organizational structure designs. Canadian health care organizations must be responsive to changes in government (provincial, territorial, and federal) policy, financing, and organization-level structural or policy changes that cause individual organizational units to be concerned with efficiencies in service delivery, redeployment of existing resources, reorganization, restructuring, and re-alignment of services through various redesign processes. In addition, patients and families expect that care will be individualized to meet their needs, which means that more decision making must be done where the care is delivered. Increased public knowledge about health issues and care programs has resulted in patients demanding more immediate access to care.

Information from Internet sources is significantly altering the expectations and behaviours of health care users. For example, Health Quality Ontario (2014) maintains a Web site where members of the public can access a searchable database that aims to provide public reporting about patient safety indicators such as hospital-associated infections, hand hygiene adherence, and hospital mortality rates in Ontario's hospitals. The Web site is designed to assist the public to become informed users of Ontario's health care system. By entering a specific indicator or a hospital name, the public can access the indicator rates by hospital and compare them with those of other hospitals in the province and the overall rate for Ontario. Changes in both facility design and care delivery systems are likely to continue as efforts are made to increase access, reduce wait times and costs, and enhance efficiencies while still striving to improve patient outcomes.

In Canada, rising health care costs, demands for quicker access to care, changes in government policy, and technological and research innovations are key factors influencing organizational structure design. These factors necessitate the re-engineering of health care structures. Whereas redesign is a process of analyzing tasks to improve efficiency (e.g., identifying the most efficient flow of supplies to a nursing unit) and restructuring entails fundamental changes to an organization to achieve greater efficiency or profit (e.g., identifying the most appropriate type and number of staff members for a particular nursing unit), re-engineering involves a total overhaul of an organizational structure. It is a radical reorganization of the totality of an organization's structure and work processes. In re-engineering, fundamentally new organizational expectations and relationships are created. An example of where re-engineering is required is technological change—particularly in information services that provide a means of individualizing care. The potential for making all information concerning a patient immediately accessible to direct care givers can have a profound positive impact on health care decision making. McGillis-Hall, Doran, and Pink (2008) showed that staff nurse participation in designing interventions explicitly aimed at improving nurses' work environments had significant positive effects on their perceptions of their work and work environment.

Regardless of the level of changes made within an organization—redesign, restructuring, or re-engineering—staff and patients alike feel the impact. Some of the changes result in improvements, whereas others may not; some of the impacts are expected, whereas others are not. It is critical, therefore, that nurse managers as well as staff nurses be vigilant for both anticipated and unanticipated results of these changes. Nurses need to position themselves to participate in change discussions and evaluations. Ultimately, it is their day-to-day work with their patients that is affected by the decisions made in response to a rapidly changing environment (Cormack, Hillier, Anderson, et al., 2007; Martin, Greenhouse, Merryman, et al., 2007; Murphy & Roberts, 2008). The Evidence section at the end of this chapter describes the impact of organizational restructuring on nurses.

EXERCISE 9-3

Arrange to interview a nurse employed in a health care organization or use your own experience to identify examples of changes taking place that necessitate re-engineering. These may include changes associated with implementation of new emergency department wait-time reduction strategies, development of policies to carry out legislative regulations related to patient information and confidentiality, or development of new community primary health care centres. Identify examples of how previous systems of communication and decision making were either adequate or inadequate to cope with these changes.

CHARACTERISTICS OF ORGANIZATIONAL STRUCTURES

The characteristics of different types of organizational structures provide a catalogue of options to consider in designing structures that fit specific situations. Knowledge of these characteristics also helps managers understand the structures in which they currently function.

Organizational designs are often classified by their characteristics of complexity, formalization, and centralization. *Complexity* concerns the division of labour in an organization, the specialization of that labour, the number of hierarchical levels, and the geographical dispersion of organizational units. *Division of labour* and *specialization* refer to the separation of processes into tasks that are performed by designated people. The horizontal dimension of an organizational chart, the graphical representation of work units and reporting relationships, relates to the division and specialization of labour functions attended by specialists. Hierarchy connotes lines of authority and responsibility. Chain of command is a term used to refer to the hierarchy depicted in vertical dimensions of organizational charts. Hierarchy vests authority in positions on an ascending line away from where work is performed and allows control of work. Staff members are often placed on a bottom level of the organization, and those in authority, who provide control, are placed in higher levels. Span of control refers to the number of individuals a supervisor manages. For budgetary reasons, span of control is often a major focus for organizational restructuring. Although cost implications arise when a span of control is too narrow, when a span of control becomes too large, supervision can become less effective. The Literature Perspective describes the effect of span of control on the perceived empowerment of staff nurses.

LITERATURE PERSPECTIVE

Resource: Lucas, V., Laschinger, H. K., & Wong, C. A. (2008). The impact of emotional intelligent leadership on staff nurse empowerment: The moderating effect of span of control. *International Journal of Nursing Management, 16*, 964–973. doi:10.1111/j.1365-2834.2008.00856.x

Multiple studies have shown that managers are critical to creating environments that empower nurses for professional practice. Still, efforts to improve efficiency and decrease costs often result in a reduction in the number of front-line managers. Using a descriptive correlational survey design, Lucas, Laschinger, and Wong tested a model to evaluate staff nurses' perceptions of their manager's emotionally intelligent (EI) leadership style and the impact of the manager's number of direct reports (their span of control). The hypothesized model was tested with staff nurses in two community hospitals in Ontario. Sixty-eight percent (n = 230) of nurses surveyed returned usable questionnaires. Managers who had higher EI leadership styles were more likely to empower nurses by ensuring access to workplace structures of opportunity, information, support, and resources. However, span of control was a significant moderator of the relationship between managers' EI behaviour and nurses' empowerment. As span of control increased, the effect of managers' EI behaviour on nurses' empowerment diminished.

Implications for Practice
During times of restructuring, administrators need to be aware of the relationship between a manager's span of control and his or her staff nurses' perceptions of empowerment and support. If an empowered nursing workforce is valued, efforts must be made to maintain a reasonable span of control for managers. Staff at all levels must be aware of this effect and actively develop plans with this correlation in mind.

Organizational size is closely related to the complexity of the organization. The stability and viability of an organization requires a certain essential base of resources. Efficiencies are often achieved when organizations increase in size, and this is often part of the rationale behind mergers of health care facilities (Smith, Klopper, Paras, et al., 2006). When organizations grow larger with more units or subdivisions and levels of decision making, they become more complex.

Geographical dispersion refers to the physical location of units. Units of work may be in one building; in several buildings in one location; spread throughout a city; or in different towns, provinces, territories, or countries. The more dispersed an organization is, the greater are the demands for creative designs that place decision making related to patient care close to the patient and, consequently, far from the central office. A similar type of complexity exists in organizations that deliver care at multiple sites in the community; for example, RHAs usually have multiple sites and types of health care facilities that previously may have been independent organizations, each with unique identities and cultures. It then becomes challenging to create a new overall culture and garner the commitment of employees, managers, and other stakeholders to a new organization (Smith et al., 2006).

Formalization is the degree to which an organization has rules, stated in terms of policies that define a member's function. The amount of formalization varies among institutions. It is often inversely related to the degree of specialization and the number of professionals within the organization.

EXERCISE 9-4
Review a copy of a nursing department's organizational chart and identify the divisions of labour, the hierarchy of authority, and the degree of formalization.

Centralization refers to the location where a decision is made. Decisions are made at the top of a centralized organization. In a decentralized organization, decisions are made at or close to the patient-care level. As organizations grow larger, they sometimes increase centralization of decision making. Highly centralized organizations often delegate *responsibility* (the obligation to perform the task) without the *authority* (the right to act, which is necessary to carry out the responsibility). For example, some hospitals have delegated both the responsibility and the authority for admission decisions to the charge nurse (decentralized), whereas others require the nurse supervisor or chief nurse executive to make such decisions (centralized).

EXERCISE 9-5
Review nursing policies in a public health department, a primary health care centre, a community care access centre, and a hospital. Are there common policies? Does one of the organizations have more detailed policies than others? Is this formalization consistent with the structural complexity of the organization?

BUREAUCRACY

Many organizational theories in use today find their basis in the works of early twentieth century theorists Max Weber, a German sociologist who developed the basic tenets of bureaucracy (Weber, 1947), and Henri Fayol, a French industrialist who crafted 14 principles of management (Fayol, 1949). Initially, bureaucracy referred to the centralization of authority in administrative bureaus or government departments. The term has come to refer to an inflexible approach to decision making or an employer encumbered by "red tape" that adds little value to organizational processes.

Bureaucracy is an administrative concept imbedded in how organizations are structured. It arose at a time of societal development when services were in short supply, workers' and patients' knowledge bases were limited, and technologies for sharing information were undeveloped. Characteristics of bureaucracy arose out of a need to control workers and were centred on the division of processes into discrete tasks. Weber proposed that organizations could achieve high levels of productivity and efficiency only by adherence to what he called "bureaucracy." Weber believed that bureaucracy, based on the sociological concept of rationalization of collective activities, provided the idealized organizational structure. Bureaucratic structures are formal and have a centralized and hierarchical command structure (chain of command). Bureaucratic structures have a clear division of labour and well-articulated and commonly accepted expectations for performance. Rules, standards, and protocols ensure uniform actions and limit individualization of services and variance in workers' performance. In bureaucratic organizations, as shown in Figure 9-1, communication and decisions flow from top to bottom. Although it enhances consistency, bureaucracy, by nature, limits employees' autonomy.

In developing his 14 principles of management, Fayol outlined structures and processes that guide how work is accomplished within an organization. Consistent with theories of bureaucracy, his principles of management include division of labour or specialization, clear lines of authority, appropriate levels of discipline, unity of direction, equitable treatment of staff, the fostering of individual initiative, and the promotion of a sense of teamwork and group pride. More than 60 years after they were described, these principles remain the basis of most organizations. Therefore,

to be effective organizational leaders, nurses need to be familiar with the theory and concepts of bureaucracy.

EXERCISE 9-6

Develop a list of decisions that you as a staff nurse would like to make to optimize care for your patients. Determine where those decisions are made in a nursing organization with which you are familiar. Consider issues such as (1) deciding on visiting schedules that meet your own, your patients', and their significant others' needs; and (2) determining a personal work schedule that meets your personal needs and your patients' needs. An example of the latter is talking to the children of a confused older adult patient during the evening because they work during the day shift, when you are on duty.

At the time that bureaucracies were developed, these characteristics promoted efficiency and production. As the knowledge base of the general population and employees grew and technologies developed, the bureaucratic structure no longer fit the evolving situation. Increasingly, employees and patients or patients functioning in bureaucratic situations complain of red tape, procedural delays, and general frustration.

The characteristics of bureaucracy can be present in varying degrees. An organization can demonstrate bureaucratic characteristics in some areas and not in others. For example, nursing staff in critical care units may be granted autonomy in making and carrying out direct patient care decisions, but they may not be granted a voice in determining work schedules or financial reimbursement systems for hours worked. One method to determine the extent to which bureaucratic tendencies exist in organizations is to assess the organizational characteristics of the following:

- Labour specialization (the degree to which patient care is divided into highly specialized tasks)
- Centralization (the level of the organization on which decisions regarding carrying out work and remuneration for work are made)
- Formalization (the percentage of actions required to deliver patient care that is governed by written policy and procedures)

EXERCISE 9-7

Analyze the decisions identified in Exercise 9-6 from a manager's perspective. Is that perspective similar to or different from the original perspective you identified?

Decision making and authority can be described in terms of line and staff functions. Line functions are

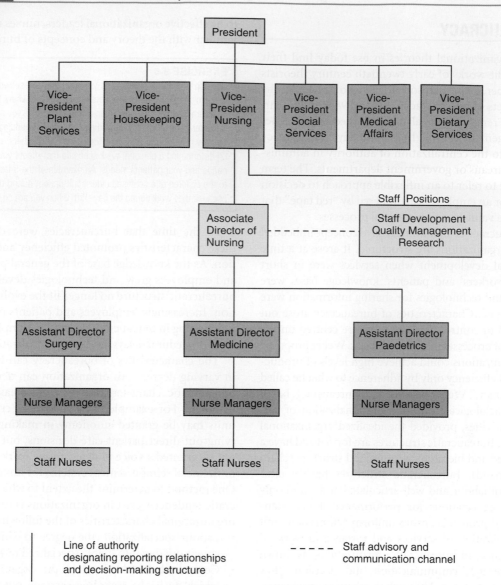

Line of authority
designating reporting relationships
and decision-making structure

– – – – – Staff advisory and
communication channel

FIGURE 9-1 A bureaucratic organizational chart depicting specialization of labour, centralization, hierarchical authority, and line and staff responsibilities.

those that involve direct responsibility for accomplishing the objectives of a nursing department, service, or unit. Line positions may include registered nurses, registered psychiatric nurses, registered practical nurses, and unregulated care providers who have the responsibility for carrying out all aspects of direct care. Staff functions are those that assist those in line positions in accomplishing the primary objectives. In this context, the term *staff positions* should not be confused with specific jobs that

include "staff" in their names, such as "staff nurse" or "staff physician." Staff positions include individuals such as staff development personnel, researchers, and special clinical consultants who are responsible for supporting line positions through activities of consultation, education, role modelling, and knowledge development, with limited or no direct authority for decision making. Line personnel have authority for decision making, whereas personnel in staff positions provide support, advice, and counsel. Organizational charts usually indicate line positions through the use of solid lines and staff positions through broken lines (reminder: in this context, the term "staff position" does not reference staff nurses). Line structures have a vertical line, designating reporting and decision-making responsibility. The vertical line connects all positions to a centralized authority (see Figure 9-1 on page 158).

To make line and staff functions effective, decision-making authority is clearly spelled out in position descriptions. Effectiveness is further ensured by delineating competencies required for the responsibilities, providing methods for determining whether personnel possess these competencies, and providing means of maintaining and developing the competencies.

EXERCISE 9-8

Organizational structures vary in the extent to which they have bureaucratic characteristics. Using observations from your current practice, place a check mark (✔) in the "Present" column beside the bureaucratic characteristics that you believe apply to the organization. What does this analysis indicate about the bureaucratic tendency of the organization? Do the environment and technologies fit the identified bureaucratic tendency? (Consider the state of development of information systems, method of care delivery, patients' characteristics, workers' characteristics, and regulatory status.)

CHARACTERISTIC	PRESENT
Hierarchy of authority	
Division of labour	
Written procedures for work	
Limited authority for workers	
Emphasis on written communication related to work performance and workers' behaviours	
Impersonality of personal contact	

TYPES OF ORGANIZATIONAL STRUCTURES

In health care organizations, the most common types of organizational structures are functional, service line, matrix, or flat. Nursing organizations often combine characteristics of several of these structures to form a hybrid structure. Shared governance is an organizing structure designed to meet the changing needs of professional nursing organizations.

Functional Structures

Functional structures arrange departments and services according to specialty. This approach to organizational structure is common in health care organizations. Departments providing similar functions report to a common manager or executive (Figure 9-2). For example, a health care organization with a functional structure would have vice-presidents for each major function: nursing, finance, human resources, and information technology.

This organizational structure tends to support professional expertise and encourage advancement. It may, however, result in discontinuity of patient-care services. Delays in decision making can occur if a silo mentality develops within groups. In fact, Lencioni (2006) points out the pitfalls of silos. That is, issues that require communication across functional groups typically must be raised to a senior management level before a decision can be made.

Service-Line Structures

In service-line structures (sometimes called *product lines*), the functions necessary to produce a specific service or product are brought together into an integrated organizational unit under the control of a single

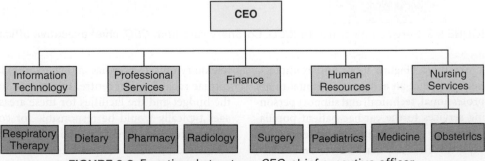

FIGURE 9-2 Functional structure. *CEO*, chief executive officer.

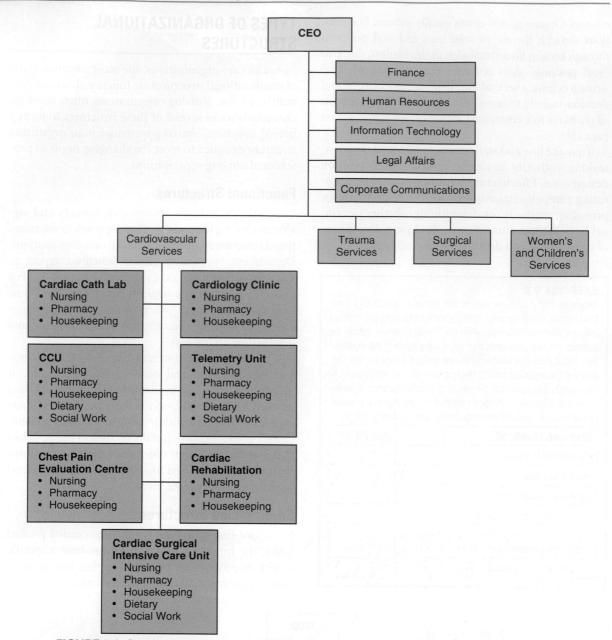

FIGURE 9-3 Service-line structure. *CCU,* Coronary care unit; *CEO,* chief executive officer.

manager or executive (Figure 9-3). For example, a cardiology service line at an acute care hospital might include all professional, technical, and support personnel providing services to the cardiac patient population. The manager or administrator in this service line would be responsible for any cardiac services situated within the emergency department, the coronary care unit, the cardiovascular surgery critical care unit, the

telemetry unit, the cardiac catheterization lab, and the cardiac rehabilitation centre. In addition to managing the budget and the facilities for these areas, the manager typically would be responsible for coordinating services for the physicians and other providers who admit and care for these patients.

The benefits of a service-line approach to organizational structure include coordination of services, an expedited decision-making process, and clarity of purpose. The limitations of this model can include increased expense associated with duplication of services, loss of professional or technical affiliation, and lack of standardization.

Matrix Structures

Matrix structures are complex and designed to reflect both function and service in an integrated organizational structure. In a matrix organization, the manager of a unit responsible for a service reports to both a functional manager and a service- or product-line manager. For example, a director of paediatric nursing could report to both a vice-president for pediatric services (the service-line manager) and a vice-president of nursing (the functional manager) (Figure 9-4).

Matrix structures can be effective in the current health care environment. The matrix design enables timely response to forces in the external environment that demand continual programming, and it facilitates internal efficiency and effectiveness through the promotion of cooperation among disciplines. However, such a structure can lead to some dispersion of accountability and potential conflict as some employees may report to more than one supervisor. Another disadvantage is that a matrix structure may lead to an increase in bureaucracy, in the form of more meetings or slower decisions where too many people are involved.

A matrix structure combines both a bureaucratic structure and a flat structure; teams are used to carry out specific programs or projects. A matrix structure superimposes a horizontal program management over the traditional vertical hierarchy. Personnel from various functional departments are assigned to a specific program or project and become responsible to two supervisors—their functional department head and a program manager. This creates an interdisciplinary team. Matrix structures permit better cross-communication among various organizational units

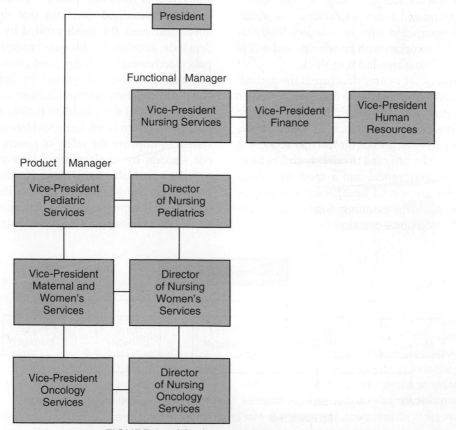

FIGURE 9-4 Matrix organizational structure.

or departments and may serve to flatten or simplify decision-making structures and allow for timely and quality responses to changes initiated by factors outside the control of the organization. Organizations that operate in a dynamic environment and need to make decisions more quickly (often bringing higher-level decision makers in contact with front-line activities) while including a broad cross-section of the organization's functional units often create structures that are reflective of matrix structures.

A line manager and a project manager must function collaboratively in a matrix organization. For example, in nursing, there may be a chief nursing executive, a nurse manager, and staff nurses in the line of authority to accomplish nursing care. In the matrix structure, some of the nurse's time is allocated to project or committee work. Nursing care is delivered in a teamwork setting or within a collaborative model. The nurse is responsible to a nurse manager for nursing care and to a program or project manager when working within the matrix overlay. Well-developed collaboration and coordination skills are essential to effective functioning in a matrix structure. The nature of a matrix organization with its complex interrelationships requires workers with knowledge and skill in interpersonal relationships and teamwork.

One example of the matrix structure is the patient-focused care delivery model that is being implemented in some facilities. Another example is the program focused on specialty services such as geriatric services, women's services, and cardiovascular services. A matrix model can be designed to cover both a patient-focused care delivery model and a specialty service. Other examples are special health care facility programs such as discharge planning, total quality management, and professional practice.

Flat Structures

The primary organizational characteristic of a *flat* structure is the delegation of decision making to the professionals doing the work. The term *flat* signifies the removal of hierarchical layers, thereby granting authority to act and placing authority at the action level (Figure 9-5). Decisions regarding work methods, nursing care of individual patients, and conditions under which employees work are made where the work is carried out. In a flat organizational structure, decentralized decision making replaces the centralized decision making typical of functional structures. In the United States, Magnet™ hospitals have recognized the benefits of decentralized decision making and its impact on both nursing satisfaction and patient outcomes (Aiken, Buchan, Ball, & Rafferty, 2008; Manojlovich, 2005). Magnet hospitals are those known for their ability to recruit and retain nurses, excellence in nursing care and patient outcomes, support for professional development, and effective leadership.

Flat organizational structures are less formalized than hierarchical organizations. A decrease in strict adherence to rules and policies allows employees to make individualized decisions that fit specific situations and meet the needs created by the increasing demands associated with government funding and policy, technological change, and public expectations. For example, work supported by Safer Healthcare Now! (http://www.saferhealthcarenow.ca), the flagship program of the Canadian Patient Safety Institute (2014), invests in front-line providers and the delivery system to improve the safety of patient care throughout Canada by implementing interventions known to reduce avoidable harm. Safer Healthcare Now! is a resource for front-line health care providers and others who want to improve patient safety and interventions. These interventions are designed to help organizations,

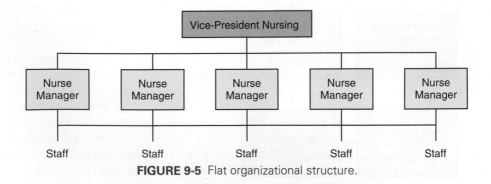

FIGURE 9-5 Flat organizational structure.

managers, and clinicians implement, measure, and evaluate patient safety initiatives made at the unit level.

Decentralized structures are not without their challenges, however. These include the potential for inconsistent decision making, loss of growth opportunities, and the need to educate managers to communicate effectively and demonstrate creativity in working within these nontraditional structures (Matthews, Spence Laschinger, & Johnstone, 2006).

The degree of flattening varies from organization to organization. Organizations that are decentralized often retain some bureaucratic characteristics. They may at the same time have units that are operating as matrix structures. A hybrid organizational structure has characteristics of several types of organizational structures.

As organizational structures change, some managers are hesitant to relinquish their traditional role in a centralized decision-making process. This reluctance, when combined with recognition of the need to move to a more facilitative role, is partially responsible for the development of hybrid structures. Managers are unsure of what needs to be controlled, how much control is needed, and which mechanisms can replace control. Fear of chaos without control predominates. Education that prepares managers to use leadership techniques that empower nursing staff to take responsibility for their work is one method of minimizing managers' fears. These fears stem from loss of centralized control as authority with its concomitant responsibilities moves to the place of interaction. The evolutionary development of shared-governance structures in nursing departments demonstrates a type of flat structure being used to replace hierarchical control.

Shared Governance

Shared governance is a flat type of organizational structure with decentralized decision making. It goes beyond participatory management by creating an organizational structure that helps nursing staff have more autonomy to govern their practice. Accountability is the foundation for shared governance. To be accountable, authority to make decisions concerning all aspects of responsibilities is essential. The need for authority and accountability is particularly important for nurses who treat the wide range of human responses to wellness states and illnesses. Organizations in which professional autonomy is encouraged have higher levels of staff satisfaction, enhanced productivity, and

improved retention (Moore & Hutchinson, 2007; Ulrich, Buerhaus, Donelan, et al., 2007).

A major cause of nurses' dissatisfaction with their work revolves around the absence of professional autonomy and accountability. An early study of Magnet™ hospitals in the United States (McClure, Poulin, Sovie, et al., 1983), which identified characteristics of hospitals successful in recruiting and retaining nurses, found that the major contributing characteristic to success was a nursing department structured to provide nurses the opportunity to be accountable for their own practice. Studies of Magnet™ hospitals demonstrate that governance structures provide nurses with accountability that will be effective in recruiting and retaining nursing staff while also meeting patients' demands and remaining competitive. These findings continue to be validated and expanded upon (Bogue, Joseph, & Sieloff, 2009; Schmalenberg & Kramer, 2007). Magnet™ characteristics are now accepted as affecting not only the quality of the work environment but also the quality of patient care (Aiken, Clarke, Sloane, et al., 2008; McGillis-Hall & Doran, 2007).

Shared or self-governance structures, sometimes referred to as *professional practice models,* go beyond decentralizing and diminishing hierarchies. In an organization that embraces shared governance, the structure's foundation is the professional workplace rather than the organizational hierarchy. Shared governance vests the necessary levels of authority and accountability for all aspects of the nursing practice in the nurses responsible for the delivery of care. The management and administrative level serves to coordinate and facilitate the work of the practising nurses. Mechanisms are designed outside of the traditional hierarchy to provide for the functional areas needed to support professional practice. These functions include areas such as quality management, competency definition and evaluation, and continuing education. Changing nurses' positions from dependent employees to independent, accountable professionals is a prerequisite for the radical redesign of health care organizations that is required to create value for patients. Doing so requires administrators, managers, and staff to abandon traditional notions regarding the division of labour in health care organizations. MacPhee, Wardrop, and Campbell's (2010) three-year participatory action research project conducted in selected sites in British Columbia showed the importance of staff nurse–nurse leader shared

BOX 9-2	SHARED-GOVERNANCE STRUCTURE EVOLUTION

Phase One

Representative staff nurses are members of clinical forums, which have authority for designated practice issues and some authority for determining roles, functions, and processes. Managers are members of the management forums, which are responsible for the facilitation of practice through resource management and location. Recommendations for action go to the executive committee, which has administrative and staff membership that may or may not be in equal proportion. The nurse executive retains decision-making authority.

Phase Two

Representative staff nurses belong to nursing committees that are designated for specific management or clinical functions. These committees are chaired by staff nurses or administrators appointed by the vice-president of nursing/chief nursing officer. The nursing committee chairs and nurse administrators make up the nursing cabinet, which makes the final decision on recommendations from the committees.

Phase Three

Representative staff nurses belong to councils with authority for specific functions. Council chairs make up the management committee charged with making all final operational organizational decisions.

decision-making teams in addressing workload issues. The structures of shared governance organizations vary. Box 9-2 shows three governance structures in progressive stages of evolution. As shown, evolution is moving structure beyond committees imposed on hierarchical structures to governance structures at the unit level.

Shared governance structures require new behaviours of all staff, not just new assignments of accountability. Particularly important are the areas of interpersonal relationship development, conflict resolution, and personal acceptance of responsibility for action. Education, experience in group work, and conflict management are essential for successful transitions.

ANALYZING ORGANIZATIONS

When an organization is analyzed, it is important to scrutinize the various systems that exist to accomplish the work of the organization. This includes delineating the processes or procedures that have been developed to coordinate the work to be done. To conceptualize how the organization functions, it is imperative to know the recruitment procedures, the method of selecting individuals for positions, the reporting relationships, the information network, and the governance structure for nurses. In a positive organization, the mission, vision,

and philosophy fit with the structure and practices. The criteria for designating hospitals as US Magnet™ facilities (American Nurses Credentialing Center, 2014), irrespective of structure, could form the basis for evaluating nursing services and is a useful reference for Canadian nurses. A US credentialing program called the Magnet Recognition Program® assesses and designates Magnet™ organizations (http://www.nursecredentialing.org/Magnet.aspx). However, in Canada, the Canadian Nurses Association (http://www.cna-nurses.ca), provincial and territorial professional nursing associations, and nurse licensing agencies set standards and guidelines for quality nursing services in organizations. Provincial nurse licensing bodies set mandatory standards of practice. Professional associations at the provincial and territorial or national levels represent nurses and work to advance the practice and profession of nursing, improve health outcomes, and influence health policy. For example, the Registered Nurses' Association of Ontario (http://www.rnao.org) has developed Best Practice Guidelines for healthy work environments on a number of topics, including nursing leadership; staffing and workload; managing workplace violence; cultural diversity; and workplace health and safety. In addition, Accreditation Canada (http://www.accreditation.ca) is a not-for-profit, independent organization that provides health care organizations with an external peer review process to assess and improve the services they provide to their patients based on standards of excellence. The accreditation program covers diverse health care services, and standards are based on research and best practices. It also addresses the management function across and throughout all levels of the organization, rather than individual or position-specific competencies. The organization's standards clarify the requirements for effective operational and performance management supports, decision-making structures, and the infrastructure needed to drive excellence and quality improvement in health care service delivery in all departments and programs, including nursing.

EMERGING FLUID RELATIONSHIPS

Under the continuum of care, when health care services occur outside of institutional parameters, different skill sets, relationships, and behavioural patterns will be required. Organizations are beginning to lose their traditional boundaries. Old boundaries of hierarchy, function, and geography are disappearing. Vertical integration aligns dissimilar but related entities such as the hospital, home care employer, rehabilitation centre, long-term care facility, insurance provider, and medical office or clinic. New technologies, fast-changing public demands for service, changes in government policy, and global competition are revolutionizing relationships in health care, and the roles that people play and the tasks that they perform have become blurred and ambiguous.

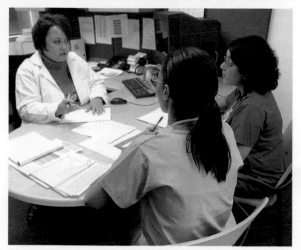

Nurses must have the ability to work with other members of the organization to design organizational models for care delivery that meet patient needs and priorities.

In the future, nurses will no longer practise in geographically limited settings but, rather, in systems of care that have extended boundaries. Reframing or changing current static organizations into vibrant learning organizations will require significant effort (Garvin, Edmondson, & Gino, 2008). A learning organization is an organization that is continually expanding its capacity to create its future and provide opportunities and incentives for its members to learn continuously over time (Senge, 2006). To be successful, nurses need to be able to participate as active members in these living-learning organizations. Nurses, whether leaders, managers, or staff, must have the ability to work with other members of the organization and with society at large to design organizational models for health care delivery that meet patient needs and priorities. It is essential to take a new look at the nature of the work of nursing and propose innovative models for nursing practice that consider emerging labour-saving assistive technologies and rapidly changing health care needs. Employee participation and learning environments go hand in hand, and work redesign needs to be regarded as a continuous process. It is essential that nurses value their and others' autonomy to deal successfully in these new structures.

A SOLUTION

Laurie's first task was to determine and establish the management structure, including how the scope of responsibility had changed for individual managers. The next step was to actively recruit for the vacant positions and ensure that effective retention strategies were implemented so that those who were already members of the team were committed to the new direction. Laurie also created a staff development coordinator position in order to involve nurse managers in the development of a vision for clinical management.

After establishing the management team, Laurie's next priority was to articulate core competencies for the clinical staff. Staff participated in identifying and designing the initial set of competencies through staff representatives from each major clinical department.

At the same time, the management team has been developing a second set of competencies that are unit-specific. The interest and enthusiasm the nurses have shown in meeting this challenge has been very gratifying. Also, the staff development coordinator has been an asset; because she has previous university teaching experience, she appreciates the importance of high standards and consistency in staff education. She has also been using her connections to develop a solid recruitment program.

Would this be a suitable approach for you? Why or why not?

THE EVIDENCE

Organizational culture plays an important role in creating a positive work environment and enhancing employee commitment and intent to stay after major organizational changes. Gregory, Way, LeFort, et al. (2007) invited 1173 front-line registered nurses working in acute care settings in Newfoundland and Labrador to participate in a survey following a restructuring and regionalization of health services in 2005. Changes in health care services included moving from a facilities-based structure to a functional-based structure with multidisciplinary teams; a change to program-based management; a 40 to 50% reduction of management and support personnel; the closure and merger of hospitals and facilities; and the dislocation of approximately 50% of nursing staff. Of the nurses surveyed, a final sample of 343 was obtained for a response rate of 29.4%. *Organizational culture* in this study was defined as satisfaction with the emotional climate of the workplace, practice issues, and collaborative relations with management and other disciplines. Although nurses were moderately satisfied with their jobs, they reported negative effects from the restructuring on organizational culture, trust in their employers, and their commitment to stay with their organization. Study findings supported the connection and impact of organizational culture on nurses' trust in their employer and job satisfaction and, ultimately, on nurses' commitment to the organization and their intent to stay.

The study also provided evidence of the impact of organizational changes on the attitudes of nurses. The researchers made recommendations on how managers might reduce the negative impact of restructuring activities. They suggested that positive leaders who are present, visible, and accessible to all staff were necessary to renew and revitalize supportive organizational cultures. Moreover, they also suggested that managers who focus on developing and implementing strategies to enrich culture (in particular, the emotional climate), control practice issues, encourage collaborative relationships, and rebuild trusting relationships with nurses could positively influence reorganizational changes. Creating a more supportive work environment requires a partnership approach with all levels of health care providers to identify and implement interventions and policies that are responsive to employee needs.

NEED TO KNOW NOW

- Know the mission, vision, and philosophy of your organization and work unit.
- Identify the expected lines of communication as presented on the formal organizational chart.
- Analyze actual workplace practices for opportunities to streamline decision making.

CHAPTER CHECKLIST

The mission, vision, and philosophy of the organization determine how nursing care is delivered in a health care organization. Changes occurring in the organization's mission affect both the culture of the workplace and the philosophies regarding the work required to accomplish the mission. Actualizing new missions and philosophies requires re-engineered organizational structures that place decision-making authority and responsibility where care is delivered. Decision-making responsibility requires staff to understand the organization's mission and to participate in the development of mission and philosophy statements.

- Five factors influencing design of an organization structure are the following:
  - The types of service performed or the product produced
  - The characteristics of the employees performing the service or producing the product
  - The beliefs and values held by the people responsible for delivering the service concerning the work, the people receiving the services, and the employees

- The technologies used to perform the service and produce the product
- The needs, desires, and characteristics of the users of the product or service
- Re-engineering, the complete overhaul of an organizational structure, is driven by the following forces:
  - Changes in government policy and funding
  - Public demand for services
  - Enhanced technology and research evidence
- Bureaucratic structures are characterized by the following:
  - A high degree of formalization
  - Centralization of decision making at the top of the organization
  - A hierarchy of authority
  - Structures can be organized along the following lines:
    - Functional
    - Service-line
    - Matrix
    - Flat

- Functional structures are characterized by the following:
  - Departments and services organized according to specialty
  - Discontinuity of patient services because of silo mentality, even when structure supports professional expertise and encourages advancement
- Service-line structures are characterized by the following:
  - Functions necessary to provide a specific service brought together under a single line of authority
- Matrix structures are characterized by the following:
  - Dual authority for product and function
  - Mechanisms such as committees to coordinate actions of product and function managers
  - Success that depends on recognition and appreciation of each other's missions and philosophies and commitment to the organization's mission and philosophy
- Flat organizations are characterized by the following:
  - Decision making concerning work performed, decentralized to the level where the work is done
  - Authority, accountability, and autonomy, as well as responsibility, provided to staff performing care
- Low level of formalization in relation to rules, with processes tailored to meet individual patient's needs
- Mission, vision, and values and beliefs (philosophy) determine the characteristics of the organizational structure by doing the following:
  - Describing patient needs and services as a prescription for the technologies and human resources needed to accomplish the defined purpose (mission)
  - Creating an ultimate state of existence (vision)
  - Citing values and beliefs that shape and are shaped by the nature of the work and the rights and responsibilities of workers and patients (philosophy)
  - Designing characteristics that support the service implementation to fulfill the mission and philosophy (structure)
- Shared governance is characterized by the following:
  - The creation of organizational structures that allow nursing staff more autonomy to govern their practice
  - Recruitment and retention of nursing staff while meeting patient needs in an effective and efficient manner

TIPS FOR UNDERSTANDING ORGANIZATIONAL STRUCTURES

- Professional nurses in staff or followership positions need to understand the mission, vision, philosophy, and structure at the organization and unit level to maximize their contributions to patient care.
- The overall mission of the organization and the mission of the specific unit in which a professional nurse is employed or is seeking employment provides information concerning the major focus of the work to be accomplished and the manner in which it will be accomplished.
- Understanding the philosophy of the organization or unit where work occurs provides knowledge of the behaviours that are valued in the delivery of patient care and in interactions with persons employed by the organization.
- Formal organizational structures describe the expected channels of communication and decision making.
- Matrix organizations usually have two persons responsible for the work, and therefore it is important to know to whom you are responsible for what.
- For a shared-governance structure to function effectively, the professionals providing the care must put mechanisms in place to promote decision making about patient care.

℮volve WEBSITE

Visit the Evolve website for Suggested Readings, Internet Resources, and additional resources related to the content in this chapter: http://evolve.elsevier.com/Canada/Yoder-Wise/leading/.

REFERENCES

Aiken, L. H., Buchan, J., Ball, J., & Rafferty, A. M. (2008). Trans-formative impact of Magnet designation: England case study. *Journal of Clinical Nursing, 17,* 3330–3337. doi:10.1111/j.1365-2702.2008.02640.x

Aiken, L. H., Clarke, S. P., Sloane, D. M., et al. (2008). Effects of hospital environment care on patient mortality and nurse outcomes. *Journal of Nursing Administration, 38,* 223–229. doi: 10.1097/01.NNA.0000312773.42352.d7

American Nurses Credentialing Center. (2014). 2014 Magnet® application manual. Washington, DC: Author. Retrieved from http://www.nursecredentialing.org/Magnet.aspx.

Bogue, R. J., Joseph, M. L., & Sieloff, C. L. (2009). Shared governance as vertical alignment of nursing group power and nurse practice council effectiveness. *Journal of Nursing Management, 17,* 4–14. doi:10.1111/j.1365-2834.2008.00954.x

Brafman, O., & Beckstrom, R. A. (2008). *The starfish and the spider: The unstoppable power of leaderless organizations.* New York, NY: Penguin Books.

Canadian Patient Safety Institute. (2014). *Safety healthcare now.* Ottawa, ON: Author. Retrieved from http://www.saferhealthcarenow.ca/EN/Pages/default.aspx.

Casida, J. (2008). Linking nursing unit's culture to organizational effectiveness: A measurement tool. *Nursing Economic$, 26*(2), 106–110.

Chen, Y. C. (2008). Restructuring the organizational culture of medical institutions: A study of a community hospital in the I-Lan area. *Journal of Nursing Research, 16,* 211–219. doi:10.1097/01.JNR.0000387308.42364.34

Cormack, C., Hillier, L. M., Anderson, K., et al. (2007). Practice change: The process of developing and implementing a nursing care delivery model for geriatric rehabilitation. *Journal of Nursing Administration, 37*(6), 279–286. doi:10.1097/01.NNA.0000277719.79876.ec

Fayol, H. (1949). *General and industrial management.* London, UK: Pitman.

Garvin, D. A., Edmondson, A. C., & Gino, F. (2008). Is yours a learning organization? *Harvard Business Review, 86*(3), 109–116.

Gregory, D. M., Way, C. Y., LeFort, S., et al. (2007). Predictors of registered nurses' organizational commitment and intent to stay. *Health Care Management Review, 32*(2), 119–127. doi:10.1097/01.HMR.0000267788.79190.f4

Health Quality Ontario. (2014). Public reporting: Patient safety. Retrieved from http://www.hqontario.ca/public-reporting/patient-safety.

Henderson, A., Cooke, M., Creedy, D.K., et al. (2012). Nursing students' perceptions of earning in practice environments: A review. *Nurse Education Today, 32,* 299–302. doi:10.1016/j.nedt.2011.03.010

Laschinger, H. K., Finegan, J., & Wilk, P. (2009). Context matters: The impact of unit leadership and empowerment on nurses' organizational commitment. *Journal of Nursing Administration, 39,* 228–235. doi:10.1097/NNA.0b013e3181a23d2b

Lencioni, P. (2006). *Silos, politics and turf wars: A leadership fable.* San Francisco, CA: Jossey-Bass.

Lucas, V., Laschinger, H. K., & Wong, C. A. (2008). The impact of emotional intelligent leadership on staff nurse empowerment: The moderating effect of span of control. *International Journal of Nursing Management, 16,* 964–973. doi:10.1111/j.1365-2834.2008.00856.x

MacPhee, M., Wardrop, A., & Campbell, C. (2010). Transforming work place relationships through shared decision making. *Journal of Nursing Management, 18,* 1016–1026. doi:10.1111/j.1365-2834.2010.01122.x

Manojlovich, M. (2005). The effect of nursing leadership on hospital nurses' professional practice behaviors. *Journal of Nursing Administration, 35*(7–8), 366–374.

Martin, S. C., Greenhouse, P. K., Merryman, T., et al. (2007). Transforming care at the bedside: Implementation and spread model for single-hospital and multihospital systems. *Journal of Nursing Administration, 37,* 444–451. doi:10.1097/01.NNA.0000285152.79988.f3

Matthews, S., Spence Laschinger, H. K., & Johnstone, L. (2006). Staff nurse empowerment in line and staff organizational structures for chief nurse executives. *Journal of Nursing Administration, 36*(11), 526–533.

McClure, M. L., Poulin, M. A., Sovie, M. D., et al. (1983). *Magnet hospitals: Attraction and retention of professional nurses.* Kansas City, MO: American Nurses Association.

McGillis-Hall, L., & Doran, D. (2007). Nurses' perceptions of hospital work environments. *Journal of Nursing Management, 15,* 264–273. doi:10.1111/j.1365-2834.2007.00676.x

McGillis-Hall, L., Doran, D., & Pink, L. (2008). Outcomes of interventions to improve hospital nursing work environments. *Journal of Nursing Administration, 18*(1), 40–46. doi:10.1097/01.NNA.0000295631.72721.17

Meagher-Stewart, D., Underwood, J., MacDonald, M., et al. (2010). Organizational attributes that assure optimal utilization of public health nurses. *Public Health Nursing, 27*(5), 433–441. doi:10.1111/j.1525-1446.2010.00876.x

Melnick, G., Ulaszek, W. R., Lin, H. J., et al. (2009). When goals diverge: Staff consensus and the organizational culture. *Drug and Alcohol Dependence, 103,* S17–S22. doi:10.1016/j.drugalcdep.2008.10.023

Moore, S. C., & Hutchinson, S. A. (2007). Developing leaders at every level: Accountability and empowerment actualized through shared governance. *Journal of Nursing Administration, 37,* 556–558. doi:10.1097/01.NNA.0000302386.76119.22

Murphy, N., & Roberts, D. (2008). Nurse leaders as stewards at the point of service. *Nursing Ethics, 15,* 243–253. doi:10.1177/0969733007086022

Richards, J. (2014a). About nursing. Retrieved from http://hapi.uhn.ca/about_uhn/nursing/site/about/index.html.

Richards, J. (2014b). Practice—Patient-centred care. Retrieved from http://hapi.uhn.ca/about_uhn/nursing/site/practice/pcc/index.html.

Saskatoon Health Region. (2014). *Saskatoon Health Region: Our vision, mission values & strategic directions.* Saskatoon, SK: Author. Retrieved from http://www.saskatoonhealthregion.ca/about_us/goals.htm.

Schmalenberg, C., & Kramer, M. (2007). Types of intensive care units with the healthiest, most productive work environments. *American Journal of Critical Care, 16*(5), 458–468.

Scott-Findlay, S., & Estabrooks, C. A. (2006). Mapping the organizational culture research in nursing: A literature review. *Journal of Advanced Nursing, 56*(5), 498–513. doi:10.1111/j.1365-2648.2006.04044.x

Senge, P. M. (2006). *The fifth discipline: The art & practice of the learning organization.* Random House Digital.

Smith, D. L., Klopper, H. E., Paras, A., et al. (2006). Structure in health agencies. In J. M. Hibberd & D. L. Smith (Eds.), *Nursing leadership and management in Canada* (3rd ed., pp. 163–198). Toronto, ON: Elsevier Canada.

Ulrich, B. T., Buerhaus, P. I., Donelan, K., et al. (2007). Magnet status and registered nurse views of the work environment and nursing as a career. *Journal of Nursing Administration, 37*(5), 212–220. doi:10.1097/01.NNA.0000269745.24889.c6

Weber, M. (1947). *The theory of social and economic organization.* Parsons, NY: Free Press.

Williams, J., Smythe, W., Hadjistavropoulos, T., et al. (2005). A study of thematic content in hospital mission statements: A question of values. *Health Care Management Review, 30*(4), 304–314. doi:10.1097/00004010-200510000-00004

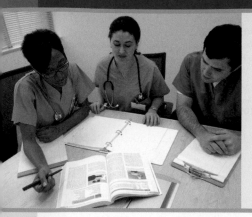

Cultural Diversity in Health Care

Karen A. Esquibel and Dorothy A. Otto
Adapted by Yolanda Babenko-Mould

This chapter focuses on the importance of cultural considerations for patients and staff. Although it does not address comprehensive details about any specific culture, it does provide guidelines for actively incorporating cultural competence into the roles of leading and managing. This chapter also presents the concepts and principles of cultural safety and emphasizes the importance of respecting diverse lifestyles. As well, it includes scenarios and exercises that promote an appreciation of cultural richness.

OBJECTIVES

- Understand the concepts of culture, cultural diversity, cultural sensitivity, cultural competence, and cultural safety in leading and managing in nursing.
- Understand how cultural diversity affects leading and managing in health care organizations.
- Describe how prejudice can interfere with quality patient care.
- Identify theoretical models that can help health care providers deliver culturally competent patient care.
- Understand individual and societal factors related to cultural diversity.
- Consider how nurse managers and leaders can design services and programs to meet the needs of culturally diverse staff and patients.

TERMS TO KNOW

cross-culturalism	cultural marginality	ethnocentrism
cultural competence	cultural safety	multiculturalism
cultural diversity	cultural sensitivity	transculturalism
cultural imposition	culture	

(?) A CHALLENGE

Dwayne is a newly graduated nurse practitioner from London, Ontario, who has been assigned to practise in an outpost community in the Northwest Territories. In addition to providing nursing care to a population of approximately 1500 individuals (most of whom are Aboriginal people), part of Dwayne's role will be to manage the small community health clinic, which is staffed by two nurses and an administrative assistant who are of Aboriginal origin. This will be Dwayne's first experience working in the Northwest Territories and in the role of a nurse manager. Given that he will work in a community with a rich heritage, Dwayne wants to ensure that he prepares himself to be culturally competent so that his associations with clinic personnel and patients are respectful.

If you were Dwayne, how might you enhance your cultural competence so that you relate well to your new staff and the community you will serve?

INTRODUCTION: CONCEPTS AND PRINCIPLES

What is *culture*? Does it exhibit certain characteristics? What is *cultural diversity*, and what do you think of when people refer to *cultural sensitivity, cultural competence,* and *cultural safety*? Are *culture* and *ethnicity* the same? Some answers to these questions appear in this chapter. Nurse managers and leaders are concerned with culture, particularly as it relates to patient care and diversity in the workplace. Culture, a social determinant of health, is defined broadly as "shared patterns of learned behaviours and values transmitted over time, and that distinguish the members of one group from another" (Canadian Nurses Association [CNA], 2004, p. 2). This view recognizes that culture helps shape us but does not define who we are as individuals; culture is dynamic and changing, and people come to understand culture by interacting with one another and developing relationships. In this chapter, culture is viewed from this constructivist perspective (Gray & Thomas, 2006), which is an understanding of culture that aligns with that of the Aboriginal Nurses Association of Canada (ANAC) (ANAC, 2009, p. 1) as noted in *Cultural Competency Framework for Nursing Education.*

The constructivist perspective moves away from a historical or *essentialist* perspective of culture. The essentialist perspective holds that culture is not changeable, that people are simply a product of their culture, and that the "norm" culture in Canada is white and moderately affluent. Any culture outside of this supposed norm is "different." The essentialist perspective can lead groups who are considered "different" to be devalued, which reinforces imbalanced power relationships. By contrast, a constructivist perspective of culture recognizes that various social, political, and economic forces have influenced or shaped an individual to a certain moment in time. Thus, each person's individual experience of culture varies and cannot be easily categorized. What this means for nurse managers, nurse leaders, and staff nurses is that they need to dedicate time to building relationships with colleagues and patients to become aware of their particular cultural beliefs, practices, values, and ways of being to avoid erroneous assumptions. It is also important for nurse managers and leaders to engage health care staff in discussions about the ways in which culture is socially constructed, so as to avoid sweeping generalizations and cultural stereotypes. The Research Perspective below illustrates that nursing students predominantly hold an essentialist understanding of culture. Gregory, Harrowing, Lee, et al. (2010) proposed that when nurse leaders and nursing staff develop an awareness of their assumptions and beliefs about culture, they are better prepared to learn about how culture shapes themselves and their colleagues. Such awareness and knowledge creates cultural competence that is important to delivering patient care and relating with patients' families.

(Q) RESEARCH PERSPECTIVE

Resource: Gregory, D., Harrowing, J., Lee, B., et al. (2010). Nursing pedagogy as contributing to essentialized understanding of culture among undergraduate nursing students. *International Journal of Nursing Education Scholarship, 7,* Article [On-Line]

In a study by Gregory, Harrowing, Lee, et al. (2010) 14 nursing and 8 non-nursing student participants were asked to define *culture* and write narratives regarding specific cultural encounters. The researchers found that of the 14 nursing students interviewed about their understanding of culture, 13 viewed culture from an essentialist perspective and only one viewed culture from a constructivist perspective. The researchers also found that of the 8 non-nursing students, 3 viewed culture from an essentialist perspective and 5 viewed culture from a constructivist perspective. According to these findings, most nursing students perceived culture as something unchanging, passed down from generation

Continued

to generation, and associated with defined behaviours. Such a view limited participants' abilities to consider culture as dynamic, related to context, and unique to each individual. By contrast, the nursing student who framed culture from a constructivist perspective wrote narratives that recognized culture as temporal or ever-evolving and not solely able to define who patients are as individuals.

Implications for Practice

Based on the study findings, nursing student participants predominantly reflected essentialist rather than constructivist perspectives of culture. The researchers affirmed that nurse educators should be aware of their perspective on culture and how culture is taught to nursing students to be able to move away from the limiting essentialist perspective.

Language clarity among nurse managers, nurse leaders, staff nurses, and nursing students is important so that everyone uses common points of reference in practice. Language clarity is also important to nurse leaders and staff nurses in relation to quality patient-care practices. When a message communicated to or by a patient is translated from one language to another, it is important to ensure linguistic equivalence, which means that the message must have the same meaning in both languages. Achieving an equivalent translation involves interpretation, which extends beyond a "word-for-word" translation. When providing care to a patient from another culture whose first language is not English, the nurse must realize that the process of translation of illness or disease conditions and treatment can be complex. Thus, a nurse who values cultural safety should advocate for and retain a translator for the patient. By doing so, the principles of equity and justice for the patient are at the forefront of how the nurse engages in the care experience.

As role models, nurse managers and leaders can demonstrate a constructivist perspective of cultural diversity through their everyday actions. It is vital to explore the idea of cultural diversity at an individual level. The International Council of Nurses (ICN) (2013) notes that diversity in nursing "means understanding that each individual is unique, and recognizing individual differences. These differences may span the dimensions of race, ethnicity, gender, sexual orientation, socio-economic status, age, physical abilities, religious beliefs, political beliefs or other ideologies"

(p. 2). The Registered Nurses' Association of Ontario (2007) proposes a similar definition, in that cultural diversity "is used to describe variation between people in terms of a range of factors such as ethnicity, national origin, race, gender, ability, age, physical characteristics, religion, values, beliefs, sexual orientation, socio-economic class, or life experiences" (p. 70). Further, Burnard and Gill (2009) suggest that culture reflects an individual's identity or sense of self. Thus, to explore individual perceptions of identity, along with what is observed, nurse managers and leaders need to interact with people from different cultures. Doing so can help them develop cultural sensitivity, which is the capacity to recognize that people from cultures other than our own are individuals who share similarities and differences.

The *Code of Ethics for Registered Nurses* of the (CNA, 2008) sets out primary nursing values (see Chapter 2, page 25) that should be applied in a way that respects the cultural diversity of health care staff, patients, and their families. For instance, nursing value six—promoting justice—requires that "nurses uphold principles of justice by safeguarding human rights, equity and fairness and by promoting the public good" (p. 21). Applying this value to nursing practice, if a nurse manager or leader does not support a nurse who seeks to provide an interpreter for a patient who cannot speak English, then the patient is not being treated fairly or equally, and the patient's human rights are essentially violated. This ethical value helps nurses recognize that health care must be provided to culturally diverse populations in Canada and globally. Although a nurse may be inclined to impose his or her own cultural values on others (patients or staff), refraining from doing so affirms the nurse's respect for and sensitivity to the values and health care practices associated with a multitude of cultures.

Effective leaders shape the cultural sensitivity of their organizational culture. Doing so demonstrates cultural competence in action (CNA, 2010). *Cultural competence* is the process of integrating values, beliefs, and attitudes different from one's own perspective in order to render effective nursing care. "Culturally competent practices are a congruent set of workforce behaviours, management practices and institutional policies within a practice setting resulting in an organisational environment that is inclusive of cultural and other forms of diversity" (Pearson, Srivastava, Craig, et al., 2007, p. 55). According to Noone (2008): "Nursing leaders at all levels are calling for a nursing workforce able to provide culturally competent patient care. Our commitment to social justice and the practical demands of the workplace call for nursing to take strong, sustained, and measurable actions to produce a workforce that closely parallels the population it serves" (p. 133).

Cultural safety relates to the acknowledgement that power difference and inequities exist in systems, including health care (ANAC, 2009). It refers to what is experienced by a patient when health care providers communicate in a respectful and inclusive way, empowering the patient in decision making and ensuring maximum effectiveness of care (National Aboriginal Health Organization, 2008). Nurse managers, nurse leaders, and staff nurses have a vital role to play in addressing issues of power and inequity through collaborative advocacy efforts and by uncovering practices that can lead to inequitable access to care or to forms of discrimination or racism that can ultimately affect the provision of care (Varcoe, 2004, as cited in ANAC, 2009). A lack of mutual understanding between people from different cultures can lead to cultural marginality, which has been defined as "situations and feelings of passive betweenness when people exist between two different cultures and do not yet perceive themselves as centrally belonging to either one" (Choi, 2001, p. 193). Therefore, it is imperative for nurse managers, nurse leaders, and staff nurses not to make assumptions about culture, and to initiate a dialogue with individuals to explore what culture means for them.

related to gender and ethnic diversity. The numbers of men recruited into the profession have risen but not to the point of creating gender equality. According to the Canadian Institute of Health Information (2009), approximately 6% of all registered nurses in Canada were male in 2009. Although stereotypes (e.g., "not smart enough for medical school") have diminished over the years, the number of men in nursing still does not approach the proportional number of men in Canada. In terms of ethnic diversity, according to the 2006 census (Statistics Canada, 2006), 1 172 790 Canadian people (3.7% of the total population) self-reported as an Aboriginal person (Inuit, Métis, First Nations). However, in 2006, 2.2% of health care providers in Canada were of Aboriginal ethnicity (Lecompte, 2012). Many Canadian nursing organizations and academic institutions are creating educational pathways to increase the number of Aboriginal nurses in practice (ANAC, 2009). Because nursing is not a particularly diverse profession, it is critical for nurse managers and leaders to provide support to those who are a minority in employment settings and to foster cultural sensitivity in the workforce.

Health care organizations can benefit from providing nursing staff with professional development opportunities in culturally competent and culturally safe patient care. In addition, they could also address these topics in relation to how health care providers from various cultural backgrounds can collaborate to develop and sustain healthy practice environments. Such environments are fundamental to advancing quality patient care.

EXERCISE 10-1

If you were to provide care to a patient from another culture in an acute care setting, in what ways could you show cultural competence and ensure cultural safety?

How would these actions be different from how you have provided care in the past or have seen care provided by others in the past?

EXERCISE 10-2

On the accompanying Evolve site under Additional Resources, complete the Cultural Competence Self-Assessment Tool for Primary Health Care Providers.

What did you learn from using the tool? In what ways might you develop additional cultural competence?

CULTURAL DIVERSITY IN HEALTH CARE ORGANIZATIONS

The demographics of the nursing profession have historically not matched general demographics

Managing in a Culturally Diverse Environment

Managing in a culturally diverse environment means managing personal thinking and helping others to think in new ways. Managing issues that involve culture—whether institutional, ethnic, gender, religious, or any other kind—requires patience, persistence, and much understanding. One way to promote this understanding is through shared stories that have symbolic power.

EXERCISE 10-3
Think of a recent event in your learning environment or workplace, such as a project, task force, or celebration. What meaning did people give to the event? What quality of the learning environment or workplace did it symbolize (e.g., effectiveness, values and beliefs, innovation)? How is cultural diversity considered?

A health care organization with a straightforward mission and clear goals, rewards, and acknowledgement of efforts leads to greater productivity and work effort from a culturally diverse staff who aspires to unity. When assessing staff diversity, the nurse manager can ask these questions:

- What is the cultural representation of individuals in the workplace?
- What kind of team-building activities are needed to create a cohesive workforce for effective health care delivery?
- How can management and staff further enhance cultural competence and cultural safety in the workplace?

Nurse managers and leaders who have a positive view of culture and its characteristics effectively acknowledge cultural diversity among staff and patients. This includes providing culturally sensitive care to patients while simultaneously balancing a culturally diverse staff.

To show their understanding and value of cultural diversity, nurse managers and leaders need to approach every staff person as an individual. Although staff members may have different cultural origins and may be diverse in appearance, values, beliefs, communication patterns, and mannerisms, they have many things in common. For example, staff members want to be accepted by others and to succeed in their jobs. With fairness and respect, nurse managers and leaders should openly support the competencies and contributions of staff members from all cultural groups with the goal of achieving quality patient care. Nurse managers and leaders hold the key to enabling the full potential of each person on the staff.

Sullivan and Decker (2009) described the importance of communication and how cultural attitudes, beliefs, and behaviour affect communication. Body movements, gestures, verbal tone, and physical closeness in communication tend to be determined by a person's culture. For the nurse manager or leader, understanding culturally specific behaviours is imperative in accomplishing effective communication in a diverse workforce. Tappen (2001) addressed differences across cultures that the nurse manager and leader need to monitor. These differences include relationships to people in authority, spatial differences, eye contact, expressions of feelings, meaning of different language versions, thinking modes, evidence-informed decision making, and preferred leadership or management style. Failure to address cultural diversity leads to negative effects on performance and staff interactions.

Nurse managers and leaders can address cultural diversity in many ways. For example, in relation to performance, a nurse manager can make sure messages about patient care are received. This might be accomplished by sitting down with a staff nurse and analyzing the situation to ensure that understanding has occurred. In addition, the nurse manager might use a communication notebook that allows the nurse to slowly "digest" information by writing down communication areas that may be unclear. For effective staff interaction, the nurse manager can also make a special effort to pair mentors and mentees who have different ethnic backgrounds.

For nurse managers and leaders, attending to cultural diversity requires being sensitive to or being able to embrace the emotions of a large multicultural group comprising staff and patients. It might mean acknowledging and respecting choices related to faith. For instance, Muslims are one of the fastest-growing populations in North America and worldwide. El Gindy (2004) addressed the need to show respect for and accommodate Muslim nurses' dress requirements and to understand the role of Islam in their lives. For example, one Muslim nurse wore her hijab and became frustrated because the infection control staff consistently asked her to wear short sleeves or to roll up the sleeves. El Gindy stated that for Muslim women, following the Islamic dress code is necessary to obey the dictate that their body must be covered in the presence of males who are not family.

Regardless of organizational setting, health care providers should be made aware of this religious belief, whether it exists among staff or patients, and respond to it in a positive way.

A nurse manager's or leader's choices, decisions, and behaviours reflect learned beliefs, values, ideals, and preferences. A nurse manager or leader who shows respect for culturally diverse individuals and groups supports the best interests of both staff and patients.

Cultural Diversity and Patient Care

In Canada, many patients in health care settings are new to this country. According to the 2011 National Household Survey, 6.8 million people, or 20.6% of the total Canadian population, were born outside the country (Statistics Canada, 2013). This was the highest proportion since 1931, when foreign-born people made up 22.2% of the population (Statistics Canada, 2003, p. 4). Further, of the 1.2 million immigrants who arrived between 2006 and 2011, 56.9% were from Asia, including the Middle East; 13.7% from Europe; 12.3% from the Caribbean, Central and South America; 12.5% from Africa; and 3.9% from the United States (Statistics Canada, 2013). New immigrants to Canada might have varied understandings about the Canadian health care system, their rights to health care through Canada's national health insurance plan, and how to navigate the health care system. Often, issues of accessibility to health care influence whether care is ever sought or provided (see, for example, the Literature Perspective in Chapter 11, page 190).

Accessibility to health care in Canada is based on the *Canada Health Act* principles of universality and accessibility (Health Canada, 2014). However, such principles are not always adequately upheld. For instance, individuals living in rural or remote areas might not have ready access to health care or might have access to limited amounts and types of care. Further, individuals who do not speak English or French as their first language may find it challenging to know how or where to access health care. Such discrepancies in Canada's health care system challenge nurse managers and leaders who seek to value, respect, and provide individualized attention to patients and staff regardless of their culture, education, geographical location, or socioeconomic status. Novice nurse managers and leaders may feel that they lack "real-life" experience

that could help them address staff and patient needs. In reality, while a lack of experience may be a slight drawback, it is by no means an obstacle to addressing individual staff and patient issues. If nurse managers and leaders understand people and their needs, they can advocate for and gain access to health care for all Canadians.

Communication and Patient Care

Nurse leaders need to ensure that clear and understandable communication takes place between health care providers and patients. Ineffective communication by staff with patients and others can lead to misunderstandings and eventual alienation. The use of a health professional interpreter can be an effective strategy when caring for non–English-speaking or limited–English-speaking patients. The current practice seems to be one of using these interpreters rather than translators when speaking with non–English-speaking patients. Why? Purnell and Paulanka (2008) advocate that trained health care providers who act as interpreters can decode words and provide the right meaning of the message. However, Purnell and Paulanka also state that interpreters might affect the reporting of symptoms if they apply their own ideas or omit information. It is important to allow time for translation and interpretation and to clarify information as needed. When patients and health care providers cannot communicate effectively, inequities in accessing needed health care services might translate into negative health outcomes.

CULTURAL DIVERSITY AND PREJUDICE

Canadian society is considered to be a "cultural mosaic" because it includes people of different ethnicities who maintain their culture and language. Given that Canada's population includes Aboriginal peoples and immigrants from all over the world, cultural diversity is the norm and ought to be respected and valued as contributing to the unique and non-homogeneous character of the country.

Based on the College of Nurses of Ontario (2009) ethical framework, nurses have an obligation to care for all patients, regardless of differences—whether they be related to culture, economic status, or gender. Providing care for a person or people from a culture other than one's own is a dynamic and complex experience. The experience according to Spence (2004) might involve "prejudice, paradox and possibility" (p. 140). Prejudices "enable us to make sense of the situations in which we find ourselves, yet they also constrain understanding and limit the capacity to come to new or different ways of understanding. It is this contradiction that makes prejudice paradoxical" (Spence, 2004, p. 163). Paradox, although it may seem incongruent with prejudice, describes the dynamic interplay of tensions between individuals or groups. It is our responsibility to acknowledge the "possibility of tension" as a potential for new and different understandings derived from our communication and interpretation. Possibility, therefore, presumes a condition for openness with a person from another culture (Spence, 2004). Using hermeneutic interpretation, Spence conducted a study that consisted of accounts from 17 New Zealand nurses who delivered nursing care to patients in acute medical and surgical wards, public health centres, mental health settings, and midwifery specialties. Spence found that prejudice was a condition that enabled or constrained interpretation based on one's values, attitudes, and actions. By talking with people outside their "circle of familiarity," the nurses enhanced their understanding of personally held prejudices. As such, the provision of patient care also became a learning opportunity, which detracted from prejudice and opened up the potential for new understanding and awareness of culture from an individual or family perspective.

> **EXERCISE 10-4**
> In a group, discuss the values and beliefs of justice and equality. As a nurse, you may have strong values and beliefs, but you may never have observed their application in health care. Consider language, skin colour, dress, and gestures of patients and staff from various cultures. How will you learn and value what individual differences exist?

CULTURE AND THEORETICAL MODELS

How do managers, leaders, and followers take all of the expanding information on cultural diversity in health care and give it a useful organizing structure that can be applied to practice? Purnell (2002), Campinha-Bacote (1999, 2002), and Giger and Davidhizar (2002) provide theoretical models to guide health care providers in delivering culturally competent patient care.

Purnell's (2002) Model for Cultural Competence provides an organizing framework (Figure 10-1). The model uses a circle with the outer zone representing global society, the second zone representing community, the third zone representing family, and the inner zone representing the person. The interior of the circle is divided into 12 pie-shaped wedges delineating cultural domains and their concepts (e.g., workplace issues, family roles and organization, spirituality, and health care practices). The innermost centre circle is black, representing unknown phenomena. Cultural consciousness is expressed in behaviours from unconsciously incompetent (being unaware of one's lack of cultural knowledge), consciously incompetent (being aware of one's lack of cultural knowledge), consciously competent (providing culturally specific interventions), to unconsciously competent (automatically providing culturally congruent care to patients). The usefulness of this model is derived from its concise structure, applicability to any setting, and wide range of experiences that can foster inductive and deductive thinking when assessing cultural domains.

Campinha-Bacote's (1999, 2002) model of cultural competence in health care delivery comprises five constructs: (1) cultural awareness, (2) cultural knowledge, (3) cultural skill, (4) cultural encounters, and (5) cultural desire. All of the constructs have an interdependent relationship, and health care providers must address or experience each of them. In doing so, health care providers cultivate greater cultural competence. Cultural awareness is the self-examination and in-depth exploration of one's own cultural and professional background. It involves the recognition of one's bias, prejudices, and assumptions about individuals from other cultures (Campinha-Bacote, 2002). "One's world view can be considered a paradigm or way of viewing the world and phenomena in it" (Campinha-Bacote, 1999, p. 204). Cultural knowledge is the process of seeking and obtaining a sound educational foundation about diverse cultural and ethnic groups. Further, obtaining cultural information about the individual patient's health-related beliefs and values will help explain how he or she interprets his or her illness and how it guides his or her thinking, doing, and being (Campinha-Bacote,

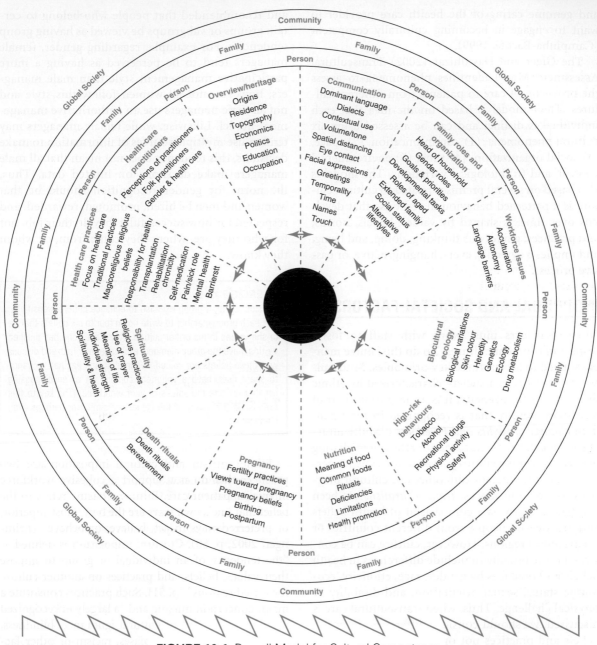

FIGURE 10-1 Purnell Model for Cultural Competence.

2002). The skill of conducting a cultural assessment is learned while assessing one's values, beliefs, and practices to provide culturally competent services. Cultural encounters are direct engagement with individuals from other cultures. This process allows the person to validate, negate, or modify his or her existing cultural knowledge. It provides culturally specific knowledge bases from which the individual can develop culturally relevant interventions. Cultural desire requires the intrinsic qualities of motivation and genuine caring of the health care provider to want to engage in becoming culturally competent (Campinha-Bacote, 1999).

The Giger and Davidhizar (2002) Transcultural Assessment Model identifies phenomena to assess the provision of care to patients from different cultures. Their model is based on the idea that each individual is distinct and can be assessed using six cultural phenomena: (1) communication, (2) space, (3) social organization, (4) time, (5) environmental control, and (6) biological variations. The model is also based on several premises related to culture: culture is a patterned behavioural response that develops over time; is shaped by values, beliefs, norms, and practices; guides our thinking, doing, and being; and implies a dynamic, ever-changing, active, or passive process.

INDIVIDUAL AND SOCIETAL FACTORS

Nurse managers must work with staff to foster respect of different cultures. To do this, nurse managers need to accept three key principles. **Multiculturalism** refers to a society characterized by ethnic or cultural heterogeneity; it is an important part of Canadian identity that is recognized in the *Canadian Charter of Rights and Freedoms* ("Multiculturalism," n.d.). **Cross-culturalism** refers to mediating between or among cultures. **Transculturalism** refers to bridging significant differences in cultural practices. In some instances, *transculturalism* has been defined narrowly as a comparison of health beliefs and practices of people from different countries or geographical regions. However, culture can be construed more broadly to include differences in health beliefs and practices by gender, race, ethnicity, economic status, sexual orientation, and disability or physical challenge. Thus, when transcultural care is discussed, we should consider differences in health beliefs and practices not only between and among nationalities but also between genders, and between and among individuals of different races, ethnic groups, and socioeconomic levels. As a result, nurses need to consider multiple factors about all individuals.

All members of a particular group or subgroup are *not* indistinguishable. Tappen (2001) described this "indistinguishable" phenomenon

and recommended that people who belong to certain groups or subgroups be viewed as having group tendencies. For example, regarding gender, female managers tend to be perceived as having a more participative management style than male managers; however, not all women follow this style and not all male managers use an authoritative management model. Likewise, while female managers may tend to use multiple sources of information to make decisions, this tendency does not mean that all male managers make decisions on limited data. Thus, the norm for gender recognition should be that women and men be hired, promoted, rewarded, and respected for how successfully they do their job, not for who they are, where they come from, or whom they know.

EXERCISE 10-5

Consider doing a group exercise to enhance cultural sensitivity. Ask each group member to write down four to six beliefs that he or she values in his or her culture. When everyone has finished writing, have the group members exchange their lists and discuss why these beliefs are valued. When everyone has had a chance to share lists, have a volunteer compile an all-encompassing list that reflects the values of your workforce. (The key to this exercise is that many of the values are similar or perhaps even identical.)

Ethnocentrism and cultural imposition are two practices that do not support a cohesive workforce or quality patient care. **Ethnocentrism** "refers to the belief that one's own ways are the best, most superior, or preferred ways to act, believe, or behave" (Leininger, 2002, p. 50). **Cultural imposition** is defined as "the tendency of an individual or group to impose their values, beliefs, and practices on another culture for varied reasons" (p. 51). Such practices constitute a major concern in nursing and "a largely unrecognized problem as a result of cultural ignorance, blindness, ethnocentric tendencies, biases, racism or other factors" (p. 51).

Although the literature has addressed the multicultural needs of patients, it is sparse in identifying effective methods for nurse managers to use when dealing with multicultural staff. Differences in education and culture can influence patient care, and uncomfortable situations may emerge from such differences. For example, staff members may be reluctant to admit language problems that hamper their written communication. They may also be reluctant to admit their lack of understanding when interpreting directions. Psychosocial skills may be problematic as well, because some non-Western cultures encourage emotional restraint. Staff may have difficulty addressing issues that relate to private family matters. The lack of assertiveness and the subservient physician–nurse relationships of some cultures are other issues that provide challenges for nurse managers. Nurse managers can help prepare staff to handle cultural work situations in two ways: by arranging unit-oriented workshops to address effective techniques and by involving family to better understand cultural differences as they apply to patient care.

Giddens (2008) has encouraged the use of multicontextual learning environments to enhance the learning of diverse students. She created a Web-based virtual community called The Neighborhood as an exemplar of such a learning environment. The Neighborhood features 30 fictional characters from different cultural and socioeconomic backgrounds with different health issues and their interactions with health care providers in various health care settings. It is designed to promote conceptual learning and offer an alternative approach to learning about diversity in undergraduate nursing programs. According to Giddens, "The Neighborhood presents nursing concepts in a rich personal and community context through stories and supplemental multimedia" (p. 78). Nurse managers can also use this innovative teaching tool to expand staff members' understanding of how to interact with diverse patients. In addition, this learning tool helps address the Institute of Medicine's (2004) finding that the lack of cultural diversity in the nursing workforce affects the quality of health care delivery.

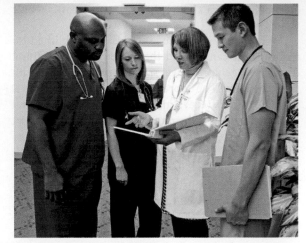

Respecting cultural diversity in the team fosters cooperation and supports sound decision making.

DEALING EFFECTIVELY WITH CULTURAL DIVERSITY

Nurse managers and leaders are the key people who must address cultural diversity in the health care workplace. They must give unwavering support to embracing diversity in the workplace rather than use a standard "cookie cutter" approach. Creating a culturally competent workplace involves a long-term vision and both financial and health care provider commitment. Nurse managers and leaders need to make the strategic decision to design services and programs to meet the needs of culturally diverse staff and patients. They need to focus first on building a knowledge base by requiring employees to attend educational sessions to become familiar with cultural practices and to achieve a culture-friendly environment (Biggerstaff & Hamby, 2004).

Nurse managers hold the key to making cultural diversity an asset. They have the position of power to create activities and programs that enrich the cultural knowledge of staff. For example, they can capitalize on the staff's personal cultural beliefs and knowledge to achieve better quality care outcomes. One way to do so is to allow staff to verbalize their feelings about particular cultures in relationship to personal beliefs. Another is to have two or three staff members of different ethnic origins present a patient-care conference, giving their views on how they would care for

---

EXERCISE 10-6

As a small group activity, reflect on previous or current clinical practice settings where you have had a clinical placement. Do these settings have professional development programs or policies related to cultural diversity in the workplace? If yes, why is that the case? What do the programs cover? What do the policies propose in regard to staff and patients? If there are no programs or policies, why do you think they have not been implemented?

a specific patient's needs based on their own ethnic values.

Mentorship programs should be established so that all staff can expand their knowledge of cultural diversity. Mentors have specific relationships with their mentees. The more closely aligned a mentor is with the mentee (e.g., similar age group, ethnicity, and primary language), the more effective the relationship. Programs that address the staff's cultural diversity should not try to make people of different cultures pattern their behaviour after the prevailing culture. Nurse managers must carefully select those mentors who ascribe to transcultural, rather than ethnocentric, values and beliefs.

A much richer staff exists when nurse managers build on the valuable culture of all staff members and when diversity is rewarded. Nurse managers are aware of the increasing shortage of nurses, the demanding work environment with its external influences, and studies indicating that new nurses have a high rate of intention to leave during their first professional nursing position because of job dissatisfaction and level of stress (Lavoie-Tremblay, O'Brien-Pallas, Gelinas, et al., 2008). The first year of a nursing position may be even more challenging for individuals whose culture differs from the predominant unit culture.

The National Quality Forum (NQF) (NQF, 2009) created a comprehensive framework for measuring and reporting cultural competency in health care settings. The 45 preferred practices the NFQ endorses fall within the following domains: leadership; integration into management systems and operations; patient–provider communication; care delivery and supporting mechanisms; workforce diversity and training; community engagement; and data collection, public accountability, and quality improvement. The NQF framework provides nurse managers, leaders, and staff with preferred practices that can enhance the delivery of culturally competent patient care.

Continuing-education programs can also help nurses learn about the care of different ethnic groups. For example, professional organizations related to cultural groups and institutions might develop or sponsor a workshop or conference on cross-cultural nursing for nursing service staff and faculty in schools of nursing who have had limited preparation in cultural care or cultural beliefs in healing.

EXERCISE 10-7

Identify a situation in which working with culturally diverse staff had positive or negative outcomes. If a negative outcome resulted, what could you have done to make it a positive one? If a positive outcome resulted, share lessons learned on how to make future interactions positive.

EXERCISE 10-8

Identify a situation involving a staff member or student nurse colleague requesting additional days of leave that required a culturally sensitive decision. What religious or ethnic practices did you learn about in regard to this request and decision?

EXERCISE 10-9

Holiday celebrations have cultural significance. Select a specific holiday such as the Chinese Lunar New Year, Araw ng mga Patay (Philippines), or Diwali (India). What is the cultural meaning of the holiday? How do staff members or students of the respective culture celebrate the festive day? Does the nursing unit or academic environment engage in recognition of special holidays?

The two scenarios described in Box 10-1 illustrate how problem-solving communication can promote mutual understanding and respect. The first scenario involves a nurse manager and a staff member from a different culture and the second scenario involves a nurse, an individual coping with a terminal illness, and the connectedness of community.

CONCLUSION

Nurses are called upon to provide quality care for a growing number of culturally diverse patients. Nurse managers and leaders who embrace diversity inspire others to do the same. They make clear that staff are valued as individual people, not as representatives of some group. By showing respect for all patients, regardless of their cultural background, nurse managers and leaders demonstrate to staff nurses that their cultural differences are also valued. It is key for nurse managers and leaders to attend to diversity issues in the nursing workforce with the same zest as they do patient issues. Promoting cultural awareness and understanding is essential to workplace harmony as well as quality, culturally competent care.

BOX 10-1 PROBLEM-SOLVING COMMUNICATION: HONOURING CULTURAL ATTITUDES

Scenario 1: A Nurse Manager and Another Staff Member

Eastern Catholics celebrate a loved one 40 days after the death. The nurse manager needs to recognize that time off for the nurse involved in this celebration is imperative. Such an occurrence had to be addressed by a nurse manager of Asian descent. The nurse manager quickly realized that the nurse, whose mother died in India, did not ask for any time off to make the necessary burial arrangements but, rather, waited 40 days to celebrate his mother's death. The celebration included formal invitations to a church service, as well as a dinner after the service. One day during early morning rounds, the nurse explained how death is celebrated by many Eastern Catholics. The Bible's description of the Ascension of the Lord into heaven 40 days after his death served as the conceptual framework for the loved one's death. The grieving family believed their loved one's spirit would stay on earth for 40 days. During these 40 days, the family held prayer sessions meant to assist the "spirit" to prepare for its ascension into heaven. When the 40 days have passed, the celebration previously described marks the ascension of the loved one's spirit into heaven. Because this particular unit truly espoused a multicultural concept, the nurses had no difficulty in allowing the Indian nurse 2 weeks of unplanned vacation so that his mother's "passage of life" celebration could be accomplished in a respectful, dignified manner.

Scenario 2: A Nurse, a Patient, the Family, and the Community

Bourque Bearskin (2011), a Cree/Métis nurse from a First Nations community, tells the story of Nicole, a 19-year-old First Nations member of a northern community, who was seriously injured in a car accident while she was the passenger of a vehicle with a drunk driver. Her injuries included a serious brain stem injury that required that she be transferred from her community to a tertiary hospital in the south. The nurses in the intensive care unit (ICU) cared for her for two days before Nicole's family were able to travel to the hospital from their northern community. Her parents and extended family, including the community Elder, arrived and requested permission to integrate traditional approaches to care along with the other aspects of nursing care for Nicole. Bourque Bearskin describes what happened:

> The Elder requested permission from the nursing staff to perform a ceremony that would include smudging (ritual cleansing) and the use of traditional medicines. However, because of the concern for the safety of other patients in the ICU, the staff denied the request, and the family members were disappointed; the deep despair on their faces was evident. They continued to make requests and incorporate their traditions in caring for Nicole. They pin a medicine pouch to the inside of the nursing gown close to the body and near the heart. They believed that the contents would protect her and guide her to the spirit world. With clear directions to the staff not to touch or remove the pouch, the family returned on numerous occasions to find that it had been removed and pinned to the wall. The staff contended that the pouch impeded their ability to provide safe care; because in their view the risk of infection was a serious concern, they had removed the pouch. Upset, the family members approached the nurses with harsh words, but the nurses labeled them difficult, uncooperative, and disrespectful of hospital policies. After several discussions the staff permitted the family to tie the pouch to Nicole's left ankle. However, on another occasion the family found the pouch tied to Nicole's left big toe. Distressed and feeling helpless, the family said nothing though they were extremely angered by the situation. To help ease the tensions with the family, the staff scheduled an interdisciplinary meeting during which the physician informed the family that Nicole would recover and that, as soon as she was stable, she would be transferred home. With this renewed hope, the family began the necessary preparations to return home to the north. They left the next day, and a day later Nicole died alone. (p. 550)

Bourque Bearskin's description of Nicole's care in the ICU highlights the importance for nurses to understand the unique cultural needs of patients and their families and illuminates the importance of honouring cultural approaches to health care. How might the nurses have incorporated cultural competence and cultural safety into their approach to Nicole's care?

💡 A SOLUTION

To increase his cultural competence, Dwayne decided that he would strive to learn more about every person—patients and colleagues—encountered in his practice. He knew cultural safety might be an important part of northern experiences and that being aware of his own cultural perspective might be the first step to understanding other cultures. Dwayne asked people to tell him about themselves and encouraged them to share their life stories. With a genuine interest in learning about northern ways and northern peoples, he listened for what people valued and how they experienced the health care system. He decided that the people he encountered held the expertise he needed to increase his knowledge of northern life and culture. Dwayne also participated in local community events, which offered him greater insight into local ideas, beliefs, and values.

Would this be a suitable approach for you? Why or why not?

THE EVIDENCE

1. Acknowledging cultural diversity in patients and staff requires leaders to be proactive.
2. Working with culturally diverse nursing organizations enhances opportunities for successful recruitment and retention.
3. Taking deliberate actions to acknowledge and celebrate culturally related events helps employees from various groups feel valued.

NEED TO KNOW NOW

- Determine what the dominant cultural groups are in your community and know what the implications for care are.
- Be aware that many subcultures exist within cultures and that each individual has his or her own perspective of culture and how it influences the health and illness experience.
- Be alert for opportunities to learn about co-workers' cultural backgrounds and practices.
- Know how to retrieve literature and research related to best practices and evidence for cultural topics in health care.

CHAPTER CHECKLIST

All potential or current nurse managers or leaders must acknowledge and address cultural diversity among staff and patients. Culture lives in each of us. It contributes to how we think, what we value, how we behave, and how we communicate with each other. In everyday work activities, the nurse manager must be able to do the following:

- Assess staff diversity and use techniques to manage a culturally diverse workforce and recognize staff members' diverse strengths. Use the strengths to benefit the unit and patients.
- Lead staff with a clear understanding of principles that embrace culture, cultural diversity, and cultural sensitivity.
- Be able to communicate effectively with staff and patients from diverse cultural backgrounds:
  - Recognize terms that have different meanings for individuals in different cultures.
  - Understand that nonverbal behaviours also carry different connotations depending on one's culture.
- Appraise factors, both individual and societal, inherent in cultural diversity:
  - Three key principles foster respect for different lifestyles:

- *Multiculturalism* refers to maintaining several different cultures simultaneously.
- *Cross-culturalism* refers to mediating bestween or among cultures.
- *Transculturalism* denotes bridging significant differences in cultural practices.
- Ethnicity, national origin, race, gender, ability, age, physical characteristics, religion, values, beliefs, sexual orientation, socioeconomic class, and life experiences are important factors to consider in dealing fairly with all cultures and staff members.
- Use tools that clarify staff cultural diversity effectively:
  - Mentoring programs can help staff expand their knowledge of cultural diversity and recognize their own biases as well as better integrate with diverse colleagues.
  - Continuing education programs can help nurses learn about caring for different ethnic groups in ways that honour patients' beliefs.
- Appreciate the cultural richness of staff and patients.
  - Print and online resources can provide nurses with valuable information on cultural topics.

■ TIPS FOR DEALING WITH CULTURAL DIVERSITY

Canadian nurse managers practise in a culturally rich country. Thus, nurse managers need to do the following:

• Describe to effective techniques for managing a culturally diverse workforce.

• Encourage programs that show appreciation for and build understanding of the cultural diversity of staff and patients.

• Help address the special cultural needs of colleagues and patients.

• Embrace three key principles relating to culture: multiculturalism, cross-culturalism, and transculturalism.

• Commit to lifelong learning about culture for their benefit and that of staff and patients.

℮volve WEBSITE

Visit the Evolve website for Suggested Readings, Internet Resources, and additional resources related to the content in this chapter: http://evolve.elsevier.com/Canada/Yoder-Wise/leading/.

REFERENCES

Aboriginal Nurses Association of Canada. (2009). *Cultural competence and cultural safety in nursing education.* Ottawa, ON: Aboriginal Nurses Association of Canada. Retrieved from http://www.anac.on.ca/Documents/Making%20It%20Happen%20Curriculum%20Project/FINALFRAMEWORK.pdf.

Biggerstaff, G., & Hamby, L. (2004). Diversity: An evolving leadership initiative. *Nurse Leader, 2*(4), 30.

Bourque Bearskin, R. L. (2011). A critical lens on culture in nursing practice. *Nurse Ethics, 18*(4), 548–559. doi:10.1177/0969733011408048

Burnard, P., & Gill, P. (2009). *Culture, communication and nursing.* Harlow, UK: Pearson Education.

Campinha-Bacote, J. (1999). A model and instrument for addressing cultural competence in health care. *Journal of Nursing Education, 38*(5), 203–207.

Campinha-Bacote, J. (2002). The process of cultural competence in a delivery of healthcare services: A model of care. *Journal of Transcultural Nursing, 13*(3), 181–184.

Canadian Institute of Health Information. (2009). Canada's health providers 2009 provincial profiles: A look at 24 health occupations. Retrieved from https://secure.cihi.ca/free_products/ProvProf2009EN.pdf.

Canadian Nurses Association. (2004). Position statement: Promoting culturally competent care. Canadian Nurses Association. Retrieved from http://www.cna-aiic.ca/sitecore%20modules/web/~/media/cna/page%20content/pdf%20fr/2013/09/05/18/06/ps73_promoting_culturally_competent_care_march_2004_e.pdf#search=%22culture%22.

Canadian Nurses Association. (2008). *Code of ethics for registered nurses (2008 centennial edition).* Toronto, ON: Author. Retrieved from http://www.cna-aiic.ca/~/media/cna/page%20content/pdf%20fr/2013/09/05/18/05/code_of_ethics_2008_e.pdf.

Canadian Nurses Association. (2010). Position statement: Promoting cultural competence in nursing. Retrieved from http://www.cna-aiic.ca/~/media/cna/page%20content/pdf%20en/2013/09/04/16/27/6%20-%20ps114_cultural_competence_2010_e.pdf.

Choi, H. (2001). Cultural marginality: A concept analysis with implications for immigrant adolescents. *Issues in Comprehensive Pediatric Nursing, 24,* 193–206.

College of Nurses of Ontario. (2009). *Practice standard: Ethics.* Retrieved from http://www.cno.org/Global/docs/prac/41034_Ethics.pdf.

El Gindy, G. (2004, Winter). Treating Muslims with cultural sensitivity in a post-9/11 world. *Minority Nurse,* 44–46.

Giddens, J. F. (2008). Online content: Achieving diversity in nursing through multicontextual learning environments. *Nursing Outlook , 56,* 78–83.

Giger, J. N., & Davidhizar, R. (2002). The Giger and Davidhizar transcultural assessment model. *Journal of Transcultural Nursing, 13*(3), 185–188.

Gray, D. P., & Thomas, D. J. (2006). Critical reflections on culture in nursing. *Journal of Cultural Diversity 13*(2), 76–82.

Gregory, D., Harrowing, J., Lee, B., et al. (2010). Nursing pedagogy as contributing to essentialized understanding of culture among undergraduate nursing students. *International Journal of Nursing Education Scholarship,* 7, Article [On-line].

Health Canada. (2014). *Canada's health care system.* Ottawa, ON: Author. Retrieved from http://www.hc-sc.gc.ca/hcs-sss/pubs/system-regime/2011-hcs-sss/index-eng.php.

Institute of Medicine. (2004). *In the nation's compelling interest: Ensuring diversity in the health-care workforce.* Washington, DC: National Academies Press.

International Council of Nurses. (2013). *Cultural and linguistic competence: Position statement.* Geneva, Switzerland: Author. Retrieved from http://www.icn.ch/images/stories/documents/publications/position_statements/B03_Cultural_Linguistic_Competence.pdf.

Lavoie-Tremblay, M., O'Brien-Pallas, L., Gelinas, C., et al. (2008). Addressing the turnover issue among new nurses from a generational viewpoint. *Journal of Nursing Management, 16*(6), 724–733.

Lecompte, E. (2012, March). Aboriginal health human resources: A matter of health. *Journal of Aboriginal Health,* 16–22. Retrieved from http://www.naho.ca/jah/english/jah08_02/08_02_health-human-resources.pdf.

Leininger, M. (2002). Essential transcultural nursing care concepts, principles, examples, and policy statements. In M. Leininger & M. R. McFarland (Eds.), *Transcultural nursing: Concepts, theories, research & practice* (3rd ed., pp. 129–130). New York, NY: McGraw-Hill Medical.

Multiculturalism. (n.d.) Historica Canada. Retrieved from http://-www.thecanadianencyclopedia.ca/en/article/multiculturalism/.

National Aboriginal Health Organization. (2008). *Cultural competency and safety: A guide for health care administrators, providers and educators.* Ottawa. ON: Author. Retrieved from http://www.naho.ca/documents/naho/publications/culturalCompetency.pdf.

National Quality Forum. (2009). *Endorsing a framework and preferred practices for measuring and reporting cultural competency.* Washington, DC: Author. Retrieved from http://www.quality forum.org/Publications/2009/04/A_Comprehensive_Framework_ and_Preferred_Practices_for_Measuring_and_Reporting _Cultural_Competency.aspx.

Noone, J. (2008). The diversity imperative: Strategies to address a diverse nursing workforce. *Nursing Forum, 43*(3), 133–143.

Pearson, A., Srivastava, R., Craig, D., et al. (2007). Systematic review on embracing cultural diversity for developing and sustaining a healthy work environment in healthcare. *International Journal of Evidence-Based Healthcare, 5*, 54–91.

Purnell, L. D. (2002). The Purnell model of cultural competence. *Journal of Transcultural Nursing, 13*(3), 193–196.

Purnell, L. D., & Paulanka, B. J. (2008). *Transcultural health care: A culturally competent approach* (3rd ed.). Philadelphia, PA: FA Davis.

Registered Nurses' Association of Ontario. (2007). *Embracing cultural diversity in health care: Developing cultural competence.* Toronto, ON: Author.

Spence, D. (2004). Prejudice, paradox and possibility: The experience of nursing people from cultures other than one's own. In K. H. Kavanaugh & V. Knowlden (Eds.), *Many voices: Toward caring culture in healthcare and healing* (pp. 140–180). Madison, WI: The University of Wisconsin Press.

Statistics Canada. (2003). *2001 Census: Analysis series. Canada's ethnocultural portrait: The changing mosaic* (Catalogue no. 96F0030XIE2001008). Ottawa, ON: Author. Retrieved from http://www12.statcan.gc.ca/access_acces/archive.action-e ng.cfm?/english/census01/products/analytic/companion/ etoimm/pdf/96F0030XIE2001008.pdf.

Statistics Canada. (2006). *Population reporting an Aboriginal identity, by age group, by province and territory (2006 census).* Ottawa, ON: Author. Retrieved from http://www.statcan.gc.ca/tables-tableaux/sum-som/l01/cst01/demo40a-eng.htm.

Statistics Canada. (2013). *Immigration and ethnocultural diversity in Canada: National Household Survey, 2011.* Ottawa, ON: Author. Retrieved from http://www12.statcan.gc.ca/nhs-enm/2011/as-sa/99-010-x/99-010-x2011001-eng.pdf.

Sullivan, E. J., & Decker, P. J. (2009). *Effective leadership and management in nursing* (5th ed.). Upper Saddle River, NJ: Prentice Hall.

Tappen, R. (2001). *Nursing leadership and management: Concepts and practice* (4th ed.). Philadelphia, PA: FA Davis.

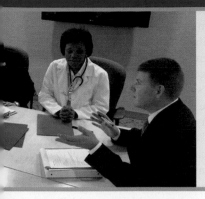

Power, Politics, and Influence

Maura MacPhee

This chapter considers how power and politics influence the roles of leaders and how leaders use power and politics to be influential. It also explores contemporary concepts of power, empowerment, types of power exercised by nurses, personal and organizational strategies for exercising power, and the power of nurses to shape health care policy.

OBJECTIVES

- Explore the types of power in relation to nursing.
- Describe the empowerment strategies used by effective leaders.
- Choose appropriate power strategies to influence the politics of the workplace, professional organizations, and government.

TERMS TO KNOW

coalitions	lobbying	politics
empowerment	network	power
influence	policy	public policy
lobby	policy process	stakeholders

❓ A CHALLENGE

Carol is a bachelor of science in nursing student and is excited about becoming a nurse. The nurse who helped her during her labour made a positive impact on her, which is why she decided that she wanted to become a nurse. When Carol was pregnant with her daughter, the pregnancy was difficult, and so too was the labour. During labour, the nurse not only guided Carol through challenges skillfully but also made Carol feel safe and confident in her care. Carol wanted to provide the same level of care to other moms and dads going through the birth experience. Most of Carol's friends are

not nurses, and at a recent birthday party, a long-time friend said that she was surprised that Carol had chosen nursing as a career. She said, "Well, it's not very challenging, is it? You just do what the doctors tell you to do. On all the TV shows I've seen, nurses aren't portrayed in a very flattering way. Aren't you worried about what others will think of you?"

How should Carol respond to this statement?

INTRODUCTION

Many definitions of *power* are context- or discipline-specific. Power in nursing practice relates to nurses' capacity to empower patients, which can have transformative, healing properties (Benner, 2001). The most common definition of *power* used in leadership and management comes from Rosabeth Moss Kanter, a business management expert from Harvard Business School. According to Kanter (1993), power "is the ability to get things done, to mobilize resources, to get and use whatever it is that a person needs for the goals he or she is attempting to meet" (p. 166).

The concept of empowerment depends on the theoretical framework in which it is considered. Three common theoretical perspectives on empowerment are critical social theory, social psychological theories, and organizational and management theories (Trus, Razbadauskas, & Doran, 2012). *Critical social theory* focuses on power and empowerment in relation to how the nursing discipline is viewed in different social or societal contexts over time. Pervasive stereotypes about nurses are promoted through the media, such as popular TV shows; for example, nurses are portrayed as sexualized, uneducated handmaidens of physicians. The Truth About Nursing is an international not-for-profit organization that seeks to increase public understanding of nursing. It monitors news articles, TV shows, movies, and songs for their portrayal of nursing. Where problems exist, the organization arranges meetings with major corporations and producers to discuss ways to improve media representation of nurses (Summers, 2014). *Social psychological theories* focus on how individuals are intrinsically motivated by the work they do. When people believe that there is meaning and significance to what they do, they report feeling more psychologically empowered in their workplace (Greco, Laschinger, & Wong, 2006). Positive psychology is one branch of social psychology that strives to understand what factors in different contexts are associated with individual feelings of happiness and engagement which, in turn, may affect how they work. Visit the University of Pennsylvania's authentic happiness Web site to measure your levels of personal empowerment and happiness (http://www.authentichappiness.sas.upenn.edu). *Organizational and management theories* focus on the distribution of power in organizations. Organizational empowerment structures in health care have a greater influence on nurses' work attitudes and behaviours than personal characteristics and socialization experiences (Trus et al., 2012). Dr. Heather Laschinger has devoted her career to studying structural empowerment and its influence on nurses, nurse managers, patients, and the workplace. Her research Web site (http://publish.uwo.ca/~hkl) chronicles the research she has conducted over the past two decades on the effect of nursing work environments on nurses' empowerment.

Policy is a specifically designated statement to guide decisions and actions. Within health care organizations, nurses are expected to adhere to organizational policies as well as procedures, which are guidelines for nurses to follow to correctly perform a task. In health care settings, policies and procedures are both "power tools" (a term coined by Kanter, 1993) because they provide nurses with legitimate power to carry out health care interventions.

Another type of policy of importance to nurses is public policy. Public policy is "a course of action that is anchored in a set of values regarding appropriate public goals and a set of beliefs about the best way of achieving those goals" (Bryant, 2009, p. 1). Public policy decisions are shaped by a variety of forces, including political, social, and economic forces. Public policy (enacted through governments' policy decisions) determines the distribution of resources that influence people's health. In Canada, many public policy decisions of importance to nurses involve the social determinants of health, or those factors that significantly influence people's health and wellness. Health Canada is the federal department that oversees the health and well-being of Canadians. Health Canada's Web site (http://www.hc-sc.gc.ca) has a wealth of information about policy activities related to Canadians' health, including information on policy actions involving the social determinants of health, such as proper housing and nutrition.

In 1999, Health Canada created the Office of Nursing Policy to "help Canadians maintain and improve their health through the development of policy which integrates the views of nurses and the nursing profession" (Health Canada, 2009). Some of the Office's functions include identifying important policy issues based on best evidence, disseminating important policy-related information, and advocating for Canadians—getting them involved in policy activities, such as policy development and consulting with key stakeholder groups. Stakeholders are considered those individuals, groups, or organizations that are influenced by an issue or invested in policy related to an issue. A recent, joint publication by the Canadian Foundation for Healthcare Improvement and the Office of Nursing Policy recommended a series of evidence-informed nurse recruitment and retention policy initiatives (McGillis Hall, MacDonald-Rencz, Peterson, et al., 2013).

Politics involves "using power to influence, persuade, or otherwise change—it is the art of understanding relationships between groups in society and using that understanding to achieve particular outcomes" (McIntyre & McDonald, 2010, p. 70). Influence is the process of using power—from the punitive power of coercion to the interactive power of collaboration. Nurses' lack of involvement in politics is sometimes associated with their discomfort with acknowledging and using power. Nursing has been a predominantly female profession, and women traditionally were not socialized to exert power. Now in the twenty-first century, nurses must exercise their power to create a strong voice for nursing. This is an era of rapid and often unplanned change with dramatic nursing shortages. Nurses must use their collective power and flex their political muscles to create a preferred future for the health care system, health care consumers, and the profession of nursing (Manojlovich, 2007).

KEY POWERFUL CANADIAN NURSE LEADERS

Canada's first nurse, Jeanne Mance (1606–1673), was an inspirational woman who helped found Montreal's first hospital, a hospital that was under her direction for 17 years. Mance procured funds and resources and recruited workers from France to support her unwavering mission to care for the sick in the New World (Canadian Biography Online, 2011). In 2011, Mance was officially recognized as Montreal's co-founder; her ability to bring money to the Ville Marie settlement (which became Montreal) through her connections in France was vital to the settlement's financial well-being ("Jeanne Mance," 2011).

Many Canadian nurses have received public acknowledgement and awards for their positive contributions to the health and well-being of Canadians. The Order of Canada, awarded through the office of the Governor General, has been presented to over 30 nurses, including Dr. Helen K. Mussallem. Dr. Mussallem received the highest level of the Order of Canada for her many contributions to society. She was the first Canadian nurse to earn a doctoral degree, and she was the first Canadian nurse to address the annual general assembly of the Canadian Medical Association (CMA). She was also a prominent policymaker and advocate as the chair for the World Health Organization Scientific Group on Research in Nursing and the Economic Council of Canada (see the Helen Mussallem biography project at http://drhkm.ca).

Another powerful nurse leader is Dr. Judith Shamian, past president of the Canadian Nurses Association (CNA) and past president and chief executive officer of the Victorian Order of Nurses. Dr. Shamian was elected as president of the International Council of Nurses (ICN) in 2013. As president of the CNA, the national professional voice of over 140 000 Canadian registered nurses (RNs), Dr. Shamian championed a collaboration between the CNA and the CMA to develop a set of principles to promote primary health care in Canada. The health care principles supported by the CNA–CMA include patient-centred care, quality care, health promotion and illness prevention, equitable care, sustainable care, and accountable care (Lankshear, 2012). The CNA–CMA has been lobbying (seeking to influence) government policymakers to have these principles guide policymaking discussions at the provincial, territorial, and federal levels.

TYPES OF POWER

Nurses often view power as if it were totally contradictory to the caring nature of nursing. However, nurses exercise power in many ways in their daily nursing practice. Nurses routinely influence patients to improve their health status, which is an essential element of nursing practice. Nurses provide health teaching to patients and their families, with the goal of changing patient (and perhaps family) behaviour to promote optimal health. Nurses seek to change the behaviour of colleagues by instructing them about a new policy being implemented in the nursing unit. Nurses coach other nurses to improve their performance. The chief nursing

THEORY BOX

Types of Power

KEY CONTRIBUTORS	KEY IDEAS	APPLICATION TO PRACTICE
Types or bases of social power were formulated by Hersey et al. (1979) to explain the personal use of power. Sullivan (2013) reorganized these types, eliminating much of the overlap in the original categories.	**Personal power:** Based on one's reputation and credibility.	The leader of a provincial or territorial nurses' association may have access to provincial or territorial government leaders based on personal power. This leader has worked with government members for many years and is known for integrity—following through on promises of support and providing useful information on matters related to health.
	Expert power: Results from the knowledge and skills one possesses that are needed by others.	An advanced practice nurse is viewed as the clinical expert on a nursing unit.
	Position power: Possessed by virtue of one's position within an organization or status within a group.	The dean of a school of nursing is viewed on campus as powerful because this dean leads the fastest-growing academic unit on campus.
	Perceived power: Results from one's reputation as a powerful person.	A nursing student seeks out a certain nurse leader as a preceptor during a senior clinical practicum because of the leader's reputation with nurses and students within the organization.
	Connection power: Gained by association with people who have links to powerful people.	At one acute care hospital during a Nurses' Week celebration, nurses take advantage of the opportunity to have extended, informal conversations with the hospital's chief nursing officer.

officer of a hospital manages a multi-million-dollar budget. All of these examples are exercises of power.

Hersey, Blanchard, and Natemeyer (1979) developed a classic formulation on the basis of social power. Sullivan (2013) revised these types of power from a nursing perspective. Examples of types of power appear in the Theory Box. These types of power are not mutually exclusive. They are often used in concert to exert influence on individuals or groups.

Nurses commonly use all of these types of power while implementing a wide range of nursing activities. Nurses who teach patients use expert power by virtue of the information they share with patients. Nurses also exercise position power because they are accorded a certain status by society. Members of a provincial or territorial nurses' association who lobby members of Parliament use expert, perceived, personal, and position power when trying to gain legislators' support for health care legislation. New

graduates, employed on probationary status until they demonstrate the initial clinical competencies of a position, may view the nurse leader as exercising both position and expert power related to their evaluation for continued employment. Nursing faculty and skilled clinicians exercise expert and perceived power as students emulate their behaviour. Connection power is evident at any social gathering in the workplace. People of high status (e.g., vice-presidents, directors, deans) within an organization may be sought out for conversation by those who want to move up the organizational hierarchy.

Having a high-status position in an organization immediately provides stature, but power depends on the ability to accomplish goals from that position. Although some may think that "knowledge is power," acting on that knowledge is where the real power lies. Sharing knowledge expands one's power and, in turn, empowers others, including colleagues and patients (Sullivan, 2013).

EXERCISE 11-1

Part A. Recall a recent opportunity in which you observed the work of an expert nurse. Think about that nurse's interactions with patients, family members, nursing colleagues, and other health care providers. What kinds of power did you observe this nurse using? What did the nurse do and say that told you, "This is a powerful person"?

Part B. Using the Types of Power Questionnaire found on the Evolve website, rate your current level of power for each of the five types of power outlined in the Theory Box (on the previous page). Think of one strategy to increase each type of power. Some people think that power is finite and must be given to them, but in actuality, power is limitless—we choose how to increase our power bases through what we do and say.

	Current Rating
	1----2----3----4----5
Type of Power	1 = Powerless,
Questionnaire	5 = Very Powerful
Personal Power	Current rating: 1----2----3----4----5
Strategy for raising personal power:	
Expert Power	Current rating: 1----2----3----4----5
Strategy for raising expert power:	
Position Power	Current rating: 1----2----3----4----5
Strategy for raising position power:	
Perceived Power	Current rating: 1----2----3----4----5
Strategy for raising perceived power:	
Connection Power	Current rating: 1----2----3----4----5
Strategy for raising connection power:	

EMPOWERMENT THEORIES AND NURSING

Empowerment is essential to nursing. It is the process of exercising one's own power. It is also the process by which we facilitate the participation of others in decision making and taking action so they are free to exercise power (Ozimek, 2007). This section focuses on three theoretical perspectives of empowerment and how they relate to nursing.

Critical Social Theories and Empowerment

Critical social theories focus on how society controls access to power based on individual characteristics such as skin colour, gender, religion, and sexual orientation. The most common critical social theories are critical race theory and feminist theory. Those groups whose freedoms and rights are restricted by socially imposed inequalities are known as *oppressed*

groups (Matheson & Bobay, 2007). Sociologists consider nursing an "oppressed group" because of its historical domination by medicine. The traditional health care hierarchy that placed medicine at the top may be related to the fact that nursing has been a predominantly female profession supervised by predominantly male physicians. Gender, class, and status no doubt have contributed to nursing's long-time subordination to medicine. One characteristic of oppressed group behaviour is that group's inability to realize that powerlessness is socially conditioned—and can be challenged. Individuals within oppressed groups tend to oppress others that they can dominate (consider the notion "nurses eat their young"). Bullying and horizontal violence are oppressed group behaviours. The following Literature Perspective provides an example of nursing student oppression and empowerment. The opposite of oppression is emancipation, and critical social theory examines ways in which social activism can be used to end oppression (Purpora, Blegen, & Stotts, 2012; Sauer, 2012; Udod, 2008).

LITERATURE PERSPECTIVE

Resource: Bradbury-Jones, C., Sambrook, S., & Irvine, F. (2011). Nursing students and the issue of voice: A qualitative study. *Nurse Education Today, 31,* 628–632.

The purpose of this qualitative study was to explore the empowerment of nursing students in clinical practice. Thirteen students were interviewed at annual intervals during their nursing program: from first year to graduation. Many first-year students felt that they were powerless to express their opinions when they had patient-care concerns. In these instances, they psychologically withdrew from these situations as a coping response. As students progressed in the program, "voice" increased among most of the students. They realized that strongly stating their opinions would be counterproductive, so they created "bridges" to carefully craft their statements between a continuum of "exit–voice." Some students said that they had to dampen their voice to avoid labels such as "cocky." Other research has shown that students are at risk for disciplinary power or ostracism if they appear too confident or assertive—even when a patient's welfare is at stake.

Implications for Practice
Students' voice may be hampered by fear of reprisal in situations where poor patient care conditions exist. Instructors and education programs need to provide safe places for students to express their concerns and collectively discuss options to address these

Continued

LITERATURE PERSPECTIVE—cont'd

power imbalances. Most organizations have confidential reporting systems where unsafe conditions or inappropriate behaviours can be documented—by students, faculty, and staff. Adequate orientation to clinical teams can also be helpful, and strong practice–academic collaborations between educational institutions and practice settings can help promote team spirit where students are considered important members of clinical teams.

From a critical social theory perspective, nurse empowerment signifies that nurses are aware of the influence of power on them and how power influences their behaviour toward others. However, nurses may exert power over others in unconscious, well-intentioned ways. One UK study found that primary care nurses unknowingly controlled their patients' decisions during asthma teaching sessions. Although the nurses said that they used shared decision making with their patients, the researchers found that the nurses only offered patients opportunities to make decisions about their inhaler devices based on the nurses' preselected recommendations. Rather than empowering patients by treating them as equal partners in decision making, these nurses tightly controlled information to conform decisions to their agenda (Upton, Fletcher, Mado-Sutton, et al., 2011).

A Canadian study examined nurses' workplace violence through a critical social theory lens (St-Pierre & Holmes, 2008). Nurses are at high risk for workplace violence, even compared with police officers and prison guards. Despite the high risk of nurses' work, nurses tend to under-report violent episodes because they view them as "part of their job." Workplace violence can contribute to stress, depression, and workplace injuries and absenteeism. Nurse absenteeism is closely tracked and monitored by supervisors; nurses know they are under surveillance, making them question their own needs—versus those of the organization. Nurses are also expected to "normalize" unsafe work conditions for the greater good of the organization. Due to cost efficiencies, everyone within the organization is expected to accept cuts in resources and proper supports. According to St-Pierre and Holmes (2008), nurses have come to accept violence as a regular occurrence and to doubt their rights with respect to a safer work environment. Workplaces need to explore what policies need to be in place to change

the culture and empower nurses to report workplace violence.

Structural Empowerment Theory

Structural empowerment theory postulates that employees of organizations become empowered when they gain access to opportunities, information, resources, and supports through informal and formal power sources. This theory is based on the ethnographic work of Kanter (1993), who observed that employee attitudes and behaviour were influenced by their access to empowerment structures within their workplaces. *Access to opportunity* refers to having professional advancement opportunities or opportunities to be involved in organizational activities beyond one's job description. *Access to information* refers to having the necessary information about aspects of organizational functioning in order to be effective in the workplace. *Access to resources* refers to having the resources needed to efficiently and effectively carry out one's work. *Access to support* involves receiving support to fulfill one's job responsibilities and engage in relevant decision making (Kanter, 1993). *Formal power* comes from an individual's position of formal authority within an organization, and *informal power* is based on networks and alliances with supervisors, peers, and other contacts within and outside the organization. The following Literature Perspective is an example of how Kanter's structural empowerment theory has been applied to theoretical understandings of nursing care.

LITERATURE PERSPECTIVE

Resource: Laschinger, H., Gilbert, S., Smith, L., et al. (2013). Towards a comprehensive theory of nurse/patient empowerment: Applying Kanter's empowerment theory to patient care. *Journal of Nursing Management, 18*, 4–13. doi:10.1111/j.1365-2834.2009.01046.x

These authors argued that a key responsibility of nurses is to empower patients for optimal health and well-being. Very little research has been done that directly links nurse activities to patient empowerment. This conceptual paper proposes a nurse/patient empowerment model that incorporates many empowerment concepts: nurse structural empowerment, nurse psychological empowerment, nurses' use of patient empowering strategies, and patient empowerment. The major proposition is that empowered nurses are better able to empower their patients. Empowered patients have increased capacity to care for themselves, access needed health services, and express satisfaction with health care delivery.

LITERATURE PERSPECTIVE—cont'd

The paper provided many examples of patient-empowering nurse behaviours that are related to Kanter's (1993) structural empowerment theory. Examples are presented in the table below.

Examples of Patient-Empowering Nurse Behaviours

Components of Kanter's (1993) Theory	
Access to information	• Respond to patients' questions in clear, understandable terms.
	• Always explain your actions before carrying them out.
Access to support	• Ask patients what you can do for them.
	• Offer encouraging remarks for meeting health goals.
Access to resources	• Facilitate access to community resources.
	• Facilitate patients' access to the health care team.
Access to opportunity	• Provide patients with opportunities to practise new skills.
Informal power	• Promote positive, trusting relationships between the patient, their family, and the team.
Formal power	• Refrain from using your formal authority to intimidate or dominate patients' decision making.

Implications for Practice

This article provides an excellent overview of important empowerment terms, and it has tables with nurse-empowering behaviours and patient-empowering behaviours. Use this article as a learning resource to gain comfort with key empowerment concepts and their applications.

As mentioned at the beginning of this chapter, Dr. Heather Laschinger at Western University (and her colleagues) has extensively studied structural empowerment with respect to empowering nurses in Canadian health care settings. Nurses' perceptions of access to organizational empowerment structures have been associated with numerous outcomes such as organizational commitment, job satisfaction, trust, and low burnout. As suggested by Kanter (1993), numerous studies have shown that structural empowerment is more predictive of nurse outcomes than personal attributes (Wagner, Cummings, Smith, et al., 2010). Laschinger (2008) conducted a study of Ontario acute care nurses and found that nurses associated effective

leadership with access to organizational empowerment structures. Effective leaders were instrumental in creating empowering work environments for their staff. In addition to enabling access to important empowerment structures, Laschinger's (2008) research showed that leaders can champion empowering work environments for nurses by promoting nurse participation in making patient care delivery decisions, ensuring staffing adequacy, and encouraging nurse–physician collaboration. In this study, nurses who reported having effective leaders and empowering work environments were more satisfied with their work, and they reported a higher quality of care delivery than those nurses in less empowered workplaces.

EXERCISE 11-2

Think about a recent clinical experience in which you empowered a patient. What did you do for and/or with the patient (and family) that was empowering? How did you feel about your own actions in this situation? How did the patient (or family) respond to your efforts? Does reading the Literature Perspective above help you think differently about your role as a nurse in relation to patient empowerment?

Social Psychological Theories and Psychological Empowerment

Psychological empowerment refers to an individual's belief of their empowerment at work. Spreitzer (2007) identified four main dimensions of empowerment: (1) *meaning*, which implies a good fit between the individual's work role and his or her beliefs, values, and behaviours; (2) *impact*, which is the degree to which an individual can make a significant difference at work; (3) *self-determination*, which is the degree to which an individual has control over what he or she does at work; and (4) *competence*, which is an individual's belief that he or she can perform work activities successfully. Empowerment comes from within, but outside catalysts can "spark" people's positive beliefs about themselves. For example, nurse leaders can catalyze nurses' belief in themselves (i.e., psychological empowerment) by providing them with organizational empowerment structures. Laschinger, Finegan, and Wilk (2009) found that the quality of nurse–nurse leader relationships and nurses' perceptions of access to empowerment structures influenced nurses' feelings of psychological empowerment that in turn enhanced their commitment to the organization. Because organizational commitment is closely tied to actual turnover, this study provides evidence that strong leaders can initiate an empowerment chain reaction among followers: strong leader–follower relationships→ ↑ nurse perceptions of structural empowerment→ ↑ feelings of psychological empowerment→ ↑ positive follower outcomes, such as organizational commitment and nurse retention. Strong leaders, especially leaders who use structural empowerment as a major organizational strategy, can raise nurses' psychological beliefs about their capacity to be valued contributors in their workplaces (Wagner et al., 2010).

Another area of study from social psychology is leaders' use of specific empowerment strategies, known as *leader empowering behaviours* (LEBs) (Greco et al., 2006). The five major LEB categories appear in Table 11-1, along with examples of each. More on these categories and supporting references can be found in Dahinten, MacPhee, Hejazi, et al. (2013). Some research has shown that LEBs are important for supporting new graduate nurses (Ulrich, Krozek, & Early, 2010).

TABLE 11-1	LEADER-EMPOWERING BEHAVIOURS (LEBs)
LEB CATEGORY	**NURSING EXAMPLE**
Enhancing the meaningfulness of work	Inspiring staff to follow the organization's vision and mission through transformational leadership
Fostering participatory decision making	Providing release time for nurses to participate in shared governance councils
Providing autonomy from bureaucratic restraints	Eliminating unnecessary policies and procedures; supporting nurses to regularly update evidence-informed protocols
Facilitating goal accomplishment	Providing educators and professional development opportunities
Expressing confidence in high performance	Publicly acknowledging nurses' professional accomplishments and contributions to interprofessional teamwork

---

EXERCISE 11-3

Part A. Observe the first-line nurse leader on your clinical unit. Write down examples of leader-empowering behaviours (LEBs) you saw (see Table 11-1). Were you able to find an example of each type of behaviour?

Part B. Since leader-empowering behaviours have a strong influence on nurses, interview a few nurses on your clinical unit. Ask them to provide examples of the leader's LEB. If the staff and you are able to provide many examples of LEB, it is likely that the work environment is an empowering one where nurses appear to work well together and to enjoy their work—even in stressful situations. If the staff and you are not able to provide examples of LEB, it is likely that the work environment is less empowering and less satisfactory to staff. Do you see evidence of the link between the leader's use of LEB and staff behaviour on the unit?

An Empowering Professional Identity

Nurses' use of power has implications for nursing practice, politics, and policy.

Power and professionalism are closely related; having a strong professional identity is important, because a lack of empowering professional identity means that others can step in and decide what nursing is and what nurses can do (Ponte, Glazer, Dann, et al., 2007). Empowered nurses demonstrate a positive and professional attitude about being a nurse to nursing colleagues, patients, and their families, other colleagues in the workplace, the public, and government. This attitude facilitates the exercise of power among colleagues while educating others about nurses and nursing. A powerful image is important because the impressions we make on people influence the way they view us now and in the future, as well as how they value what we do and say.

EXERCISE 11-4

How do you routinely introduce yourself to patients, families, physicians, and other colleagues? A powerful and positive approach involves making eye contact with each individual, shaking hands, and introducing yourself by saying, "I'm Ted Carvalho, a registered nurse [or nursing student]." If you do not currently use this technique, try it out. Note any difference in the responses of people whom you meet using this technique in comparison with a less formal approach. How are you contributing to a powerful, professional identity for nursing?

Professional identity arises through a socialization process whereby individuals learn the behaviours, attitudes, and values associated with their profession. Professional nursing socialization often begins in nursing programs where students learn about professional standards of practice and codes of ethics (Chapter 6). Entry into the workplace can cause a significant clash between learned ideals and actual nursing practice: "reality shock" is a term originally coined by Kramer (1974) to describe this values clash. Another more recent term in the literature is "transition shock" (Duchscher, 2009). New nurse socialization is an ongoing concern. In a Quebec survey study, new nurses said they were considering leaving the profession due to high psychological demands, job strain, and lack of social support (Lavoie-Tremblay, O'Brien-Pallas, Gelinas, et al., 2007). Dr. Heather Laschinger is conducting a Canada-wide study of new nurse graduates to document their intentions of leaving their job and their profession, and this study is also examining those work environment factors that are most strongly influencing intent to leave decisions (see "Starting Out" at http://publish.uwo.ca/~hkl/chair/starting _out.html). To retain and support new nurses, the literature emphasizes the importance of providing mentorship, peer alliances, support networks, and comprehensive orientation during new nurse transition to the work environment.

Identity development and the work environment are closely intertwined (Vessey, DeMarco, Gaffney, et al., 2009). This finding has important ramifications for nurse leaders. As we have noted in our previous discussion of leader-empowering behaviours, leaders have the capacity to empower staff and shape the quality of the work environment. In one US study on bullying (Vessey et al., 2009), nurses did not seem to know how to access organizational supports to manage bullying events. Other literature has noted a lack of trust between staff and leadership, and the presence of organizational structures (such as power hierarchies) that even promote caste systems and bullying cultures (Laschinger et al., 2010). Nurses who report bullying are more likely to report negative perceptions of their work environment, less job satisfaction, and higher levels of anxiety and depression (Quine as cited in Laschinger et al., 2010). In a survey study of newly graduated nurses ($N = 415$) in Ontario acute care settings, one-third of respondents reported exposure to bullying behaviours (Laschinger, Grau, Finegan, et al., 2010). Leaders, therefore, need to advocate for and role model the right way of

doing things—including the implementation of "no tolerance" policies and sanctions against behaviours that oppress others. Canadian researchers Smith, Andrusyszyn, and Laschinger (2010) provide examples of leader-empowerment strategies directed specifically at new graduate retention. One strategy that is particularly important to new nurses is professional development opportunities, such as access to specialty certification programs. New graduate retention is also influenced by adequate staffing levels, inclusion in committee work, mentoring supports, ongoing feedback, and positive reinforcement and praise for achievements.

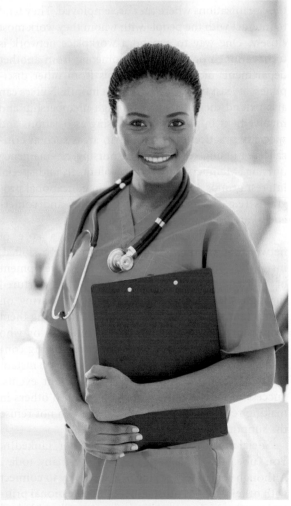

A powerful professional identity is essential for successful political efforts in the workplace, the profession, and the public policy arena.

POWER STRATEGIES

Networking and coalition building are additional power strategies used by nurse leaders that are effective at different levels: from intra-organizational to provincial or territorial and federal levels.

Networking

Networking is an important power strategy and political skill. A network is the result of identifying, valuing, and maintaining relationships with a system of individuals who are sources of information, advice, and support (MacPhee, Jackson, & Suryaprakash, 2009). Many nurses have relatively limited networks within the organizations where they are employed. They tend to interact with the people with whom they work most closely. One way to expand a workplace network is to have lunch or coffee with someone from another department, including individuals from other disciplines, at least two or three times a month. Nurses can also extend their networks through membership and involvement in professional nursing associations and specialty practice organizations in areas such as critical care nursing, cardiovascular nursing, or emergency nursing. Membership in civic, volunteer, and special interest groups, and participation in educational programs (e.g., formal academic programs and conferences) are other ways to network.

The successful networker identifies a core of networking partners who are particularly skilled, insightful, and eager to support the development of colleagues. These partners need to be nurtured through strategies such as information sharing on topics that relate to their interests; introducing them to persons who have comparable interests or who are connected with others of influence; staying connected through notes, e-mail, phone calls, or instant messages; and meeting them at important events. Successful networkers are not a burden to others in making requests for support, and they do not refuse the support that is provided.

Social media such as Facebook, Twitter, LinkedIn, YouTube, and Instagram are used by many today. Although social networking is a great way to connect with others, nurses must adhere to professional principles of social networking. Some well-publicized examples of Facebook gone "afoul" include three US students who were temporarily suspended from their program for posting a picture of themselves with a human placenta. A nurse in the United Kingdom was professionally investigated by her regulatory body for posting this comment on Facebook: "Euthanasia for gingers, the elderly and those with bad toenails." Although the nurse intended this as humour, other nurses on Facebook were offended by this posting and reported her (Smith, 2012).

The College of Registered Nurses of Nova Scotia (2012) has developed the recommendations outlined in Table 11-2 for the appropriate use of social media by nurses, nursing students, employers and nurse educators.

TABLE 11-2   RECOMMENDATIONS FOR THE APPROPRIATE USE OF SOCIAL MEDIA

1. **RNs and nursing students** using social media tools:
   a. abide by organizational policies concerning personal and professional social media tools;
   b. protect personal identity by reading, understanding, and using the strictest privacy settings in order to maintain control over access to personal information;
   c. maintain privacy and confidentiality of clients and co-workers or fellow students' information and immediately report any breach to their employer or faculty;
   d. maintain professional nurse-client professional boundaries and avoid engaging in personal social media relationships with clients;
   e. refrain from posting any client information or image(s) unless it is related to employer expectation for client care;
   f. never post unprofessional or negative comments about clients, co-workers, other students or employers;
   g. avoid using social media sites to vent or discuss work/school-related events and refrain from commenting on posts of this nature made by others;
   h. maintain a professional manner in postings, photos and/or videos;
   i. never speak on behalf of a health care organization unless authorized to do so;
   j. keep work/school related social media activities separate from personal social media activities;
   k. create strong passwords and change them frequently. Do not share passwords with others; and
   l. avoid offering health-related advice in response to posted comments or questions; if relied upon, such advice could trigger professional liability (CNPS, 2010) and/or a complaint to the College.

College of Registered Nurses of Nova Scotia, Position Statement: Social Media., Retrieved from https://www.crnns.ca/documents/PositionStatement_SocialMedia.pdf

The CNA *Code of Ethics for Registered Nurses* (see Chapter 6) provides a framework for ethical decision making, and this framework can provide guidance with respect to nurses' use of social media. Chapter 29 also addresses elements of professional practice in using electronic communications.

Coalition Building

The exercise of power is often directed at creating change. Although an individual can often be effective at exercising power and creating change, certain changes require collective action. Coalition building is an effective political strategy for collective action. Coalitions are groups of individuals or organizations that join together temporarily around a common goal. Coalitions of professionals and consumers can be particularly powerful in influencing public policy related to health care. During the Severe Acute Respiratory Syndrome (SARS) outbreak in Toronto, the Community Coalition Concerned about SARS was formed to quickly disseminate information about SARS, fight against potential ethnic group discrimination through advocacy work, and organize fundraising events to support front-line workers and SARS research. The coalition included 63 Chinese-Canadian businesses, community, cultural, religious, and professional organizations. Other Asian ethnic groups worked with the coalition, including Japanese, Korean, Sri Lankan, and Filipino groups. One of the most outstanding coalition actions was the rapid mobilization of user-friendly, linguistically and culturally appropriate telephone support lines. Over 100 volunteers were available to answer calls and provide emotional and informational support (Dong, Fung, & Chan, 2010).

Nursing organizations often use coalition building when dealing with government policymakers. As mentioned above, Dr. Judith Shamian's CNA–CMA collaboration on the development of health care principles for legislators' consideration is an example of a coalition.

Coalitions can develop into more permanent partnerships or even lobbies. A *lobby* is a group of people who seek to influence government policymakers on a particular issue. The Health Action Lobby (HEAL) is one example (see http://www.healthactionlobby.ca). This lobby was formed in 1991, and represents 35 national health organizations (including the CNA) with a cross-section of stakeholder groups, including health care providers, health regions, institutions, and facilities. HEAL is particularly concerned with upholding the unique qualities of the Canada Health Act (see Chapter 1). The purpose of HEAL is to influence health care policy at the federal level. HEAL was very active during the 2011 federal election campaign, calling on the major political party candidates to "clearly articulate their views on the role of the federal government when it comes to the future of health and health care in Canada" (HEAL, 2011).

EXERCISING POWER AND INFLUENCE: POLICY AND POLITICS

Previous sections have provided examples of how nurses can use different power strategies or sources of power to influence change. This section provides a more in-depth look at policy and political action.

The Policy Process and Politics

The policy process involves developing, implementing, and evaluating policy on the basis of the best evidence available. Within health care settings, policies enforce specific structures and processes that are associated with quality, safe outcomes. They are considered organizational standards that must be followed. Hand hygiene policy, for instance, is based on the best available evidence of how to prevent infection transmission. Employees, patients, and visitors in health care settings are expected to comply with this policy, and health care settings have quality and safety departments that monitor and document adherence rates. When policies are not followed, that may put people at risk. In health care organizations, nurses typically play a key role in reviewing best evidence and updating policies on a regular basis. Nurses' involvement in policy work may take place within unit-based or hospital-wide shared-governance councils.

A controversial nursing policy is mandatory nurse-to-patient ratios. Nurse-to-patient ratios are one way to define nurses' workloads. Ratio legislation is based on a large body of research evidence that shows that as nurses' workloads increase, patient morbidity and mortality rates increase, and nurses are at greater risk for injury and emotional burnout (Berry & Curry, 2012). In California and two states in Australia, legislation exists that requires acute care hospitals to maintain specific nurse-to-patient ratios. Hospitals have policies in place that ensure that a minimum number of nurses are available at all times to care for a set number of patients (e.g., 1 nurse to every 4 patients on medical and surgical units). Since ratio legislation and hospital policies were enacted in California, nurses have reported better job satisfaction, less burnout, and better quality care delivery (Aiken, Sloane, Cimiotti, et al., 2010). Ratio policies must be enforced, but some policy experts believe that this approach to safe staffing limits hospital administrators' capacity to respond to patient population needs in a flexible, cost-effective fashion (Buerhaus, 2009).

Public policy is intended to ensure effective, equitable service and resource distribution for the public. Public policy, however, is closely intertwined with politics. Politics is based on the use of power to control or manipulate policy decisions. Politicians typically represent different values-based approaches to making decisions that influence the distribution of public resources, such as those associated with the social determinants of health (e.g., housing, transit, education). The competitive values-based positions of politicians and the complexity of public health often result in policies that do not adequately address fundamental inequities in society (Fafard, 2008). In Canada, the federal government is accountable for raising funds for public health needs, but the provincial governments are primarily responsible for making health policy. The fact that two levels of government are involved in health resource management and decision making adds to the complexity of Canadian health policy (and politics). Take, for example, planning for the health human resources (HHR) supply in Canada. Although many actors are involved in this policy area, no pan-Canadian HHR policy exists to "smooth" the distribution of health care providers across the country. "Many have called for a health human resources process or table at which policy discussions encompassing all health professions could take place. We do not have such a process in Canada; instead, we have a variety of actors attempting to react to current and perceived future pressures" (Wilson, 2013, p. 30).

EXERCISE 11-5

1. Take a look at the websites of the Canadian Nurses Association (https://www.cna-aiic.ca/en) and the Canadian Federation of Nurses Unions (https://nursesunions.ca). What policy work is underway? What political activities are posted on the websites? You may consider getting involved around an issue of significance to you.

2. Another source of information about nurses' involvement in policy and politics is the website of your provincial or territorial nursing association. Use the "search" field to look up "policy" or "position statements" on the association website. As one example, the Registered Nurses' Association of Ontario website (http://rnao.cahttp://www.rnao.org/) contains many resources on political action along with health and nursing policy, toolkits, and position statements.

3. After viewing the websites of national and provincial or territorial nursing associations and unions, select a topic of interest to you. Within your own sphere of influence (e.g., your peers at work, friends, and family), what can you do to raise awareness about this topic?

4. One way to get involved in policy development within your organization is through committee work or shared governance councils. Political awareness begins with nurses' knowledge of opportunities to participate in policymaking within their own units, departments, and organizations. Scope out opportunities to engage in policymaking at different levels within your organization. This is the first step toward making a commitment to action.

A basic policymaking framework appears in Figure 11-1. An assumption about public policy is that good data will lead to good policy. As depicted in Figure 11-1, the process begins with the *synthesis* of best available evidence. *Knowledge translation* involves the packaging of evidence in a clear, succinct format for policymakers. This linear model often ignores *other policy inputs* that have a significant influence on policymaking. Other policy inputs include economic considerations, interest group lobbying, and election pressures. According to Moloughney (2012), researchers who typically generate the evidence have a naive understanding of how decisions are actually made. An example used by Fafard (2008) is tobacco policy. Scientific evidence clearly demonstrates how smoking and second-hand smoke negatively influence health. Despite numerous attempts to transfer this knowledge to policymakers, over many years, other considerations (inputs) were weighted more heavily by policymakers. Other overriding inputs included lobbying by

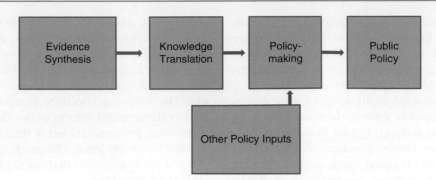

FIGURE 11-1 A basic policymaking framework.

Aboriginal peoples (cultural concerns) and small businesses, such as restaurants and pubs. The knowledge translation box, therefore, makes a critical difference in how evidence is transferred to policymakers and how it is weighted in relation to other policy inputs. Does scientific evidence even appear on some policymaking agendas? According to Fafard (2008), "how a given issue is framed can also have an enormous impact on the place of evidence and what evidence is considered relevant" (p. 10). One way that researchers have been able to gain policymaker attention is by aligning themselves with other stakeholder groups (e.g., working with coalitions) and creating a sense of urgency.

The *policymaking* box represents a process of (1) setting an agenda, (2) formulating a policy, (3) adopting the policy, (4) implementing the policy, and (5) evaluating policy outcomes. Government agendas, which influence policymaking, typically consist of three distinct streams. The "problem" stream deals with issues that have immediacy and public attention (e.g., teen suicide and cyber-bullying). The "policy" stream deals with public ideals that are more abstract, and more difficult to understand and to act upon; these agenda items may be outside public awareness or have limited public awareness (e.g., a comprehensive cancer care strategy). The "political" stream consists of priorities for re-election; these agenda items often overlap with those of problem streams because they have public appeal (e.g., an official Family Day). Government agenda items, therefore, depend on salient social, ethical, and political implications—that often supersede the evidence (Howlett & Ramesh, 2003).

During the policy formulation phase, policymakers often consult with interest groups, academics, and other governments. A range of possible policy actions are drafted to address the agenda issue. Childhood obesity is an example of a problem stream issue. Policy actions depend on how this issue is framed. If obesity is considered an individual behaviour problem, for instance, policy actions might include policies aimed at changing individual behaviours such as diet and exercise regimens. The government, for instance, might formulate policy to remove vending machines with junk food and high sugar drinks from schools. Another policy might be family tax breaks for children's recreational and sports program fees. Policy formulations are rarely clear or straightforward, and they are typically tempered by sociocultural and political forces that carry greater weight than the scientific evidence. When technical or knowledge experts are invited to participate in policy formulation, nurse experts have an opportunity to promote evidence-informed practices. Nurses often serve as experts on public health and health care services policies. One Canadian nurse policy expert is Dr. Gail Tomblin Murphy. Dr. Tomblin Murphy's area of expertise is HHR planning. Throughout the world, there are notable shortages of nurses and doctors. Evidence-informed HHR planning and policy development ensure that the number of health care providers is adequate to meet the burgeoning demands of aging populations. Dr. Tomblin Murphy is director of the World Health Organization/Pan American Health Organization (WHO/PAHO) Collaborating Centre on Health Workforce Planning and Research, Dalhousie University. She has served as a technical expert for WHO/PAHO policy development, and she has advised Canadian policymakers at provincial and federal levels. According to Dr. Tomblin Murphy, HHR planning in Canada has been based on historical and political factors rather than the needs of populations. In many instances, HHR policies are reactive—based on perceived deficiencies—rather than systematic, proactive plans for the future (Tomblin Murphy & MacKenzie, 2013).

After assembling information from diverse groups on a range of possible actions, decisions have to be made about what action(s) to take. *Public policy* decision making may involve hundreds of people (e.g., Cabinet decision making) and decision-making rounds to "chunk" decisions on complex issues. Public policy rarely arises from one discrete decision. Some policy decisions include regulation, public expenditures, and tax measures. Policy research on the role of evidence in government decision making indicates that research evidence is not always used or sought out. The following Literature Perspective illustrates how evidence might inform policy development. In many cases, policymakers justify their decisions (after the fact) with evidence: "Research is assembled in order to justify a decision that has already been taken" (Fafard, 2008, p. 11).

LITERATURE PERSPECTIVE

Resource: Asanin, J., & Wilson, K. (2008). "I spent nine years looking for a doctor": Exploring access to health care among immigrants in Mississauga, Ontario, Canada. *Social Science & Medicine, 66*(6), 1271–1283. doi:10.1016/j.socscimed.2007.11.043

In Canada, approximately 20% of the total population consists of immigrants, and every year, about 250 000 new immigrants arrive in Canada, accounting for two-thirds of annual population growth. Although these immigrants make significant economic and social contributions to our society, research suggests that immigrants have difficulty receiving social benefits and health care. This qualitative study explored access to health care among immigrants in one Canadian neighbourhood. This research approach was chosen because most research on access to care in Canada is done with national-level survey data that do not provide detailed insights into subpopulation groups like immigrants. In many instances, public policy decisions are based on these high-level data. Focus group interviews generated three categories of accessibility that were concerning for immigrant participants: geographical, sociocultural, and economic. In this immigrant neighbourhood, access to primary care was rarely obtainable. Several participants said that they were not comfortable leaving their neighbourhood to seek out medical care (geographical accessibility). Participants reported language difficulties with expressing their health concerns in English and interpreting medical directions in English. For many cultural and religious reasons, the Canadian biomedical model of care was deemed inappropriate by the majority of participants. There were notable differences in conceptions of health and healing between immigrants and the Canadian health care system (sociocultural accessibility). Cost was a barrier for immigrants requiring prescription medications, and in some instances, the medicare 3-month waiting period was an issue for recent immigrants, particularly immigrants with young children (economic accessibility). Some participants felt that foreign-trained physicians and nurses might aid their situation.

Based on the research findings, the authors made policy recommendations for local, provincial, and national levels. A summary of these recommendations follows:

Policy Recommendations
Local Policy Recommendations
- Involve community agencies in assisting immigrants with physician access
  - Provide community centre transportation (e.g., a van).
  - Arrange for physicians to come to the community centre on specified dates.
  - Offer translation services through neighbourhood volunteers.

Provincial Policy Recommendations
- Re-assess the 3-month waiting period in provinces that require it (e.g., British Columbia). This waiting period appears to legally contradict the "accessibility" principle of the *Canada Health Act*.
- Speed up the process by regulatory bodies to access the qualifications of foreign-born doctors and nurses.

Federal Policy Recommendations
- Review the national Skilled Worker Program to ensure its adequacy for meeting public needs. Large numbers of foreign-trained health care providers are unemployed or in unskilled jobs, highlighting the ineffectiveness of the current program.
- Re-evaluate the *Canada Health Act* principles (25 years old) to determine whether they accurately reflect the needs of current immigrants.
- Include immigrants ("local experts") in commissioned studies on public health policy (this point is important at every level).

Implications for Practice
Although this was a formal study, it portrayed a way that health care providers can make better connections with priority and vulnerable populations such as immigrants, Aboriginal peoples, individuals with mental health and addiction issues, and people with chronic health conditions. One-on-one conversations and informal focus groups can be organized at community centres and not-for-profit agencies in neighbourhoods where these populations are located. Making genuine inquiries about subpopulation needs is an important way for health care providers to build a trusting relationship with the community. Accurate portrayals of population needs come from the "local experts." Individuals or focus group participants can also be engaged to offer possible solutions for existing problems and influence policy.

The actual implementation of policy may involve a complex series of additional decisions, often related to funding. Imagine that a provincial Minister of Health, in response to the issue of childhood obesity, declares a policy that physical activity will be increased in public schools. This broad policy may even include the transfer of funds to school boards. Although the policy must be implemented, the specifics on how to do so will rest with school boards, schools, teachers, and families. Clearly, a high-level decision can initiate a domino effect of subsequent decisions. The implementation phase may be the policy phase most in need of research evidence to operationalize actions at the local level. At the local level, it is particularly critical during this phase for nurses to collaborate with other stakeholders in designing and implementing an evidence-informed program that truly meets the needs of the affected community or population (Fafard, 2008). Depending on the complexity of the policy, implementation may take place over a prolonged period of time and go through multiple adaptations.

Public policy evaluation involves examining the effectiveness of policies at different governmental levels. Macro-policy or broad policy evaluation is particularly difficult because of all the variables involved, the length of time it takes to enact broad policies, and the multiple decisions associated with one policy. With respect to a tobacco production control program in the United States, many evaluations were conducted to determine which federal policies had the biggest impact on tobacco producers—regulatory or taxation policies (see the BeTobaccoFree Web site at http://betobaccofree.hhs.gov/laws/). Public policy research has had its biggest successes with respect to program evaluation at the local level. In Canada, the Social Research and Demonstration Corporation (SRDC) evaluates existing social programs. The mission of SRDC is to help policymakers and practitioners identify those programs that can improve the well-being of Canadians, particularly disadvantaged or marginalized populations. A secondary goal is to identify research designs and methods that are most suited to public policy evaluation (see the SRDC Web site at http://www.srdc.org).

The Cochrane Collaboration (health policy) and the Campbell Collaboration (social policy and education) are international examples of not-for-profit organizations that critically evaluate the evidence available to inform policy decisions. The Cochrane Library has over 5000 systematic reviews on health-related topics. Most universities have subscriptions to the Cochrane Library. Cochrane Library publications are considered a gold standard for making policy decisions related to health care.

EXERCISE 11-6

Visit the Cochrane Collaboration website at http://www.cochrane.org. Check out the website's features. Go to the "About us" page and click on "Newcomer's guide" to find out more about the organization. Go to the Cochrane Summaries website at http://summaries.cochrane.org.

1. Search a health term of interest to you and locate a summary to share with your class or your peers. You may also choose to share what you have learned by listening to a podcast under Cochrane Summaries.
2. Consider the public policy implications of your topic. Recommend one broad policy action based on Cochrane Summaries information.

POLICY ADVOCACY AND NURSING

Policy advocacy refers to nurses' capacity as individuals or members of professional associations and coalitions to influence policymakers. As discussed above, other policy inputs from key stakeholder groups can significantly impact the policymaking process, and an understanding of the formal government process of policy development helps nurses know when and how to present evidence, voice their concerns, and recommend potential policy actions.

Other forms of policy advocacy include monitoring, alleviating and preventing, and bringing about social change (Cohen & Reutter, 2007). Policy advocacy often begins with raising public awareness of the issue(s). An example is the social determinants of health and the inequities that exist within certain populations. Nurses provide care to at-risk populations in different settings (e.g., acute care, home care, public health clinics), and they are ideally placed to collect and share stories of people's lives that can raise awareness about health inequities. In the United Kingdom, public health nurses, in particular, monitor or profile the living conditions of their patients. This practice is common in the United Kingdom where public health nurses are assigned to monitor and report on unsafe or unhealthy conditions. Nurse experiences can help validate existing research evidence on health inequities among certain populations (Cohen & Reutter, 2007). Advocacy roles related to alleviating and preventing involve nurses' use of expert power to obtain access to needed health and social services for patients. The

Research Perspective on p. 200 provides an example of these nurse advocacy roles in Canada. In the United States, nurses in case management roles often screen patients for risk factors related to poor quality of life and make referrals to welfare advocates (Cohen & Reutter, 2007). Monitoring and alleviating and preventing roles are typically carried out by individual nurses. Bringing about social change is more effective as collective action. Whenever possible, nurses should work through their professional associations or in collaboration with not-for-profit organizations. Canadian nurses have many opportunities to formally influence public policy by participating in advocacy activities that are sponsored through national and provincial or territorial nursing associations, such as the Canadian Nurses Association, the Registered Nurses' Association of Ontario, and the Association of Registered Nurses of British Columbia. Visit your nursing association's Web site for ideas on how to get involved.

RESEARCH PERSPECTIVE

Resource: MacDonnell, J. (2009). Fostering nurses' political knowledges and practices: Education and political activation in relation to lesbian health. *Advances in Nursing Science, 32*(2), 158–172. doi:10.1097/ANS.0b013e3181a3ddd9

Nursing has always supported vulnerable groups through unions, professional organizations, and educational institutions. This article explores the career trajectories of nurse political activists advocating for the sexual health needs of lesbians. The purpose of the study was to determine the antecedents or life circumstances leading to this type of nurse advocacy. Ten nurses from Ontario who are publicly known for their lesbian health advocacy were interviewed for the study. These nurses came from diverse nursing backgrounds ranging from rural health to critical care in a large urban area. All the nurses, however, had developed strong knowledge bases related to sexual diversity, and they had all been involved in other advocacy work. Their advocacy work began at the bedside level but quickly broadened after recognizing the social and political forces influencing the health and health care delivery of vulnerable populations. "A variety of collective initiatives have shaped these nurses' politics whether their nursing practice involves community or hospital settings and participation during their workplace hours or on their own time. They describe ties to street outreach teams and woman abuse projects and affiliations with boards of community agencies, professional organizations and political parties" (p. 162).

Nursing education influenced all of these nurses—either positively or negatively. Some nurses had wonderful role models and stimulating class discussions, while others endured stigmatizing class conditions that raised their awareness of the oppressive nature of "invisibility and silence." All of the nurses, however, recognized the importance of education as an advocacy tool to increase others' awareness of lesbian health and sexual diversity.

Over time, these nurses increased their capacity to advocate for lesbian health through education and by building their professional credibility. They also created networks among key stakeholder groups, including politicians. "These nurses, networks and coalitions are interdisciplinary or intersectoral in nature. Consistent with an upstream strategy to address root causes of health and social inequities for marginalized groups with the collaboration of individuals and groups beyond the health sector, this approach creates opportunities to sustain changes at the institutional and community levels" (p. 168).

Implications for Practice

These nurses became political through a quest to know more. Their political knowledge is based on personal, ethical, and empirical knowledge gained through formal education and clinical experience. They all recognized inequities and made a choice to do more than advocate for change at the clinical or bedside level. "Sociopolitical knowing [is a] focus on ethics and a critical analysis of structures of power and domination and their effects on individuals and communities" (p. 169). Each nurse has the choice to "do just a job" or choose to know and do more. Political knowledge is gained through education, networking, and engaging with others to address the nature of power dynamics that create inequities in health within our Canadian society.

EXERCISE 11-7

A model of political activism proposed by Leavitt, Chaffee, & Vance (2007) can be applied to the political development and activism of individual nurses in both professional and legislative political arenas. Assess yourself to see where you fit within this model—from apathy to leading the way. Based on where you fall within this model of political activism, consider two things you can do right now in your health care organization to move yourself further along this model's continuum.

1. *Apathy:* no membership in professional organizations; little or no interest in legislative politics as they relate to nursing and health care
2. *Buy-in:* recognition of the importance of activism within professional organizations (without active participation) and legislative politics related to critical nursing issues
3. *Self-interest:* involvement in professional organizations to further one's own career; the development and use of political expertise to further the profession's self-interests
4. *Political sophistication:* high level of professional organization activism (e.g., holding office at the municipal or provincial level) moving beyond self-interests; recognition of the need for activism on behalf of the public and the profession
5. *Leading the way:* serving in elected or appointed positions in professional organizations at the provincial or federal level; providing true leadership on broad health care interests in legislative politics, including seeking appointment to policymaking bodies and election to political positions.

A SOLUTION

Carol was taken aback by what her friend said, but then she reflected on the types of shows that are on TV—and most do not portray nurses as intelligent, autonomous practitioners. So she decided to change her friend's view of nursing. Carol started by telling her friend about the life-changing experience she had during labour in which the nurse's help led to the safe delivery of her daughter. Having a professional there to coach and reassure them was essential to Carol's partner as well. Carol told her friend about a few of the expert nurses she knows from clinical experiences. She gave her friend examples of how nurses use their knowledge and skills to make a difference in the quality and safety of care delivery every day. Telling stories makes a difference. Carol's experiences had a powerful effect on her friend. She apologized for not knowing more about nursing and for making assumptions. Perhaps a number of people have the same ideas. Carol was glad for the apology but decided to go further. She went online to The Truth About Nursing Web site (http://www.truth aboutnursing.org) to learn more about how she could help improve nursing's image. The founder and executive director of The Truth About Nursing, Sandy Summers, discovered the hard truth about the public's perceptions of nursing when she was a graduate student at Johns Hopkins School of Nursing. Sandy and her fellow graduate students banded together to create a not-for-profit organization to support a positive professional image of nurses. Their work has included campaigns to change the image of nurses on shows such as *Grey's Anatomy*. The Truth About Nursing has given TV shows that positively portray nurses, such as *Call the Midwife*, its award of excellence for showing the full range of what nurses do. The Web site gave Carol additional ways to take collective action to change how others think about nursing. Carol is proud to be entering the nursing profession and plans to speak to everyone she knows about the value of nursing. She will also keep a log of all those occasions when her care has made a positive difference for someone—and hopes to have a very large log! Carol and a group of nursing students at her school have contacted their provincial professional association to offer help in scanning the media for negative portrayals of nurses—so that they can collectively mount campaigns against media that undervalue or disrespect nursing. This situation led Carol to think about ways that she can use the power she has to make a difference for her new profession.

What approach might work for you in a similar situation? Have a look at Chapter 25; does it offer any information that might help with this kind of situation?

THE EVIDENCE

Laura Eggertson (2011) examined the impact of emotional abuse and bullying in the workplace on nurses. The statistics in this article are staggering. A 2005 National Survey of the Work and Health of Nurses showed that 44% of female nurses and 50% of male nurses in Canada reported being exposed to hostility or conflict by people they work with. (Conflict management and workplace violence are discussed in Chapters 23 and 25.) The article also discusses the findings of a 2010 study by Claire Mallette and colleagues on horizontal violence at the University Health Network in Toronto. This study found even higher levels of horizontal violence: 95% of nurses had observed horizontal violence and 71% identified themselves as targets. As part of their research, Mallette and colleagues created an online curriculum that included a role-playing scenario where nurses could choose avatars to represent them in a virtual world. This allowed the nurses to safely role play different responses to bullying scenarios.

Eggertson concludes: "A genuine investment in coaching and mentoring nurses on how to value and respect one another will pay off, not only for nurses, but also for the patients they serve" (p. 20). Moreover, she states that "changing the workplace culture also requires managers and their supervisors to act immediately if nurses report bullying to them, and to back up nurses who have been hurt" (p. 20).

NEED TO KNOW NOW

- Select positive and powerful role models.
- Form alliances with other new nurses: create your own support network.
- Join committees in your institution and/or professional nursing organizations.
- Contribute your talents to a topic of importance to you.

- Stay informed. What are current nursing policies in your organization? What are health policies at local, provincial or territorial, and national levels? Are they evidence-informed?

CHAPTER CHECKLIST

- Power is not finite: it expands by sharing it with others.
- Leaders can empower nurses and others by providing access to organizational empowerment structures (opportunities, information, supports, resources).
- Access to these empowerment structures (also called "power tools") is a catalyst for psychological empowerment—how nurses feel about themselves in their workplace.
- Psychological empowerment has four main dimensions: (1) meaning, (2) impact, (3) self-determination, and (4) competence.
- Nurses who are structurally and psychologically empowered are more satisfied and less likely to burn out or leave the organization.
- Another way to catalyze nurses' belief in themselves is through leader-empowering behaviours. Empowering leaders express confidence in their staff; they publicly value nursing; they involve nurses in making important decisions about health care delivery; and they support nurses in reaching their professional goals.

- Empowering work environments are known for strong nurse leadership at all levels, positive nurse–physician relationships, safe staffing, professional development opportunities, and giving nurses more control over practice. Some theorists and scholars consider nursing an oppressed behaviour group due to socialization practices that treat nurses as inferior. Passive-aggressive behaviours and bullying are associated with oppressed cultures.
- Nurses can build powerful professional identities by accentuating why they are irreplaceable. For instance, nurses make a positive difference in better, safer patient outcomes.
- Power strategies include networking and coalition building.
- The policy process should be based on best evidence, but other policy inputs, such as lobbying by special interest groups, can diminish the use of evidence during policymaking. However, evidence is important in every phase of the policy process.
- Policy engagement and political activism begin with nurses' desire to make a difference.

TIPS FOR USING INFLUENCE

- Make nursing your career, not just a job.
- Develop a powerful professional identity.
- Invest in your nursing career by continuing your education.

- Develop networking skills.
- Engage in policy advocacy by finding out what you can do through your provincial or territorial and national professional nursing associations.

evolve WEBSITE

Visit the Evolve website for Suggested Readings, Internet Resources, and additional resources related to the content in this chapter: http://evolve.elsevier.com/Canada/Yoder-Wise/leading/.

REFERENCES

Aiken, L., Sloane, D., Cimiotti, J., et al. (2010). Implications of the California nurse staffing mandate for other states. *Health Services Research, 45*(4), 904–921.

American Nurses Association. (2011). *Principles for social networking and the nurse.* Silver Spring, MD: Author.

Asanin, J., & Wilson, K. (2008). "I spent nine years looking for a doctor": Exploring access to health care among immigrants in Mississauga, Ontario, Canada. *Social Science & Medicine, 66*(6), 1271–1283. doi:10.1016/j.socscinied.2007.11.043

Benner, P. (2001). *From novice to expert: Excellence and power in clinical nursing practice* (commemorative ed.). Upper Saddle River, NJ: Prentice Hall Health.

Berry, L., & Curry, P. (2012). *Nursing workload and patient care: Understanding the value of nurses, the effects of excessive workload, and how nurse-patient ratios and dynamic staffing models can help.* Ottawa, ON: Canadian Federation of Nurses Unions. Retrieved from http://nursesunions.ca/sites/default/files/cfnu_workload_paper_pdf.pdf.

Bradbury-Jones, C., Sambrook, S., & Irvine, F. (2011). Nursing students and the issue of voice: A qualitative study. *Nurse Education Today, 31*, 628–632.

Bryant, T. (2009). *An introduction to health policy.* Toronto, ON: Canadian Scholars' Press.

Buerhaus, P. (2009). Avoiding mandatory hospital nurse staffing ratios: An economic perspective. *Nursing Outlook, 57*(2), 107–112.

Canadian Biography Online. (2011). *Jeanne Mance.* Retrieved from http://www.biographi.ca/en/bio/mance_jeanne_1E.html.

Cohen, B., & Reutter, L. (2007). Development of the role of public health nurses in addressing child and family poverty: A framework for action. *Journal of Advanced Nursing, 60*(1), 96–107. doi:10.1111/j.1365-2648.2006.04154.x

Dahinten, S., MacPhee, M., Hejazi, S., et al. (2013). Testing the effects of an empowerment-based leadership development programme: Part 2—staff outcomes. *Journal of Nursing Management, 22*(1), 16–28. doi:10.1111/jonm.12059

Dong, W., Fung, K., & Chan, K. (2010). Community mobilisation and empowerment for combating a pandemic. *Journal of Epidemiology and Community Health, 64*, 182–183. doi:10.1136/jech.2008.082206

Duchscher, J. E. (2009). Transition shock: The initial stage of role adaptation for newly graduated registered nurses. *Journal of Advanced Nursing, 65*(5), 1103–1113. doi:10.1111/j.1365-2648.2008.04898.x

Eggertson, L. (2011). Targeted: The impact of bullying, and what needs to be done to eliminate it. *Canadian Nurse, 107*(6), 16–20.

Fafard, P. (2008). *Evidence and healthy public policy: Insights from health and political sciences.* Ottawa, ON: National Collaborating Centre for Healthy Public Policy/Canadian Policy Research Networks. Retrieved from http://www.ncchpp.ca.

Greco, P., Laschinger, H., & Wong, C. (2006). Leader empowering behaviours, staff nurse empowerment and work engagement/burnout. *The Canadian Journal of Nursing Leadership, 19*(4), 41–56.

HEAL. (2011, April 6). HEAL calls on federal political parties to focus on health system during election [News release]. Retrieved from http://www.newswire.ca/en/story/776657/heal-calls-on-federal-political-parties-to-focus-on-health-system-during-election.

Health Canada. (2009). Office of nursing policy. Retrieved from http://www.hc-sc.gc.ca/ahc-asc/branch-dirgen/spb-dgps/onp-bpsi/index-eng.php.

Hersey, P., Blanchard, K., & Natemeyer, W. (1979). Situational leadership, perception and impact of power. *Group and Organizational Studies, 4*, 418–428.

Howlett, M., & Ramesh, M. (Eds.). (2003). *Studying public policy: Policy cycles and policy subsystems* (2nd ed.). Don Mills, ON: Oxford University Press.

Jean Mance to be named Montreal co-founder. (2011, March 8). *CBC News.* Retrieved from http://www.cbc.ca/news/canada/montreal/jeanne-mance-to-be-named-montreal-co-founder-1.1035017.

Kanter, R. M. (1993). *Men and women of the corporation* (2nd ed.). New York, NY: Basic Books.

Kramer, M. (1974). *Reality shock: Why nurses leave nursing.* Saint Louis, MO: Mosby.

Lankshear, S. (2012). *Primary health care summit summary report; January 25–26, 2012, Ottawa, Ontario.* Ottawa, ON: Canadian Nurses Association and the Canadian Medical Association. Retrieved from http://www.cna-aiic.ca/~/media/cna/page%20content/pdf%20en/2013/07/31/10/00/primary_health_care_report_e.pdf.

Laschinger, H. (2008). Effect of empowerment on professional practice environments, work satisfaction and patient care quality: Further testing the nursing worklife model. *Journal of Nursing Care Quality, 23*(4), 322–330. doi:10.1097/01.NCQ.0000318028.67910.6b

Laschinger, H., Finegan, J., & Wilk, P. (2009). Context matters: The impact of unit leadership and empowerment on nurses' organizational commitment. *The Journal of Nursing Administration, 39*(5), 228–235.

Laschinger, H., Gilbert, S., Smith, L., et al. (2013). Towards a comprehensive theory of nurse/patient empowerment: Applying Kanter's empowerment theory to patient care. *Journal of Nursing Management, 18*, 4–13. doi:10.111/j.1365-2834.2009.01046.x

Laschinger, H., Grau, A., Finegan, J., et al. (2010). New graduate nurses' experiences of bullying and burnout in hospital settings. *Journal of Advanced Nursing, 66*(12), 2732–2742. doi:10.1111/j.1365-2648.2010.05420.x

Lavoie-Tremblay, M., O'Brien-Pallas, L., Gelinas, C., et al. (2008). Addressing the turnover issue among new nurses from a generational viewpoint. *Journal of Nursing Management, 16*(6). 724–733. doi:10.1111/j.1365-2934.2007.00828.x

Leavitt, J. K., Chaffee, M. W., & Vance, C. (2007). Learning the ropes of policy and politics. In D. J. Mason, J. K. Leavitt, & M. W. Chaffee (Eds.), *Policy & politics in nursing and health care* (5th ed., pp. 34–46). St. Louis, MO: Saunders.

MacDonnell, J. (2009). Fostering nurses' politic knowledges and practices: Education and political activation in relation to lesbian health. *Advances in Nursing Science, 32*(2), 158–172. doi:10.1097/ANS.0b013e3181a3ddd9

MacPhee, M., Jackson, C., & Suryaprakash, N. (2009). Online knowledge networking: What leaders need to know. *Journal of Nursing Administration, 39*(10), 415–422. doi:0.1097/NNA.0b013e3181b9221f

Manojlovich, M. (2007). Power and empowerment in nursing: Looking backward to inform the future. *Online Journal of Issues in Nursing, 12*(1), Manuscript 1. doi:10.3912/OJIN.Vol12No01Man01

Matheson, L. K., & Bobay, K. (2007). Validation of oppressed group behaviors in nursing. *Journal of Professional Nursing, 23*, 226–234.

McGillis Hall, L., MacDonald-Rencz, S., Peterson, J., et al. (2013). *Moving to action: Evidence-based retention and recruitment policy initiatives for nursing.* Ottawa, ON: Canadian Foundation for Healthcare Improvement and Office of Nursing Policy. Retrieved from http://www.cfhi-fcass.ca/sf-docs/default-source/reports/Moving-to-Action-McGillis-Hall-E.pdf?sfvrsn=0.

McIntyre, M., & McDonald, C. (2010). *Realities of Canadian nursing: Professional, practice, and power issues.* Philadelphia, PA: Wolters Kluwer Health.

Moloughney, B. (2012). The use of policy frameworks to understand public health-related public policy processes: A literature review. Retrieved from https://www.peelregion.ca/health/library/pdf/Policy_Frameworks.PDF.

Ozimek, R. W. (2007). Taking action: Distributed campaigns—Using the Internet to empower activism. In D. J. Mason, J. K. Leavitt, & M. W. Chaffee (Eds.), *Policy & politics in nursing and health care* (5th ed., pp. 171–176). St. Louis, MO: Saunders.

Ponte, P. R., Glazer, G., Dann, E., et al. (2007). The power of professional nursing practice: An essential element of patient and family centered care. *Online Journal of Issues in Nursing, 12*(1), Manuscript 3. doi:10.31912/OJIN.Vol12No01Man03

Purpora, C., Blegen, M., & Stotts, N. (2012). Horizontal violence among hospital staff nurses related to oppressed self or oppressed group. *Journal of Professional Nursing, 28*(5), 306–314.

Sauer, P. (2012). Do nurses eat their young? Truth and consequences. *Journal of Emergency Nursing, 38*(1), 43–46.

Smith, B. (2012). Social networking and professional pitfalls. *International Journal of Orthopaedic and Trauma Nursing, 16*, 63–64. doi:10.1016/j.ijotn.2012.03.001

Smith, L. A., Andrusyszyn, M. A., & Laschinger, H. (2010). Effects of workplace incivility and empowerment on newly-graduated nurses' organizational commitment. *Journal of Nursing Management, 18*(8), 1004–1015. doi:10.1111/j.1365-2834.2010.01165.x

Spreitzer, G. (2007). Taking stock: A review of more than twenty years of research on empowerment at work. In J. Barling & C. Cooper (Eds.), *The Sage handbook of organizational behavior, Volume 1: Micro approaches* (pp. 54–73). Los Angeles, CA: Sage.

St-Pierre, I., & Holmes, D. (2008). Managing nurses through disciplinary power: A Foucauldian analysis of workplace violence. *Journal of Nursing Management, 16*, 352–359. doi:10.1111/j.1365-2834.2007.00812.x

Sullivan, E. J. (2013). *Becoming influential: A guide for nurses* (2nd ed.). Upper Saddle River, NJ: Pearson Education.

Summers, S. (2014, January). Changing how the world thinks about nursing. *Canadian Nurse*, 26–30.

Tomblin Murphy, G., & MacKenzie, A. (2013). Using evidence to meet population healthcare needs: Successes and challenges. *Healthcare Papers, 13*(2), 9–21.

Trus, M., Razbadauskas, A., & Doran, D. (2012). Work-related empowerment of nurse managers: A systematic review. *Nursing and Health Sciences, 14*(3), 412–420.

Udod, S. (2008). The power behind empowerment for staff nurses: Using Foucault's concepts. *The Canadian Journal of Nursing Leadership, 21*(2), 77–92.

Uhlrich, B., Krozek, C., & Early, S. (2010). Improving retention, confidence, and competence of new graduate nurses: Results from a 10-year longitudinal database. *Nursing Economics, 28*, 448–462.

Upton, J., Fletcher, M., Mado-Sutton, H., et al. (2011). Shared decision making or paternalism in nursing consultations? A qualitative study of primary care asthma nurses' views on sharing decisions with patients regarding inhaler device selection. *Health Expectations, 14*(4), 374–382. doi:10.1111/j.1369-7625.2010.00653.x

Vessey, J., DeMarco, R., Gaffney, D., et al. (2009). Bullying of staff registered nurses in the workplace: A preliminary study for developing personal and organizational strategies for the transformation of hostile to healthy workplace environments. *Journal of Professional Nursing, 25*(5), 299–306.

Wagner, J., Cummings, G., Smith, D., et al. (2010). The relationship between structural empowerment and psychological empowerment for nurses: A systematic review. *Journal of Nursing Management, 18*, 448–462.

Wilson, R. (2013). Policy and evidence in Canadian health human resources planning. *Healthcare Papers, 13*(2), 28–31.

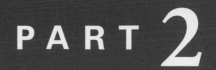

Managing Resources

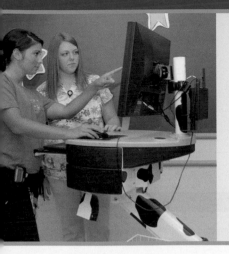

Caring, Communicating, and Managing with Technology

Janis B. Smith and Cheri Hunt
Adapted by Kathy L. Rush

This chapter describes current biomedical technology with an emphasis on information technology that allows nurses to use data gathered at the point of care effectively and efficiently. Nurses are knowledge workers who use biomedical and information technology to care for patients. This chapter includes sections on biomedical, information, and knowledge technology with subsections that discuss informatics competencies, standardized terminologies, information systems hardware, the science of informatics, evidence-informed practice, and patient-care safety and quality. Nurses build knowledge for practice by comparing and contrasting not only current patient data with previous data for the same patient but also data across patients with the same diagnosis. Information tools and skills are essential for these decision-making processes now and in the future.

OBJECTIVES

- Describe three types of health care information technology trends.
- Apply one structured nursing terminology to a nursing scenario.
- Analyze three types of technology for capturing data at the point of care.
- Describe the core components of informatics: data, information, knowledge, and wisdom.
- Evaluate a model to change accepted practice into evidence-informed practice.
- Articulate the role of several new technologies in patient safety.
- Discuss decision support systems and their impact on patient care.
- Explore the issues of patient safety, ethics, and information security and privacy within information technology.
- Understand the value and limitations of the Internet for health care information.

TERMS TO KNOW

biomedical technology
blog
clinical decision support (CDS)
clinical decision support systems
  (CDSSs)
communication technology
data
database

electronic health record (EHR)
electronic medical record (EMR)
evidence-informed practice
informatics
information
information technology
knowledge
knowledge broker

knowledge brokering
knowledge technology
knowledge worker
nursing minimum data set
  (NMDS)
speech recognition (SR)
telehealth
wisdom

⑦ A CHALLENGE

Hollary is a registered practical nurse in a small, rural hospital. The nursing leadership in her hospital is collaborating with the information systems leadership, medical staff, and allied health leadership on a pilot project to implement a clinical information system to create a "safe hospital of the future." Key electronic systems to be implemented included nursing documentation, bedside medication verification, and physician ordering. During the design phase of the project, Hollary was asked to consult with her colleagues and offer input on the following questions:

- How can the new clinical information system support the nursing workflow and patient-centred care?
- How can nurses who will be affected by the new system be involved in the decision-making process?

- What types of hardware are most appropriate in your care setting?
- To what degree is standardized terminology required for consistent, meaningful data interpretation?
- How can the new system enhance the quality and safety of health care delivery?

Hollary and her colleagues need to offer prudent and future-minded input.

What do you think you would do if you were Hollary?

INTRODUCTION

Technology surrounds us! Intravenous pumps are "smart," biomedical monitoring is no longer exclusively an intensive care practice, and computers are used at the bank, at the grocery checkout, in our cars, and in almost every other aspect of daily living, including the provision of health care. Health care is both a technology- and an information-intensive business; therefore, the success of nurses using biomedical technology, information technology, and knowledge technology will contribute to their personal and professional development and career achievement.

Technology is critical to the quality and safety of Canadian health care. Compared with six other countries (Australia, Germany, the Netherlands, New Zealand, the United Kingdom, and the United States), Canadian adults had the third-highest self-reported

medical, medication, and laboratory errors at 17%, which translates into 4.25 million affected Canadians (O'Hagan, MacKinnon, Persaud, et al., 2009). Self-reported errors were associated with a combination of system, provider, and patient risk factors, and proactively addressing these factors is essential to enhancing the safety of Canada's health care system. Many leaders in health care see technology as a means to facilitate decision making, improve efficacy and efficiency, enhance patient safety and quality care, and decrease health care costs (Hannah, 2005; Romanow, 2002). But a leader's vision of technology must engage followers in partnership so that these benefits can be realized. If appropriately implemented and fully integrated, technology has the potential to improve the practice environment for nurses as well as patients and their families. Good decision making for patient care requires good information. Nurses are knowledge workers who need data and information to provide effective and efficient patient care. Technology plays an important role in supporting nurses in their knowledge work (Mathieu, 2007). Data and information must be accurate, reliable, and presented in an actionable form. Currently, information systems support nurses in collecting data but not in the more complex functions of knowledge use and development (Mathieu, 2007).

TYPES OF TECHNOLOGIES

As nurses, we commonly use and manage three types of technologies: biomedical technology, information technology, and knowledge technology. **Biomedical technology** involves the use of equipment in the clinical setting for diagnosis, physiological monitoring, testing, and administering therapies to patients. **Information technology** is the use of computer hardware and software to process data into information to solve problems. **Knowledge technology** is the use of expert systems by clinicians to make decisions about patient care. In nursing, these systems are designed to mimic the reasoning of nurse experts in making patient-care decisions.

Biomedical Technology

Biomedical technology is used for: (1) physiological monitoring, (2) diagnostic testing, (3) intravenous fluid and medication dispensing and administration, and (4) therapeutic treatments.

Physiological Monitoring. Physiological monitoring systems measure heart rate, blood pressure, and other vital signs. They also monitor cardiac rhythm; measure and record central venous, pulmonary wedge, intracranial, and intra-abdominal pressures; and analyze oxygen and carbon dioxide levels in the blood.

Patient surveillance systems are designed to provide early warning of a possible impending adverse event. One example is a system that provides wireless monitoring of heart rate, respiratory rate, and attempts by a patient at risk for falling to get out of bed unassisted; this monitoring is via a mattress coverlet and bedside monitor.

Innovative technology is increasingly being deployed to meet the needs of populations in remote areas. Telemonitoring and teletriage are two telehealth approaches that provide enhanced patient follow-up.

Telemonitoring is the remote observation of patients' physiological parameters and therapeutic regimen readjustments, while *teletriage* is the evaluation of a patient's health status and the formulation of recommendations relative to treatment and follow-up (Côté, 2007).

Intracranial pressure (ICP) monitoring systems monitor the cranial pressure in critically ill patients with closed head injuries or postoperative craniotomy patients. The ICP, along with the mean arterial blood pressure, can be used to calculate perfusion pressure. This allows assessment and early therapy as changes occur. When the ICP exceeds a set pressure, some systems allow ventricular drainage. Similarly, monitoring pressure within the bladder has recently been demonstrated to accurately detect intra-abdominal hypertension as measures of maximal and mean intra-abdominal pressures and abdominal perfusion pressure are made. Intra-abdominal hypertension occurs with abdominal compartment syndrome and other acute abdominal illnesses. Routine intra-abdominal pressure (IAP) monitoring has been recommended for those critically ill patients subjected to shock and subsequent resuscitation (Kirkpatrick, DeWaele, Ball, et al., 2007).

Continuous dysrhythmia monitors and electrocardiograms (ECGs) provide visual representation of electrical activity in the heart and can be used for surveillance and detection of dysrhythmias and for interpretation and diagnosis of the abnormal rhythm. Although they are not new technology, these systems have grown increasingly sophisticated. More important, integration with wireless communication technology permits new approaches to triaging alerts to nurses about cardiac rhythm abnormalities. The need for wireless approaches to decrease response time to dysrhythmia alarms was demonstrated in a study of remote cardiac telemetry nurses, who detected a valid rhythm disturbance an average of 72% of the time but required physically checking alarms every 2.1 to 6.2 minutes while simultaneously carrying their patient load (Billinghurst, Morgan, & Arthur, 2003).

Biomedical devices for physiological monitoring can be interfaced with clinical information systems. Monitored vital signs and invasive pressure readings are downloaded directly into the patient's electronic medical record, where the nurse confirms their accuracy and affirms the data entry.

Diagnostic Testing. Dysrhythmia systems can also be diagnostic. The computer, after processing and analyzing the ECG, generates a report that is confirmed by a trained professional. ECG tracings can be transmitted over telephone lines from remote sites (such as the patient's home) to the physician's office or clinic. Patients with implantable pacemakers can have their cardiac activity monitored without leaving home.

Other systems for diagnostic testing include blood gas analyzers, pulmonary function systems, and ICP monitors. Contemporary laboratory medicine is virtually all automated. In addition, point-of-care testing devices extend the laboratory's testing capabilities to the patient's bedside or care area. In critical care areas, for example, blood gas, ionized calcium, hemoglobin, and hematocrit values are often measured from unit-based "stat labs." Point-of-care blood glucose monitors can download results of bedside testing into an automated laboratory results system and the patient's electronic medical record. Results can be communicated quickly and trends analyzed throughout patients' hospital stays and at ongoing ambulatory care visits. Results can calculate the necessary insulin doses based on evidence for tight blood glucose control and evoke electronic orders for administration. This example integrates diagnostic test results with the appropriate orders-based intervention.

Intravenous Fluid and Medication Dispensing and Administration. Intravenous (IV) fluid and medication distribution and dispensing via Automated Dispensing Cabinets (ADCs) were introduced in the 1980s. ADCs can decrease the wait time for medications on patient-care units, ensure greater protection of medications (especially controlled substances), and efficiently and accurately capture medication charges. Most important, ADCs can reduce the risk of medication errors, but only when safeguards are available and used. The Institute for Safe Medication Practices Canada (ISMP Canada) has developed a set of recommendations for the appropriate use of ADCs that highlight the pharmacist's role in reviewing medication orders, the process for retrieving medications, stocking and restocking, and staff education (Institute for Safe Medication Practices Canada, 2007).

IV smart pumps are used to deliver fluids, blood and blood products, and medications either continuously or intermittently at rates between 0.1 and 999 mL per hour. Twenty-first-century pumps offer safety features, accuracy, advanced pressure monitoring, ease of use, and versatility. These pumps have rate-dependent pressure detection systems, designed to provide an early alert to IV cannula occlusion with real-time display of the patient-side pressure reading in the system. Smart pumps can be programmed to calculate medication doses and medication infusion rates, as well as determine the volume and duration of an infusion. Smart syringe pumps can be used in environments such as the intensive or critical care unit and in anesthesia where precise delivery of concentrated medications is required. Infusion rates as small as 0.01 mL per hour can be delivered.

Therapeutic Treatments. Treatments may be administered via implantable infusion pumps that administer medications at a prescribed rate and can be programmed to provide boluses or change doses at set points in time. These pumps are commonly used for hormone regulation, treatment of hypertension, chronic intractable pain, diabetes, venous thrombosis, and cancer chemotherapy.

Therapeutic treatment systems may be used to regulate intake and output, regulate breathing, and assist with the care of the newborn. Intake and output systems are linked to infusion pumps that control arterial pressure, medication therapy, fluid resuscitation, and serum glucose levels. These systems calculate and regulate the IV drip rate.

Increasingly sophisticated mechanical ventilators are used to deliver a prescribed percentage of oxygen and volume of air to the patient's lungs and to provide a set flow rate, inspiratory-to-expiratory time ratio, and various other complex functions with less trauma to lung tissue than was previously possible. Computer-assisted ventilators are electromechanically controlled by a closed-loop feedback system to analyze and control lung volumes and alveolar gases. Ventilators also provide sophisticated, sensitive alarm systems for patient safety.

In the newborn and intensive care nursery, computers monitor the heart and respiratory rates of the babies there. In addition, newborn nursery systems can regulate the temperature of the infant's environment by sensing his or her temperature and the air of the surrounding environment. Alarms can be set to notify the nurse when pre-set physiological parameters are exceeded. Computerized systems monitor fetal activity before delivery, linking the ECGs of the mother and baby and the pulse oximetry, blood pressure, and respirations of the mother.

Biomedical technology affects nursing as nurses provide direct care to patients treated with new technologies: monitoring data from new devices, administering therapy with new techniques, and evaluating patients' responses to care and treatment. Nurses must be aware of the latest technologies for monitoring patients' physiological status, diagnostic testing, medication administration, and therapeutic treatments. It is important to identify the data to be collected, the information that might be gained, and the many ways that these data might be used to provide new knowledge. More important, nurses must remember that biomedical technology supplements but does not replace the skilled observation, assessment, and evaluation of the patient.

Nurse leaders must be aware of how these technologies fit into the delivery of patient care and the strategic plan of the organization in which they work. They must have a vision for the future and be ready to suggest solutions that will assist nurses across specialties and settings to improve patient-care safety and quality.

EXERCISE 12-1

List the types of biomedical technology available for patient care in your organization. List ways that you currently use the data and information gathered by these systems. How do these types of technology help you care for patients? Can you think of other ways to use biomedical technology? Can you think of other ways to use the data or information? For example, data from biomedical devices might be sent directly to the electronic health record (EHR), negating the need for transcription of a result into the patient's chart. Nurses spend many hours learning to use biomedical devices and to interpret the data gained from them. Have we come to rely too heavily on technology rather than on our own judgement?

Information Technology

Health care is an information and knowledge-intensive enterprise. In the landmark Romanow (2002) report *Building on Values: The Future of Health Care in Canada*, information was seen to be key in finding cures to illnesses, giving health care providers access to new treatments and medications, improving health care system quality and safety, and empowering patients to self-manage health. Information is only effective if it

can be accessed. Access involves four facets: *discovery*—knowing whether the required information is available and where to find it; *connectivity*—the ability to obtain the resource where and when it is needed; *language*—agreement between the provider and user on the meaning of terminology; and *permission*—consent to use the information, which gets into issues of privacy (Goddard, Mowat, Corbett, et al., 2004). Information technology can help health care providers access, manage, analyze, and disseminate both information and knowledge. Health care in the twenty-first century should be safe, effective, patient-centred, timely, efficient, and equitable (White, 2007).

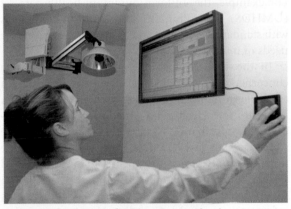

Patient data displayed with computerized systems to provide meaningful information and trends.

Computers offer the advantage of storing, organizing, retrieving, and communicating digital data with accuracy and speed. Patient-care data can be entered once, stored in a database, and then quickly and accurately retrieved many times and in many combinations by health care providers and others. A **database** is a collection of data elements organized and stored together. Data processing is the structuring, organizing, and presenting of data for interpretation as information. For example, vital signs for one patient can be entered into the computer and communicated on a graph; many patients' blood pressure measurements can be compared with the number of doses of antihypertensive medication. Vital signs for male patients between selective ages, such as 40 and 50 years, can be correlated and used to show relationships with age, ethnicity, weight, presence of co-morbid conditions, and so on.

Humans process data continuously, but in an analogue form. Computers process data faster, in a digital form and more accurately than humans, and provide a method of storage so that data can be retrieved as needed. Box 12-1 describes the development of information management skills from novice to expert.

Structured Nursing Terminologies. Collecting a set of basic data from every patient at every health care encounter makes sense because comparisons can be made among many patients, institutions, or countries, almost in any combination imaginable, as well as for individual patients and patient groups across time. Structured terminologies define the standardized data elements necessary for a clinical information system. For example, the uniform minimum health data set (UMHDS) is a minimum set of information items with standard definitions and categories that meets the needs of multiple data users.

In the 1980s, Canadian nursing leaders became concerned about the absence of nursing information available in national databases such as the Canadian Institute for Health Information's (CIHI) management information system (MIS) and Discharge Abstract Database (DAD), thus making invisible nursing's contribution to patient, organizational, and system outcomes (Doran, Mildon, & Clark, 2011; Kleib, Sales, Doran, et al., 2011). To address this information gap, the Canadian Nurses Association (CNA) convened the first nursing minimum data set (NMDS) conference in the early 1990s to promote the entry, accessibility, and retrievability of nursing data (Canadian Nurses Association, 2000; Haines, 1993). The resulting NMDS—a system that collects essential nursing data in a standardized manner—was named the Health Information: Nursing Components (HI:NC). Additional data elements were recommended at the conference, but consensus was not achieved for coding these elements. The additional data elements included nursing care elements (patient status, nursing interventions, and patient outcome); principal nurse provider (using nurse identifier); and nursing intensity (Doran et al., 2011, p. 8). Since CNA's (2006b) adoption of the International Classification for Nursing Practice (ICNP®) and the development of standardized terminology, coding for nursing care data elements now exists and work has begun on coding nursing workload data (Doran et al., 2011). Four data elements in the NMDS are unique to nursing: nursing diagnosis, nursing intervention, nursing outcome, and intensity of nursing care. Box 12-2 lists the five nursing care elements included in the NMDS. Doran et al. (2011, p. 7) summarized the purposes of the NMDS:

1. To ensure the availability, accessibility, and retrievability of standardized nursing data (CNA, 2000).
2. To enable comparison of nursing data among patient populations, settings, geography, and time (Butler, Treacy, Scott, et al., 2006).
3. To describe nursing care; identifying or projecting trends related to nursing care and resources (MacNeela, Scott, Treacy, et al., 2006).
4. To promote nursing research (Werley, Devine, Zorn, et al., 1991).

BOX 12-1 DEVELOPMENT OF INFORMATION MANAGEMENT SKILLS: NOVICE TO EXPERT PRACTICE

Novice nurses focus on learning what data to collect, the process of collecting and documenting the data, and how to use this information. They learn what clinical applications are available for use and how to use them. Computer and informatics skills focus on applying concrete concepts.

As nurses grow in expertise, they look for patterns in the data and information. They aggregate data across patient populations to look for similarities and differences in response to interventions. Expert nurses integrate theoretical knowledge with practical knowledge gained from experience.

Expert nurses know the value of personal professional reflection on knowledge and synthesize and evaluate information for discovery and decision making.

BOX 12-2 NURSING CARE ELEMENTS INCLUDED IN THE NURSING MINIMUM DATA SET

1. Patient status
2. Nursing interventions
3. Patient outcome
4. Nursing intensity
5. Primary nurse identifier

Doran, D., Mildon, B., & Clarke, S. (2011). *Toward a national report card in nursing: A knowledge synthesis.* Toronto, ON: Nursing Health Services Research Unit (Toronto site) and Lawrence S. Bloomberg Faculty of Nursing, University of Toronto.

5. To provide data to "facilitate and influence clinical, administrative and health policy decision-making" (Kleib et al., 2011, p. 489), including evaluating the appropriateness of nursing care (Butler et al., 2006).

6. To differentiate nursing care from that of other health care providers and thus making it visible (Butler et al., 2006; MacNeela et al., 2006).

Nursing classification systems and standardized nursing terminology contributed to NMDS development (Doran et al., 2011). From NMDS data, nursing-sensitive outcome databases have evolved and are international in scope. In Ontario, Health Outcomes for Better Information and Care (HOBIC) is an initiative that collects information on nursing in acute care, home care, long-term care, and complex continuing care settings. It measures a number of generic nurse-sensitive outcomes: functional status/activities of daily living; symptom status (pain, nausea, dyspnea, fatigue); safety outcomes (pressure ulcers, falls); and therapeutic self-care. Patient satisfaction was added as a nurse-sensitive outcome to the Canadian HOBIC (C-HOBIC), an expansion of HOBIC for application in long-term care settings in Manitoba and Saskatchewan. The data on nursing-related outcomes collected by HOBIC and C-HOBIC provide nurse leaders and administrators with valuable information about their organization's performance as well as decisional support to enhance improved outcomes.

An action learning study of a HOBIC early adopter site showed that HOBIC implementation required more than mastery of the technology; nurses required ongoing support to help them adapt their daily practice to maximize HOBIC's functionality (Tregunno, Gordon, Gardiner-Harding, 2010). The authors offered the following suggestions to enhance HOBIC implementation:

- Nursing records must be integrated with other records so that patient information is integrated and can be communicated among the health care team.
- Clinical nursing experts are needed to work with terminology experts to develop standard language in areas of nursing not yet adequately developed.
- Nurse leaders must advocate for use of structured nursing terminologies with the creators and vendors of information systems.

EXERCISE 12-2

Examine the nursing care elements of the NMDS. Which of them would be collected by patient registration? What information do you as a nurse need to collect? For example, in an acute care setting, you have provided care to a postoperative patient today, administering pain medication several times. The nursing diagnosis was Acute Pain. You charted the medication administration and the patient's pain rating 30 minutes after the medication was given. Which of the nursing care elements of the NMDS have you documented?

Standardized, computerized nursing terminology allows nurses to collect, aggregate, and analyze patient data for decision support, quality improvement, and research. Data from within and across patient populations are needed to build evidence from practice and to use evidence in practice. These data are also needed to quantify and describe nursing practice and its impact on the quality of care provided and on patient outcomes.

INFORMATION SYSTEMS

A patient information system can be manual or computerized—in fact, we have collected and recorded information about patients and patient care since the dawn of health care. Computer information systems manage large volumes of data, examine data patterns and trends, solve problems, and answer questions. In other words, computers can help translate data into information. Ideally, data are recorded at the point in the care process where they are gathered and are available to health care providers when and where they are needed. Data access is accomplished, in part, by networking computers both within and among organizations to form larger systems. These networked systems might link inpatient care units and other departments, hospitals, clinics, hospices, home health agencies, and/or physician practices. Data from all patient encounters with the health care system are stored in one or more data repositories and can be accessed by clinicians according to their scope of practice from anywhere in the world. These provide the potential for automated patient records, which contain health data from birth to death.

Adopting the technology necessary to computerize patient care information systems is complex and must be accomplished in stages. The Health Information

TABLE 12-1   ELECTRONIC MEDICAL RECORD ADOPTION MODEL

STAGE	DESCRIPTION
7	• The health care organization has a paperless electronic medical record (EMR) environment. • Clinical information can be shared via electronic transactions with all entities within the health information network (i.e., other hospitals, clinics, subacute settings, employers, and patients). • The health care organization can share and use health and wellness information with consumers and providers. • Data warehousing and mining technologies are used to capture and analyze care data and improve care protocols via decision support.
6	• Full physician documentation using structured templates is implemented for at least one patient care service area. • A full complement of all radiology images (digital and film) is available to health care providers via an intranet or other secure network.
5	• Closed-loop medication administration is fully implemented in at least one patient care service area. • The electronic medication administration record (e-MAR) and bar coding or other auto-identification technology (e.g., radio frequency identification [RFID]) are implemented and integrated with computerized physician order entry (CPOE) and pharmacy to maximize point-of-care patient safety processes for medication administration.
4	• CPOE is implemented and available for use by health care providers. • Second-level clinical decision support (related to evidence-informed protocols) is implemented.
3	• Clinical documentation (on vital signs, flow sheets, nursing notes, care planning, the e-MAR, etc.) is implemented and integrated with the clinical data repository for at least one service in the organization. • First-level clinical decision support for error checking with order entry (e.g., drug/drug, drug/allergy, drug/food, drug/lab conflict checking) is implemented. • Some radiology images from picture archive and communication systems (PACS) can be accessed by health care providers via a secure network.
2	• Major ancillary clinical systems feed data to a clinical data repository that provide health care providers access for retrieving and reviewing results. • The data repository contains a controlled medical vocabulary and the rules and clinical decision support system for rudimentary conflict checking.
1	• Major ancillary (laboratory, radiology, and pharmacy) clinical systems are installed.
0	• Some clinical automation may exist. • Laboratory and/or pharmacy and/or radiology clinical systems are not installed.

Adapted from Health Information Management Systems Society. (2008). The premier EMR adoption assessment tool. Retrieved from http://www.himssanalytics .org/docs/emram.pdf.

and Management Systems Society (HIMSS) has described seven stages of adoption—the seventh of which marks achievement of a fully electronic health care record. The seven stages of adoption are listed and described in Table 12-1. A recent HIMSS survey of Canadian hospitals revealed that fewer than 30% of Canadian hospitals have achieved stage three (compared with 50% of US hospitals), while just 1% have achieved ratings at stage four or higher (Webster, 2010).

Nurses care for patients in acute care, ambulatory, and community settings, as well as in patients' homes. In all settings, nurses focus not only on managing acute illnesses but also on health promotion, maintenance, and education; care coordination and continuity; and monitoring chronic conditions. Ideally, information systems support the work of nurses in all settings.

Communication networks are used to transmit data entered at one computer and received by others in the network. These networks can reduce the clerical functions of nursing. They can provide patient demographic and census data, results from tests, and lists of medications. Nursing policies and procedures can be linked to the network and accessed, when needed, at the point of care. Links can be provided between the patient's home, hospital, and/or physician's office with computers, handheld technologies, and point-of-care devices. Day-to-day events can be recorded and downloaded into the patient record remotely in community nursing settings or at the point of care in the hospital or clinic.

EXERCISE 12-3
Select a health care setting with which you are familiar. What information systems are used? Make a list of the names of these systems and the information they provide. How do they help you in caring for patients or in making management decisions? Think about the communication of data and information among departments. Do the systems communicate with each other? If you do not have computerized systems, think about how data and information are communicated. How might a computer system help you be more efficient?

As an example, assume that an abdominal magnetic resonance imaging (MRI) with contrast has been ordered. In a paper-based system, handwritten requisitions are sent to nutrition services, pharmacy, and the radiology department. With a computerized system, the MRI is ordered and the requests for dietary changes, bowel preparation medications, and the diagnostic study itself are automatically sent to the appropriate departments. Radiology would compare its scheduled openings with the patient's schedule and automatically place the date and time for the MRI on the patient's automated plan of care. The images and results of the diagnostic procedure are available online.

Nurses caring for patients in home health care and hospice must complete documentation necessary to meet government and billing requirements. Computers assist with direct entry of all required data in the correct format. Portable computers are used to download files of the patients to be seen during the day from a main database. During each visit, the computer prompts the nurse for vital signs, assessments, diagnosis, interventions, long-term and short-term goals, and medications based on previous entries in the medical record. Nurses enter any new data, modifications, or nursing information directly. Entries can be transmitted by a secured data line or Internet connection to the main computer at the office or downloaded from the device at the end of the day. This action automatically updates the patient record and any verbal order entry records, home visit reports, required treatment plans, productivity and quality improvement reports, and other documents for review and signature. Portable and wireless computers have made recording patient-care information more efficient and have improved personnel productivity and adherence with necessary documentation.

Placing computers or handheld devices "patient-side" permits nurses to enter data once, at the point of care. Documentation of patient assessments and care that are provided patient-side saves time, gives others more timely access to the data, and decreases the likelihood of forgetting to document vital information. Point-of-care devices and systems that fit with nurses' workflow, personalize patient assessments, and simplify care planning are available. Patient-care areas with point-of-care computers have improved the quality of patient care by decreasing errors of omission, providing greater accuracy and completeness of documentation, reducing medication errors, providing more timely responses to patient needs, and improving discharge planning and teaching. These systems can eliminate redundant charting and facilitate patient hand-offs from shift to shift or between care areas.

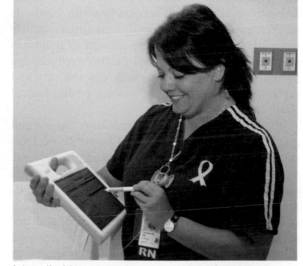

A handheld computer permits point-of-care documentation.

EXERCISE 12-4
Think about the data you gather as you care for a patient through the day. How do you communicate information and knowledge about your patient to others? Does the information system support the way you need this information organized, stored, retrieved, and presented to other health care providers? For example, if a patient's pain medication order is about to expire and you want to assess the patient's use and response to the pain medication during the past 24 hours, can the information system generate a graph for this patient comparing the time, dose, and pain score for this period? If your assessment is that the medication order needs to be renewed, how do you communicate that message to the prescriber?

Information Systems Quality and Accreditation

Quality management and measuring patient-care efficiency, effectiveness, and outcomes are necessary for accreditation and licensing of health care organizations. This attention to quality management is demonstrated through the documentation of patient-care processes and outcomes. The plan of care outlines patient care that needs to occur. Orders are entered to prescribe the needed care and documentation confirms that the care was provided. Computers can capture and aggregate data to demonstrate both the processes of care and the patient outcomes achieved.

Accreditation Canada is a not-for-profit, independent organization that provides over 1000 health care organizations with an external peer review to assess the quality of their services based on standards of excellence. Accreditation Canada fosters quality in health care services; adherence with its standards and Required Organizational Practices reduces the potential for adverse events within health care and service organizations (http://www.accreditation.ca/about-us/).

Further information on Accreditation Canada and quality improvement is found in Chapter 21. Accreditation Canada's Governance Standards include the following categories: building knowledge through information, which describes the gathering and production of knowledge and information; the assessment of information needs; the appropriateness of available information; and the dissemination of information throughout the organization (Denis, Champagne, & Pomey, 2005).

All nurses, including nurse leaders, share responsibility to ensure that cost-effective, high-quality patient care is provided. Nursing administrative databases containing both clinical and management data support decision making for these purposes. Administrative databases assist in the development of the organization's information infrastructure, which ultimately allows for links between management decisions (e.g., staffing or nurse–patient ratios), costs, and clinical outcomes.

Selection of a clinical information system and software partner may be one of the most important decisions of a chief nursing officer and the nursing leadership team (Hannah, 2005). This decision may

---

BOX 12-3   ELEMENTS OF THE IDEAL HOSPITAL INFORMATION SYSTEM

- Data are standardized and use structured terminology.
- The system is reliable—minimal scheduled or unscheduled downtime.
- Applications are integrated across the system.
- Data are collected at the point of care.
- The database is complete, accurate, and easy to query.
- The infrastructure is interconnected and supports accessibility.
- Data are gathered by instrumentation whenever possible so that only minimal data entry is necessary.
- The system has a rapid response time.
- The system is intuitive and reflective of patient care delivery models.
- The location facilitates functionality, security, and support.
- Screen displays can be configured by user preference.
- The system supports outcomes and an evidence-informed approach to care delivery.
- The system supports interprofessional care planning.

---

require that leaders become followers and take their direction from the front-line staff that will ultimately ensure the success and sustainability of the technology. Nurse leaders and direct care nurses must be members of the selection team, participate actively, and have a voice in the selection decision. Remember, nurses are knowledge workers who require data, information, and knowledge to deliver effective patient care. The information system must make sense to the people who use it and fit effectively with the processes for providing patient care. The involvement of a team of professionals in care provision requires that the information system have the capacity for interprofessional care planning. Box 12-3 identifies key elements of an ideal clinical information system that can guide the decision making necessary for selecting or developing health information software. It is imperative to make site visits at organizations already using the software being considered for selection. Discussions at site visits include both the utility and performance of the software and the customer service and responsiveness of the vendor.

Information Systems Hardware

Placing the power of computers for both entering and retrieving data at the point of patient care is a major thrust in the move toward increased adoption of clinical information systems. Many hospitals and clinics are using a number of computing devices in the clinical setting—desktop, laptop, or tablet computers, and personal digital assistants (PDAs)—as we learn about both the possibilities and limitations of different hardware solutions. Theoretically, nurses may work best with robust mobile technology. Installing computers on mobile carts, also known as *Workstations on Wheels*, or *WOWs*, may create work efficiency and time savings. However, if the cart is cumbersome to move around or if concern about infection risk is associated with moving the cart from one room to another, some organizations favour keeping one cart stationed in each patient-care room.

Wireless Communication

Wireless communication is an extension of an existing wired network environment and uses radio-based systems to transmit data signals through the air without any physical connections. Telemetry is a clinical use of wireless communication. Nurses can communicate with other health care team members, departments, and offices and with patients using pagers, cellphones, PDAs, and wireless computers. Nurses can send and receive e-mail, clinical data, and other text messages. Wireless communication allows nurses to document assessments and update care plans at point of care. Nurses can also access the Internet on many of these devices.

Wireless systems are used by emergency medical personnel to request authorization for the treatments or medications needed in emergency situations. Laboratories use wireless technology to transmit laboratory results to physicians; patients awaiting organ transplants are provided with wireless pagers so that they can be notified if a donor is found; and parents of critically ill children carry wireless pagers when they are away from a phone. Visiting nurses using a home-monitoring system employ wireless technology to enter vital signs and other patient-related information. Inpatient nurses can send messages to the admissions department when a patient is being transferred to another unit without having to wait for someone to answer the phone. Increasingly, whole hospitals are using wireless technology to deploy their information systems at the point of patient care.

New hardware for patient information systems has both advantages and disadvantages. Purchasing a few portable devices, such as PDAs and tablet computers, is less expensive than placing a stationary computer in each patient room. In addition, each caregiver on a shift can be equipped with a portable device. Portable devices allow access to information at the point of care, both for retrieval of information and entry of patient data. The disadvantages of handheld technology stem from their size and portability. They have a small display screen, which limits the amount of data that can be viewed on the screen and the size of the font. They can be put down, forgotten, dropped and broken, and are a target for theft. In addition to these disadvantages, Garrett and Klein (2008) found that one of advanced practice nurses' biggest concerns related to the security of wireless data transmissions. Portable devices must also be stored in a convenient and safe location when they are not in use and have their batteries recharged as needed. Moreover, wireless technology may not always operate with the speed required by busy health care workers in fast-paced environments.

Management of the hardware designed to host clinical information system software is important. Nurse leaders must make knowledgeable decisions about the type of hardware to use, the education needed to use it effectively, and the proper care and maintenance of the equipment. Important questions to ask include the following: What data and information do we need to gather? When and where should it be gathered? How difficult is the equipment to use? Has the hardware been tested sufficiently to ensure the purchase of a dependable product?

COMMUNICATION TECHNOLOGY

Communication technology is an extension of wireless technology that enables hands-free communication among mobile hospital workers. Hospital staff members wear a pendant-like badge around their neck and, by simply pressing a button on the badge, can be connected to the person with whom they wish to speak by stating the name or function of the person.

Voice technology may also enhance the use of computer systems in the future. Speech recognition (SR) refers to electronic devices and programs that permit data entry by human speech (also known as *computer speech recognition*). The term *voice recognition* is also used to refer to speech recognition, but that term is less accurate. SR converts spoken words to machine-readable input. SR applications in everyday life include voice dialling (e.g., "Call home"), call routing (e.g., "I would like to make a collect call"), and simple data entry (e.g., stating a credit card or account number). In health care, SR can be used to prepare structured documents, such as radiology reports, or order tests. In all of these examples, the computer gathers, processes, interprets, and executes audible signals by comparing the spoken words with a template in the system. If the patterns match, recognition occurs and a command is executed by the computer. Voice technology allows untrained personnel or those whose hands are busy to enter data in an SR environment without touching the computer. Voice technology also allows quadriplegic and other physically challenged individuals to function more efficiently when using a computer. SR systems recognize a large number of words but are still in their infancy. The speaker must use staccato-like speech, pausing between each clearly spoken word; and an SR system must be programmed for each user so that it recognizes each user's voice patterns.

Automating the health care delivery process is not an easy task. Patient-care processes are often not standardized across settings, and most software vendors cannot customize software for each organization. Some current versions of the electronic patient record have merely automated the existing schema of the chart rather than considering how computers could allow data to be viewed or used differently from manual methods. The complexity of decision making about health information systems software and hardware has given rise to the science of informatics.

INFORMATICS

Informatics is the use of technology and information systems to support improvements in patient care and health care administration. It is "a science that combines domain science, computer science, information science, and cognitive science" (Hunter, 2001, p. 180). Health care informatics, however, is truly interdisciplinary, focusing on the care of patients rather than on a specific discipline (Hannah, Ball, & Edwards, 2006). Although specific bodies of knowledge exist for each health care profession (e.g., nursing, dentistry, dietetics, pharmacy, medicine), they interface at the level of the patient. Working with integrated clinical information systems demands interdisciplinary collaboration at a high level.

The term *nursing informatics* seems to have originated with Canadian nursing informatics specialist Dr. Katherine Hannah during an International Medical Informatics Association (IMIA) conference in 1985. Hannah (1985) originally defined *nursing informatics* as "the use of information technologies in relation to those functions within the purview of nursing that are carried out by nurses when performing their duties" (p. 181). Since then, the definition has evolved. In 2001, the CNA introduced a definition of *nursing informatics*, formulated by the National Nursing Informatics Project working group. "Nursing Informatics (NI) is the application of computer science and information science to nursing. NI promotes the generation, management and processing of relevant data in order to use information and develop knowledge that supports nursing in all practice domains" (p. 1). In 2009 at their Helsinki general meeting, the Nursing Informatics Special Interest Group of the IMIA, of which Canada is a member, adopted a new definition of *nursing informatics* as "science and practice [that] integrates nursing, its information and knowledge and their management with information and communication technologies to promote the health of people, families, and communities world wide" (International Medical Informatics Association News, 2009).

Nursing informatics is now a thriving subspecialty of nursing that combines nursing knowledge and skills with computer expertise. Like any knowledge-intensive profession, nursing is greatly affected by the explosive growth of both scientific advances and technology. Nurse informatics specialists manage and communicate nursing data and information to improve decision making by consumers, patients, nurses, and other health care providers. In 2001, the Canadian Nursing Informatics Association (CNIA) received emerging group status from CNA and in 2003 was granted full associate status. Its mission is to be the voice for nursing informatics in Canada. Since its inception, CNIA has completed a national study of the informatics educational needs of Canadian nurses and launched the *Canadian Journal of Nursing Informatics*.

The informatics educational needs of nursing students and faculty across Canada have been a priority for CNIA for over a decade, beginning with a national study of informatics opportunities, preparedness, and information and communications technology (ICT) infrastructure and support (Canadian Nursing Informatics Association, 2003). For the past two decades Canadian nursing informatics leaders have been visioning a nationwide nursing informatics strategy, which culminated in an e-nursing strategy commissioned by CNA (2006a). The CNA's (2006a) e-nursing strategy identified the need for integrating ICT competencies in undergraduate, graduate, and continuing nursing education as one of its top goals. In May 2011, the Canadian Association of Schools of Nursing (CASN) announced a three-year funded initiative in partnership with Canada Health Infoway to integrate ICT in the curriculum of 91 nursing degree–granting colleges and universities across Canada. The program will engage educators, informatics experts, and students in the preparation of future health care providers for practice in modern, technology-enabled clinical environments. Although this initiative is still in progress, CASN (2011) has defined three entry-to-practice nursing informatics competencies under the domains of information and knowledge management, professional and regulatory accountability, and the use of ICTs.

Data, information, knowledge (CNA, 2001), and wisdom (Matney, Brewster, Sward, et al., 2011) are the foundation of nursing informatics and all nursing communication. The core of this model (Figure 12-1) is the transformation of data into information and then into knowledge for use at the point of care, or what has been called *practice-based evidence*. It requires access to real-time clinical data housed in comprehensive repositories such as EHR systems with robust analytical tools (Remus & Kennedy, 2012). Having actionable data available at the point of care enhances the credibility of information used to direct and coordinate patient-centric care. Data are discrete entities that describe or measure something without interpretation. Numbers are data; for example, the number *30*, without interpretation, means nothing. Information consists of defined, interpreted, organized, or structured data. The number *30* defined as millilitres, minutes, or hours has meaning. Knowledge refers to information that is combined or synthesized so that interrelationships are identified. For example, the number *30*, when included in the statement "All patients who had indwelling bladder catheters for longer than 30 days developed infections," becomes knowledge, something that is known. Wisdom, the appropriate use of knowledge to manage and solve human problems (American Nurses Association, 2008), occurs when the nurse chooses a specific, tailored means of preventing urinary tract infections in patients with long-term catheter use. The transformation of data into knowledge facilitates decision making, new discoveries, and the creation of designs. Wisdom allows for the application of designs in addressing clinical problems.

In practice, skilled clinicians synthesize data and information quickly, interpreting and comparing new data with previous information about the patient to reach knowledgeable conclusions. Much of the data's potential value is lost, however, if not stored where others can retrieve and use them in a timely manner to synthesize new information and knowledge. Box 12-4 illustrates combining and interpreting data to provide information, which, when synthesized, provides new knowledge.

Data from many patients analyzed and synthesized in scientific studies are combined to provide evidence for best practices in patient care. Either evidence-informed practice reassures us that our approach to patient care is correct or the evidence redirects our thinking. Technology has influenced both the availability and the applicability of evidence for practice.

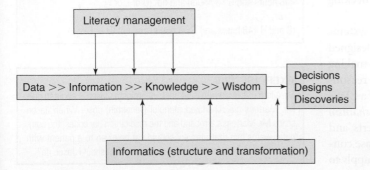

FIGURE 12-1 Nursing informatics conceptual model.

BOX 12-4   USING THE INFORMATION TRIAD

Several patients in the cardiac care unit had fallen at night in the previous 3 weeks. These events were very unusual because patients with heart conditions do not usually become disoriented at night. The newly assigned charge nurse became concerned about these events and began to look for commonalities among the patients who had fallen. She found that they were all taking the same sleeping medication. She mentioned this information at a meeting and found that several other nurses had noticed the same situation. Together, they contacted the pharmacist, who contacted the pharmaceutical representative. He found that the medication dosage had been tested on college students and that the dose was too high for older, less healthy individuals. The result was a change in medication dosage. This example shows that combining data to provide information and processing that data lead to new knowledge and wisdom that can be applied to effectively address a problem.

Knowledge Technology

Knowledge technology consists of systems that generate or process knowledge and provide **clinical decision support (CDS)**. Defined broadly, CDS is a clinical computer system, computer application, or process that helps health care providers make clinical decisions to enhance patient care. The clinical knowledge embedded in computer applications or work processes can include simple facts and relationships to best practices for managing patients with specific disease states, new health knowledge from clinical research, and other types of information. Among the most common forms of CDS are medication-dosing calculators—computer-based programs that calculate appropriate doses of medications after a clinician inputs key data (e.g., patient weight or the level of serum creatinine). These calculators are especially useful in managing the administration of medications with a narrow therapeutic index. Allergy alerts, dose range checking, drug–drug interaction, and duplicate order checking are other common applications of CDS.

Clinical (or diagnostic) **decision support systems (CDSSs)** are interactive computer programs designed to assist health care providers with decision-making tasks by mimicking the inductive or deductive reasoning of a human expert. The basic components of a CDSS include a knowledge base and an *inferencing mechanism* (usually a set of rules derived from the experts and evidence-informed practice). The knowledge base contains the knowledge that an expert nurse would apply to

data entered about a patient and information to solve a problem. The inference engine controls the application of the knowledge by providing the logic and rules for its use with data from a specific patient.

Box 12-5 illustrates the use of an expert system for determining the maximum dose of pain medication that can safely be given to a patient after an invasive procedure. The knowledge base contains eight items that are to be considered when giving the maximum dose. The inference engine controls the use of the knowledge base by applying logic that an expert nurse would use in making the decision to give the maximum dose. This decision frame states that if pain is severe (A) or a painful procedure is planned (B), and there is an order for pain medication (C) and the time since surgery is less than 48 hours (H) and the time since the last dose is greater than 3 hours (G), and there are no contraindications to the medication (D) or history of allergy (E) or contraindication to the maximum dose (F), then the "decision" would be to give the dose of pain medication. The rules are those that expert nurses would apply in making the decision to give pain medication.

BOX 12-5   EXPERT DECISION FRAME FOR "GIVE MAXIMUM DOSE OF PAIN MEDICATION"

The Knowledge Base
A. Pain score
B. Invasive procedure scheduled
C. Opiate analgesic ordered
D. Contraindications to the medication
E. History of allergic reaction to opiate analgesics
F. Contraindication to maximum dose of opiate analgesic
G. Time since last dose of opiate analgesic administered
H. Time since surgical procedure

The Inference Engine
Give the maximum dose of pain medication if (A or B) and (C and H <48 hours and G >3 hours) and not (D or E or F)
   or:
(C and H <48 hours and G >4 hours) and not (D or E or F)

EXERCISE 12-5
Mr. Martens's heart rate is 54 beats per minute. Jason is about to give Mr. Martens his scheduled atenolol (Tenormin) dose. When Jason scans Mr. Martens's armband and the medication bar codes, the computer warns him that atenolol should not be given to a patient with a heart rate less than 60 beats per minute. What should Jason do?

One of the advantages of CDSSs is that they permit the novice nurse to benefit from the decision-making expertise and judgement of experts. Nurse leaders must be aware of the usefulness of decision support systems for nursing and that the development of CDSSs applicable to nursing practices is just beginning. Clinical experts are needed to develop both the knowledge in the database and the logic used to develop the rules for its application to a particular patient in a particular circumstance. Advanced critical-thinking skills are needed to develop logic and rules. When these are in place, patient-care quality can be standardized and improved.

A critical use of information has been in the area of the medication management process. This process involves high-risk and high-volume activities (Saginur, Graham, Forster, et al., 2008). Although new applications have been developed to provide support for all aspects of the process, uptake of the various technologies has been shown to vary significantly (Saginur et al., 2008).

Saginur et al. (2008) conducted a cross-sectional survey of the uptake of medication safety technologies by 100 of Canada's largest acute-care hospitals. The survey studied the major technologies from a Canadian Agency for Drugs and Technology in Health (CADTH) systematic review. The most commonly used technologies were clinical pharmacy services (97%), followed in descending order by pharmacy-based intravenous admixture services (81%), computerized decision support modules for pharmacy order entry systems (77%), unit-dose medication distribution systems (75%), computerized medication administration records (MARs) (67%), and automated dispensing (56%). Computerized physician order entry (CPOE), computerized decision support systems (CDSS) for CPOE, and bar-coding for medication dispensing and medication administration were used in less than 10% of hospitals. Although hospitals used less of the technologies with less evidence of effectiveness, these technologies were high relative priorities for uptake.

EVIDENCE-INFORMED PRACTICE

Evidence-informed practice (EIP) is a systematic approach to clinical decision making that provides the most consistent and best possible care to patients.

EIP integrates current research findings that define best practices, clinical expertise, and patient values to optimize patient outcomes as well as their quality of life (Sackett, Straus, Richardson, et al., 2005). It also involves acknowledging and considering the myriad factors beyond evidence, such as local indigenous knowledge, cultural and religious norms, and clinical judgement. The skills necessary to provide an evidence-informed solution to a clinical dilemma include (1) defining the problem, (2) conducting an efficient search to locate the best evidence, (3) critically appraising the evidence, and (4) considering that evidence and its implications in the context of patients' circumstances and values (DiCenso, 2003, p. 21). In Chapter 22, the process of translating research into practice is explained. Despite the value of evidence for informing practice, a substantial gap exists between evidence from research findings and practice. Research use remains low among front-line nurses. The scarcity and low quality of studies included in their systematic review led Canadian researchers to conclude that insufficient evidence exists to either support or refute a specific intervention aimed at increasing research use in nursing (Thompson, Estabrooks, Scott-Findlay, et al., 2007). Technology holds promise as a way to enhance evidence-informed practice made up of the four key elements examined below.

Ask a Clinical Question

To acquire evidence for nursing practice, nurses must realize they have an information need. Precisely articulating a clinical question is the first step in the process. For example, nurses might ask, "What is the most reliable method for measuring temperature in an infant younger than 60 days?"

Acquire and Appraise the Evidence

Clinicians can access electronic evidence summaries via Web-based resources such as Clinical Evidence (http://www.clinicalevidence.bmj.com), systematic reviews of evidence from the literature about health care practices through use of the Cochrane Library (http://www.thecochranelibrary.com) or relevant articles and studies from other relevant electronic databases (CINAHL, EMBASE, MedLine, OVID, PubMed, and PsycINFO). Clinical librarians can be of great assistance in fine-tuning a clinical question and literature search. Technology can expedite evidence acquisition. In one study, researchers found that nurses using mobile information technology in a variety of settings (acute to long-term care) reported that having access to electronically accessible resources supported their information or learning needs (Doran, Haynes, Kushniruk, et al., 2009). Mobile technology allows access to online appraisal tools (http://www.cebm.net/?o=1040) for assessing the literature that can make this time-consuming process more efficient.

Apply the Evidence

When clinicians identify information that answers a clinical question, a practice change may be required. Practice changes require use of the appropriate internal channels to revise policies, procedures, and standards of care and communicate to the end user (aspects of leading change are discussed in Chapter 18). Clinical information systems with appropriate CDS can support the application of evidence-informed practice to direct patient care. For example, if a patient is at risk for the development of a pressure ulcer, nurses complete and document a standardized risk assessment and the software suggests the most appropriate interventions to maintain skin integrity. Communities of practice have emerged as an important knowledge transfer strategy to reduce gaps between research and practice. For example, the interactive and information exchange capacities of Web 2.0 can help practitioners shift from using the Internet for the sole purpose of accessing knowledge to becoming involved in a community of practice that enhances translating the knowledge into practice (David, Poissant, & Rochette, 2012).

Assess the Outcomes

Measuring process and outcome changes is a key step in the evidence-informed practice model. Information systems play a key role in this process. Across health care settings, technology allows for ongoing measurement of daily practice against evidence-informed guidelines, standards, or protocols. Real-time reports can detect variation from recommended practice by a service, a department, or an individual practitioner. A regular evaluation must take place of these findings to determine the reasons for and approaches to addressing the variation.

Like other health care providers, nurses cannot read or retain all the information needed to act effectively for patients. Information technology can provide real-time access to clinical information and integrate evidence-informed clinical guidelines in standardized plans for patient care. Nurses across many settings who used PDAs showed a significant ($p < 0.05$) improvement in research awareness and values that was accompanied by a significant reduction in organizational and technological barriers to research use (Doran et al., 2009). In their qualitative study, David et al. (2012) found that health care providers involved in stroke care perceived technology, such as Web 2.0, as a support to evidence-informed practice and knowledge transfer but described lack of time as influencing their intention to use it.

Easily accessed information about best care practices makes positive patient outcomes more likely than relying on either the nursing interventions learned in basic educational programs or traditional practice experience. Patients' clinical data can be linked to reference literature and medication information, as well as to organizational policies, procedures, patient education materials, and the like.

PATIENT SAFETY

The patient-care environment is complex and associated with adverse events (Baker, Norton, Flintoft, et al., 2004). Approximately 8% of patients admitted to Canadian acute care hospitals were found to experience one or more adverse events. Of these patients, 36.9% were judged to have highly preventable adverse events (Baker et al., 2004). As the largest health care provider group, nurses have a significant understanding of the risks to patient safety and are in the best position to implement preventive measures (Nicklin & McVeety, 2002). In addition to physical challenges, resource challenges, and interruptions characteristic of nursing work, nurses are challenged by inconsistencies and breakdowns in care communication. Communication and information difficulties are among the most common nursing workplace challenges and are frustrating and potentially dangerous for patients. Mistakes in the nurse–patient process, a failure to know the patient, and a lack of patient involvement in decision making threaten patient safety (Bournes & Flint, 2003; MacDonald, 2008; O'Hagan et al., 2009). For example, O'Hagan et al. (2009) found twice as many self-reported medical errors among Canadian adults who perceived lack of involvement in decision making about their care compared with those who perceived involvement. Followers have the opportunity to upwardly influence a culture of safety by actively advocating for listening to and knowing patients, and involving patients in decisions about their own care.

Information technology is an essential tool for advancing patient safety (Canada Health Infoway, 2005). Nurses and other health care providers rely increasingly on information technology to improve patient safety by reducing medical errors, enhancing clinical decision making and management, and promoting patient-centric care. In a national Canadian study of staff nurses and senior nurse managers across health care delivery sectors, researchers studied the factors that affected nurses' adoption of technologies and their perceptions of confidence and efficiency in using technologies (Wang, Nagle, Li, et al., 2004). Technologies were grouped into the following categories: communication tools, information system, diagnostic devices, and therapeutic devices. Researchers found that nurses in direct care used communication tools and information systems less than non-direct care nurses, and older nurses were less confident in the use of these tools and systems. Confidence in using technology was associated with the adequacy of training, regardless of age, education level, or area of practice. Clinical information systems and automated medication-dispensing systems were perceived as efficient or useful by about 60% of practical nurses and registered nurses and less than half of psychiatric nurses (Wang et al., 2004).

The introduction of technology has the potential to increase nurses' productivity. MacDonald (2008) describes technology as a way to support knowing the patient, training in state-of-the art technology can save time that nurses consistently report as a barrier to knowing the patient. Home health care nurses who perceived the usefulness of wireless PDAs incorporated for 1 month in their daily activities were more likely to adopt the technology (Zhang, Cocosila, & Archer, 2010).

Documentation to meet organizational, accreditation, regulatory, professional practice standards and requirements, as well as to provide information needed by other health care providers, imposes a heavy demand on nurses' time. Documentation requirements lessen nursing time for direct contact with patients and families. Reduced nursing availability affects patient safety and care quality. A diary study of home-care nursing visits with Ontario Community Care Access Centres (CCACs) showed that considering all nursing activities and duties, approximately 60% of nursing time with the traditional paper-based system was spent on communications, documentation, and related duties (Zhang et al., 2010).

IMPACT OF CLINICAL INFORMATION SYSTEMS

Good decision making requires good information. Clinical information systems that provide access to patient information and provide clinical decision support can reduce errors and inefficiencies (Nagle & Catford, 2008).

Patient information in an electronic clinical information system is organized and legible. Nurses see all of the medications prescribed for a patient in one location; doses are written clearly, and medication names are spelled correctly. The patient problem list shows acute and chronic health conditions and complete allergy information. Abnormal findings are highlighted and can be graphed and compared with interventions. Alerts signal nurses that critical information has been entered in the electronic record. For example, critical test results signal the need for provider notification and intervention. An alert that a patient is at risk for falling signals the need for additional monitoring and interventions to ensure safety.

When standards for care are not being followed, clinical information systems can generate alerts, reminders, or suggestions. Rules remind health care providers to perform required care. When documentation is not recorded for medication administration, IV tubing change, or wound care, for example, the system generates a reminder based on rules that have been agreed to by providers. Evidence-informed practices are integrated in the process of care as providers are guided to select the most appropriate course of action.

Errors are avoided by eliminating the problem of illegible handwriting. Computerized order entry also eliminates the nursing time required for clarification of illegible and incomplete orders. Transcription is no longer required, orders are sent directly to the performing department, and patient-care needs are communicated more clearly and quickly to all clinicians. Computerized decision-making support has been shown to significantly reduce the rate of initiation of inappropriate prescriptions involving drug–disease contraindications, drug–age contraindications, and excessive duration of therapy and therapeutic duplication prescriptions (Tamblyn, Huang, Perreault, et al., 2003).

Impact on Communication

Integrated information systems allow all members of the interdisciplinary patient-care team to see pertinent patient information and plan care based on what is currently happening and what should occur in the future. Everyone knows who is responsible for the patient and who needs to communicate about the patient's care. Clinical information systems provide multiple users with simultaneous, real-time access to patient records. Patient-care hand-offs are safer when information is available or not lost in the process. Patient-care processes are facilitated and treatment delays are decreased. The patient's care experience is also improved by decreasing redundant data collection by multiple members of the care team.

Impact on Patient-Care Documentation

Nurses spend much time documenting patient-care activities. Clinical documentation in an electronic information system improves access to patient information and increases documentation efficiency and organization (Canada Health Infoway, 2005). This should allow nurses to spend more time in direct patient care, but no clear link has been made between electronic nursing documentation systems and the resulting time spent in direct patient-care activities (Detwiller, 2006). In a study in which electronic documentation was introduced in a small rural hospital, 75% of respondents agreed that nurses have less time to give hands-on care with the use of the electronic system (Detwiller, 2006). Detwiller (2006) noted that many variables can affect time, including the design of the system, policies and procedures, and the experience of the staff. In a critical care unit setting, automatic downloads of patient vital signs, ventilator settings, and IV intakes remove the need to record these items by hand and provide time savings for nurses. An integrated clinical information system eliminates the need to collect certain patient information (such as chronic conditions, allergies, or previous medical history) more than once because it is readily accessible in the system. As a result,

nursing time is not spent searching for this information or asking the patient the same questions multiple times.

Impact on Medication Administration Processes

A Canadian study reported that 7.5% of patients who were admitted to hospital during 2000 experienced one or more adverse events, with medications and injectable solutions found to be the second most common causes of adverse events (Baker et al., 2004). Technologies that are used to automate medication dispensing and administration may decrease this source of error, improve quality of care, and reduce associated costs. These technologies include automated medication-dispensing devices, bar-coding verification for medication dispensing and administration, and electronic medication administration records (Perras, Jacobs, Boucher, et al., 2009).

Automated medication administration systems can ensure that the right patient gets the right medication, in the correct dose, by the appropriate route, and at the specified time. However, it is imperative that this new information technology not impede nurses' care of patients. Wulff, Cummings, Marck, et al. (2011) conducted a mixed methods systematic review of research evidence evaluating relationships between medication administration technologies (MATs) use and incidence of medication administration incidents (MAIs) and preventable adverse drug events (ADEs). They concluded from their review of 12 studies, including one from Canada, that findings were generally positive about MATs and MAIs on patient safety but noted that the level of evidence overall was equivocal. A concern raised in the review was the development of problematic workarounds when introducing MATs that could compromise patient safety. During the introduction of an automatic medication-dispensing system in a larger Canadian tertiary care centre, workarounds emerged to fill the gap between prescribed and actual work practices, activities, and processes (Balka, Kahnamoui, & Nutland, 2007). Workarounds develop when new technologies hinder workflow (Perras et al., 2009). Further, the technologies carry the potential for introducing different types of medication errors, such as completing tasks with minimal reflection and less checking due to overreliance on a machine.

Closed-loop electronic prescribing, dispensing, and bar-code patient identification systems reduce prescribing errors and adverse drug events and increase confirmation of patient identity before administration. A clinical and economic impact study of technologies for medication dispensing and administration in Canadian hospitals found inconsistent results in the time spent on medication-related tasks by pharmacists and nurses (Perras et al., 2009).

SUCCESSFULLY IMPLEMENTING HEALTH INFORMATION TECHNOLOGY

The successful implementation of a clinical information system is related to a combination of individual, group, and organizational factors (Nagle & Catford, 2008). If any one of the people, processes, or technology is not adequately addressed, a clinical information system implementation has a high risk of failure. Leadership, engagement, communication, process redesign, and support must be considered in the acquisition and implementation of information systems.

Relying too heavily on health information technology can negatively affect patient safety and care quality (Canadian Nurses Association and University of Toronto, Faculty of Nursing, 2004). It adds to the complexity of care, and overreliance may contribute to nurses attending more to the technology and less to the patient's signs and symptoms, which undervalues the patient's voice. Although improved access and better organized information can eliminate nurses' locating information for other nurses and physicians, information technology

will never eliminate the need for personal communication and teamwork (Bournes & Flint, 2003).

Successful development and implementation of nursing information technology depends on nurses working in partnership with organizational leadership, information systems vendors, and systems analysts to create tools that truly benefit nurses. Patient safety and care may be affected when nurses are not involved in decisions related to the development and implementation of new technology or fail to receive adequate pre-implementation training (CNA and University of Toronto, Faculty of Nursing, 2004). The technologically savvy Millennial nurse has the potential to contribute know-how and experiential insights to decisions about technology that earlier generations of nurses may lack. Nurses need to have the systems and tools to provide patient care effectively, efficiently, and safely. Direct care nurses must work with informatics nurses and information system developers and programmers in systems development, implementation, and ongoing improvement. Nurses should be key partners in every phase of the clinical information life cycle (Benham-Hutchins, 2009). By combining computer and information science with nursing science, the goals of supporting nursing practice and the delivery of high-quality nursing care can be achieved (Delaney, 2007). The Literature Perspective identifies areas of success and lack of success in Canada's implementation of electronic health information technology (HIT).

📖 LITERATURE PERSPECTIVE

Resource: Rozenblum, R., Jang, Y., Zimlichman, E., et al., (2011). A qualitative study of Canada's experience with the implementation of electronic health information technology. *Canadian Medical Association Journal, 183*(5), E281–E288. http://dx.doi.org/10.1503/cmaj.100856

Although many Canadian provinces have made some progress toward the implementation of information technologies and Canada Health Infoway has invested almost $1.6 billion in e-health initiatives over the past decade, Canada has lagged behind other Western countries in its uptake of EHRs. To address this situation, Canadian researchers conducted a case study to assess areas of achievement/success and lack of success/effectiveness in adoption of EHRs. The study involved a review of Canada Health Infoway documents and the completion of interviews with national and provincial stakeholder groups. Successful aspects of the e-strategy included its comprehensive national approach to the standards for health information technology, which allowed for interoperability

across jurisdictions and a framework for collaboration and idea sharing; successful lobbying for health information technology, and the acquisition of political and financial support; and successful health information technology applications, namely digital imaging technology and provincial patient registries. Less successful aspects included the absence of an e-health policy that would foster effective adoption strategies by clinicians; a lack of meaningful engagement of clinicians; a lack of alignment of the e-health plan with needs of clinicians; a lack of flexibility in incorporating change; and a focus on national rather than regional interoperability.

Implications for Practice

One recommendation to improve the adoption of EHRs was more effective engagement of clinicians. As a leader, how would you address clinician engagement in your organization? What might you do to facilitate some "quick wins" for clinicians? What strategies would help ensure an alignment of EHR adoption with the needs of clinicians?

Imagine that a patient you are caring for complains of light-headedness and nausea. When documenting vital signs, you note that the blood pressure measurement is lower than it was the day before. Graphing the values across several days illustrates a steady decline in the readings. Reviewing the medication list, you note that he is receiving hydralazine (Apresoline). Processing the data that you have collected, you implement "fall precautions," send a communication order to monitor his blood pressure and other symptoms frequently, and notify the physician if the situation has not changed.

> **EXERCISE 12-6**
> Think about the data that you gather and document every day: vital signs, intake and output, laboratory and test results, and the patient's responses to care. What data did you automatically combine or reorganize to help you make a decision regarding patient care? How did you use this information to improve your patient's outcome? How and with whom did you communicate the data and information? How did technology combine or organize data?

FUTURE TRENDS AND PROFESSIONAL ISSUES

Biomedical Technology

In Canada's decentralized health care system, where each of the ten provinces and three territories is responsible for the delivery of health care, variability exists in the adoption, diffusion, and reimbursement of health care technologies within and across jurisdictions (A. Morrison, personal communication, August 24, 2011). Demographic composition often drives the adoption of health care technologies, which means that more highly populated regions are better resourced to support them.

CADTH is a national, not-for-profit, organization that provides Canada's federal, provincial, and territorial health care decision makers with evidence, analysis, advice, and recommendations about the effectiveness and efficiency of new and emerging health technologies. Since 1997, CADTH's Early Awareness Service has identified upcoming health technologies likely to have a significant impact on the delivery of health care in Canada (in alignment with national health priorities). The implementation of new health technologies consumes approximately a quarter of Canada's

total health care budget (Murtagh & Foerster, 2009). CADTH provides timely information on the efficiency and effectiveness of health technologies so that health care leaders can make informed decisions about technology investments. In its first decade, the program exclusively identified new and emerging health technologies (e.g., medications, medical devices, diagnostics equipment, and medical and surgical procedures), including those that are two to three years from launch. In 2007, CADTH services expanded to include identifying and monitoring significant jurisdictional health policy issues. The goals are for CADTH to be able to align innovative health technologies with the most pressing jurisdictional health care priorities and to prepare policymakers for new developments in health care (A. Morrison, personal communication, August 24, 2011).

The Canadian Network for Environmental Scanning in Health (CNESH) was established in 2011. It is the first collaboration of academics, researchers, clinical experts, and health care decision makers from across Canada actively involved in identifying and sharing information on innovative health technologies (A. Morrison, personal communication, August 24, 2011). CADTH is associated with CNESH.

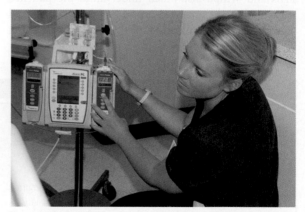

Twenty-first-century IV pumps offer safety features, accuracy, advanced pressure monitoring, ease of use, and versatility.

Information Technology

In 2000, health information and communications technologies were identified by a First Ministers' agreement as health care priorities. In response, the federal government committed to immediately invest in Canada Health Infoway, an independent not-for-profit corporation. Over the subsequent four years, more than $1 billion were allocated to Canada Health Infoway for the development and adoption of modern systems of information technology and standards to govern and ensure interoperability of the health infostructure (Canada Health Infoway, 2010).

In order to interoperate, Canada's EHR systems must use pan-Canadian standards to exchange health data. Standards-based EHRs offer benefits to patients, health care providers, and service delivery organizations including reduced wait times and fewer duplicate tests; newer tools to manage chronic conditions; better overall care; safer medication prescribing; and better infectious disease outbreak control (Canada Health Infoway, n.d.). Infoways' Standards Collaborative supports and sustains pan-Canadian health information standards and fosters collaboration to accelerate their implementation. Infoway has invested in over 20 standards-development projects (which are completed or in progress) and has dedicated funding to continue this support. It has also developed a number of pan-Canadian standards that are critical to achieving interoperability across EHRs: Client Registry Standard, Provider Registry Standard, Diagnostic Imaging Standard, Laboratory Messaging Standards, Interoperable EHR Standard, Immunization Standard, and Drug Standard.

Electronic Patient Care Records. Multiple terms have been used to define electronic patient care records, with overlapping definitions. Both the electronic health record (EHR) and the electronic medical record (EMR) have gained widespread use, with some health informatics users assigning the term *EHR* to a global concept and *EMR* to a discrete localized record. An EHR is "a complete health record under the custodianship of a health care provider(s) that holds all relevant health information about a person over their lifetime" (Hodge & Giokas, 2011). An EMR is "a partial health record under the custodianship of a health care provider(s) that holds a portion of the relevant health information about a person over their lifetime" (Hodge & Giokas, 2011). The EHR is a longitudinal electronic record of patient health information generated across encounters in any care delivery setting. EHR systems coordinate the storage and retrieval of individual records with the aid of computers. The EHR is most often accessed on a computer, often over a network, and may include EMRs from many locations and/or sources. Among the many forms of data often included in EHRs are patient demographics, health history, progress and procedure notes, health problems, medication and allergy lists (including immunization status), laboratory test results, radiology images and reports, and advanced directives.

The personal health record (PHR), or an online health record that is initiated and maintained by an individual patient, is beginning to gain attention in Canada (Office of the Privacy Commissioner of Canada, 2009). Patient portals are another model in which a patient's information is maintained under the control of a provincial or territorial health system, physician, hospital, or insurance company. The implementation of computer-based health information systems leads to computer networks that store health records across local, provincial, territorial, national, and international boundaries. Patients are mobile and consult many practitioners, with the potential for fragmentation of their records. Therefore, patient participation in maintaining their health information will help coordinate care; improve quality-of-care decisions; and reduce risk, waste, and duplication of effort. A pan-Canadian survey of privacy officers and managers of Health Records and Health Information Services employed in general and acute care hospitals reported financial resources, patient computer literacy, and clinician buy-in as the most important barriers to providing patients access to their EHR (Urowitz, Wiljer, Apatu, et al., 2008).

Data Privacy and Security. Privacy is a fundamental right of individuals and a growing area of concern in health care with advances in information technology and the increased adoption of EHRs across the country. Privacy is a core value of nursing and is at the heart of CNA's *Code of Ethics for Registered Nurses* (2008), which states "informational privacy is the right of individuals to determine how, when, with whom and for what purposes any of their personal information will be shared" (p. 27). Quality health care depends on individuals trusting that their personal health information will be kept private and confidential as they interact with the health system. In a large telephone survey of Canadians (n = 2469), 87% reported that they felt it was difficult for health care providers to provide quality care without timely and easy access to patient information, yet only 39% believed that their health information was safe and secure (EKOS Research Associates, 2007).

Canada's *Privacy Act* has been in force since 1983, and in 2000 the *Personal Information Protection and Electronic Documents Act* (PIPEDA) (2000) came into effect. PIPEDA governs the collection, use, and disclosure of personal information, including personal health information. PIPEDA requirements include the following: individual informed consent; the protection of personal information with appropriate security safeguards; individual rights to hold consent, to access their personal information and have it corrected; and mechanisms for dealing with privacy breaches and complaints. Chapter 5 contains additional details on important legislation governing privacy, security, and confidentiality.

Data protection, systems' security, and patient privacy are concerns with EHRs. However, patients' rights to privacy of their data must be maintained whether recorded in a manual or automated system. With computerized data, any person with the proper permission may access the information anywhere in the world, and multiple people can do so simultaneously. Data can also be inadvertently sent to the wrong individual or site. Information security and privacy are and will continue to be important concerns as the number of health care organizations that have electronic health information systems grows.

A firewall protects the information in the central data repository from access by unauthorized users. It is a network security measure that keeps electronic intruders from accessing an organization's data on its private network while allowing members of the organization to reach the Internet. Organizational policies on the use, security, and accuracy of data must be developed and monitored for adherence.

Communication Technology

Telecommunications. Telecommunications and systems technology facilitate clinical oversight of health care via telephone or cable lines, remote monitoring, information links, and the Internet. Telehealth is the use of telecommunications and information technologies for the provision of health care to individuals at a distance and the transmission of information to provide that care. Telehealth employs two-way interactive videoconferencing and high-speed telephone lines, fibre optic cable, and satellite transmissions. Patients

sitting in front of the teleconferencing camera can be diagnosed, treated, monitored, and educated by nurses and physicians. ECGs and radiographs can be viewed and transmitted. Sophisticated electronic stethoscopes and dermascopes allow nurses and physicians to hear heart, lung, and bowel sounds and to look closely at wounds, eyes, ears, and skin. Ready access to expert advice and patient information is available no matter where the patient or information is located. Patients in rural areas and prisons especially benefit from this technology. In 2010, Canada had 5710 telehealth systems in place in at least 1175 communities, servicing the 21% of the Canadian population who live in rural or remote areas (Praxia Information Intelligence and Gartner Incorporated, 2011). Not only did patients experience significant savings in terms of travel time and costs as a result of these services, but more than 80% reported satisfaction, better capability to manage their care, and measurable improvements in clinical outcomes and hospitalizations. A telepsychiatry project in southern Ontario that delivered mental health crisis interventions to patients at multiple locations in the province yielded positive outcomes, but leadership, team dynamics, and the involvement of front-line staff were critical to the success of the project (Bhandari, Tiessen, & Snowdon, 2011).

Telecommunications also supports distance learning with enhanced opportunities to engage students in online classrooms. With online or "virtual" classrooms, students from anywhere in the world with computer access can log into a university's online learning system via the Internet. The Internet, which can provide health education and other health information, fosters communication, collaboration, resource sharing, and information access. It is a multicultural library that is open 24 hours a day, every day to ordinary computer users.

In addition to formal distance education possibilities, the Internet provides access to peer-reviewed e-journals reporting the latest research. Many hospital libraries provide staff with access to databases such as EBSCO-host, ProQuest, CINAHL, EMBASE, MedLine, OVID, PubMed, and PsycINFO in addition to hospital intranets and Web sites. Using the Internet to seek answers to specific questions, promote high-level thinking, and develop problem-solving skills is the objective of WebQuest (Dodge, 1995). A WebQuest is "an inquiry-oriented lesson format in which most or all the information that learners work with comes from the web" (WebQuest.org, n.d.). Students develop inquiry-based skills and information technology literacy through WebQuests (Lahaie, 2007). Table 12-2 lists websites of interest to nurses.

TABLE 12-2	HEALTH-RELATED WEBSITES
DESCRIPTION	**URL**
Accreditation Canada	http://www.accreditation.ca
Canada Health Infoway	http://www.infoway-inforoute.ca
Canadian Agency for Drugs and Technology in Health	http://www.cadth.ca
Canadian Health Care	http://www.canadian-healthcare.org
Canadian Health Coalition	http://healthcoalition.ca
Canadian Healthcare Network	http://www.canadianhealthcare network.ca
Canadian Best Practices Portal	http://cbpp-pcpe.phac-aspc.gc.ca
Canadian Institute of Health Information	http://www.cihi.ca
Canadian Nurses Association	https://www.cna-aiic.ca
Canadian Nursing Informatics Association	http://www.cnia.ca
Canadian Public Health Association	http://www.cpha.ca
CTF: Canadian Telehealth Forum	http://coachorg.com
First Nations and Inuit Health: eHealth	http://www.hc-sc.gc.ca/fniah-spnia/services/ehealth-esante/index-eng.php
McMaster's Best Evidence for Nursing Care	http://plus.mcmaster.ca/NP/Default.aspx
Nursing and Environmental Health	https://www.cna-aiic.ca/en/download-buy/nursing-and-environmental health
Women's Health Matters	http://www.womenshealthmatters.ca

Although reliable and high-quality information can be found via the Internet, Web users need to evaluate the quality of websites related to health and the credentials of the author(s) of the information or website Table 12-3 lists criteria for evaluating Internet sources. In addition to recognizing these criteria when evaluating their own Web searches, nurses can share this information with patients to improve patient use of health information websites.

E-mail use is also pervasive in health care. E-mails of particular interest may be obtained by subscribing to a listserv or blog. A *listserv* is a group of people who have similar interests. Subscribers to a listserv become part of the "conversation." All messages sent to the listserv are forwarded to all subscribers, who can then read and respond to them. A blog (a contraction of the term *weblog*) is a type of Web site, usually maintained by an individual, with regular entries of commentary, descriptions of events, images, and videos. Many blogs provide commentary or news on a particular subject, including health care topics. A typical blog combines text, images, and links to other blogs and other media related to its topic. The ability for readers to leave comments in an interactive format is an important part of many blogs.

E-mail is becoming a preferred communication method between some health care providers and patients. This asynchronous mode of communication allows timely responses to non-emergent health care issues at the convenience of both the patient and provider. It prevents "telephone tag" and avoids the interruptions often encountered when paging health care providers. E-mail can be a very effective means of delivering health care services to people and may be especially effective with patients and families managing chronic illness. The value of technology-based health programs has been documented. In one study, Chinese Canadian caregivers for family members with Alzheimer's disease were found to benefit from receiving professional support via asynchronous e-mails and a dedicated information website. Those who used the support experienced a significant reduction in caregiver burden compared with those who did not (Chi, Marziali, Colantonio, et al., 2009). E-mail provides documentation on patient–provider communication and gives the patient instructions in writing. E-mails can have embedded links to information from a variety of websites the provider recognizes as legitimate sources of sound information. Box 12-6 presents guidelines for the use of e-mail between patients and providers; Chapter 29 also contains valuable suggestions for email communications.

Social media (or Web 2.0) is a group of Internet-based applications and technologies that allow "real-time" online interactions and collaborations among users in the creation and sharing of information, ideas, and opinions (CNA, 2012). Social media sites such as Facebook, Twitter, Blog.com, LinkedIn, and YouTube have increasingly entered the health care arena and

TABLE 12-3   CHECKLIST FOR EVALUATING INTERNET SOURCES

1. **Authority**—Source of Information	Is there a clearly identifiable author?
	What are the author's credentials and organizational affiliations?
	Is e-mail address or contact information provided?
	What does the domain tell you about the source? (e.g., .ca—Canadian-based website; .org—organization or special interest group)
2. **Accuracy**—Reliability of the Information	Is the information correct? Reliable? Credible?
	Can information be verified by other sources (e.g., footnotes, bibliographies)
	Has the information been refereed?
	Does the information include citations?
	Has the information been edited?
	Are data presented in graphs and charts clearly labelled?
	Is the top-level domain .edu, .com, .gov, .org, .net, or .info?
3. **Currency**—Timeline of the Information	When was the website created?
	When was the last update, revision, or edit?
	Is the website maintained on a regular basis?
	How current are the links, and do they work?
	Is the information considered current for your topic/research?
4. **Purpose**—Possible bias present in the information	What is the purpose of the website Is it clearly stated? (e.g., to teach, market, or entertain)
	Is the website a comprehensive or selective resource?
	Does the information appear objective and impartial or does it display a certain bias or perspective?
	Do advertisements appear at the website and are they separated from the content?
	What other websites are linked to this one?
5. **Relevance**—Depth, importance, and coverage of information	Does the information relate to your topic or answer your question?
	Who is the intended audience? What is the intended age or academic level?
	Is the website complete or still under construction?
	Does the website claim to be comprehensive, and does it meet these claims?
	How does the website compare with other related websites? With other related print sources?
	Is the information unique, or is it available in other forms?

Queen's University. (2011, March 30). Evaluating Web sources. Retrieved from http://library.queensu.ca/inforef/tutorials/qcat/evalint.htm; University of Alberta. (2011, August 5). Critical evaluation of Internet resources. Retrieved from http://guides.library.ualberta.ca/eval_internet; University of British Columbia. (2011, April 6). Evaluating Internet sources. Retrieved from http://help.library.ubc.ca/researching/evaluating-internet-sources/.

BOX 12-6   PATIENT–PROVIDER E-MAIL COMMUNICATION GUIDELINES

Patient Responsibilities and Expectations
- Include the patient's name in the body of the e-mail.
- Include the category or type of message in the subject line.
- Review the e-mail to make sure it is clear and that all relevant information is provided before sending to the provider.
- Follow up with the provider as needed to determine whether the intended recipient received the e-mail and when the recipient will respond.
- Take precautions to preserve the confidentiality of the e-mail.
- Inform the provider of e-mail address changes.
- Inform the provider of the types of information the patient does not want to be sent by e-mail.

Provider Responsibilities and Expectations
- Use an encrypted security system.
- Obtain informed consent from the patient before using e-mail communication.
- Establish acceptable types of e-mail messages, and provide clear guidelines regarding emergency subject matter.
- Develop a system for integrating e-mail contact into the patient's record.
- Establish an expected response time for messages.

have been used successfully to share information and keep Canadians up to date on the latest developments related to their chronic illnesses. For example, a number of organizations have Facebook pages, including the Canadian Patient Safety Institute (http://www.facebook.com/PatientSafety) and the Canadian Arthritis Patient Alliance (https://www.facebook.com/CAPA.Aca). At the same time, social media provide patients with a way to voice concerns while contributing their unique solutions (Read & Giustini, 2011).

Most social media sites were not developed as professional practice tools but as venues for open and immediate sharing of personal information. Consequently, their use within the context of health care raises concerns about privacy and confidentiality. Information posted on social media becomes part of the public domain and is completely removed from the user's control. When the personal crosses into the professional and information about patient or workplace situations are inadvertently shared through social media, issues of privacy and confidentiality arise (CNA, 2012). A breach in privacy and confidentiality can result in professional disciplinary or legal action and can even result in loss of employment.

Creating social media policies is a major part of addressing this blurring of personal and professional boundaries. Bacigalupe (2011) suggests that social media policies be written before specific Internet-based applications are implemented and should address issues of privacy, control of information, accountability, accuracy, and transparency. Writing effective policies in health care requires knowledge about social media and an awareness of how risks associated with information leakage can be minimized. As with the use of any communication device, nurses should follow social media etiquette by adhering to certain guidelines (Schaffner, 2010) including the following:

- Frame your posts and responses in a respectful and professional manner as the information is easily accessible by others, who can go on to share it in various ways.
- Consider carefully if social media sites are the best way to share the information. Such communication cannot replace in-person professional interactions.
- Restrict the personal use of social media sites at work as you would personal phone calls.
- Maintain the privacy of patients, their families, and other staff.

- Adjust privacy settings to limit access by others to your communications and information—but remembering that doing so in no way guarantees complete privacy.
- Keep in mind that sometimes messages meant for one person or a specific group may be better sent by e-mail or in person.

EXERCISE 12-7

You go on Facebook at the end of the day and discover a new nurse graduate friend of yours sharing her unbelievable day at work—one where "everything that could go wrong went wrong." She shares details that you think go over the line and leave you concerned about privacy and confidentiality. What do you do?

Informatics

Many opportunities exist to improve the safety, efficiency, and effectiveness of nursing care. The goal of direct care nurses, informatics nurses, and nurse leaders is to use information technology to ensure that critical information is available to caregivers at the point of care to make health care safer and more effective while improving efficiency. Achieving this goal requires interconnected and integrated health care technology across hospitals, health care systems, and geographical regions. Standards for data systems that operate efficiently with one another (called "interoperability") and attention to data security and patient privacy are necessary.

Despite the fundamental value and impact of informatics in advancing evidence-informed, patient centred health care, nurse leaders have not adopted nursing informatics competencies as widely as expected (Remus & Kennedy, 2012). Nurse executives need to supplement traditional roles with nursing informatics competencies if they are to provide leadership that transforms health care. Nurses are working as leaders in several national initiatives to lay the groundwork and guide progress toward the goal of a nationwide health information network. Every nurse can embrace technology to improve nursing practice. Some strategies to accomplish this objective include (1) having clinicians partner with their information technology staff so that they drive EHR initiatives; (2) involving nurses in decisions about the process, design, and workflow in health IT integration initiatives; (3) investing in training nurses in EHR systems; and (4) levering opportunities to use information technology to enable quality improvement (Nagle & Catford, 2008).

Knowledge Technology. Technology has the potential to shorten the many years that currently exist between the development of new knowledge for patient care and the application of that knowledge in real-time practice with patients. It is more important than ever to inform nurses of the best knowledge regarding clinical phenomena that are the focus of nursing care: medication management, activity intolerance, immobility, risk for falls and actual falls, risk for skin impairment and pressure ulcer, anxiety, dementia, sleep, prevention of infection, nutrition, incontinence, dehydration, smoking cessation, pain management, patient and family education, and self-care.

Leaders need to support the transfer of useful knowledge to those making decisions. **Knowledge brokering** has grown in importance as a means of facilitating the exchange of knowledge between those who know and those who need to know (Goddard et al., 2004). Ultimately, knowledge brokering is about supporting evidence-informed decision making in the organization, management, and delivery of health care services and has an important role in implementing health technology assessment (Scott Findlay, 2003). **Knowledge brokers** are go-betweens who facilitate communication and exchange between knowledge producers and users. Knowledge brokers have the following skills:

- The ability to bring people together and facilitate their interaction
- The ability to find research-based and other evidence to shape decisions
- The ability to assess evidence, interpret it, and adapt it to circumstances
- A knowledge of marketing, communication, and Canadian health care
- The ability to identify emerging management and policy issues which research could help to resolve (Canadian Health Services Research Foundation, 2003, p. i)

Professional, Ethical Nursing Practice and New Technologies

Technology has and will continue to transform the health care environment and the practice of nursing. Nurses are professionally obligated to maintain competency with a vast array of technological devices and systems. Baseline informatics competencies are required for all nurses to function in the twenty-first century.

Because of the increasing ability to preserve human life with biomedical technology, questions about living and dying have become conceptually and ethically complex. Conceptually, it becomes more difficult to define extraordinary treatment and human life because technology has changed our concepts of living and dying. A source of ethical dilemmas is the use of invasive technological treatment to treat patients with extraordinary means and to prolong life for patients with limited or no decision-making capabilities. Nurses are concerned with individual patient welfare and the effects of technological intervention on the immediate and long-term quality of life for patients and their families. Patient advocacy remains an important function of the professional nurse.

Safeguarding patients' welfare, privacy, and confidentiality is another obligation of nurses. Security measures are available with computerized information systems, but it is the integrity and ethical principles of system end users that provide the final safeguard for patient privacy. System users must never share the passwords that allow them access to information in computerized clinical information systems. Each password uniquely identifies a user to the system by name and title, gives approval to carry out certain functions, and provides access to data appropriate to the user. When a nurse signs on to a computer, all data and information that are entered or reviewed can be traced to that password. Every nurse is accountable for all actions taken using his or her password. All nurses must be aware of their responsibilities for the confidentiality and security of the data they gather and for the security of their passwords.

Nurse leaders must promote ethical practice in the use of technology. One way is to make use of an ethics committee in their institutions and to assign knowledgeable nurses to serve on these committees. Nurse managers must ensure that policies and procedures for collecting and entering data and the use of security measures (e.g., passwords) are established to maintain the confidentiality of patient data and information. Nurse managers must also be knowledgeable patient advocates in the use of technology for patient care by referring ethical questions to the organization's ethics committee.

EXERCISE 12-8

Think about the use of the Internet in health care. How do you use it to look up health care information? How would you advise a patient to select appropriate websites?

SUMMARY

Biomedical, information, communication, and knowledge technology will become increasingly connected in the future, linking people and information together in the rapidly changing world of health care. With new technology comes the need for a new set of competencies. By participating in designing this exciting future, nurses will ensure that their unique contributions to patient and family health and illness care are clearly and formally represented.

💡 A SOLUTION

The leadership in Hollary's organization understands that technology by itself does not improve quality and safety; a project that introduces technology must also consider the people and processes impacted. The new clinical information system must support clinical processes, and nurses are integral to ensuring this outcome. Without nurses' involvement, the new system would not be aligned with patient-care processes, would not deliver the anticipated benefits, and would not be successful.

To ensure nurses are involved in the decision-making process, Hollary requested that a nurse specialist from the hospital was brought onto the project full-time. This nurse engaged clinicians through all the stages of the project. Initially, nursing staff created a storyboard that outlined their perspective on how a clinical information system could support their practice to deliver safe, quality care. Nursing staff were involved in reviewing and providing feedback for the system build, device selection, process and workflow redesign impacted by the system, and training and implementation.

Hollary requested that nursing staff trial the hardware and recommend the type, number, and location of the devices required to support an efficient workflow. As nurses used the clinical information system to plan and document care, as well as administer medications, they noted that a variety of devices and carts were required. Wireless technology was implemented to support clinical staff and physicians in using systems at the point of care. Nursing staff provided ongoing feedback for improvements to the software, hardware, and wireless technology.

A significant change for nurses was the introduction of a standardized documentation methodology. Prior to the implementation of electronic documentation, nursing staff did not follow a specific charting methodology. In order to trend information and to easily view information over time, a standardized documentation methodology was introduced. While this was a significant change for nurses, it was one that was well accepted once staff made the transition. An evaluation post-implementation indicated that the quality of nursing documentation improved with the electronic clinical documentation system. Nursing documentation is now more consistent, comprehensive, and accurate. Information from previous visits is easier to access electronically, which helps improve continuity of care.

The clinical information system introduced at this hospital has helped improve the quality and safety of health care delivery, not only through improved documentation, but also through the introduction of electronic clinical decision support. The system provides clinicians with prompts, tools, and information at the point of care, supporting clinicians to provide the right care. The use of electronic bedside medication verification alerts nurses to times when medication should not be given to a patient. Electronic physician ordering prevents the errors that arise when health care providers need to decipher poor handwriting; it also standardizes physician ordering to incorporate evidence-informed order sets.

Would this be a suitable approach for you? Why or why not?

■ THE EVIDENCE

Kennedy & Hannah (2007) undertook a retrospective qualitative analysis of nursing records across multiple Canadian practice settings (acute care, inpatient mental health care, home care, long-term care) to examine the effectiveness of the International Classification for Nursing Practice (ICNP®) Beta Version in representing nursing practice. Nursing records were coded according to nursing phenomena, actions, and outcomes as found in the ICNP® classification system. With the exception of home care, the ICNP® achieved either a Match or a Conceptual Match for Nursing Phenomena and Nursing Actions in more than 60% of nursing records. The findings highlighted the need for more complete and visible nursing documentation to fully assess according to ICNP® standards.

NEED TO KNOW NOW

- Use the biomedical technology frequently required for patient care in your clinical practice area.
- Access the clinical information systems you will need to find information about the patients assigned to your care and enter data about their status, interventions you provide, the plan of care, and their responses to care.
- Know the standards for information privacy and confidentiality required within your organization.

CHAPTER CHECKLIST

Nurses are the key personnel in the health care system to mediate the interaction among science, technology, and the patient because of their unique holistic viewpoint and the "24/7" role of vigilant health care providers who preserve the patients' humanity, optimal functioning, and promotion of health. The challenge for the profession is to continue to provide patient-centred care in a technological society that strives for efficiency and cost-effectiveness. Nurse administrators, managers, and staff must provide leadership in managing information and technology to meet the challenge.

- Informatics is the transformation of data into knowledge. It consists of four core components: data, information, knowledge, and wisdom.
- Nurses commonly manage three types of information technology: biomedical technology, information technology, and knowledge technology.
- Biomedical technology includes the following:
  - Physiological monitoring
  - Diagnostic testing
  - Medication administration
  - Therapeutic interventions
- Information technology refers to computers and programs that are used to manage data and information.
- The goals of information management are as follows:
  - To obtain, manage, and use information to improve patient outcomes
  - To improve individual and organizational performance in patient care
  - To improve performance in other organizational processes
- Information systems can be used for the following:
  - Reducing clerical nursing
  - Providing patient census and location
  - Obtaining test results and lists of medications
  - Accessing nursing policies and procedures
  - Coordinating patient care
  - Monitoring chronic conditions
  - Managing statistical reporting
- Placement of computers at the patient's side or using handheld devices has many advantages, including the following:
  - Saves time
  - Improves communication by providing more timely access by others
  - Decreases likelihood of documentation omission
  - Adapts to nurse's workflow
  - Personalizes patient assessment
  - Simplifies care planning
- Knowledge technology involves decision support systems that are used to mimic the informational processing of an expert nurse.
- Evidence-informed practice involves both the application of evidence to practice and the building of evidence from practice.
- The electronic health record (EHR) contains health care information for an individual from birth to death, allowing immediate access to comprehensive health information.
- Future trends in biomedical, information, and knowledge technology will occur rapidly and demand that nurses remain involved in their development and implementation.
- Privacy and security issues have become important with increased access to and therefore potential broad misuse of patient-care data.
- Ethical decision making in health care becomes more complex with an increase in the use of medical technology.

TIPS FOR MANAGING INFORMATION AND TECHNOLOGY

- Create a vision for the future.
- Match your vision to the institution's mission and strategic plan.
- Learn what you need to know to fulfill the vision.
- Join initiatives that are moving in the direction of your vision.

- Be prepared to initiate, implement, and support new technology.
- Use an automated dispensing system.
- Use biometric technology.
- Never stop learning, or you will always be behind.

evolve WEBSITE

Visit the Evolve website for Suggested Readings, Internet Resources, and additional resources related to the content in this chapter: http://evolve.elsevier.com/Canada/Yoder-Wise/leading/.

REFERENCES

Statutes

Personal Information Protection and Electronic Documents Act. (2000). SC 2000, c. 5. Retrieved from http://laws.justice.gc.ca/en/P-8.6/.

Texts

American Nurses Association. (2008). *Nursing informatics: Scope and standards of practice.* Silver Spring, MD: Nursesbooks.org.

Bacigalupe, G. (2011). Is there a role for social technologies in collaborative healthcare? *Families Systems & Health, 29*(1), 1–14. doi:10.1037/a0022093

Baker, G. R., Norton, P. G., Flintoff, V., et al. (2004). The Canadian Adverse Events Study: The incidence of adverse events among hospital patients in Canada. *Canadian Medical Association Journal, 170*(11), 1678–1686. doi:10.1503/cmaj.1040498

Balka, E., Kahnamoui, N., & Nutland, K. (2007). Who is in charge of patient safety? Work practice, work processes, and utopian views of automatic drug dispensing systems. *International Journal of Medical Informatics, 76S*, S48–S57. doi:10.1016/j.ijmedinf.2006.05.038

Benham-Hutchins, M. (2009). Frustrated with HIT? Get involved! *Nursing Management, 40*(1), 17–19. doi:10.1097/01.NUMA.0000343977.08258.80

Bhandari, G., Tiessen, B., & Snowdon, A. (2011). Meeting community needs through leadership and innovation: A case of virtual psychiatric emergency department. *Behaviour & Information Technology, 30*(4), 517–523. doi:10.1080/0144929X.2011.553745

Billinghurst, F., Morgan, B., & Arthur, H. M. (2003). Patient and nurse-related implications of remote cardiac telemetry. *Clinical Nursing Research, 12*(4), 356–370. doi:10.1177/1054773803258998

Bournes, D. A., & Flint, F. (2003). Mis-takes: Mistakes in the nurse-person process. *Nursing Science Quarterly, 16*(2), 127–130. doi:10.1177/0894318403251787

Butler, M., Treacy, M., Scott, A., et al. (2006). Towards a nursing minimum data set for Ireland: Making Irish nursing visible. *Journal of Advanced Nursing, 55*(3), 364–375. doi:10.1111/j.1365-2648.2006.03909.x

Canada Health Infoway. (n.d.). *Standards collaborative guide.* Retrieved from https://www.infoway-inforoute.ca/flash/lang-en/scguide/docs/StandardsCatalogue_en.pdf.

Canada Health Infoway. (2005). Pan-Canadian electronic health record: Quantitative and qualitative benefits. Retrieved from https://www2.infoway-inforoute.ca/Admin/Upload/Dev/Document/VOL1_CHI%20Quantitative%20&%20Qualitative%20Benefits.pdf.

Canada Health Infoway. (2010). Electronic Health Records 2015: Canada's next generation of health care at a glance. Retrieved from https://www2.infoway-inforoute.ca/Documents/Vision_Summary_EN.pdf.

Canadian Association of Schools of Nursing. (2011, May 19). Re: Education of next generation of nurses to include effective clinical use of information and communication technologies [Web log message]. Retrieved from http://www.casn.ca/en/Whats_new_at_CASN_108/items/104.html.

Canadian Health Services Research Foundation. (2003). The theory and practice of knowledge brokering in Canada's health system. Retrieved from http://www.cfhi-fcass.ca/migrated/pdf/Theory_and_Practice_e.pdf.

Canadian Nurses Association. (2000). *Collecting data to reflect nursing impact: A discussion paper.* Ottawa, ON: Author. Retrieved from http://www.cna-aiic.ca/CNA/documents/pdf/publications/collct_data_e.pdf.

Canadian Nurses Association. (2001). What is nursing informatics and why is it so important? *Nursing Now: Issues and Trends in Canadian Nursing, 11*, 1–4.

Canadian Nurses Association. (2006a). E-nursing strategy for Canada. Ottawa, ON: Author. Retrieved from http://www.cna-nurses.ca/CNA/documents/pdf/.../E-Nursing-Strategy-2006-e.pdf.

Canadian Nurses Association. (2006b). Position statement: Nursing information and knowledge management. Ottawa, ON: Author. Retrieved from http://www.cna-aiic.ca/CNA/documents/pdf/publications/PS87-Nursing-info-knowledge-e.pdf.

Canadian Nurses Association. (2008). *Code of ethics for registered nurses (centennial edition)*. Ottawa, ON: Author. Retrieved from http://www.cna-aiic.ca/~/media/cna/files/en/codeofethics.pdf.

Canadian Nurses Association. (2012). When private becomes public: The ethical challenges and opportunities of social media. Ottawa, ON: Author. Retrieved from http://www2.cnaaiic.ca/CNA/documents/pdf/publications/Ethics_in_Practice_Feb_2012_e.pdf.

Canadian Nurses Association and University of Toronto, Faculty of Nursing. (2004). Nurses and patient safety: A discussion paper. Retrieved from http://www.cna-nurses.ca/CNA/.../pdf/.../patient_safety_discussion_paper_e.pdf.

Canadian Nursing Informatics Association. (2003). *Assessing the informatics education needs of Canadian nurses educational institution component: Educating tomorrow's nurses—Where's nursing informatics?* Retrieved from http://www.cnia.ca/documents/OHIHfinal.pdf.

Chi, T., Marziali, E., Colantonio, A., et al. (2009). Internet-based caregiver support for Chinese Canadians taking care of a family member with Alzheimer disease and related dementia. *Canadian Journal on Aging, 28*(4), 323–336. doi:10.1017/S0714980809990158

Côté, J. (2007). Using interactive health communication technology in a renewed approach to nursing. *Canadian Journal of Nursing Research, 39*(1), 135–136.

David, I., Poissant, L., & Rochette, A. (2012). Clinicians' expectations of Web 2.0 as a mechanism for knowledge transfer of stroke best practices. *Journal of Medical Internet Research, 14*(5). doi:10.2196/jmir.2016

Delaney, C. (2007). Nursing and informatics for the 21st century. *Creative Nursing, 12*(2), 4–6.

Denis, J. L., Champagne, F., & Pomey, M. P. (2005). *Toward a framework for the analysis of governance in health care organizations and systems*. Montreal, QC: Université de Montréal. Retrieved from http://www.accreditation.ca/accreditation-programs/qmentum/standards/sustainable-governance/on.

Detwiller, M. (2006). *Enhancing the quality of health care delivery through the use of electronic clinical documentation* (Unpublished master's thesis). Royal Roads University, Victoria, BC.

DiCenso, A. (2003). Evidence-based nursing practice: How to get there from here. *Nursing Leadership, 16*(4), 20–26. doi:10.12927/cjnl.2003.16257

Dodge, B. (1995). Some thoughts about WebQuest. Retrieved from http://webquest.sdsu.edu/about_webquests.html.

Doran, D., Haynes, B., Kushniruk, A., et al. (2009). *Evaluation of mobile information technology to improve nurses' access to and use of research evidence*. Toronto, ON: Ministry of Health and Long-Term Care.

Doran, D., Mildon, B., & Clarke, S. (2011). *Toward a national report card in nursing: A knowledge synthesis*. Toronto, ON: Nursing Health Services Research Unit (Toronto site) and Lawrence S. Bloomberg Faculty of Nursing, University of Toronto.

EKOS Research Associates. (2007). Final report: Electronic health information and privacy survey: What Canadians think. Retrieved from https://www2.infoway-inforoute.ca/Documents/EKOS_Final%20report_EN.pdf.

Garrett, B., & Klein, G. (2008). Value of wireless personal digital assistants for practice: Perceptions of advanced practice nurses. *Journal of Clinical Nursing, 17*, 2146–2154. doi:10.1111/j.1365-2702.2008.02351.x

Goddard, M., Mowat, D., Corbett, C., et al. (2004). The impacts of knowledge management and information technology advances in public health decision-making in 2010. *Health Informatics Journal, 10*(2), 111–120. doi:10.1177/1460458204042233

Haines, J. (1993). *Leading in a time of change: The challenge for the nursing profession. A discussion paper*. Ottawa, ON: Canadian Nurses Association. Retrieved from http://trove.nla.gov.au/version/36478507.

Hannah, K. J. (1985, May). Current trends in nursing in informatics: Implications for curriculum planning. In K. J. Hannah, E. J. Guillemin, & D. N. Conklin (Eds.), *Nursing uses of computers and information science: Proceedings of the IFIP/IMIA International Symposium on Nursing Uses of Computers and Information Science* (Calgary, AB) (pp. 181–187). Amsterdam, The Netherlands: Elsevier.

Hannah, K. J. (2005). Health informatics and nursing in Canada. *Health Care Information Management and Communications in Canada, 19*(3), 45–51.

Hannah, K. J., Ball, M. J., & Edwards, K. J. (2006). *Introduction to nursing informatics* (3rd ed.). New York, NY: Springer-Verlag.

Health Information Management Systems Society. (2008). The premier EMR adoption assessment tool. Retrieved from http://www.himssanalytics.org/docs/emram.pdf.

Hodge, T., & Giokas, D. (2011, April 7). EMR, EHR, and PHR—Why all the confusion? [Web log message]. Retrieved from http://infowayconnects.infoway-inforoute.ca/blog/electronic-health-records/374-emr-ehr-and-phr-%E2%80%93-why-all-the-confusion/.

Hunter, K. M. (2001). Nursing informatics theory. In V. K. Saba & K. A. McCormick (Eds.), *Essentials of computers for nurses: Informatics for the new millennium* (pp. 179–190). New York, NY: McGraw-Hill.

Institute for Safe Medication Practices Canada. (2007). Automated dispensing cabinets in the Canadian environment. *ISMP Canada Safety Bulletin, 7*(3), 1–3.

International Medical Informatics Association News. (2009, August 24). IMIA-NI definition of nursing informatics updated. Retrieved from http://imianews.wordpress.com/2009/08/24/imia-ni-definition-of-nursing-informatics-updated/.

Kennedy, M. A., & Hannah, K. (2007). Representing nursing practice: Evaluating the effectiveness of a nursing classification system. *Canadian Journal of Nursing Research, 39*(1), 58–79.

Kirkpatrick, A. W., DeWaele, J. J., Ball, C. G., et al. (2007). The secondary and recurrent abdominal compartment syndrome. *Acta Clinica Belgica, 62*(Suppl.), 60–65.

Kleib, M., Sales, A., Doran, D. M., et al. (2011). Nursing minimum data sets. In D. M. Doran (Ed.), *Nursing outcomes: State of the science* (2nd ed., pp. 487–512). Sudbury, MA: Jones & Bartlett.

Lahaie, U. (2007). WebQuests: A new instructional strategy for nursing education. *CIN: Computers, Informatics, Nursing, 25*(3), 148–156. doi:10.1097/01.NCN.0000270051.83152.78

MacDonald, M. (2008). Technology and its effect on knowing the patient: A clinical issue analysis. *Clinical Nurse Specialist, 22*(3), 149–155. doi:10.1097/01.NUR.0000311695.77414.f8

MacNeela, P., Scott, P. A., Treacy, M. P., et al. (2006). Nursing minimum data sets: A conceptual analysis and review. *Nursing Inquiry, 13*(1), 44–51. doi:10.1111/j.1440-1800.2006.00300.x

Mathieu, L. (2007). Nursing informatics: Developing knowledge for nursing practice. *Canadian Journal of Nursing Research, 39*(1), 15–19.

Matney, S., Brewster, P. J., Sward, K. A., et al. (2011). Philosophical approaches to the nursing informatics data-information-knowledge-wisdom framework. *Advances in Nursing Science, 34*(1), 6–18.

Murtagh, J., & Foerster, V. (2009). *Managing technology diffusion: A discussion paper*. Ottawa, ON: Canadian Agency for Drugs and Technologies in Health. Retrieved from http://www.cadth.ca/en/policy-forum/discussion-papers/managing-technology-diffusion.

Nagle, L. M., & Catford, P. (2008). Toward a model of successful electronic health record adoption. *Healthcare Quarterly, 11*(3), 84–91.

Nicklin, W., & McVeety, J. E. (2002). Canadian nurses' perceptions of patient safety in hospitals. *Canadian Journal of Nursing Leadership, 15*(3), 11–21.

Office of the Privacy Commissioner of Canada. (2009). The promise of personal health records. Retrieved from http://www.priv.gc.ca/media/nr-c/2009/res_090910_eh_e.asp.

O'Hagan, J., MacKinnon, N. J., Persaud, D., et al. (2009). Self-reported medical errors in seven countries: Implications for Canada. *Healthcare Quarterly, 12*, 55–61.

Perras, C., Jacobs, P., Boucher, M., et al. (2009). *Technologies to reduce errors in dispensing and administration of medication in hospitals: Clinical and economic analyses* (Technology report no. 121). Ottawa, ON: Canadian Agency for Drugs and Technologies in Health.

Praxia Information Intelligence and Gartner Incorporated. (2011). Telehealth benefits and adoption: Connecting people and providers across Canada: A Study Commissioned by Canada Health Infoway. Retrieved from https://www2.infoway-inforoute.ca/Documents/telehealth_report_summary_2010_en.pdf.

Queen's University. (2011, March 30). Evaluating Web sources. Retrieved from http://library.queensu.ca/inforef/tutorials/qcat/evalint.htm.

Read, K., & Giustini, D. (2011). Social media for health care managers: Creating a workshop in collaboration with the UBC Centre for Health Care Management. *Journal of the Canadian Health Librarians Association, 32*, 157–163.

Remus, S., & Kennedy, M. A. (2012). Innovation in transformative nursing leadership: Nursing informatics competencies and roles. *Nursing Leadership, 25*(4), 14–26. doi:10.12927/cjnl.2012.23260

Romanow, R. J. (2002). *Building on values: The future of health care in Canada—Final report*. Ottawa, ON: Commission on the Future of Health Care in Canada. Retrieved from http://www.cbc.ca/healthcare/final_report.pdf.

Rozenblum, R., Jang, Y., Zimlichman, E., et al. (2011). A qualitative study of Canada's experience with the implementation of electronic health information technology. *Canadian Medical Association Journal, 183*(5), E281–E288. doi:10.1503/cmaj.100856

Sackett, D. L., Straus, S. E., Richardson, W. S. et al. (2005). *Evidence-based medicine: How to practice and teach EBM* (3rd ed.). New York, NY: Churchill Livingstone.

Saginur, M., Graham, I. D., Forster, A. J., et al. (2008). The uptake of technologies designed to influence medication safety in Canadian hospitals. *Journal of Evaluation in Clinical Practice, 14*(1), 27–35. doi:10.1111/j.1365-2753.2007.00780.x

Schaffner, M. (2010). Networking or not working? *Gastroenterology Nursing, 33*(5), 379–380. doi:10.1097/SGA.0b013e3181f5059f

Scott Findlay, S. (2003). *Knowledge brokers: Linking researchers and policy makers*. Edmonton, AB: Alberta Foundation for Medical Research. Retrieved from http://www.ihe.ca/documents/HTA-FR14.pdf.

Tamblyn, R., Huang, A., Perreault, R., et al. (2003). The medical office of the 21st century (MOXXI): Effectiveness of computerized decision-making support in reducing inappropriate prescribing in primary care. *Canadian Medical Association Journal, 169*(6), 549–556.

Thompson, D. S., Estabrooks, C. A., Scott-Findlay, S., et al. (2007). Interventions aimed at increasing research use in nursing: A systematic review. *Implementation Science, 2*, 15. doi:10.1186/1748-5908-2-15

Tregunno, D., Gordon, S., & Gardiner-Harding, P. (2010). Implementing Health Outcomes for Better Information and Care (HOBIC): Lessons from an early adopter site. *Nursing Leadership, 23*(3), 56–68. doi:10.12927/cjnl.2010.21942

University of Alberta. (2011, August 5). Critical evaluation of Internet resources. Retrieved from http://guides.library.ualberta.ca/eval_internet.

University of British Columbia. (2011, April 6). Evaluating Internet sources. Retrieved from http://help.library.ubc.ca/researching/evaluating-internet-sources/.

Urowitz, S., Wiljer, D., Apatu, E., et al. (2008). Is Canada ready for patient accessible electronic health records? A national scan. *BMC Medical Informatics and Decision Making, 8*, 33. doi:10.1186/1472-6947-8-33

Wang, S., Nagle, L., Li, X., et al. (2004). *Building the future: An integrated strategy for nursing human resources in Canada: Technological change*. Ottawa, ON: The Nursing Sector Study Corporation. Retrieved from https://www.cna-aiic.ca/~/media/cna/page%20content/pdf%20fr/2013/09/05/19/20/technological_change_e.pdf.

WebQuest.org. (n.d.) Welcome. Retrieved from http://webquest.org.

Webster, P. C. (2010). Canadian hospitals make uneven strides in utilization of electronic health records. *Canadian Medical Association Journal, 182*(11), E487–E488. doi:10.1503/cmaj.109-3288

Werley, H. H., Devine, E. C., Zorn, C. R., et al. (1991). The nursing minimum data set: Abstraction tool for standardized, comparable, essential data. *American Journal of Public Health, 81*(4), 421–426.

White, J. L. (2007). Adverse event reporting and learning systems: A review of the relevant literature. Canadian Patient Safety Institute. Retrieved from http://www.docstoc.com/docs/44079864/Adverse-Event-Reporting-and-Learning-Systems-A-Review-of.

Wulff, K., Cummings, G. G., Marck, P., et al. (2011). Medication administration technologies and patient safety: A mixed-method systematic review. *Journal of Advanced Nursing, 697*(10), 2080–2095. doi:10.1111/j.1365-2648.2011.05676.x

Zhang, H., Cocosila, M., & Archer, N. (2010). Factors of adoption of mobile information technology by homecare nurses. *CIN: Computers, Informatics, Nursing, 28*(1), 49–56. doi:10.1097/NCN.0b013e3181c0474a

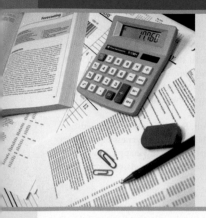

Managing Costs and Budgets

Trudi B. Stafford
Adapted by Arden Krystal

This chapter focuses on methods of financing health care and specific strategies for managing costs and budgets in patient-care settings. As well, it explores factors that escalate health care costs, sources of health care financing, cost-containment and health care reform strategies, and their implications for nursing practice. Various budgets and the budgeting process are explained. In addition to clinical competency and caring practices, nurses must understand the cost issues in health care delivery and the ethical implications of financial decisions to contribute fully to the health and healing of patients and populations.

OBJECTIVES

- Explain the major factors that are escalating the costs of health care.
- Evaluate different approaches to health care funding and their implications.
- Differentiate between variable and fixed costs, revenue, and expenditures in relation to a specified unit of service, such as a hospital visit, a hospital stay, or a procedure.
- Provide examples of cost considerations for nurses working in clinical environments.
- Discuss the purpose of and relationship between the operating and capital budgets.
- Explain the budgeting process.
- Identify variances on monthly expense reports and what they indicate.
- Understand how to develop a basic full-time equivalent (FTE) labour budget.

TERMS TO KNOW

budget	fixed costs	revenue
budgeting process	full-time equivalent (FTE)	unit of service
capital budget	nonproductive hours	utilization
case mix groups (CMGs)	operating budget	variable costs
cost	price	variance
cost centre	productive hours	variance analysis
expenditures	productivity	

❓ A CHALLENGE

The Fraser Health Authority is one of the fastest-growing health authorities in Canada, comprising over one-third of the entire population of British Columbia. Its emergency department visits grow by at least 5 to 6% year over year, despite a provincial and regional focus on preventive strategies and community alternatives to acute care. One of its largest sites is the Surrey Memorial Hospital, which sees close to 95 000 emergency department visits annually. Rajesh works at Surrey Memorial Hospital as a nurse manager in the emergency department. Although Rajesh has made some progress in filling vacancies and reducing overtime in the department, he continues to struggle with vacancy rates in the 8% range. Provincial revenues are not growing fast enough to keep pace with the demand for health care services. As a consequence, Rajesh needs to find ways to improve efficiency in his department, reduce less value-added expenditures (such as overtime), and meet the demand for emergency services while still staying on budget.

What would you do if you were Rajesh?

INTRODUCTION

Health care costs in Canada continue to rise at a rate greater than general inflation (Canadian Institute for Health Information [CIHI], 2013b). In 2011, total health expenditure in Canada was over 11% of the gross domestic product (GDP), an increase of over 2% since 2000 (CIHI, 2013b, p. 10). Drug expenditures have almost doubled during that same time frame and account for approximately 17% of total spending (CIHI, 2013b). In 2011, Canada spent $200.1 billion on health care, or an average of $5803 per capita (CIHI, 2013a, p. xiii). Approximately 70% of total health expenditure is financed by the public sector, and the rest is financed by the private sector. By comparison, health care spending in the United States reached $2.8 trillion in 2012, or $8915 per capita (Centers for Medicare & Medicaid Services, 2014).

The significant portion of the GDP spent on health care can potentially pose problems to the economy. Public-sector funds may need to be diverted from needed social programs such as child care, housing, education, transportation, and the environment.

WHAT ESCALATES HEALTH CARE COSTS?

Total health care costs are a function of the prices and the utilization rates of health care services (Costs = Price × Utilization) (Table 13-1). Price is the rate that health care providers set for the services they deliver, such as the hospital rate or physician fee as well as the unit prices of medications and supplies. Utilization refers to the quantity or volume of services provided, such as the number of diagnostic tests provided or the number of patient visits.

Price inflation in medications and supplies as well as growing labour costs are leading contributors to increasing prices for health care services. In recent decades, the rise in health care prices has dramatically outpaced general inflation. Examples of factors that stimulate price inflation are physician incomes that rise faster than average worker earnings and the high prices and utilization of prescription medications. Many provinces are moving to group purchasing of medications and supplies as a method to control costs. Group purchasing organizations (GPOs), which purchase goods in high volumes to obtain discounts, are able to deliver lower unit prices and savings to their members. In order to achieve the best economy of scale, health care organizations who are members of GPOs must standardize supplies and drug formularies as much as possible.

Several interrelated factors contribute to an increased utilization of medical services. These include a lack of appropriateness or effectiveness of some type

TABLE 13-1	RELATIONSHIP OF PRICE AND UTILIZATION RATES TO TOTAL HEALTH CARE COSTS			
PRICE	×	UTILIZATION RATE =	TOTAL COST	% CHANGE
$1.00		100	$100.00	0
$1.08*		100	$108.00	+8.0%
$1.08		105†	$113.40	+13.4%
$1.08		110‡	$118.80	+18.8%

*8% increase for inflation.
†5% more procedures done.
‡10% more procedures done.

of care, consumer beliefs and attitudes, health care financing, pharmaceutical usage, and changing population demographics and disease patterns. For example, a review of trends in health care utilization in British Columbia indicated that while only 5% of the population represented those with high complexity chronic conditions or those who were frail in residential care, this group represented over 42% of total health care expenditure in the province (British Columbia Ministry of Health, 2010). Inappropriate or ineffective medical procedures are also prevalent and have led to national initiatives to demonstrate the efficacy of interventions and to decrease variations in physician practice. The Canadian Agency for Drugs and Technologies in Health (CADTH) reviews the effectiveness of medical devices and medications annually and provides health care decision makers with evidence-based information on those that provide the best value.

Our attitudes and behaviours as consumers of health care also contribute to rising costs. In general, we prefer to "be fixed" when something goes wrong rather than practise prevention. When we need "fixing," expensive high-tech services typically are perceived as the best care. Many of us still believe that the physician knows best, so we do not seek much information related to costs and effectiveness of different health care options. When we do seek information, it may not be readily available, accurate, or understandable. Also, we are not accustomed to using other, less costly health care providers, such as nurse practitioners.

The way health care is financed in Canada may contribute to rising costs. Since a large portion of health care spending is financed through taxation and not directly by consumers, users of the system are less aware of the direct costs involved with even something as simple as a visit to the emergency department. Effectively, no direct disincentive exists for overutilization. Physicians are largely paid through a fee-for-service model, which can provide incentive for a physician to do more rather than less work. Most physicians are connected to the health care system not as employees but as independent contractors who drive the utilization of services such as diagnostic tests, procedures, and in-hospital bed days. Physicians are not directly accountable for the costs borne by a health region, hospital network, or a community care environment.

Changing population demographics are increasing the volume of health services needed as well. For example, chronic health problems increase with age, and the number of older adults in Canada is rising. In 2011, 5 million Canadians were 65 or older, a number that is expected to double in the next 25 years (Employment and Social Development Canada, n.d.)

HOW IS HEALTH CARE FINANCED?

Health care in Canada is financed through a mix of public and private funding. Approximately 70% of health care services are publicly financed, and approximately 30% are financed by third-party insurance plans and private pay situations, or out-of-pocket (Makarenko, 2010). Private health care delivery in Canada is heavily regulated and tends to apply to less acute or noncore services as opposed to basic health care services (Makarenko, 2010). Although each province and territory determines the services its public plan provides, those services must comply with the principles of the *Canada Health Act*, which are as follows:

- Comprehensiveness: all necessary physician and hospital services are covered
- Universality: services are available to all insured citizens
- Accessibility: citizens have access to all covered health care services under uniform terms and conditions, regardless of ability to pay
- Public administration: the government is the single payer for all covered services
- Portability: citizens are covered across the country (Canadian Nurses Association [CNA], 2009, p. 2)

Examples of publicly funded services include hospital admissions, emergency department visits, general practitioner visits, and most home health and public health services, such as immunizations and vaccines. Private health insurance is the second major source of health care funding in Canada. Many Canadians have some form of private health insurance to complement their publicly funded basic insurance. Examples of third-party or private financing include those services reimbursed through extended health plans and private corporate insurance plans, such as eyewear and some eye exams, and selected physiotherapy and massage therapy services. Individuals who are nonresidents of the province or territory in which they are treated also pay directly for health care services when they do not have insurance. Costs paid by individuals are called *out-of-pocket expenses* and include deductibles, additional fees, and co-insurance typically related to services such as dental care and prescription medications.

EXERCISE 13-1

As a student nurse, how aware are you of the costs and financing of health care in Canada? What kinds of strategies could be employed to increase the awareness of consumers and health care providers about the subject? As a health care provider, what can you do to contribute to ensuring a cost efficient and effective system?

APPROACHES TO HEALTH CARE FINANCING

In Canada, the primary source of funding for hospitals and health regions is a fixed, global budget transfer from the provincial or territorial government. The annual amount is typically based on historical spending, inflation, and politics rather than a zero-based assessment (e.g., where previous expenditures are not considered and budgets are based on starting from zero) of the type and volume of services provided (Sutherland, 2011). The advantages of this approach to funding include predictability and autonomy to move resources from one priority to another based on demand. A major disadvantage is that global budgets often do not grow to the same degree as demand, which can lead to longer wait times for services and other gaps in service.

Activity-based funding (ABF), although commonly used internationally, has just recently gained prominence in the Canadian health care context. ABF funds health care organizations based on the type and quantity of services provided, paid at a set unit price. While the money is still provided by the provincial or territorial government, this mechanism has been shown in some settings to create a powerful incentive to find efficiencies because organizations are able to retain the difference in funding between the payment and the actual cost of delivering the service (Sutherland, 2011). Many provinces have adopted a mixed funding approach that combines global funding and ABF to reduce wait times yet still control health care spending.

Most health care organizations do not pay their physicians directly, with some exceptions. As mentioned

earlier, most physicians are paid based on a fee-for-service model. Although common in Canada, other jurisdictions (e.g., the United Kingdom) have moved away from this payment method since it may perpetuate inefficient utilization (Li, 2006).

Pay-for-performance (P4P) is another funding method that is becoming more common in Canada. As opposed to ABF, which funds organizations based on the volume of procedures, P4P provides funding incentives based on a predetermined set of quality outcomes (e.g., wait times) and outcome measures (e.g., hemoglobin A1C testing) (Sutherland, 2011). In British Columbia, the Emergency Department Decongestion P4P program is reported to have decreased emergency department wait times (Ministry of Health Services, Fraser Health, and Vancouver Coastal Health, 2009). This approach to funding can lead to innovation in care delivery, provided that the incentives are large enough to fund improvements on a cost-neutral basis.

Direct billing to the consumer is a form of financing that is less common in the public health sector in Canada. Most direct billing occurs as a consequence of nonresidents of a province or territory who are underinsured or not insured. As an example, in Canada, new immigrants are often not granted public health insurance without a required waiting period. In 2004, Canada admitted 204 000 landed immigrants and 31 000 refugees; delays to access to the public system can mean that these individuals never receive coverage or can wait up to two years (Caulford & Yasmin, 2006). Should a health care facility need to provide services that require direct billing, collecting payment can at times be very challenging.

Major health care financing approaches are summarized in Box 13-1. Researchers do not agree on the exact effects of these approaches on cost and quality (Sutherland, 2011). However, consideration of these effects is important because changes in payment systems have implications for how care is provided in health care organizations.

EXERCISE 13-2

A provincial government has set up an ABF system for hip arthroplasty. The health organization's current actual cost to provide the surgery is an average of $12 000. The Ministry of Health is paying $10 500. What strategies can the nurse administrator explore to make this a cost-neutral or surplus situation?

BOX 13-1	HEALTH CARE FINANCING APPROACHES
METHOD	**KEY POINTS**
Global funding	A set amount of funding distributed to a health care organization annually, not directly tied to volume or types of services
Activity-based funding (ABF)	Funding that is based on a set price for a specific service and distributed based on volume
Fee-for-service	Funding for every service provided based on a set fee
Pay-for-performance (P4P)	Funding incentives provided for a specific quality outcome, such as reduced waiting time
Direct billing	Direct billing of patients for the services provided

USING ACTIVITY TO INFORM THE BUDGET

Case mix groups (CMGs) represent a patient classification system used to group the types of inpatients a hospital treats. The CMG system is modelled after American Diagnosis Groups (DRGs) and was developed by the Canadian Institute for Health Information (CIHI) (Manitoba Centre for Health Policy, 2010a). CMGs are assigned after a person is discharged from hospital, at which time the patient chart is reviewed and coded. The abstract produced from the review is sent to CIHI, which uses a computer algorithm to sort cases into CMGs. CMGs can either be categorized as typical or atypical, such as long-stay outliers. Most provinces and territories have been sending data to CIHI for inclusion in the discharge abstract database (DAD) since at least the mid-1990s. CMGs can be a useful source of data for nurse managers to use in determining the types of services and resources required to care for patients within their portfolio. For example, a general medical unit may appear to care for a large range of medical problems, but after evaluating the CMGs, it may become evident that as few as three or four CMGs actually make up the majority of the patient population. This information allows nurse managers to plan resources more accurately to meet the specific needs of patients.

Although CMGs can help categorize patients' health problems more accurately, the need to understand the level of resources required for those patients is important. As a result, CIHI established resource intensity weights (RIWs). Each CMG is assigned a weight that represents the relative value of resources that cases within that CMG are expected to consume. Generally, it is reasonable to assume that the more acute the patient, the higher the RIW (such as a critical care unit patient). However, the RIW is not always a good proxy for acuity, especially when we consider a rehabilitation patient. In this case, the patient is no longer acutely ill but requires high levels of resources and so would be assigned a relatively high RIW (Manitoba Centre for Health Policy, 2010b). Age and other co-morbidities also play a factor in RIW calculation, as these factors can have a major effect on the resources required to care for different patients with the same diagnosis.

> **EXERCISE 13-3**
> If a nurse manager is developing a staffing model (including nursing, allied health, and unregulated staff) for a new unit, how could he or she use CMGs and RIWs to guide decisions regarding the makeup of the care team?

THE CHANGING HEALTH CARE ECONOMIC ENVIRONMENT

Health care is a major public concern, and rapid changes are occurring in an attempt to reduce costs and improve the health and wellness of Canadians. As shown in Box 13-2, strategies shaping the evolving

BOX 13-2	HEALTH CARE DELIVERY REFORM STRATEGIES
STRATEGIES	**KEY FEATURES**
Primary health care reform	Focus on nonhospital, early treatment of health problems, with an emphasis on prevention to reduce overall costs
PFF or ABF	A system whereby an organization gets reimbursed at a set price per case based on agreed-upon outcomes, such as wait time targets.
Regionalization	An operating model where several health entities are merged into one organizational structure with the intent of reducing overhead and creating efficiencies

health care delivery system include primary health care reform, patient-focused funding (PFF) or activity-based funding (ABF), and regionalization. These strategies affect both the cost and utilization of health care services.

BENDING THE COST CURVE

With health care spending accounting for close to 40% of many provincial and territorial budgets in Canada (CIHI, 2013b), the concept of "bending the cost curve" has never been more prevalent. The demand for health care services rises every year, as do the associated costs. As a consequence, most jurisdictions in Canada are exploring new ways of providing services to maximize efficiencies and, most important, to reduce demand. The emphasis on primary health care is an attempt to reduce the burden of hospitalization, particularly for people with multiple chronic illnesses. By reducing demand at the front door, the need to expand services and build new capital infrastructure is reduced, avoiding costs that otherwise would be borne by taxpayers. Primary health care clinics and providers can treat many people for the same cost as a single overnight hospital stay.

PFF and ABF are gaining some acceptance in many provinces and territories, although their true impact on efficiency has elicited mixed reviews (Sutherland, 2011). It is assumed that by paying per case or unit of service, hospitals and health care providers will strive for efficiencies that will increase outputs (e.g., inpatient services) and reduce waste (and garner more payments). Another related hypothesis is that health care organizations will work hard to be more efficient on a case to provide the service at less than the unit cost allocated, allowing for the residual amount to be retained by the provider organization. In both cases, the drive for greater efficiency has been the primary motivator for jurisdictions to experiment with this approach.

Regionalization is an organizational structure many provinces have gone to in an effort to reduce overhead and administrative costs, drive standardization, and create clinical efficiencies. When several hospitals and community care services operate under one umbrella, the need for separate support services such as human resources, finance, and procurement of goods and services is significantly reduced, which, in theory, lowers costs to the system (Church & Barker, 1998). As consumers of health care demand more value for money, the push to further consolidate back office or overhead functions continues to grow.

WHAT DOES THE HEALTH CARE ECONOMIC ENVIRONMENT MEAN FOR NURSING PRACTICE?

Although the health care economic environment is ever-changing, nurses must value themselves as health care providers and think of their practice within a context of organizational viability and quality of care. To do this, they must add "financial thinking" to their repertoire of nursing skills, and they must determine whether the services they provide add value for patients. Services that add value are of high quality, affect health outcomes positively, and minimize costs. The following sections help develop financial thinking skills and ways to consider how nursing practice adds value for patients by minimizing costs.

COST-CONSCIOUS NURSING PRACTICES
Knowing and Controlling Costs

Understanding what is required for a department or employer to remain financially sound requires that nurses think about not only the costs associated with individual patients but also revenue and expenses more globally, while actively considering how to control costs to the system as a whole.

As direct caregivers and case managers, nurses are constantly involved in determining the type and quantity of resources used for patients. Resources include supplies, personnel, and time. Nurses need to know what costs are generated by their decisions and actions. They also need to know what items cost and how they are paid for in an organization so that they can make cost-effective decisions. For example, nurses need to know per-item costs for supplies so that they can appropriately evaluate lower-cost substitutes.

Although nurses must develop and implement their plans of care with full knowledge of the cost implications, cost alone does not drive care. Nurses are expected to continue to advocate for patients while working within cost and contractual constraints. Moreover, when nurses understand the funding practices of their organization, they can help patients maximize the resources available to them.

In hospitals, the cost of nursing care usually is not calculated or billed separately to patients; instead, it is part of the general per-diem fee allocated per bed day, which is either paid for by the global budget (using tax dollars) or billed directly to the patient who is underinsured or not insured.

Using Time Efficiently

The adage that time is money is fitting in health care and refers to both the nurse's time and the patient's time. When nurses are organized and efficient in their care delivery and in scheduling and coordinating patients' care, the organization will save money. Doing as much as possible during each episode of care is particularly important to decrease repeat visits and unnecessary service utilization. Because length of stay (LOS) is the most important predictor of hospital costs (Finkler, Kovner, & Jones, 2007), patients who stay extra days cost the hospital a considerable amount and increase congestion. Decreasing LOS also makes room for other patients, thereby potentially increasing patient volume and reducing wait times. Nurses can become more efficient and effective by evaluating their major work processes and eliminating areas of redundancy and rework. Automated clinical information systems that support integrated practice at the point of care will also increase efficiency and improve patient outcomes.

An important element of efficiently managing nursing resources is the concept of appropriate scheduling. Nurse staffing and scheduling represent a significant human and financial resource issue in health care organizations. Nurse managers must consider many elements when determining appropriate staffing decisions. These decisions could be categorized into three general areas: strategic, logistical, and tactical decision making (College and Association of Registered Nurses

of Alberta, 2008). Strategic decisions refer to judgements that result in overall approaches to nursing care delivery (such as skill mix) and models of care delivery (see also Chapter 14). Logistical decisions refer to decisions in overall staffing directions at the unit and team level relative to baseline staffing in order to achieve appropriate patient care and management objectives. These encompass decisions around replacement staffing methods (e.g., float pools, relief lines, developing algorithms) and scheduling approaches and methods (e.g., self-scheduling and 7.5-hour shifts). Tactical decisions refer to those judgements made on a shift-to-shift basis that result in changes to schedules to safely meet the needs of patients in light of patient acuity or staffing availability (College and Association of Registered Nurses of Alberta, 2008). Coupled with appropriate staffing decisions is the need to ensure that scheduling decisions are made in accordance with any collective agreements and organizational policies (such as overtime policy).

Many public health care institutions also use managerial tools such as Lean and Six Sigma to reduce inefficiencies. Lean is a process redesign method used to reduce waste through process-improvement tools such as value stream mapping and five S (Liker, 2003). Six Sigma is focused on improving the quality of processes and reducing errors (Keller & Pyzdek, 2009). Many provinces have begun using techniques such as Lean. For example, Saskatchewan is the first province to introduce Lean across its entire health system (Government of Saskatchewan, 2012). As at writing, the province had over one-quarter of its 40 000 health sector workforce trained in Lean methodology (Accreditation Canada, 2013).

Discussing the Cost of Care with Patients

Talking with patients about the cost of care is important, although it may be uncomfortable. Moreover, although the discussions occur at a macro level in Canada due to our single-payer, tax-funded health care system, it is important that all consumers of health care understand the implications of their choices on the system as a whole.

Discovering during a clinic visit that a patient cannot afford a specific medication or intervention is preferable to finding out several days later in a follow-up call that the patient has not taken the medication. Such information compels the clinical management team to explore optional treatment plans or to find resources to cover the costs. Talking with patients about costs is important in other ways; it involves the patients in the decision-making process and increases the likelihood that treatment plans will be followed. Patients also can make informed choices and better use the resources available to them if they have appropriate information about costs.

EXERCISE 13-5

A new patient visits the clinic and is given prescriptions for three medications that will cost about $120 per month. You check her chart and discover that she has no insurance coverage for medications and may not be able to afford all of the medications. How can you determine whether she has the resources to buy this medicine each month and if she is willing to buy it? If she cannot afford the medications, what are some options?

Meeting Patient Rather Than Provider Needs

Developing an awareness of how feelings about patients' needs influence decisions can help nurses better manage costs. A nurse administrator in a home health agency recently related the story of a nurse who continued to visit a patient for weeks after the patient's health problems had resolved. When questioned, the nurse said she was uncomfortable terminating the visits because the patient continued to tell her he needed her help. Later, the patient revealed that he had not needed nursing care for some time, although he had continued telling the nurse he did because he thought she wanted to keep visiting him. This illustrates how nurses need to verify whose needs are being met with nursing care.

Evaluating the Cost-Effectiveness of New Technologies

The adoption of new technologies can present dilemmas in managing costs. In the past, if a new piece of equipment was easier to use or benefited the patient in any way, nurses were apt to want to use it for everyone, no matter how much more it cost. Now they are forced to make decisions regarding which patients really need the new equipment and which ones will have good outcomes with the current equipment. Essentially, nurses are analyzing the cost effectiveness of the new equipment with regard to different types of patients to allocate limited resources. This new and sometimes

difficult way of thinking about patient care may not always feel like a caring way of nursing. However, such decisions conserve resources without jeopardizing patients' health and thus create the possibility of providing additional health care services.

EXERCISE 13-6

Last year, a new positive-pressure, needleless system for administering IV antibiotics was introduced. Because the system was so easy to use and convenient for patients, the nurses in the contracted home IV therapy agency ordered it for everyone. Typically, patients get their IV antibiotics four times each day. The minibags and tubing for the regular procedure cost the agency $22 a day. The new system costs $24 per medication administration, or $96 a day. The agency receives the same per-diem (daily) payment for each patient. Discuss the financial implications for the agency if this practice is continued. Generate some optional courses of action for the nurses to consider. How should these options be evaluated? What secondary costs (e.g., the cost of treating fewer needle-stick injuries) should be included?

Predicting and Using Nursing Resources Efficiently

Because health care organizations are service institutions, typically the largest part of their operating budget is labour. For hospitals, in particular, nurses are the largest group of employees and often account for most of the labour budget. Staffing is the major area nurse managers can influence in managing costs, and supply management is the secondary area. To understand why this is so, it is helpful to understand the concepts of fixed and variable costs.

The total fixed costs in a unit are those costs that do not change as the volume of patients changes. In other words, with either a high or a low patient census, expenses related to facilities costs, such as heat and light, support costs, administrative salaries, and salaries of the minimum number of staff to keep a unit open must be paid. Variable costs are costs that vary in direct proportion to patient volume or acuity. Examples include nursing and direct care staff, supplies, and medications. In hospitals and community health care agencies, patient classification systems are often used to help managers predict nursing care requirements (see also Chapter 14). These systems differentiate patients according to acuity of illness, functional status, and resource needs. Some nurses do not like these systems because they believe the systems do not capture the essence of nursing. However, we need to remember that these tools help managers predict resource needs. It is not necessary for them to describe all nursing activities and judgements to be good predictors. Misguided efforts to sabotage classification systems by incorrectly or inaccurately coding patient care with the hope for better staffing work primarily to prevent the development of tools to better manage practice. Used appropriately, patient classification systems can help evaluate changing practice patterns and patient acuity levels as well as provide information for budgeting processes.

EXERCISE 13-7

Given the definitions for fixed and variable costs, why do you think nurse managers have the greatest influence over costs through management of staffing and supplies?

Managing staffing and utilization can achieve the most immediate reductions in costs. Hospitals and health regions strive to lower costs so that they can afford to meet the increasing demand for service without a large increase to the overall budget. Therefore, staffing methods and patient-care-delivery models are being closely scrutinized. Work redesign, a process for changing the way to think about and structure the work of patient care, is the predominant strategy for developing systems that better utilize high-cost professionals and improve service quality. Increased staff retention, patient safety, and positive patient outcomes result from effective work redesign processes.

Using Research to Evaluate Standard Nursing Practices

Nurses use research to restructure their work to ensure they add value for patients. Koelling, Johnson, Cody, et al. (2005) studied the effect of patient education by a nurse educator on the clinical outcomes of patients with heart failure. In this randomized, controlled trial, one group of patients received standard discharge information, and the other group of patients received standard discharge information plus 1 hour of one-on-one education from a nurse educator. All patients were followed by telephone after discharge to collect data concerning post-hospitalization clinical events, symptoms, and self-care practices. Patients who received the additional 1-hour teaching session with the

---

BOX 13-3   STRATEGIES FOR COST-CONSCIOUS NURSING PRACTICE

1. Knowing and controlling costs
2. Using time efficiently
3. Discussing the cost of care with patients
4. Meeting patient rather than provider needs
5. Evaluating the cost-effectiveness of new technologies
6. Predicting and using nursing resources efficiently
7. Using research to evaluate standard nursing practices

---

nurse educator showed improved clinical outcomes, increased adherence to self-care management, and reduced costs of care because of a reduction in rehospitalizations. The costs of care, including the costs associated with the additional education session, resulted in a savings of $2823 per patient in the education group as compared with the control group. The findings from this economic evaluation support the implementation of nursing education programs for patients with chronic heart failure as evidenced by improved patient outcomes and reduced costs. Box 13-3 summarizes some cost-conscious strategies for nursing practice. Further, the Literature Perspective below describes the need for business cases.

LITERATURE PERSPECTIVE

Resource: Jones, C. B., & Gates, M. (2007). The costs and benefits of nurse turnover: A business case for nurse retention. *Online Journal of Issues in Nursing, 12*(3), Manuscript 4.

Nurse turnover is a continual concern for nurse administrators and nurse managers, particularly in times of nursing shortages. The authors of this article presented a review of the literature related to the costs and benefits associated with nurse turnover. They found that the widely held belief is that the cost of nurse turnover exceeds the benefits of hiring new staff. However, the literature does not quantify the actual costs associated with nurse turnover as related to the economic benefits associated with nurse retention.

In their review of the literature, the authors determined that the cost of nurse turnover ranges from US$22 000 to over US$64 000 per nurse. In general, however, the authors found that the cost is typically estimated at 1.3 times the salary of the departing nurse. Determining the actual cost of nurse turnover is inherently difficult because it is challenging to calculate indirect costs (such as productivity loss or loss of organizational knowledge) or the costs associated with retaining nurses (such as ongoing education or

📖 LITERATURE PERSPECTIVE—cont'd

rewards and recognition events). The authors' review of the literature determined that nurse turnover costs include advertising and recruitment costs, vacancy costs (i.e., agency nurses, overtime), hiring and orientation costs, decreased productivity, termination costs, potential patient errors, poor work environment and culture, loss of organizational knowledge, and additional turnover. The authors indicated that the quantification of the benefits of nurse turnover is largely ignored in the literature. Some of the benefits include the reduced salaries and benefits for newly hired nurses, savings from bonuses, the new ideas and innovations brought by new nurses, and the elimination of poor performers.

The authors call for a business case to be made for nurse retention to determine the actual associated costs and benefits. A business case provides information about the value of a project or investment based on a cost-benefit analysis. According to the authors, a formal review would require that *all* costs and *all* benefits be considered, which, they underscore, is very difficult. Moreover, the authors noted that all nurse turnover is not equal, meaning that the turnover of one nurse may be welcomed, while the turnover of another may result in considerable loss of knowledge and experience.

Implications for Practice

This literature review demonstrates the challenges of attempting to quantify the actual costs of nurse turnover. It highlights the value of developing a robust business case as a means of determining the associated costs and benefits. Such a business case has the potential to drive organizational human resource practices in the areas of nurse recruitment and nurse retention programs.

EXERCISE 13-8

A community nursing organization performs an average of 36 intermittent catheterizations each day. A prepackaged catheterization kit costs the organization $17, but not every component of the kit is used each time. The four items in the kit, purchased separately, cost $5 each. What factors should be considered in evaluating the cost effectiveness of the two sources of supplies?

BUDGETS

The basic financial document used in most health care organizations is the budget—a detailed financial plan for carrying out the activities an organization wants to accomplish for a certain period. An organizational budget is a formal plan that is stated in terms of dollars and includes proposed revenue (money received for providing goods or services) and expenditures (money spent on goods and services). The budgeting process is an ongoing activity in which plans are made and revenues and expenditures are managed to meet or exceed the goals of the plan. The management functions of planning and control are tied together through the budgeting process.

A budget requires managers to plan ahead and establish explicit program goals and expectations. Changes in health care practices, payment methods, technology, demographics, and regulatory factors must be forecast to anticipate their effects on the organization. Planning encourages an evaluation of different options and helps achieve a more cost-effective use of resources.

Different types of interrelated budgets are used by health care organizations in Canada. The major budgets discussed in this section are the operating budget and the capital budget. Managers also use long-range notional budgets to help them plan for the future. Often, these future-oriented budgets are referred to as *strategic plans* (Finkler & McHugh, 2007).

Operating Budget

The operating budget is the financial plan for the day-to-day activities of the organization. The expected revenues and expenditures generated from daily operations, given a specified volume of patients (the activity budget), are stated in it. Preparing and monitoring the operating budget, particularly the expenditure portion, is often the most time-consuming financial function of nurse managers.

The expenditure part of the operating budget consists of a labour budget and a supply and expense budget for each cost centre. A cost centre is an organizational unit for which costs can be identified and managed. The labour budget is the largest part of the operating budget for most nursing units. (See The Evidence on page 253.)

Before the labour budget can be established, the volume of work predicted for the budget period must be calculated. A unit of service, which is a measure of the work being produced by the organization, is used. Units of service may be, for example, patient days, clinic or home visits, hours of service, admissions, deliveries, or treatments. Another factor needed to calculate the workload is the patient acuity mix. The formula for calculating the workload or the required patient-care hours for inpatient units is as follows: Workload volume = Hours of care per patient day × Number of patient days (Table 13-2).

TABLE 13-2   WORKLOAD CALCULATION (TOTAL REQUIRED PATIENT-CARE HOURS)

PATIENT ACUITY LEVEL*	HOURS OF CARE PER PATIENT DAY (HPPD)†	×	PATIENT DAYS‡	=	WORKLOAD§
1	3.0		900		2 700
2	5.2		3 100		16 120
3	8.8		4 000		35 200
4	13.0		1 600		20 800
5	19.0		400		7 600
Total			10 000		82 420

* *1*, low; *5*, high.
†HPPD is the number of hours of care on average for a given acuity level.
‡1 patient per 1 day = 1 patient day.
§Total number of hours of care needed based on acuity levels and numbers of patient days.

In many organizations, the workload is established by the financial office and given to the nurse manager. In some organizations, nurse managers forecast the volume. To forecast the volume, nurse managers usually start with a baseline of last year's actual workload statistics and predict whether the volume in the upcoming year is expected to rise above or fall below that baseline. Nurse managers should inform administration about any factors that might affect the accuracy of the forecast, such as changes in physician practice patterns, new treatment modalities, or changes in inpatient versus outpatient treatment practices.

The next step in preparing the labour or labour budget is to determine how many staff members will be needed to provide care. (This topic is also discussed in Chapter 15.) Because some people work full-time and others work part-time, **full-time equivalents (FTEs)** are used in this step rather than positions. Generally, one FTE can be equated to working 37.5 hours per week, 52 weeks per year, for a total of 1950 hours of work paid per year. One-half of an FTE (0.5 FTE) equates to 18.75 hours per week. The number of hours per FTE varies among provinces and territories and sometimes by type of nurse depending on collective agreements in place, so it is important to check this information prior to preparing any labour budgets.

The 1950 hours paid to an FTE in a year consist of both productive hours and nonproductive hours. **Productive hours** are paid time that is worked. **Nonproductive hours** are paid time that is not worked, such as vacation, statutory holidays, orientation, education, and sick time. Before the number of FTEs needed for the workload can be calculated, the number of productive hours per FTE is determined by subtracting the total number of nonproductive hours per FTE from total paid hours. Alternatively, payroll reports can be reviewed to determine the percentage of paid hours that are productive for each FTE. Finally, the total number of FTEs needed to provide the care is calculated by dividing the total patient-care hours required by the number of productive hours per FTE (Box 13-4).

BOX 13-4   PRODUCTIVE HOURS CALCULATION

Method 1: Add all nonproductive hours/FTE and subtract from paid hours/FTE

Example:	Vacation	20 days
	Holiday	7 days
	Average sick time	4 days
	TOTAL	37 days

37 × 7.5* hours = 277.5 nonproductive hours/FTE
1950 – 277.5 = 1672.5 productive hours/FTE

Method 2: Multiply paid hours/FTE by percentage of productive hours/FTE

Example: Productive hours = 85.8%/FTE
(1672.5 productive hours of total 1950 = 85.8%)
1950 × 0.858 = 1672.5 productive hours/FTE

Total FTE Calculation

Required Patient-Care Hours ÷ Productive Hours Per FTE = Total FTEs Needed
82 420 ÷ 1672.5 = approximately 49 FTEs

FTE, Full-time equivalent.
*Based on a 7.5-hour shift pattern or 37.5 hours/week.

The total number of FTEs calculated by this method represents the number needed to provide care 24/7 each year (including relief). It does not reflect the number of positions or the number of people working each day. In fact, the number of positions may be much higher, particularly if many part-time nurses are employed. On any given day, some nurses may be scheduled for their regular day off or vacation and others may be off because of illness. Also, some positions that do not involve direct patient care, such as nurse managers or unit secretaries, may not be replaced during nonproductive time. Only one FTE is budgeted for any position that is not covered with other staff when the employee is off.

EXERCISE 13-9

Change the number of patient hours per day at each acuity level listed in Table 13-2, either up or down, but keep the total number of patient days the same. Recalculate the required total workload. Discuss how changes in patient acuity affect nursing resource requirements.

The next step is to prepare a daily staffing plan (ratios for day, evening, and night shifts) and to establish positions through the development of a rotation or annual schedule (see also Chapter 15). Once this plan is established, the labour costs that comprise the labour budget can be calculated. Factors that must be addressed include straight-time hours, overtime hours, differentials and premiums, raises, and benefits (Finkler & McHugh, 2007). Differentials and premiums are extra pay for working specific times, such as evening shifts, night shifts, or holidays. Benefits usually include health and life insurance, Canada Pension Plan payments, and retirement plans. Benefits often cost an additional 23 to 27% of a full-time employee's salary.

EXERCISE 13-10

If the percentage of productive hours per FTE is 80%, how many worked or productive hours are there per FTE? If total patient-care hours are 82 420, how many FTEs will be needed?

The supply and expense budget includes a variety of items used in daily unit activities, such as medical and office supplies, minor equipment, and books and journals; it also includes orientation, training, and travel. Each expense category generally has its own budget line and expense code. Although different methods are used to calculate the supply and expense budget, usually the previous year's expenses are used as a baseline. Ideally, this baseline is adjusted for projected patient volume and specific circumstances known to affect expenses, such as predictable staff turnover, which increases orientation and training expenses; a percentage factor would also be added to adjust for inflation. However, the reality in many Canadian jurisdictions is that budgets rarely grow as quickly as actual expenses, and managers are expected to find efficiencies to arrive at a balanced budget.

The final component of the operating budget is the revenue budget. The revenue budget projects the revenue from a variety of sources that the organization will receive for providing patient care. Historically, nurses have not been directly involved in developing the revenue budget, although this is beginning to change. In most hospitals, the revenue budget is established by the financial office and given to nurse managers. The anticipated revenues are calculated according to the specifics of the nursing area or program. Data about the volume and types of patients and funding streams (i.e., global funding, ABF) are necessary to project revenues in any health care organization. Even when nurse managers do not participate in developing the revenue budget, learning about the organization's revenue base is essential for good decision making.

Capital Budget

The capital budget reflects expenses related to the purchase of major capital items such as equipment and physical plant. A capital expenditure must have a useful life of more than 1 year and must exceed a cost level specified by the provincial or territorial government. The minimum cost requirement for capital items in health care organizations is usually from $2000 to $5000, although some organizations have different levels. Anything below that minimum is considered a routine operating cost.

Capital expenses are separated from the operating budget because their high cost would make the costs of providing patient care appear too high during the year of purchase. To account for capital expenses, the costs of capital items are depreciated. This means that each year, over the useful life of the equipment, a portion of its cost is allocated to the operating budget as an expense. This procedure is required as part of the generally accepted accounting principles governing each province, but it does not affect the bottom line of the manager's budget.

Organizations usually set aside a fixed amount of money for capital expenditures each year, and they may also rely on charitable foundations to raise money for much-needed equipment and facility upgrades. In many provinces and territories, the Ministry of Health allocates funds for specific operational and capital expenditures. Complete well-documented justifications for new resources must be provided to the associated Ministry of Health because the competition for limited resources is stiff. Such justifications should include the projected amount of use; any services that will be duplicated or replaced; safety considerations; the need for space, personnel, or building renovations; the effect on operational revenues and expenses; and the resource's contribution to the strategic plan.

THE BUDGETING PROCESS

The phases in the budgeting process are similar in most health care organizations, although the budgeting period, budget timetable, and level of manager and employee participation vary. Budgeting is done annually and in relation to the organization's fiscal year. A fiscal year exists for financial purposes and can begin at any point on the calendar, but it is generally from April 1 to March 31. The major phases in the budgeting process include gathering information and planning, developing unit and departmental budgets, negotiating and revising, and using feedback to evaluate budget results and improve future plans (Finkler & McHugh, 2007). Each health care organization develops a timetable with specific dates for implementing the budgeting process. The timetable may be anywhere from 3 to 9 months. The widespread use of computers for budgeting is reducing the time span for budgeting in many organizations. Box 13-5 outlines the budgeting process.

Gathering Information and Planning

The information-gathering and planning phase provides nurse managers with data essential for developing their individual budgets. This phase begins with an environmental assessment that helps the organization understand its position in relation to the entire community. The assessment includes, for example, the changing health care needs of the population, influential economic factors such as inflation and unemployment, differences in payment, and patient satisfaction.

Next, the organization's long-term goals and objectives are reassessed in light of the organization's mission and the environmental assessment. Doing so helps nurse managers situate the budgeting process for

BOX 13-5	OUTLINE OF THE BUDGETING PROCESS

1. Gathering information and planning
   - Environmental assessment
   - Mission, goals, and objectives
   - Program priorities
   - Financial objectives
   - Assumptions (employee raises, inflation, volume projections)
2. Developing unit and departmental budgets
   - Operating budgets
   - Capital budgets
3. Negotiating and revising
4. Evaluating
   - Analysis of variance
   - Critical performance reports

Modified from Finkler, S. A., Kovner, C. T., & Jones, C. (2007). *Financial management for nurse managers and executives* (3rd ed.). St. Louis, MO: Saunders.

their individual units in relation to the whole organization. At this point, programs are prioritized so that resources can be allocated to programs that best help the organization achieve its long-term goals.

Specific, measurable financial objectives are then established, and the budgets must meet these objectives. The financial objectives might include limiting expenditure increases or making reductions in labour costs by designated percentages. Nurse managers also set operational objectives for their units that are in concert with the rest of the organization. At this point, units or departments interpret what effect the changes in operational activities will have on them. For instance, how will using case managers and care maps for selected patients affect a particular unit? Establishing unit-level objectives is also a good way to involve staff nurses in setting the future direction of the unit.

Along with the specific organizational and unit-level operating objectives, nurse managers need to know the organization-wide assumptions that underpin the budgeting process. Explicit assumptions regarding salary increases, inflation factors, and volume projections for the next fiscal year are essential.

Developing Unit and Departmental Budgets

Based on the information gathered, nurse managers can develop operating and capital budgets for their units or departments with their financial managers. These budgets are often developed in tandem because each affects the other. For instance, purchasing a new monitoring system will have implications for the supplies used, staffing, and staff training.

Negotiating and Revising

The negotiating and revising phase is an important part of the budgeting process that may or may not take place at the nurse manager level. This phase is complex because changes in one budget usually require changes in others. Learning to defend and negotiate budgets is an important skill for nurse managers. Nurse managers who successfully negotiate budgets know how costs are allocated and are comfortable speaking about what resources are contained in each budget category. They also can clearly and specifically depict what the effect of not having that resource will be on patients, nurses, and organizational outcomes.

EXERCISE 13-11

Seek an interview with a nurse manager and ask him or her to review the budgeting process with you. Ask specifically about the budget timetable, operating objectives, and organizational assumptions. What was the level of involvement for nurse managers and nurses in each step of budget preparation? Is there a budget manual?

Evaluating, the final and ongoing phase of the budgeting process, relates to the control function of management. Feedback is obtained regularly so that organizational activities can be adjusted to maintain efficient operations. Variance analysis, the major control process used, involves determining differences between projected and actual costs. A variance is the difference between the projected budget and the actual performance for a particular account. For expenses, a favourable, or positive, variance means that the budgeted amount was greater than the actual amount spent. An unfavourable, or negative, variance means that the budgeted amount was less than the actual amount spent. Positive and negative variances cannot be interpreted as good or bad without further investigation. For example, if fewer supplies were used than were budgeted, this difference would appear as a positive variance, showing that the unit saved money. This variance would be good news if it meant that supplies were used more efficiently and patient outcomes remained the same or improved. However, this variance would suggest a problem if using fewer or less-expensive supplies led to poorer patient outcomes.

This variance might also indicate that exactly the right amount of supplies was used but that the patient census (the average number of patients per day or other time period) was less than budgeted. To help managers interpret and use variance information better, some institutions use flexible budgets that automatically account for variances in patient census.

MANAGING THE UNIT-LEVEL BUDGET

At a minimum, nurse managers are responsible for meeting the fiscal goals related to the personnel and the supply and expense part of the operations budget for their unit of operation. Typically, monthly expense reports of operations (see Table 13-3) are sent to nurse managers, who then investigate and explain the underlying cause of variances greater than 5% (depending on the size of the budget). Many factors can cause budget variances, including patient census, patient acuity, vacation time and benefits, illness, orientation, staff meetings, workshops, staff mix, salaries, and staffing levels. To accurately interpret budget variances, nurse managers need reliable data about patient census, acuity, and LOS; payroll reports; and unit productivity reports.

Nurse managers can control *some* but not all of the factors that cause variances. After the causes of variances are determined and if they are controllable by the nurse manager, steps are taken to prevent the variance from occurring in the future. However, even uncontrollable variances that increase expenses might require actions by nurse managers. For example, if supply costs rise drastically because a new technology is being used, the nurse manager might have to look for other areas where the budget can be cut. Information learned from analyzing variances is also used in future budget preparations and management activities. The Research Perspective shows that a review of the literature can help determine the cost impact of implementing certain practices.

EXERCISE 13-12

Examine Table 13-3 and identify major budget variances for the current month. Are the variances favourable or unfavourable? What additional information would help you explain the variances? What are some possible causes for each variance? Are the causes you identified controllable by the nurse manager? Why or why not? Is a favourable variance on expenses always desirable? Why or why not?

TABLE 13-3   BALANCE SHEET, CURRENT MONTH

DESCRIPTION	ACTUAL ($)	BUDGET ($)	VARIANCE ($)	VARIANCE (%)
	REVENUES			
Contributions from the province/territory	167 615	163 635	3 980	2
Patients	206 865	194 624	12 241	6
Recoveries and other revenue	131 559	161 522	(29 963)	–19
Total	**506 039**	**519 781**	**(13 742)**	**–11**
	EXPENSES			
Salaries and wages	8 179 882	8 105 135	(74 747)	–1
Benefit compensation	1 564 280	1 555 934	(8 346)	–1
Sick and severance pay	304 621	312 878	8 257	3
Purchasing services	121 327	15	(121 312)	–808 747
Physician fees	48 422	60 412	11 990	20
Medical supplies	535 945	543 799	7 854	1
Sundry and other expenses	330 694	302 152	(28 542)	–9
Health service provider	115 714	122 443	6 729	5
Total	**11 200 885**	**11 002 768**	**(198 117)**	**–2**
Excess/(deficiency) of revenue over expenses before amortization	**(10 694 846)**	**(10 482 987)**	**(211 859)**	**—**
	AMORTIZATION			
Net invested in capital assets	126 348	123 689	–2 659	–2
Total	**126 348**	**123 689**	**–2 659**	**–2**
Excess/(deficiency) of revenue over expenses after amortization	**(10 821 194)**	**(10 606 676)**	**(214 518)**	**—**

RESEARCH PERSPECTIVE

Resource: Brooks, J. M., Titler, M. G., Ardery, G., et al. (2009). Effect of evidence-based acute pain management practices on inpatient costs. *Health Services Research, 44*(1), 245–263.

A randomized study was undertaken to estimate hospital cost changes associated with the implementation of "translating research into practice" (TRIP) acute pain management practices and to estimate the direct effect that these practices had on inpatient costs. The program was designed to increase the use of evidence-based pain management practices for patients hospitalized with hip fractures. The average cost of implementing the TRIP intervention within a hospital was US$17 714, which included the increased cost of nursing services, special operating rooms, and therapy services. The cost savings per inpatient stay were over US$1500. This study concluded that hospitals treating more than 12 patients with hip fractures can expect to lower their overall cost by implementing the TRIP intervention.

Implications for Practice
The findings from this economic evaluation support the implementation of evidence-based or evidence-informed practices of pain management for patients with hip fractures because the practices will more than pay for themselves in hospitals that treat more than 12 patients with hip fractures.

In addition, nurse managers monitor the productivity of their units. Productivity is the ratio of outputs to inputs; that is, productivity equals output/input. In nursing, outputs are nursing services and are measured by hours of care, number of home visits, and so forth. The inputs are the resources used to provide the services, such as personnel hours and supplies. Only decreasing the inputs or increasing the outputs can increase productivity. Hospitals often use hours per patient day (HPPD) as one measure of productivity. For example, if the standard of care in a critical care unit is 12 HPPD, then 360 hours of care are required for 30 patients for 1 day. When 320 hours of care are provided, the productivity rating is 113% (360 ÷ 320 = 1.13), which means either productivity increased or needed care was not delivered. One must consider the quality component in any productivity model related to care. In home health care, the number of visits per day per registered nurse is one measure of productivity. If the standard is 5 visits per day but the weekly average was 4.8 visits per day, then productivity was decreased. Variances in productivity are not inherently favourable or unfavourable and thus require investigation and explanation before judgements can be made about them. For example, an explanation of the variance (4.8 visits per day) might include the fact that one visit took twice the amount of time normally spent on a home visit because of client needs, thus preventing the nurse from making the standard 5 visits per day. The extra time spent on one client was productive time but not adequately accounted for by this measure of productivity (visits per day).

Although they are not directly accountable for the budget, staff nurses play an important role in meeting budget expectations. Many nurse managers find that routinely sharing the unit's budget and budget-monitoring activities with staff nurses fosters an appreciation of the relationship between cost and the mission to deliver high-quality patient care. Having access to cost and utilization data allows staff nurses to identify patterns and participate in selecting appropriate, cost-effective practice options that work for both staff and patients. Nurse managers and staff nurses who work in partnership to understand that cost versus care is a dilemma to manage rather than a problem to solve will develop innovative, cost-conscious nursing practices that produce good outcomes for patients, nurses, and the organization.

A SOLUTION

Rajesh started by reviewing his staffing clerks and front-line nurse leaders' processes in scheduling vacation and relief, and their decision making regarding overtime approval. He met with the patient care coordinators (PCCs) and staffing clerks and reinforced the approval processes and the policy on vacation scheduling. All overtime would need to be approved by Rajesh, and he would review the overtime report on a monthly basis. He calculated that he needed an additional four full-time equivalents (FTEs) for regular relief positions to fill short-term vacancies and vacation leave at straight-time. He discovered that when the staffing clerk was stressed and busy, she sometimes went directly to the staff member she knew was available, even if doing so resulted in overtime. Thus, Rajesh developed a casual clerk position to assist the staffing clerk on a periodic basis so that more time was available to go through casual call lists to find short-term replacements at straight time. He also cleaned up the casual call list to ensure that people who weren't actually available

were taken off the list. This made the staffing and casual clerks' jobs more efficient by dramatically reducing the calls required to find someone. Rajesh ensured that the vacation scheduling policy was adhered to, which meant that all vacations were scheduled by December of the preceding year so that relief workers could be pre-booked well in advance. He worked with the PCCs and their manager on decision-making algorithms that could make better decisions regarding whether extra staff were required when patient volumes were high. All of these efforts appear to be reaping dividends; the emergency department's overtime rate has dropped by 30%, and Rajesh anticipates further reductions.

Would this be a suitable approach for you? Why or why not?

THE EVIDENCE

Nursing services are a major cost component of health care delivery in Canada. Nurse staffing and scheduling are a critical part of maintaining effective health care services. They also represent a major cost component of health care delivery. Handled effectively, they are an integral part of managing delivery costs. Innovative approaches to nurse staffing and scheduling were explored in a multi-site, collaborative study at four health care organizations (pediatric hospital, continuing care health centre, pediatric rehabilitation hospital, and a community-based hospital) in Ontario (Moreau, Maxwill, Sorfleet, et al., 2010). The

study focused on developing "evaluative strategies and tools for identifying and optimizing promising nurse staffing and scheduling practices" (p. 139). The nurses and those responsible for nurse staffing and scheduling were either interviewed or participated in focus groups for the study. Data from the interviews and focus groups were analyzed to create logic models and evaluation frameworks for each site's nurse staffing and scheduling model, as well as to answer five "evaluability" questions related to the design, implementation, and evaluation of each model (p. 139). The study provided the participating health care organizations

THE EVIDENCE—cont'd

with tools, resources, and knowledge to conduct effective evaluations of nursing staff and scheduling models. The researchers found that evaluability assessments can be catalysts for change and improvements in nurse staffing and scheduling models; evaluability assessments can provide effective tools for stakeholder collaborations; and evaluation is an essential tool for improving nurse staffing and scheduling models.

NEED TO KNOW NOW

- Determine the most commonly used equipment and how much it costs so that you know that aspect of care.
- Know the costs and charges (if applicable) of the 20 most frequently used supplies on your unit.

- Know how to retrieve literature related to best practice in staffing according to patient acuity and patient census.
- Know how to retrieve literature related to cost savings in nursing practice.

CHAPTER CHECKLIST

Financial-thinking skills are the cornerstone of cost-conscious nursing practice and are essential for all nurses. Nurses must also determine whether the services they provide add value for patients. Services that add value are of high quality, positively affect health outcomes, and minimize costs.

Understanding what constitutes costs and why organizations must remain cost conscious to provide sustainable services is basic to financial thinking in health care. Knowing what is included in operating and capital budgets; how they interrelate; and how they are developed, monitored, and controlled is also important. Considering the ethical implications of financial decisions and collectively managing the cost–care dilemma are imperative for cost-conscious nursing practice.

- Total health care costs are a function of the prices and the utilization rates of services.
- In Canada, the government is the major source of funding for health care services, followed by private insurance companies. Individuals are the third major payer.

- Health care is financed through a range of mechanisms, including a global budget transfer from the provincial and territorial governments, activity-based funding, fee-for-service, pay-for-performance, and direct billing.
- Nurses and nurse managers directly influence an organization's ability to remain on budget.
- Cost-conscious nursing practices include the following:
  - Knowing and controlling costs
  - Using time efficiently
  - Discussing the cost of care with patients
  - Meeting patient rather than provider needs
  - Evaluating cost-effectiveness of new technologies
  - Predicting and using nursing resources efficiently
  - Using research to evaluate standard nursing practices
- Nurse managers have the most influence on costs in relation to managing personnel and supplies.
- Variance analysis is the major control process in relation to budgeting.

TIPS FOR MANAGING COSTS AND BUDGETS

- Know the major changes in the organization and how they might affect the organization's budget.
- Analyze the supplies you use in providing care and what is commonly missing as one way to make recommendations about supply needs.
- Evaluate what each of your patients would find most helpful during the time you will be caring for them.

- Decide which of your actions create costs for the patient or the organization.
- Be aware of how changes in patient acuity and patient census affect staffing requirements and the unit budget.
- Examine the upsides and downsides of the cost–care dilemma thoughtfully.

evolve WEBSITE

Visit the Evolve website for Suggested Readings, Internet Resources, and additional resources related to the content in this chapter: http://evolve.elsevier.com/Canada/Yoder-Wise/leading/.

REFERENCES

Statutes

Canada Health Act, RSC 1985, c. C-6 (Canada).

Texts

Accreditation Canada. (2013). Saskatchewan Lean Management System (LMS). Retrieved from http://www.accreditation.ca/saskatchewan-lean-management-system-lms.

British Columbia Ministry of Health. (2010, October 8). Presentation to the Health Operations Committee.

Brooks, J. M., Titler, M. G., Ardery, G., et al. (2009). Effect of evidence-based acute pain management practices on inpatient costs. *Health Services Research*, 44(1), 245–263.

Canadian Institute for Health Information. (2013a). *Drug expenditure in Canada, 1985 to 2012*. Ottawa, ON: Author. Retrieved from https://secure.cihi.ca/free_products/Drug_Expenditure_2013_EN.pdf.

Canadian Institute for Health Information. (2013b). *National health expenditure trends 1975 to 2013*. Ottawa, ON: Author. Retrieved from https://secure.cihi.ca/free_products/NHEXTrendsReport_EN.pdf.

Canadian Nurses Association. (2009, September). Position statement: Financing Canada's health system. Retrieved from http://www.nanb.nb.ca/PDF/CNA_FinancingCanadas_Health_System_2009_E.pdf.

Caulford, P., & Yasmin, V. (2006). Providing health care to medically uninsured immigrants and refugees. *Canadian Medical Association Journal*, 174(9), 1253–1254.

Centers for Medicare & Medicaid Services. (2014). National health expenditures 2012 highlights. Retrieved from http://www.cms.gov/Research-Statistics-Data-and-Systems/Statistics-Trends-and-Reports/NationalHealthExpendData/Downloads/highlights.pdf.

Church, J., & Barker, P. (1998). Regionalization of health services in Canada: A critical perspective. *International Journal of Health Services: Planning, Administration, Evaluation*, 28(3), 467–486.

College and Association of Registered Nurses of Alberta. (2008). Evidence-informed staffing for delivery of nursing care: Guidelines for registered nurses. Retrieved from http://www.nurses.ab.ca/Carna-Admin/Uploads/Evidence_Nursing_Care.pdf.

Employment and Social Development Canada. (n.d.). Canadians in context—Aging population. Retrieved from http://www4.hrsdc.gc.ca/.3ndic.1t.4r@-eng.jsp?iid=33.

Finkler, S. A., Kovner, C. T., & Jones, C. (2007). *Financial management for nurse managers and executives* (3rd ed.). St. Louis, MO: Saunders.

Finkler, S. A., & McHugh, M. (2007). *Budgeting concepts for nurse managers* (4th ed.). St. Louis, MO: Saunders.

Government of Saskatchewan. (2012). Introduction to Lean. Retrieved from http://www.health.gov.sk.ca/lean-introduction.

Jones, C. B., & Gates, M. (2007). The costs and benefits of nurse turnover: A business case for nurse retention. *Online Journal of Issues in Nursing*, 12(3), Manuscript 4.

Keller, P., & Pyzdek, T. (2009). *The six sigma handbook* (3rd ed.). n.p.: McGraw-Hill Education.

Koelling, T. M., Johnson, M. L., Cody, R. J., et al. (2005). Discharge education improves clinical outcomes in patients with chronic heart failure. *Circulation*, 111, 179–185.

Li, S. (2006, December). Health care financing policies of Canada, the United Kingdom and Taiwan. Retrieved from http://www.legco.gov.hk/yr06-07/english/sec/library/0607rp02-e.pdf.

Liker, C. (2003). *The Toyota way: 14 management principles from the world's greatest manufacturer*. New York, NY: McGraw-Hill Professional.

Makarenko, J. (2010, October 22). Canada's health care system: An overview of public and private participation. Retrieved from http://www.mapleleafweb.com/features/canada-s-health-care-system-overview-public-and-private-participation#elements.

Manitoba Centre for Health Policy. (2010a). Concept: Case mix groups (CMG™)—Overview. Retrieved from http://mchp-appserv.cpe.umanitoba.ca/viewConcept.php?conceptID=1094.

Manitoba Centre for Health Policy. (2010b). Term: Resource Intensity Weights (RIW™). Retrieved from http://mchp-appserv.cpe.umanitoba.ca/viewDefinition.php?definitionID=103807.

Ministry of Health Services, Fraser Health, and Vancouver Coastal Health. (2009, March 2). Innovation reduces ER congestion in lower mainland [Press release]. Retrieved from http://www2.news.gov.bc.ca/news_releases_2005-2009/2009HSERV0019-000256.htm.

Moreau, K., Maxwill, H., Sorfleet, C., et al. (2010). Innovative approaches to staffing and scheduling [Special Issue]. *Nursing Leadership*, 23, 138–139. doi:10.12927/cjnl.2010.21758

Sutherland, J. M. (2011, March). *Hospital payment mechanisms: An overview and options for Canada*. Ottawa, ON: Canadian Health Services Research Foundation. Retrieved from http://www.cfhi-fcass.ca/Libraries/Hospital_Funding_docs/CHSRF-Sutherland-HospitalFundingENG.sflb.ashx.

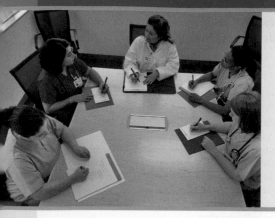

Care Delivery Strategies

Susan Sportsman
Adapted by Heather MacMillan

This chapter presents the nursing care delivery models used in health care organizations. It explores the historical development and structure of the case method; functional nursing; team nursing; primary nursing, including hybrid forms of this approach; and nursing case management. The chapter also summarizes the benefits and disadvantages of each model and describes the roles of nurse manager and staff nurse in each model. In addition, the chapter reviews care strategies that influence care delivery, such as disease management, differentiated practice, and "transforming care at the bedside."

OBJECTIVES

- Define the nursing care delivery models used in health care.
- Describe the role of the nurse manager and the staff nurse in each model.
- Describe disease-management programs.
- Summarize the differentiated nursing practice model and related methods to determine competencies of nurses who deliver care.
- Consider the impact of Transforming Care at the Bedside (TCAB) on the delivery of care in a nursing unit.

TERMS TO KNOW

case management model	functional nursing	staff mix
case manager	nursing care delivery model	Synergy Model
case method	nursing case management	team nursing
charge nurse	outcome criteria	total patient care
clinical nurse leader (CNL)	partnership model	Transforming Care at the Bedside
clinical pathway	patient-focused care model	(TCAB)
differentiated nursing practice	patient outcomes	unregulated care providers
disease management	primary nurse	(UCPs)
expected outcomes	primary nursing	variance

A CHALLENGE

The charge nurses in a newly built 25-bed medical unit were finding it increasingly difficult to make patient assignments because of the layout and design of the 1800-square-metre unit. Furthermore, throughout the shift, the nursing staff were having problems remaining engaged with the activities on the unit because of the distance between bedside stations. Also, the design of the unit made it difficult for a nurse to ask for help when needed. After occupying the unit for several months and trying numerous methods to enhance teamwork and communication among the staff, it was apparent that a more formal process was needed to resolve these problems. As the patient care manager (PCM) and registered nurse, Adeyele was tasked with resolving the problems.

What would you do if you were Adeyele?

INTRODUCTION

A nursing care delivery model is the method used to provide care to patients. Because nursing care is viewed by some as a cost rather than a method of cost savings, it is logical for institutions to evaluate their method of providing patient care for the purpose of saving money while still providing quality care. In this chapter, various models of nursing care delivery are discussed, including the case method (total patient care); functional nursing; team nursing; primary nursing, including hybrid forms; and nursing case management. In addition, the influence of disease-management programs, differentiated nursing practice, and Transforming Care at the Bedside are discussed.

Each nursing care delivery model has advantages and disadvantages, and none is ideal. Some models are conducive to large institutions, while others work better in smaller settings. Managers in any organization must examine the organizational goals, the unit objectives, patient population, staff availability, and the budget when selecting a care delivery model. A historical overview of the common care models is designed to convey the complexity of how care is delivered. Each of these models is still used within the broad range of health care organizations. In addition, these models often serve as the foundation for new and innovative care delivery models.

CASE METHOD (TOTAL PATIENT CARE)

The case method, or total patient care method, of nursing care delivery is the oldest model of providing care to patients. This model should not be confused with *nursing case management*, which is introduced later in the chapter.

The premise of the case method is that one nurse provides total care for one patient during the entire work period. This method was used in the era of Florence Nightingale (1820–1910), when patients received total care in the home. Today, total patient care is used in critical care settings where one nurse provides total care to one or two critically ill patients. Nurse educators often select this method of care when students are learning to care for patients. Variations of the case method exist, and it is possible to identify similarities among them after reviewing other models of care delivery described later in this chapter.

Model Analysis

During an 8- or 12-hour shift, the patient receives consistent care from one nurse. The nurse, patient, and family usually trust one another and work together toward specific goals. Usually, the care is patient-centred, comprehensive, continuous, and holistic. But the nurse may choose to deliver this care with a task orientation that negates the holistic perspective (Shirey, 2008). Because the nurse is with the patient during most of the shift, even subtle changes in the patient's status are easily noticed (Figure 14-1).

In today's costly health care environment, total patient care provided by one nurse is very expensive. Is it realistic to use a highly skilled and extremely knowledgeable professional nurse to provide all the care required in a unit that may have 20 to 30 patients? Who would oversee the care coordination in a 24-hour period (Shirey, 2008)? In times of nursing shortages, there may not be enough nurses to use this model.

Nurse Manager's Role

When using the case method, the nurse manager must consider the expense of the system. He or she must weigh the expense of a registered nurse (RN) or registered psychiatric nurse (RPN) versus the

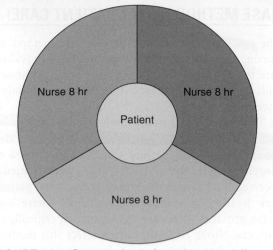
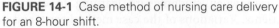

FIGURE 14-1 Case method of nursing care delivery for an 8-hour shift.

expense of licensed or registered practical nurses and **unregulated care providers (UCPs)** in the context of the outcomes required. See Chapter 5 for the differences between regulated and unregulated health care workers. UCPs, as the name connotes, are caregivers who are not licensed as health care providers and are known by many titles, including *home support workers, personal support workers, resident aides,* and *health care aides* (Harris & McGillis Hall, 2012). When a patient requires 24-hour care, a nurse manager must decide the type of nurse to be deployed to best meet the needs of the patient and whether supervised UCPs might be used.

Staff Nurse's Role

In the case method, the staff nurse provides holistic care to a group of patients during a defined work time. The physical, emotional, and technical aspects of care are the responsibility of the assigned nurse. This model is especially useful in the care of very complex patients who need active symptom management provided by an RN or specially educated nurse, for example, a patient in an acute pain management setting or a critical care unit. The staff nurse who is assigned to total patient care must complete the complex functions of care, such as assessment and teaching the patient and family, as well as the less complex functions of care, such as personal hygiene. Some nurses find satisfaction with this model of care

because no aspect of nursing care is delegated to another nurse, thus eliminating the need for supervision of others (Shirey, 2008).

FUNCTIONAL NURSING

Functional nursing became popular during World War II, when there was a severe shortage of nurses (Shirey, 2008). At the time, many nurses joined the armed forces to care for the soldiers. To provide care to patients at home, hospitals began to increase the number of practical nurses and UCPs.

Functional nursing is a model for providing patient care in which each regulated and unregulated member of the care team performs specific tasks for a large group of patients. These tasks are in part determined by the scope of practice defined for each type of caregiver. For example, an RN may be responsible for all assessments, and practical nurses and UCPs may be responsible for collecting data that can be used in assessments. Regarding treatments, one RN may administer all intravenous (IV) medications, a licensed practical nurse may provide oral medications, and two special care aides may do all hygiene tasks, check supplies, and take all vital signs (Figure 14-2).

Nursing comprises regulated nurses (RN, licensed practical nurse, registered practical nurse) who have specialized nursing skills, and advanced nursing skills, which means that the functional division of nursing work among qualified personnel can become complicated. In this model, the division of nursing work is similar to the division of work used in assembly-line systems in manufacturing. Just as an auto worker

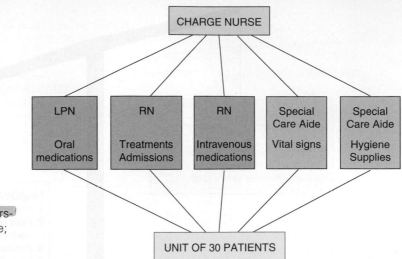

FIGURE 14-2 Functional model of nursing care delivery. *RN*, registered nurse; *LPN*, licensed practical nurse; *SCA*, special care aide.

becomes an expert in attaching fenders to a new vehicle, the staff nurse becomes an expert in the specific tasks associated with his or her role in functional nursing. A **charge nurse** is an RN responsible for delegating and coordinating patient care and staff on a specific unit. The charge nurse may ultimately be the only person familiar with all the needs of any individual patient.

Model Analysis

Functional nursing has several advantages. First, each nurse becomes efficient at specific tasks, and much work can be done in a short time. Another advantage is that UCPs can be trained to perform one or two specific tasks very well. The organization benefits financially from this model because care can be delivered to a large number of patients by mixing a small number of regulated nurses and a larger number of UCPs.

Although financial savings may be the impetus for organizations to choose the functional nursing model, the disadvantages may outweigh the savings (Figure 14-3). A major disadvantage is the fragmentation of care. The physical and technical aspects of care may be met, but the psychological and spiritual needs of care may be overlooked. Patients can become confused about who they should consult because many different health care providers care for them per shift. Moreover, the different staff members may be so busy with their assigned tasks that they may not have time to communicate with one another about the patient's progress.

Because no one care provider oversees patient care from beginning to end, the patient's response to care is difficult to assess. Critical changes in patient status may go unnoticed. Fragmented care and ineffective communication can lead to patient and family dissatisfaction and frustration. Exercise 14-2 provides an opportunity to imagine how a patient would react to the functional method and also to imagine how the nurse may feel.

EXERCISE 14-2

Imagine that your mother is a patient at a hospital that uses the functional model of patient-care delivery. She just had her knee replaced, and when you ask the practical nurse for pain medication, she says, "I'll tell the medication nurse." The medication nurse comes to the room and says that your mother's medication is to be administered intravenously and that the IV nurse will need to administer it. The IV nurse is busy starting an IV on another patient and cannot give your mother the medication for at least 10 minutes. This whole communication process has taken 40 minutes, and your mother is still in pain. Discuss your perception of the effectiveness of the functional method of patient care in this situation. How effective do you think communication among staff is when a patient has a problem? What could be done to improve this situation?

Nurse Manager's Role

In the functional model, the nurse manager must be sensitive to the quality of patient care delivered and the institution's budgetary constraints. Because staff members are responsible only for their specific tasks,

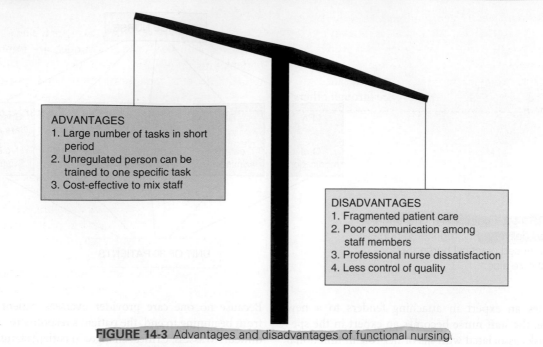

FIGURE 14-3 Advantages and disadvantages of functional nursing.

the role of achieving patient outcomes (the result of patient goals that are achieved through a combination of medical and nursing interventions with patient participation) becomes the nurse manager's responsibility.

Staff members can view this system as autocratic and may become discontented with the lack of opportunity for input. By using effective management and leadership skills, the nurse manager can improve the staff's perception that they lack independence. The manager can rotate assignments among staff within the legal limits of their role and as appropriate to each person's skill set to alleviate boredom with repetition. Staff meetings should be conducted frequently. They give staff the opportunity to express concerns and communicate about patient care and unit functions.

Staff Nurse's Role

The staff nurse becomes skilled at the tasks that are assigned to them, usually by the charge nurse. Clearly defined policies and procedures are used to complete the physical aspects of care in a safe, efficient, and economical manner. However, the functional model of nursing may leave the professional nurse feeling frustrated because of the task-oriented role. Nurses are educated to care for the patient holistically, and

providing only a fragment of care to a patient may result in the unmet personal and professional expectations of nurses.

> **EXERCISE 14-3**
>
> After 6 months of working on a unit that accommodates patients who have had general surgery, you realize that you are bored and frustrated with the functional model of delivering care. You have been administering all the IV medications and pain medications for your assigned patients. You have minimal opportunity to interact with the patients and learn about them, and you cannot be innovative in your care. Discuss strategies you could use to resolve this dissatisfaction with the functional model of nursing care delivery.

The functional model of nursing care delivery works well in emergency and disaster situations. Each health care provider knows the expectations of the assigned role and completes the tasks quickly and efficiently. Subacute care units, extended care facilities, and ambulatory clinics often use the functional model to deliver care quickly.

TEAM NURSING

After World War II, the nursing shortage continued. Many female nurses who were in the military came home to marry and have children instead of returning to the workforce. Because of criticisms of the functional model (discussed earlier), a new system of team nursing (a modification of functional nursing) was devised to improve nurse and patient satisfaction (Harris & McGillis Hall, 2012). "Care through others" is the hallmark of team nursing. This type of nursing care delivery remains in use, particularly when nursing shortages have resulted in organizations changing the staff mix (the proportion of regulated nurses and UCPs in a specific setting) and increasing the ratio of unregulated to regulated care providers.

In team nursing, a nurse team leader is responsible for coordinating a group of regulated and unregulated personnel to provide patient care to a group of patients. The team leader should be a highly skilled leader, manager, and practitioner who assigns each member specific responsibilities according to role, licensure, education, ability, and the complexity of the care required. The members of the team report directly to the team leader, who then reports to the charge nurse or unit manager (Figure 14-4 provides an illustration of this model). Each unit has several teams, and patient assignments are made by each team leader.

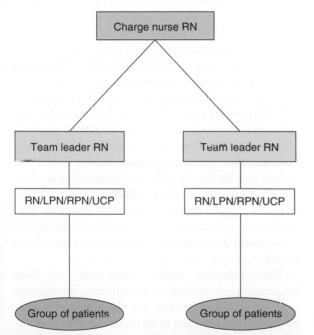

FIGURE 14-4 Team nursing model. *RN*, registered nurse; *LPN*, licensed practical nurse; *RPN*, registered practical nurse; *UCP*, unregulated care provider.

Model Analysis

Some advantages of team nursing, particularly when compared with the functional model, are improved patient satisfaction, decision making by staff nurses (which enhances their satisfaction), and cost-effectiveness for the employer. Many institutions and community health agencies currently use the team nursing method. Inpatient facilities may view team nursing as a cost-effective system because it works with a higher ratio of unregulated to regulated personnel. Thus, the organization has greater numbers of personnel for a designated amount of money.

Team nursing has one major disadvantage, which arises if the team leader has poor leadership skills. The team leader must have excellent communication skills, delegation and conflict-management abilities, strong clinical skills, and effective decision-making abilities to provide a working "team" environment for the members. The team leader must be sensitive to the needs of patients and, at the same time, be responsive to the needs of the staff providing direct care (Fairbrother, Jones, & Rivas, 2010; Shirey, 2008). When the team leader is not prepared for this role, the team nursing method becomes a miniature version of the functional model, and the potential for fragmentation of care is high. For more details on developing leadership skills, see Chapter 3.

EXERCISE 14-4

Think of a time when you worked with a group of four to six people to achieve a specific goal or accomplish a task (perhaps in school you were grouped together to complete a project). How did your group achieve the goal? Was one person the organizer or leader? How was the leader selected? Do you see yourself as a leader? Do you see yourself as a follower? Who assigned each member a component, or did you each determine what skills you possessed that would most benefit the group? Did you experience any conflict while working on this project? How did the concepts of group dynamics and leadership skills affect how your group achieved its goal? What similarities do you see between the team nursing system of providing patient care and your group involvement to achieve a goal?

Nurse Manager's Role

The nurse manager, charge nurse, and team leader must have management skills to effectively implement the team nursing method of nursing care delivery. In addition, the nurse manager must determine which nurses are skilled and interested in becoming a charge nurse or team leader. Because the basic education of baccalaureate-prepared RNs emphasizes critical thinking and leadership concepts, they are likely candidates for such roles. The nurse manager should also provide an adequate staff mix and orient team members to the team nursing system by providing continuing education about leadership, management techniques, delegation, and team interaction (see Chapters 1, 3, 4, 18, and 26). By addressing these factors, the nurse manager is helping the teams function optimally.

The charge nurse functions as a liaison between the team leaders and other health care providers because nurse managers are often responsible for more than one unit and/or have other managerial responsibilities that take them away from the unit. The charge nurse provides support to the teams on a shift-by-shift basis. Appropriate support from the charge nurse may include encouraging each team to solve its problems independently.

The team leader plans the care, delegates the work, and follows up with members to evaluate the quality of care for the patients assigned to his or her team. Ideally, the team leader updates the nursing care plans and facilitates patient-care conferences. Time constraints during the shift may prevent scheduling daily patient-care conferences or prevent some team members from attending those that are held.

The team leader must also face the challenge of changing team membership on a daily basis. Diverse work schedules and nursing staff shortages may result in daily changes in the staff mix of a team and a daily assignment change for team members. The team leader assigns the regulated and unregulated care providers to the type of patient care they are best prepared to deliver. Therefore, the team leader must be knowledgeable about the legal limits of their scope of practice and associated skill sets of each role.

Staff Nurse's Role

Team nursing uses the strengths of each caregiver. Staff nurses, as members of the team, develop expertise in care delivery. Some members become known for their expertise in the psychomotor aspects of care. If one nurse is skilled in starting IVs, she will start all IVs for her team of patients. If another nurse is skilled in motivating postoperative patients to use the incentive spirometer and ambulate, he would be assigned to the surgical patients. Under the guidance and supervision of the team leader, the collective efforts of the team become greater than the functions of the individual caregivers.

PRIMARY NURSING

A cultural revolution occurred in Canada and the United States during the 1960s. The revolution emphasized individual rights and independence from existing societal restrictions. This revolution also influenced the nursing profession because nurses were becoming dissatisfied with their lack of autonomy and began to focus more on professionalism and accountability (Shirey, 2008). In addition, the hierarchical nature of communication in team nursing caused further frustration. Institutions were also aware of the declining quality of patient care. The search for autonomy and quality care led to the primary nursing model, which increases nurse accountability for patient outcomes.

Primary nursing, an adaptation of the case method, was developed by Marie Manthey as a model for organizing patient-care delivery in which one nurse functions autonomously as the patient's primary nurse throughout the hospital stay (Manthey, Ciske, Robertson, et al., 1970). Primary nursing brought the nurse back to direct patient care. The primary nurse is a registered nurse who is responsible for planning and delivering care to a consistent group of patients. The primary nurse is accountable for patients' care 24 hours a day from admission through discharge. As well, the primary nurse plans, collaborates, communicates, and coordinates all aspects of patient care with other nurses as well as other disciplines (Shirey, 2008). Conceptually, primary nursing care provides the patient and the family with coordinated, comprehensive, continuous care (Shirey, 2008). Care is organized using the nursing process (e.g., assess, diagnose, plan, implement, and evaluate). Advocacy and assertiveness are desirable leadership attributes for this care delivery model.

The primary nurse, preferably at least baccalaureate-prepared, is accountable for meeting outcome criteria (criteria are the result of patient goals that are expected to be achieved) and communicating with all other health care providers about the patient (Figure 14-5). These criteria are the result of patient goals that are expected to be achieved through

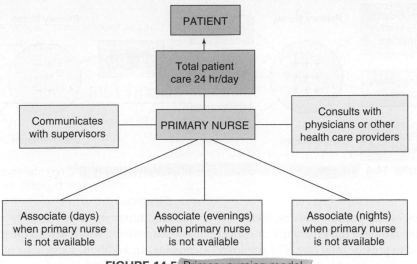

FIGURE 14-5 Primary nursing model.

a combination of nursing and medical interventions. For example, a patient with pulmonary edema is admitted to a medical unit. His primary nurse admits him and then provides a written plan of care. When his primary nurse is not working, an associate nurse implements the plan. The associate nurse is a nurse who is a member of the primary nursing team and provides care to the patient according to the plan of care. If the patient develops additional complications, the associate nurse notifies the primary nurse, who has 24-hour accountability and responsibility. The associate nurse provides input to the patient's plan of care, and the primary nurse makes the appropriate alterations.

Model Analysis

Tiedeman and Lookinland (2004) cited numerous studies that speak to the quality of care and patient satisfaction with primary care. Some studies found that primary care resulted in increased quality of care and patient satisfaction, whereas others found that the model made no difference to these parameters when compared with team nursing. More recently, some findings suggest that while the use of primary care is favoured, and that there are some improvements in staff outcomes and patient well-being, more research is needed (Butler, Collins, Drennan, et al., 2011; Hodgkinson, Haesler, Nay, et al., 2011). Nurses practising primary nursing must possess a broad knowledge base

and have highly developed nursing skills. Professionalism is promoted in this system of care delivery. Nurses experience job satisfaction because they can use their education to provide holistic and autonomous care to patients. The high level of accountability for patient outcomes encourages nurses to further their knowledge and refine their skills to provide optimal patient care. If the primary nurse is not motivated or feels unqualified to provide holistic care, job satisfaction may decrease.

In primary nursing, patients and families are typically satisfied with the care they receive because they establish a relationship with the primary nurse and identify the caregiver as "their nurse." Because the patient's primary nurse communicates the plan of care, the patient can move away from the sick role and begin to participate in his or her own recovery. By considering the sociocultural, psychological, and physical needs of the patient and family, the primary nurse can plan the most appropriate care with and for the patient and family.

A professional advantage of the primary nursing model is a decrease in the number of unregulated personnel. The ideal primary nursing system requires an all-nurse staff. The nurse can provide total care to the patient, from bed baths to patient education, even both at the same time! Unregulated personnel are not qualified to provide this level of inclusive care (Figure 14-6).

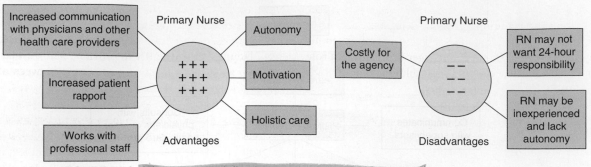

FIGURE 14-6 Advantages and disadvantages of primary nursing. *RN*, registered nurse.

A disadvantage of the primary nursing method is that the nurse may not have the experience or educational background to provide total care. The employer needs to educate staff for an adequate transition from the previous role to the primary role. In addition, one has to ask whether the primary nurse is ready, willing, and capable of handling the 24-hour responsibility for patient care.

EXERCISE 14-5

Mr. Faulkner is admitted to the medical unit with exacerbated congestive heart failure. Mohamed, RN, BSN, is Mr. Faulkner's primary nurse and will provide total care to Mr. Faulkner. Mohamed notes that this is Mr. Faulkner's third admission in 6 months for congestive heart failure–related symptoms. This is the first admission for which Mr. Faulkner has had a primary nurse. What do you think might be different about this admission, with Mohamed providing primary nursing to Mr. Faulkner? Do you think any difference will occur in the continuity of care? How involved do you think Mr. Faulkner will be with his own care in the primary nursing system?

In times of nursing shortages, primary nursing may not be the model of choice. This model will not be effective if a unit has a large number of part-time nurses who are not available to assume the primary nurse role (which assumes 24-hour responsibility). In addition, with the arrival of managed care in the 1990s, patients' hospital stays were shorter than in the 1970s, when primary nursing became popular. Expedited stays make it challenging for primary nurses to adequately provide the depth of care required by primary nursing. If the patient is admitted on Monday and discharged on Wednesday, the primary nurse has a difficult time meeting all patient needs before discharge if he or she is not working on Tuesday. The

primary nurse must rely heavily on feedback from associate nurses, which defeats the purpose of primary nursing. In addition, reductions in health care funding caused administrators to consider ways to reduce the cost of care delivery. Because labour costs are the largest expense in health care delivery and nursing staff represent the largest portion of labour costs, attention was given to reducing these costs with changes to the model of care delivery.

EXERCISE 14-6

Imagine that you are a primary nurse at an inpatient psychiatric facility. The patients you are assigned to are usually suicidal. How would you feel about the added responsibility for patients when you were not at work? Is it realistic to expect a nurse in this facility to assume the role of primary nurse with 24-hour responsibility? How would this responsibility affect your personal life? How would you make decisions about the patients and your home life?

Nurse Manager's Role

The primary nursing model can be modified to meet patient, nursing, and budgetary demands while maintaining the positive components that spawned its conception. The nurse manager needs to determine the desire of staff to become primary nurses and then train them accordingly. The associate nurses and all other health care providers need clearly defined roles. They also need to be aware of the primary nurse's role and the importance of communicating concerns directly to that nurse.

The nurse manager who implements this care delivery model experiences some benefits. Primary nursing provides the nurse manager an opportunity to demonstrate leadership capabilities, clinical competencies, and teaching abilities. In addition, the nurse manager roles of budget controller and unit quality manager remain. The traditional roles of delegation and decision making must be relinquished to the autonomous primary nurse. The nurse manager functions as a role model, advocate, coach, and consultant.

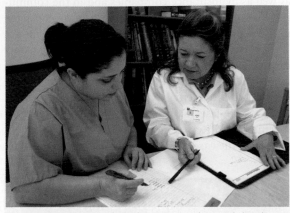

The nurse manager functions as a role model, advocate, coach, and consultant.

Staff Nurse's Role

The primary nurse uses many facets of the professional nursing role—caregiver, advocate, decision maker, teacher, collaborator, and manager. Because primary nurses cannot be present 24 hours a day, they must depend on associate nurses to provide care when they are not available. The associate nurse provides care using the plan of care developed by the primary nurse. Changes to the plan of care can be made by the associate nurse in collaboration with the primary nurse. This model provides consistency among nurses and shifts. To function effectively in this setting, staff nurses need experience and opportunities to be mentored in this role.

Because it usually is not financially possible for an employer to employ only highly qualified nurses, true primary nursing rarely exists. Some institutions have modified the primary nursing concept and implemented a partnership model to incorporate their current staff mix.

Primary Nursing Hybrid: Partnership Model

In the partnership model (or *co-primary nursing model*) of nursing care delivery, an RN is paired with another nurse (e.g., a technical assistant). The partner works with the RN consistently. When the partner is unregulated, the RN allows the assistant to perform basic nursing functions consistent with the provincial or territorial nursing regulatory body policy on delegation. Doing so frees the RN to provide "semi-primary care" to assigned patients. A partnership between an RN and a licensed practical nurse allows the latter to take more responsibility because the scope of practice for a licensed practical nurse is greater than that of a UCP. In some settings, the partnership is legitimized with an official contract to formalize the relationship. Rehabilitative care settings often use the partnership model to deliver care.

EXERCISE 14-7

You are a primary nurse in a surgical critical care unit of a small hospital. The unit you work on uses a registered nurse–licensed practical nurse partnership to decrease the number of RNs required per shift. You and your partner are assigned four surgical patients. Mr. Joyce had a lobectomy 5 hours ago and is on a ventilator; Mrs. Martinez had a quadruple cardiac bypass 14 hours ago; Mr. Tam had a nephrectomy 2 days ago and is receiving continuous peritoneal dialysis; and Mr. Tremblay has a fractured pelvis and is comatose from a motor vehicle accident 24 hours ago. How would you distribute the staff to provide primary care to these four patients? Do you think it is possible to provide primary care in this situation? What responsibilities would you assume as the primary nurse, and what could you share with the licensed practical nurse?

Primary Nursing Hybrid: Patient-Focused Care

Another view of primary care is the care delivered in a patient-focused care model. Developed in the mid-1980s and 1990s, the patient-focused care model is a team-based approach to care incorporating principles of patient-centred care (PCC) (Hobbs, 2009) with the goals of (1) improving patient satisfaction and other patient outcomes, (2) improving worker job satisfaction, and (3) increasing efficiencies and decreasing costs (Seago, 1999). This model integrates principles from business and industry and features decentralized, efficient, coordinated, and integrated care (Pelzang, 2010). The multidisciplinary team formulates the plan of care after the primary nurse and the physician have assessed the patient.

Patient-focused care units require a change in the physical environment where care is delivered. Services such as laboratory and X-rays are decentralized to the bedside (Hobbs, 2009). Original models of a patient-focused care unit included an RN paired with a cross-trained technician who provided patient-side care, including respiratory therapy, phlebotomy, and electrocardiographs. Modifications in this nurse-managed model include team members who provide direct care activities such as recording vital signs, drawing blood, and bathing patients.

In a patient-focused care unit, the role and scope of the nurse manager expand. No longer is the individual just a manager of nurses. Now the nurse manager assumes the accountability and responsibility to manage nurses and staff from other, traditionally centralized departments. Because the care is focused on the needs of the patient and not the needs of the department, the role of the nurse manager becomes more sophisticated. The nurse manager orchestrates all the care activities required by the patient and family during the hospitalization. Implementing this philosophy and model of care requires building a culture of patient-centredness and developing a new understanding about one's beliefs, attitudes, and practices toward providing care (Pelzang, 2010).

NURSING CASE MANAGEMENT

Nursing case management, another nursing care delivery model, involves a complex set of expectations. Case management is the process of coordinating health care by planning, facilitating, and evaluating interventions across levels of care to achieve cost containment and quality outcomes.

The model first appeared in the early 1900s; it was used by social workers and public health nurses working in the public sector to identify and obtain resources for the needy. In the 1970s, when a variety of factors forced health care costs upward, contemporary nursing case management began to be utilized in an effort to assure quality outcomes and cost containment (White & Hall, 2006).

In the United States during the mid-1980s, when acute care hospitals began to be reimbursed based on certain diagnoses, nursing case management became a popular and effective method to manage shortened lengths of stay for patients and to prevent expensive hospital re-admissions. In Canada, pieces of the case management model were adopted as length of stay and costs in health care settings were scrutinized; however, this change occurred primarily in community settings at

first (Cawthorn, 2005). The nursing case management process can take place "within the walls" or "beyond the walls" of the hospital. This model has been applied successfully in all health care settings, including acute, subacute, ambulatory settings, and long-term care facilities, as well as by insurance companies and in the community (Cawthorn, 2005). Table 14-1 identifies some of the service settings that use this nursing care delivery model.

The case management model maintains quality care while streamlining costs. It also requires the active involvement of the patient, the family, and diverse health care providers. Health care organizations have tailored the case management system to meet their specific needs. Key elements of the case management model are the case manager and the clinical pathway.

TABLE 14-1	NURSING CASE MANAGEMENT SERVICE AREAS
CATEGORY	**SERVICE SETTING**
Acute	Orthopedics, cardiovascular, critical care, high-risk perinatal, oncology, emergency department
Subacute	Skilled long-term care facilities, rehabilitation units
Ambulatory	Physicians' offices, clinics
Long-term care	Long-term care homes, group homes, assisted-living facilities
Insurance companies	Provincial workers' compensation agencies
Community	Nurse-managed health centres, home health care agencies, urgent care centres, schools, rural settings, mental health centres

Adapted from Cohen, E., & Cesta, T. (2004). *Nursing case management: From essentials to advanced practice applications* (4th ed.). St. Louis, MO: Mosby; Curtis, K., Lien, D., Chan, A., et al. (2002). The impact of trauma case management on patient outcomes. *Journal of Trauma, 53*(3), 477–482; Huber, D. (2010). *Leadership and nursing case management* (4th ed.). St. Louis, MO: Saunders.

Case Manager

Nurses, social workers, and other disciplines may work as case managers, bringing with them their discipline-specific skills and knowledge. Regardless of preparation, the National Case Management Network of Canada (2009) has identified the following six core standards to guide case manager practice.

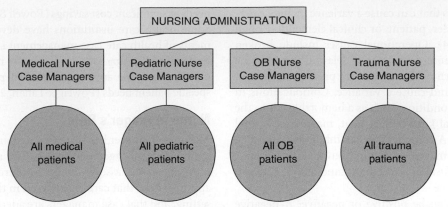

FIGURE 14-7 Nursing case management model in which all patients are assigned to a case manager. *OB,* Obstetric.

1. *Client identification and eligibility for case management services:* Clients who meet the eligibility criteria for case management services are identified.
2. *Assessment:* In conjunction with the client, the case manager conducts and documents an individualized assessment using a structured process.
3. *Planning:* Client goals and priorities are documented and are reflected in the strategy for action agreed upon between the client and the case manager.
4. *Implementation:* Planned services, resources, and supports are initiated, coordinated, and adjusted as necessary.
5. *Evaluation:* A periodic reassessment is conducted to identify the client's current needs and to monitor progress within the client's individualized plan.
6. Transition: A process that supports disengagement or shift in the mechanisms for achieving client goals (pp. 10–15)

Although there is inconsistency among nursing professional associations about the education required for case managers, many prefer master's degree–prepared clinical nurse specialists who have advanced practice with the specific populations being served. Case managers are patient focused and outcome oriented. Their goal is to provide cost-effective care by integrating financial thinking into clinical services. In addition, case managers serve as advocates for the patient and the family. The National Case Management Network of Canada (http://www.ncmn.ca) has developed principles to guide case management. Case managers support client rights, are purposeful, are collaborative, support accountability, and strive for cultural competency (National Case Management Network of Canada, 2009).

Depending on the facility, several case managers may be engaged to coordinate care for all patients or one case manager may be assigned to a specific high-risk population (Figure 14-7). A case manager may be responsible for coordinating care for up to 20 patients. It is essential for the case manager to have frequent interaction with patients and health care providers to achieve and evaluate expected outcomes.

Clinical Pathways

Many case managers use a clinical pathway to achieve patient outcomes. Also referred to as *multidisciplinary care pathways, integrated care pathways, critical pathways, care maps,* or *collaborative care pathways,* these patient-focused documents describe the clinical standards, necessary interventions, and expected outcomes for the patient at each stage of the treatment process or hospital stay. Clinical pathways are not appropriate for all patients and cannot replace professional clinical judgement; however, they do facilitate coordinated and well-organized care that links best available evidence to clinical practice (Rotter, Kinsman, James, et al., 2010).

Clinical pathways are grids that outline the critical or key events expected to happen each day of a patient's hospitalization (D'Entremont, 2009). If a patient's progress deviates from the normal path, a variance is indicated. A variance alters the patient's progress through the normal clinical pathway. An analysis of variance is essential for effective utilization of a path.

Circumstances that can cause a variance include operational, provider, patient, or clinical elements (Cohen & Cesta, 2004). Operational causes include broken equipment or interdepartmental delays. Changes in the practice pattern of the health care provider can affect the pathway and cause a variance. Complications in the patient's condition, such as a hemorrhage into the joint after total knee replacement, may increase total hospital days. A complication can inhibit the ability of the patient to meet a clinical indicator, and a patient's or family's refusal of a specific component of care can create a variance.

Variances can be positive or negative. A negative variance is an undesired outcome, whereas a positive variance is an outcome that is achieved before it is expected (Cohen & Cesta, 2004). A patient undergoing a second hip replacement who attended preoperative classes and engaged in activities to "ready himself" for the surgery may actually leave the hospital sooner than predicted in a clinical path. The case manager on the orthopedic unit would view this outcome as a positive variance, as typically would the patient.

Model Analysis

Nursing case management is geared to providing comprehensive care for those with complex health problems. It delivers a well-coordinated multidisciplinary care experience that can improve the care outcome, decrease the length of stay, and use services efficiently. Families and patients receive care across a continuum of settings, often from diverse institutions. Case managers can often break down invisible institutional barriers for the patient. Nurses receive a sense of satisfaction knowing that the patient and family received coordinated, quality care in a cost-effective manner across the spectrum of the illness or injury.

However, major obstacles exist in the implementation of case management services. Financial barriers, lack of administrative support, human resource inequities, turf battles, and a lack of information support systems have been identified as hurdles in the implementation of case management services (Powell & Tahan, 2010). Case management minimizes costs for those case types that have the potential of high resource consumption. Collaborative models of health care management that incorporate nurses, social workers, respiratory therapists, and physical or occupational therapists as case managers have demonstrated the ability to meet specific patient needs at significant cost savings (Powell & Tahan, 2010). Some health care institutions have developed departments of health care case management so that the professional background of each nurse case manager can be matched with the appropriate patient population and specific patient needs (Powell & Tahan, 2010).

Nurse Manager's Role

The nurse manager has increased demands when leading the case management system. The nurse manager must constantly assess whether resources are utilized appropriately, that care is delivered in the appropriate setting, and that case managers are adequately managing their caseloads—with particular attention to length of stay and cost (Cawthorn, 2005). Health care funding or institutional budgets for the care delivered can be tied to effective planning and care delivery within the case management process (e.g., incentives may be provided to meet specific targets, such as reducing infection rates). The nurse manager must also evaluate patient satisfaction, a measure of quality. Low patient satisfaction might be indicative of other service issues and could impact institution accreditation.

Communication among all departments involved in a patient's care must be coordinated. Because the case manager works with various departments, the nurse manager may need to facilitate interdepartmental communication. Educating the staff of other departments about the case manager's role and responsibilities will increase the effectiveness of the case management process.

Staff Nurse's Role

The staff nurse working with a patient who has a case manager as the coordinator of care provides patient care according to the case manager's specifications and must know the extent of the case manager's role. Effective communication to facilitate care is the responsibility of both the case manager and the staff nurse.

CARE STRATEGIES THAT INFLUENCE CARE DELIVERY

Disease Management

Disease management has been in existence for many decades. However, in the late 1990s, disease management became a model of care that coordinates health care interventions and communication for those individuals whose self-care needs are significant (Lukewich, Edge, Vandenkerkhof, et al., 2014). Those with chronic conditions who are high consumers of health care dollars are the recipients of disease-managed care. Disease-management programs for patients dealing with chronic illness build on the relationship with the health care team to prevent exacerbations and complications using evidence-informed guidelines and patient empowerment techniques to improve the overall health and well-being of the patient and family. The focus of this model of care is wellness: living well with a chronic disease. Determining the barriers to self-care is an essential element of successful disease-management programs.

Disease-management programs consist of assessment to identify a specific population, comprehensive patient and family self-management education, use of evidence-informed practice guidelines, medical management based on treatment algorithms, and focused visits with the health care team in an ambulatory setting to assist with adherence to the treatment protocol (Powell & Tahan, 2010). Case managers often decide whether a patient meets the specific criteria for a disease-managed program.

Differentiated Nursing Practice

One factor that makes the development and implementation of any nursing care delivery model difficult is the variation in the level of education and experience of each nurse. Over the past 50 years, as multiple entry points to nursing (e.g., registered nurse, licensed practical nurse, bachelor of science in nursing) have grown and more is known about the length of time required for a nurse to move from novice to competent nurse (Benner, 2001), efforts have been made to document and validate differentiated nursing practice (Canadian Nurses Association [CNA], 2012b; Harris & McGillis Hall, 2012; McGillis Hall, Doran, & Pink, 2004; Needleman, Buerhaus, Mattke, et al., 2002).

Background of Differentiated Practice. Differentiated nursing practice is a model of clinical nursing practice that recognizes the difference in each nurse's level of education, expected clinical skills or competencies, job descriptions, pay scales, and participation in decision making (American Association of Colleges of Nursing [AACN], 1995).

Nurses with a bachelor of science in nursing (BSN) operate across time from pre-admission to postdischarge. BSN-prepared nurses respond to the unusual and often unpredictable responses of patients that go beyond the needs addressed in professional standards or clinical pathways. They also collaborate with other disciplines, departments, and agencies and help design and facilitate a comprehensive, well-prepared discharge plan based on the unique needs of the patient and family (AACN, 2009).

Advanced nursing practice (ANP) (MacDonald, Schrieber, & Davis, 2005) and advanced practice nurses (APN) (DiCenso, Bryant-Lukosius, Martin-Misener, et al., 2010) have been in existence in Canada for more than 40 years. In most provinces and territories, a master's degree is required to achieve these designations. APNs function as clinical nurse specialists (CNS) or nurse practitioners (NP) (DiCenso et al., 2010). The ANP has in-depth education in physiology, physical assessment, and pharmacology, and has a broad health care systems perspective. The CNS/NP may create and define protocols and clinical pathways and help develop standards for emerging health care phenomena. The CNS/NP is not bound by a particular health care setting but, instead, provides a continuum of care across all settings, working with the patient and family throughout wellness or illness or until death (MacDonald, Schrieber, & Davis, 2005).

The varied educational backgrounds and philosophies of the nurses implementing a model of practice have a significant impact on the success of care delivery and the satisfaction of nurses and patients. This variation is further complicated by the experience of the nurse in the practice arena. Benner (2001), based on the Dreyfus model of skill acquisition, identified five stages of clinical competence for nurses: novice, advanced beginner, competent, proficient, and expert. Benner suggested that competence is typified by a nurse who has been on the job in the same or similar situations for 2 to 3 years. It follows that nurses who are either new graduates or in a new area of clinical practice may require more assistance than those with more experience. A group of nurses who are all at the novice or advanced beginner stage would be less likely than their more experienced counterparts to implement any type of delivery model effectively.

The competencies entry-level nurses need to meet requirements for safe and effective nursing practice are measured by national exams or entry to practice exams. For example, RN students across Canada write the

National Council Licensure Examination (NCLEX) to assess their entry-level nursing practice competencies.

Differentiated Practice in the Clinical Setting. As the complexity of health care increases and the pressures of managed care rise, communication and critical thinking in nursing has become paramount. Differentiated practice in nursing can respond to changing health care systems, changing funding strategies, health human resource challenges, and rising acuities and complex health care needs in patients and their families.

Incentives for implementing differentiated practice include the following (Bellack & Loquist, 1999):

1. The ability to identify the differences in preparation of nurses by level of education
2. The ability to use different levels of nurses to meet the total needs of the patient
3. Improved clinical outcomes that are cost-effective
4. Enhanced prestige of nursing through the identification of different levels of nursing to the public and health care administration
5. Effective utilization of nursing resources to meet the diverse needs of managed care
6. Career satisfaction with equitable compensation.

However, despite a variety of efforts to differentiate the roles and competencies of nurses with various educational backgrounds and experience, the demands of the workplace, the chronic shortage of nurses, and the greater use of technology have made it difficult to differentiate nursing practice in many clinical settings.

Clinical Nurse Leader. In response to a lack of differentiated practice in many health care settings and the increased emphasis on patient safety, clinical nurse leader (CNL) role emerged in the early 2000s in Canada and is modelled on the American Association of Nursing description of the role. The CNL is a highly skilled master's degree–prepared nurse who has completed advanced studies in clinical care with a focus on the improvement of quality outcomes for specific patient populations at the point of care. The CNL coordinates and supervises the care provided by interdisciplinary team members. Like other leadership roles, the CNL role includes development of skills in preceptoring, mentoring, and coaching. The CNL may oversee the lateral integration of care for a distinct group of patients and may actively provide direct patient care in complex situations. The CNL uses evidence-informed practice to ensure that patients benefit from the latest innovations in care delivery. The CNL collects and evaluates patient outcomes, assesses cohort risk, and has the decision-making authority to change care plans when necessary. This nurse functions as part of the interprofessional team by communicating, planning, and implementing care directly with other health care providers including physicians, pharmacists, social workers, clinical nurse specialists, and nurse practitioners. The CNL is a leader in the health care delivery system in all settings in which health care is delivered, and implementation of the role may vary across settings (AACN, 2008). Box 14-1 outlines the fundamental aspects of the CNL role, as defined by the AACN white paper on the clinical nurse leader (AACN, 2013).

BOX 14-1   FUNDAMENTAL ASPECTS OF THE CLINICAL NURSE LEADER (CNL)

- Leadership in the care of the sick in and across all environments
- Design and provision of health-promotion and risk-reduction services for diverse populations
- Provision of evidence-based practice
- Population-appropriate health care to individuals, clinical groups/units, and communities
- Clinical decision making
- Design and implementation of plans of care
- Risk anticipation
- Participation in identification and collection of care outcomes
- Accountability for the evaluation and improvement of point-of-care outcomes
- Mass customization of care

- Patient and community advocacy
- Education and information management
- Delegation and oversight of care delivery and outcomes
- Team management and collaboration with other health professional team members
- Development and leverage of human, environmental, and material resources
- Management and use of patient-care and information technology
- Lateral integration for specified groups of patients

American Association of Colleges of Nursing. (2013). Competencies and curricular expectations for clinical nurse leader education and practice. Retrieved from http://www.aacn.nche.edu/cnl/CNL-Competencies-October-2013.pdf.

The Synergy Model

Similar to the work of the AACN in developing the CNL, the American Association of Critical-Care Nurses adopted the Synergy Model as the framework for nursing practice as well as for the certification examination for the critical care nurse and the clinical nurse specialist. Some health care organizations have adopted this model as their model of care. However, the Synergy Model identifies patient characteristics as "drivers" of the necessary competencies for nurses. When there is a match between the competencies of the nurse and the characteristics of the patient, the best patient outcomes and safe passage through a hospital stay will be achieved (Kaplow & Reed, 2008).

The Synergy Model describes the following eight patient characteristics: resiliency, vulnerability, stability, complexity, resource availability, participation in care, participation in decision making, and predictability. The eight nurse competencies are clinical judgement, advocacy and moral employer, caring practices, facilitation of learning, collaboration, systems thinking, response to diversity, and clinical requirement (Kaplow & Reed, 2008). Each of the competencies is essential in providing holistic care to the patient. Depending on the acuity of the patient, some competencies emerge as priorities whereas others are used to a lesser extent (MacPhee, Wardrop, Campbell, et al., 2011). When there is synergy between the patient characteristics and the competency of the nurse, patient care is optimized (Brewer, Wojner-Alexandrov, Triola, et al., 2007). The American Association of Critical-Care Nurses Web site (http://www.aacn.org) provides information on the Synergy Model and its application in diverse care settings. While the Synergy Model has been predominantly utilized in the United States, its use in Canada as a professional practice model has been explored in a pilot project in British Columbia. Preliminary results of the pilot project were positive, including enhanced communication among regulated and unregulated care providers and nursing leadership (British Columbia Nurses Union, 2010; MacPhee, Wardrop, Campbell, et al., 2011).

Transforming Care at the Bedside

The variety of care delivery models and the complexity of patient needs, organizational structures, and technological advances require individual action to improve practice patterns in specific units. In 2003, the Robert Wood Johnson Foundation (http://www.rwjf.org) and the Institute of Healthcare Improvement (http://www.ihi.org) joined forces to create, test, and implement changes to dramatically improve care on medical and surgical units and enhance staff satisfaction (Rutherford, Moen, & Taylor, 2009). The result was Transforming Care at the Bedside (TCAB), an initiative focused on redesigning the work environment and work processes of nurses to improve care for patients. Rutherford, Phillips, Coughlan, et al. (2008) developed TCAB's conceptual framework to guide the implementation efforts of participating hospitals. They emphasize that TCAB initiatives engage front-line staff in deciding on and implementing strategies that improve patient outcomes, facilitate collaborative team work, and support professional nursing practice.

The TCAB initiative is based on a set of five premises (Box 14-2) that serve as the underpinnings of four key design themes (Box 14-3). According to Viney, Batcheller, Houston, et al. (2006), both the premises and the themes serve as a framework for teams charged with changing care processes.

The TCAB initiative was initially implemented at three pilot hospitals in the United States and was subsequently implemented in other hospitals across the United States and eventually Canada (Lavoie-Tremblay, O'Conner, Harripaul, et al., 2013). The team members involved in implementation in each hospital began by asking "What do we know?" about each design theme. The group then was encouraged to tell stories about their work environment consistent with this theme. After storytelling, the team members participated in a brainstorming session to come up with as many innovations as possible that

---

BOX 14-2 TRANSFORMING CARE AT THE BEDSIDE (TCAB) PREMISES

- Patient-centred work redesign can create value-added care processes and result in better clinical outcomes and reduced costs
- Effective care teams can have a positive impact on patient outcomes
- Management practices and organizational culture have a significant impact on the work environment
- Matching staff's knowledge and capabilities with work responsibilities enhances job satisfaction
- Eliminating inefficiencies through work redesign enhances staff satisfaction and morale

Viney, M., Batcheller, J., Houston, S., et al. (2006). Transforming Care at the Bedside: Designing new complex systems in an age of complexity. *Journal of Nursing Care Quality, 21*(2), p. 146.

could contribute to each theme. Innovations requiring minimal time and resources were then prioritized and selected for a rapid cycle trial. The CNA categorizes TCAB as an initiative for "improving work processes and optimizing the work of nurses" (CNA, n.d.).

Critical to practice changes, a rapid cycle trial is a process that encourages testing creative change on a small scale while determining potential impact (see Chapter 18 for more information on leading change). The process involves four stages—Plan-Do-Study-Act (PDSA). During the *plan phase*, the team defines the objectives and predicts how the identified change would contribute to design, how the change would occur, and what data collection methods would be needed. During the *do phase*, the team focuses on whether the change occurred as expected and, if not, what interfered with the plan. During the *study phase*, the team determines whether the innovation worked as predicted and what knowledge was gained. During the *act phase*, the team plans next actions.

The team and staff participating in the study rate the innovation in terms of adoption, adaptation, or discontinuation. The innovation is implemented for a short period (from a day to several weeks) at least twice during the prototype testing phase and the pilot testing phase. If the outcome of testing the innovation is positive, the new design can be easily spread to other participating sites.

CONCLUSION

Each nursing care delivery model identified in this chapter has strengths and weaknesses. There is no perfect method for delivering nursing care to all groups of patients and their families. Because of the variety of settings and organizational sizes, no one model addresses all needs. In addition, in times of local or national emergencies, the typical model of care may be replaced with one designed to best fit the emergency. Table 14-2 provides examples of organizational structures and processes that might influence the delivery of care used.

TABLE 14-2	STANDARDIZED SET OF ORGANIZATIONAL CRITERIA	
ORGANIZATIONAL STRUCTURES	**ORGANIZATIONAL PROCESSES**	**PATIENT CARE DESCRIPTORS**
Governance	Care planning	Case mix severity
Teaching status	Patient assessment/ monitoring	Intensity of service/skills
Aggregated units	Documentation	Length of stay
Technology level	Policies/procedures	
Case mix	Patient education	
Operating budget	Supplies	
Nursing hours/day	Implementation of physicians' orders	
Skill mix	Patient/family communication	
Nurse–patient ratio	Symptom management	
Use of temporary staff	Staff communication	
Nursing education/experience	Medication administration	
Support for professional development	Standards of care	
Continuing education	Unit activities	
Expert resources		
Support personnel		
Physical layout		

Adapted from Deutschendorf, A. (2003). From past paradigms to future frontiers: Unique care delivery models to facilitate nursing work and quality outcomes. *Journal of Nurse Administration, 33*(1), 51–58.

This chapter describes the traditional nursing care delivery models that have been used since the 20th century. The complexity of the current health care system, the shortage of health care providers, and the pressures to ensure patient safety and cost-effective care have led many organizations to explore alternative models to deliver patient care. The CNA (2011, p. 21) suggests that "nursing care delivery model design and staff-mix decision-making" is central to the future of health care and nursing in Canada. Furthermore, Ginette Rodger, past president of the CNA, stated that given the current state of interprofessional collaboration in health care settings, understanding the differences between "organizational" and "nursing care" delivery models is necessary and that specific, well-developed models of nursing care delivery need to exist (CNA, 2011, p. 4). Emerging nursing care delivery models, which are variations of traditional models of care, are being considered and tested in Canada, and efforts are being made to gain a better understanding of the principles needed to guide the development of nursing care delivery models as demonstrated by the Literature Perspective and the Research Perspective below.

LITERATURE PERSPECTIVE

Resource: Wells, J., Manuel, M., & Cunning, G. (2011). Changing the model of care delivery: Nurses' perceptions of job satisfaction and care effectiveness. *Journal of Nursing Management, 19,* 777–785.

Wells, Manuel, and Cunning (2011) describe the implementation and evaluation of an adaptation of a total patient care (TPC) model in two acute care nursing units. Reports from nurses and administration that the traditional team nursing model of care contributed to inconsistent patient care and blurred lines of responsibility and accountability, and that patient confidentiality and privacy were at risk, prompted the exploration for alternative models of care. The authors used Lewin's change model (see Chapter 18) to support the implementation of the new TPC model of care. The authors initially asked the nursing staff what components they would like to see in the new model of care. Based on the suggestions from the nursing staff, TPC seemed to be the model most fitting. In the next phase, the physical environment of the nursing units was changed to facilitate the new model of care (e.g., centralized nursing station, separate medication room). Furthermore, educational sessions were offered to all nursing staff that provided an overview of the gaps between the old and new existing models of care, the potential benefits to nurses and patients of using TPC, and a review of the processes related to TPC (which included highlighting the nursing roles and scopes of practice of those working within the TPC, such as RNs, licensed practical nurses, or patient care coordinators). As the implementation proceeded, efforts were made to ensure that those involved in the transition between models of care were part of the decision-making process regarding nursing practice issues.

This model of care was implemented in two acute nursing units with 52 beds and 78 permanent full-time staff in a regional health care facility. Job satisfaction was measured using the Index of Work Satisfaction (IWS) scale, empowerment was measured using the two subscales of responsibility and participation from the Perception of Empowerment Instrument (PEI), and the Care Delivery Effectiveness (CDE) tool was used to measure nurses' perception of the effectiveness of the provision of care. Data were collected prior to the change, and again at 3 and 6 months after the change from nurses who had been on the unit for at least 6 months. While adding to the limited and somewhat conflicting body of literature on TPC, the results suggested that TPC or a modification of it was more effective than the team nursing model previously used in the units; however, job satisfaction levels remained the same.

Implications for Practice

Although the study was undertaken in only one hospital over a discrete period of time, the results suggest that TPC is perceived by nurses to be a more effective nursing care delivery model than team nursing. The results also suggest that when planned change in nursing practice is being considered, involving and engaging the nursing staff and having organizational support is key. This is congruent with the guiding principles for nursing care delivery models outlined by the CNA (2012a).

RESEARCH PERSPECTIVE

Resource: Canadian Nurses Association. (2012a). *Nursing care delivery models: Canadian consensus on guiding principles.* Ottawa, ON: Author. Retrieved from https://www.cna-aiic.ca/~/media/cna/page%20content/pdf%20en/2013/07/26/10/41/nursing_care_delivery_models_e.pdf.

The aim of this project was to gain consensus on guiding principles for decision making regarding nursing care delivery models. The project built upon three previously completed initiatives by the CNA related to nursing care delivery models and staff mix. These initiatives included an invitational round table discussion (CNA, 2011), a comprehensive literature review (Harris & McGillis Hall, 2012), and newly developed core principles for staff mix decision making (CNA, 2012b), all of which endeavoured to improve the transfer of knowledge into the practice setting related to nursing care delivery models and staff mix.

Continued

RESEARCH PERSPECTIVE—cont'd

The article describes research undertaken to obtain a Pan-Canadian consensus on overarching principles that could guide decision making about nursing care delivery models. Expert nurses from across the country were asked to rate and comment on 18 guiding principles, based on the above-mentioned initiatives. The survey results provided a prioritized list of ten guiding principles for which consensus had been achieved:

1. Responding to the health care needs of patients, families, and communities is integral to the nursing care delivery model.
2. Staff competencies (knowledge, skills, abilities, attitudes) are a part of the nursing care delivery model.
3. The nursing care delivery model reflects an organization's patient population, best practices, professional standards and research evidence.
4. Front-line nursing staff and nursing management are engaged in decision making about the nursing care delivery model.
5. The nursing care delivery model promotes quality and safe care, which is cost-effective and sustains the system.
6. Systematically collected data about patient outcomes and nursing human resources inform decisions about the nursing care delivery model.
7. A formal plan for the nursing care delivery model, including communication and educational strategies, considers patient and staff needs as well as the organizational mission.
8. Organizational structure and leadership across all levels support the nursing care delivery model.
9. Staff mix based on patient care needs is a component of the nursing care delivery model.
10. Technology is a required component for implementing the nursing care delivery model. (CNA, 2012b, p. 17)

In addition to the need to consider all ten guiding principles in the design of nursing care delivery models, the project's researchers also identified key messages from their research, which included involving front-line staff in the development of nursing care delivery models, that nursing care delivery models cannot be designed in isolation and need to consider the interdisciplinary nature of health care, and that nursing care delivery models must be flexible to meet individual patient needs.

Implications for Practice

While the CNA's report highlights the principles needed to underpin nursing care delivery models, in a number of provinces, new "blended" models of care are being implemented. The blended models have aspects of traditional nursing care models but include elements of collaborative and patient-centred care to address current trends (Harris & McGillis Hall, 2012) while also responding to changes in funding, technology, and characteristics of patients cared for in health care organizations.

In Canada, examples of innovative nursing care delivery models being developed, implemented, and tested include the following:

1. Collaborative Nursing Practice (CNP) Acute Model (Vancouver Coastal Health Authority)
2. Nursing Demonstration Project: Building Better Nursing Care Delivery Models (Sunnybrook Health Sciences Centre)
3. Model of Care Initiative in Nova Scotia (a joint initiative for acute inpatient care)
4. Community Health Nursing Practice Models (Community Health Nurses of Canada)
5. The Ottawa Hospital's Inter-Professional Model of Patient Care (IPMPC) (CNA, 2011)

A SOLUTION

As a patient care manager (PCM), Adeyele is responsible for ensuring the delivery of excellent patient care to patients admitted to a medical unit. The nurses on the unit were committed to this approach but encountered communication challenges. Collaborating with other members of the leadership team, receiving input from the staff nurses, and seeking out best practices from her colleagues in the health care community provided her with a solution. They initiated a sit-down report for all nurses called the "practice huddle" and established a "nurse buddy" system. The "practice huddle" occurs at the beginning of the shift after each nurse has obtained the report from the nurse on the previous shift and has had the opportunity to review each patient's plan of care. The nurses are paged and notified that the "practice huddle" will occur. The charge nurse who surveys each nurse on his or her workload and the projected times he or she would need assistance with patient care facilitates the "practice huddle."

The "nurse buddy" system was initiated to provide the patient-side nurse with an immediate resource—someone other than the charge nurse. These two nurses provide each other with support on an "as-needed" basis. The "buddy" is assigned at the time the patient assignments are created and is in close proximity.

The staff response has been very positive. The charge nurse has a better understanding of the status of the patients, families, and staff. Staff nurses state they are more engaged, and thus better able to be involved with the unit's operational needs for the day. Patient care is planned collaboratively so that each nurse is available to the "buddy" when needed. Overall, teamwork and communication have been enhanced.

Would this be a suitable approach for you? Why or why not?

THE EVIDENCE

Wolf and Greenhouse (2007) recognized the need for health care system change and the importance of a well-developed care delivery model in addressing these changes. They suggested that it is not necessary to "start from scratch" in developing a model; many valuable lessons, learned from experience and scientific evidence, can be incorporated into new models. They also suggested three factors beyond the experience of the past should be considered in developing a new model. First, major health care trends, such as changes in patients, health care providers, information technology, and financing, as well as medical advances, must be considered. Second, what patients want and need should be identified. Some patient needs identified by the authors were traditionally expected, such as wanting a competent provider to meet their physical, emotional, and spiritual needs. However, others were not, such as wanting a provider to help sort through available information to find a solution that would be effective for them. Third, Wolf and Greenhouse (2007) suggested that developers must make structural (Who will do what?), process (How will it get done?), and outcome (What difference will it make?) decisions to ensure that the new model is in strategic alignment with the organization, sustainable over time, and can be replicated. The authors provide specific questions that can be helpful in making these structural, process, and outcome decisions.

NEED TO KNOW NOW

- Consider the model of nursing care delivery used by an organization when selecting a position for employment.
- Anticipate that a national or local emergency could alter normal care delivery.

- Determine whether there are experienced nurses who provide clinical leadership in specific settings.

CHAPTER CHECKLIST

The roles of the nurse manager and staff nurse vary with each nursing care delivery model. Regardless of the model, the nurse manager must have strong leadership and management skills for the model to be effective. Numerous issues must be considered when a care delivery model is implemented. Without a competent manager, none of the discussed models would be effective.

- A nursing care delivery model is the method nurses use to provide care to patients.
- Five models of nursing care delivery were presented, along with their advantages and disadvantages:
  - The case method focuses on total patient care for a specific time period.
    - The nurse manager must consider the expense of this system and identify the level of education and communication skills of all staff members.
  - Functional nursing emphasizes task-oriented care for a large group of patients.

  - The nurse manager is responsible for achieving patient outcomes, whereas staff members are responsible only for their specific tasks.
  - The functional model is most often used in subacute care facilities.
- In the team nursing model, a small team provides care to a group of patients.
  - The nurse manager needs strong management, critical thinking, and leadership skills.
  - The nurse manager functions as role model, advocate, coach, consultant, budget controller, and unit quality manager.
  - The partnership model pairs an RN with a partner (e.g., a technical assistant).
  - The patient-focused care unit employs a primary nurse and multi-skilled team members.
- In the primary nursing model a registered nurse working with a team is responsible for planning and delivering care for a consistent group of patients.

- The primary nurse is accountable for the patients' care 24 hours a day, from admission through discharge.
- The primary nurse plans, collaborates, communicates, and coordinates all aspects of patient care with other nurses as well as other disciplines.
- When the primary nurse is not working, an associate nurse implements the plan to provide care to the patient according to the primary nurse's specifications.
- The ideal primary nursing system requires an all-nurse staff.
- The nursing case management model is outcome-focused and is facilitated by a case manager, who directs unit-based care using a clinical pathway.
  - The nurse manager faces increased demands to move the patient through the system as quickly as possible.
  - Managed care is a way of organizing patient-care delivery with cost savings as the main goal.
  - The case manager plays a vital role in the management of care.

- The nurse manager and charge nurse are responsible for directing patient care, regardless of the nursing care delivery system. They apply the following key leadership and management concepts when directing patient care:
  - Accountability
  - Delegation
  - Critical thinking
  - Communication
  - Promotion of autonomy
  - Collaboration
- The disease management model of care assists those with chronic illnesses to manage their self-care to achieve optimal health.
  - The concept of differentiated nursing practice emphasizes two levels of nursing practice: technical and professional.
  - Each type of nurse has a specific role and particular responsibilities based on the nurse's education, experience, and clinical expertise.
  - All the nursing roles complement one another.
- Emerging models of professional nursing practice continue to evolve.

TIPS FOR SELECTING A CARE DELIVERY MODEL*

- Look at the organization and the population being served when selecting a care delivery model.
- Consider the organizational structure and processes when selecting the care delivery model.
- Understand that all models have advantages and disadvantages, and none is ideal.
- Know that every model has specific expectations for both managers and staff.
- Determine whether there are experienced nurses who provide clinical leadership in specific settings.

*These tips are also useful for new graduate nurses evaluating employment opportunities.

evolve WEBSITE

Visit the Evolve website for Suggested Readings, Internet Resources, and additional resources related to the content in this chapter: http://evolve.elsevier.com/Canada/Yoder-Wise/leading/.

REFERENCES

American Association of Colleges of Nursing. (1995). *A model for differentiated nursing practice.* Washington, DC: Author.
American Association of Colleges of Nursing. (2008). CNL frequently asked questions. Retrieved from http://www.aacn.nche.edu/CNL/faq.htm.
American Association of Colleges of Nursing. (2009). DNP fact sheet. Retrieved from http://www.aacn.nche.edu/DNP/index.htm.
American Association of Colleges of Nursing. (2013). Competencies and curricular expectations for clinical nurse leader education and practice. Retrieved from http://www.aacn.nche.edu/cnl/CNL-Competencies-October-2013.pdf.
Bellack, J. P., & Loquist, R. S. (1999). Employer responses to differentiated nursing education. *Journal of Nursing Administration, 29*(9), 4–8, 32.

Benner, P. (2001). *From novice to expert: Excellence and power in clinical nursing practice.* Upper Saddle River, NJ: Prentice Hall.

Brewer, B. B., Wojner-Alexandrov, A. W., Triola, N., et al. (2007). AACN Synergy Model's characteristics of patients: Psychometric analyses in a tertiary care health system. *American Journal of Critical Care, 16*(2), 158–167.

British Columbia Nurses Union. (2010). *Provincial nursing workload project: Final report.* Burnaby, BC: Author. Retrieved from https://www.bcnu.org/ProfessionalPractice/PNWP_Report.pdf.

Butler, M., Collins, R., Drennan, J., et al. (2011). Hospital nurse staffing models and patient and staff-related outcomes. *Cochrane Database of Systematic Reviews, 7.* doi:10.1002/14651858.CD007019.pub2

Canadian Nurses Association. (n.d.) Fact sheet: Nurses offer solutions for cost-effective health care. Retrieved from https://www.cna-aiic.ca/~/media/cna/page%20content/pdf%20fr/2013/09/05/19/00/roi_solutions_cost_fs_e.pdf.

Canadian Nurses Association. (2011). *Invitational round table. Nursing care delivery models and staff mix: Using evidence in decision-making.* Ottawa, ON: Author. Retrieved from http://www.nurseone.ca/docs/NurseOne/KnowledgeFeature/StaffMix/Roundtable_Report_Evidence_Decision_e.pdf.

Canadian Nurses Association. (2012a). *Nursing care delivery models: Canadian consensus on guiding principles.* Ottawa, ON: Author. Retrieved from https://www.cna-aiic.ca/~/media/cna/page%20content/pdf%20en/2013/07/26/10/41/nursing_care_delivery_models_e.pdf.

Canadian Nurses Association. (2012b). *Staff mix decision-making framework for quality nursing care.* Ottawa, ON: Author. Retrieved from http://www.clpna.com/wp-content/uploads/2013/02/doc_CNA_Staff_Mix_Framework_2012.pdf.

Cawthorn, L. (2005). Online exclusives: Discharge planning under the umbrella of advanced nursing practice case manager. *Nursing Leadership, 18*(4). Retrieved from http://www.longwoods.com/content/19033.

Cohen, E., & Cesta, T. (2004). *Nursing case management: From essentials to advanced practice applications* (4th ed.). St. Louis, MO: Mosby.

Curtis, K., Lien, D., Chan, A., et al. (2002). The impact of trauma case management on patient outcomes. *Journal of Trauma, 53*(3), 477–482.

D'Entremont, B. (2009). Clinical pathways: The Ottawa Hospital experience. *Canadian Nurse, 105*(5), 8–9.

Deutschendorf, A. (2003). From past paradigms to future frontiers: Unique care delivery models to facilitate nursing work and quality outcomes. *Journal of Nurse Administration, 33*(1), 51–58.

DiCenso, A., Bryant-Lukosius, D., Martin-Misener, R., et al. (2010). Factors enabling advanced practice nursing role integration in Canada [Special issue]. *Nursing Leadership, 23,* 211–238. doi:10.12927/cjnl.2010.22279

Fairbrother, G., Jones, A., & Rivas, K. (2010). Changing model of nursing care from individual patient allocation to team nursing in the acute inpatient environment. *Contemporary Nurse, 35*(2), 202–220.

Harris, A., & McGillis Hall, L. (2012). *Evidence to inform staff mix decision-making: A focused literature review.* Ottawa, ON: Canadian Nurses Association. Retrieved from http://www.cna-aiic.ca/~/media/cna/page%20content/pdf%20en/2013/07/26/10/41/staff_mix_literature_review_e.pdf.

Hobbs, J. L. (2009). A dimensional analysis of patient-centered care. *Nursing Research, 58*(1), 52–62.

Hodgkinson, B., Haesler, E. J., Nay, R., et al. (2011). Effectiveness of staffing models in residential, subacute, extended aged care settings on patient and staff outcomes. *Cochrane Database of Systematic Reviews, 6.* doi:10.1002/14651858.CD006563.pub2

Huber, D. (2010). *Leadership and nursing case management* (4th ed.). St. Louis, MO: Saunders.

Kaplow, R., & Reed, K. (2008). The AACN Synergy Model for patient care: A nursing model as a force of magnetism. *Nursing Economics, 26*(1), 17–25.

Lavoie-Tremblay, M., O'Conner, P., Harripaul, A., et al. (2013). The effect of Transforming Care at the Bedside initiative on healthcare teams' work environments. *Worldviews on Evidence-Based Nursing, 11*(1), 16–25. doi:10.1111/wvn.12015

Lukewich, J., Edge, D. S., Vandenkerkhof, E., et al. (2014). Nursing contributions to chronic disease management in primary care. *Journal of Nursing Administration, 44*(2), 103–110. doi:10.1097/NNA.000000000000033

MacDonald, M., Schrieber, R., & Davis, L. (2005). *Exploring new roles for advanced nursing practice: A discussion paper.* Ottawa, ON: Canadian Nurses Association. Retrieved from https://www.cna-aiic.ca/~/media/cna/page%20content/pdf%20en/2013/07/26/10/23/exploring_new_roles_anp-05_e.pdf.

MacPhee, M., Wardrop, A., Campbell, C., et al. (2011). The synergy professional practice model and its patient characteristics tool: A staff empowerment strategy. *Nursing Leadership, 24*(3), 42–56. doi:10.12927/cjnl.2011.22600

Manthey, M., Ciske, K., Robertson, P., et al. (1970). Primary nursing: A return to the concept of "my nurse" and "my patient." *Nursing Forum, 9,* 65–83.

McGillis Hall, L., Doran, D., & Pink, G. H. (2004). Nursing staff mix models, nursing hours and patient safety outcomes. *Journal of Nursing Administration, 34*(1), 41–45.

National Case Management Network of Canada. (2009). *Canadian standards of practice for case management.* n.p.: Author.

Needleman, J., Buerhaus, P., Mattke, S., et al. (2002). Nurse-staffing levels and the quality of care in hospitals. *New England Journal of Medicine 346*(22), 1715–1722.

Pelzang, R. (2010). Time to learn: Understanding patient-centered care. *British Journal of Nursing, 19*(4), 912–917.

Powell, S. K., & Tahan, H. A. (2010). *Case management: A practical guide for education and practice* (3rd ed.). Philadelphia, PA: Wolters Kluwer.

Rotter, T., Kinsman, L., James, E. L., et al. (2010). Clinical pathways: Effects on professional practice, patient outcomes, length of stay and hospital costs (Review). *Cochrane Database of Systematic Reviews, 7.* doi:10.1002/14651858.CD006632.pub2

Rutherford, P., Moen, R., & Taylor, J. (2009). TCAB: The "how" and the "what." *American Journal of Nursing, 109*(11, Suppl.), 5–17.

Rutherford, P., Phillips, J., Coughlan, P., et al. (2008). *Transforming care at the bedside how-to guide: Engaging front-line staff in innovation and quality improvement.* Cambridge, MA: Institute for Healthcare Improvement. Retrieved from http://www.IHI.org.

Seago, J. (1999). Evaluation of a hospital work redesign: Patient-focused care. *Journal of Nursing Administration, 29*(11), 31–38.

Shirey, M. R. (2008). Nursing practice models for acute and critical care: Overview of care delivery models. *Critical Care Nursing Clinics of North America, 20*(4), 365–373.

Tiedeman, M., & Lookinland, S. (2004). Traditional models of care delivery: What have we learned? *Journal of Nursing Administration* (electronic version), *34*(6), 291–297.

Viney, M., Batcheller, J., Houston, S., et al. (2006). Transforming Care at the Bedside: Designing new care systems in an age of complexity. *Journal of Nursing Care Quality, 21*(2), 143–150.

Wells, J., Manuel, M., & Cunning, G. (2011). Changing the model of care delivery: Nurses' perceptions of job satisfaction and care effectiveness. *Journal of Nursing Management, 19*, 777–785.

White, P., & Hall, M. E. (2006). Mapping the literature of case management nursing. *Journal of the Medical Library Association, 94*(2, Suppl.), E99–E106.

Wolf, G., & Greenhouse, P. (2007). Blueprint for design: Creating models that direct change. *Journal of Nursing Administration, 37*(9), 381–387.

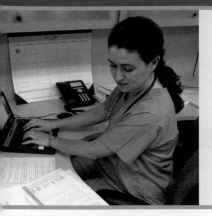

Staffing and Scheduling

Susan Sportsman
Adapted by Deb A. Gordon

This chapter explores research regarding the relationship between staffing and various nurse and patient outcomes. It considers the interrelationship between the personnel budget and staffing plan. It also discusses measures for evaluating unit productivity and the impact of various staffing and scheduling strategies on overall staff satisfaction and continuity of patient care. These key points are critical to nurse managers' ability to deliver safe and effective care in their areas of responsibility while maintaining a high degree of employee satisfaction in the unit. Understanding the impact of nursing-sensitive indicators on patient outcomes helps managers control the unit's labour expenses. The ability to use this information and communicate about staffing to employees is critical to effectively managing productive services and being a valuable member of the leadership team.

OBJECTIVES

- Evaluate the impact of patient and hospital factors, nurse characteristics, nurse staffing, nurse outcomes, and other organizational factors that influence staff and patient outcomes.
- Relate how casual staff, float pools, overtime, mandatory overtime, and the use of supplemental agency staff affect nursing staff satisfaction and patient-care outcomes.
- Integrate current research into principles on effectively managing staff.
- Understand that scheduling seeks to meet patients' needs, nurses' personal scheduling needs, and budgetary needs in a balanced and fair manner.
- Understand and be able to evaluate activity reports on a unit's staffing and productivity.

TERMS TO KNOW

average daily census (ADC)	fixed full-time equivalent (FTE)	mandatory overtime
average length of stay (ALOS)	forecast	nonproductive hours
cost centre	full-time equivalent (FTE)	nurse outcomes
direct care hours	indirect care hours	nursing productivity
factor evaluation system	labour cost per unit of service	overtime

TERMS TO KNOW—cont'd

patient outcomes	scheduling	variable full-time equivalent
percentage of occupancy	staffing	(FTE)
productive hours	staffing plan	variance report
prototype evaluation system	unit of service	workload

? A CHALLENGE

Samantha is the nurse manager of a 39-bed neonatal intensive care unit (NICU) in a large regional hospital. The region is faced with severe capacity constraints, particularly for the most acutely ill neonates. However, preparations are underway for a new NICU at the local children's hospital, which will be completed in 3 years. A significant service gap exists because the local children's hospital currently has no NICU.

Samantha has been asked to help plan the new NICU at the local children's hospital. Some of the challenges to developing neonatal intensive care beds at the children's hospital include identifying the appropriate number of beds needed by considering the volume of patients locally and in the referral area. Moreover, the medical staff need to develop and approve admission and discharge criteria for these new beds. New equipment needs must be

identified. A number of other elements must be determined, such as the staff competencies necessary to provide appropriate care to neonatal intensive care patients, staff education programs, and a staffing plan. Communication to nurses and all other staff will be critical throughout the new NICU development process; some staff at Samantha's NICU fear that they will lose their jobs because patients would be relocated to the children's hospital, and others are concerned about the impact to them and their work environment because the short-term plan for extra capacity is to utilize space in the existing pediatric intensive care unit (PICU) within the regional hospital.

What would you do if you were Samantha?

INTRODUCTION

Health care costs are escalating at a furious pace, and operational funding continues to be constrained. Health care organizations have recognized that controlling labour costs is critical for overall cost reduction. Because salaries constitute some of the major drivers of labour costs in a health care organization, health care leaders are increasingly challenged to tightly manage both staffing and scheduling within assigned cost centres. Staffing, which involves planning for recruiting, hiring, deploying, and retaining qualified human resources to meet the needs of a group of patients, is a primary responsibility of the nurse manager. It is also a major way in which a nurse in a leadership role can influence quality of care. Scheduling, by contrast, is the implementation of the staffing plan by assigning unit personnel to work specific hours and days of the week.

Nurse managers must make skilled staffing and scheduling decisions to ensure that safe and cost-effective

care is provided by the appropriate level of caregiver. No matter the practice setting—acute care, home care, continuing care, or community care—nurse managers are accountable for establishing and monitoring effective and efficient staffing systems.

THE STAFFING PROCESS

A Nurse Staffing Model

Because of the emphasis in health care on patient safety and ensuring positive patient outcomes—the result of patient goals that are achieved through a combination of medical and nursing interventions with patient participation—research to define "best practices" in staffing has been a high priority for more than 20 years. Consistently over that period, observational studies suggest that increasing the number of registered nurses (RNs) results in many positive benefits to patients, such as a reduction in hospital-related morbidity and mortality as well as failure to rescue, both nursing-sensitive outcomes (Kane, Shamliyan, Mueller, et al., 2007).

However, none of these studies demonstrated a causal relationship. Further, hospitals with an overall commitment to high-quality care through sufficient staffing also invest in other actions that improve quality of care (Kane et al., 2007). Recently, Tourangeau (2008) and Estabrooks, Midodzi, Cummings, et al. (2011) demonstrated that hospital nursing characteristics including education level, skill mix, staffing numbers and levels, the proportion of casual or temporary positions, staff burnout, leadership support, and nurse–physician relationships are as important in efforts to reduce the risk of 30-day mortality of patients.

A recently published meta-analysis by Kane et al. (2007) assessed the relationship between nursing and patient outcomes and economic outcomes. Based on the relevant research, Kane et al. (2007) developed a conceptual framework (Figure 15-1) illustrating the complex relationships between nurse staffing and the quality of patient care. The framework was used to consider the impact of patient and hospital factors, nurse staffing, nurse characteristics, nurse outcomes,

medical care, and organizational factors on patient outcomes. Hyun, Bakken, Douglas, et al. (2008) suggested that although the data available to decide how to effectively allocate scarce nursing resources in practice are still limited, existing principles, frameworks, and guidelines provide a foundation for evidence-informed nurse staffing. So, despite the complex relationships apparent in Kane et al.'s (2007) framework, it can be useful not only for further research but also for nurse managers to develop "best practices" for staffing.

The Canadian Nurses Association (CNA, 2003) has issued a position statement related to safe nursing care. Also, in collaboration with other professional nursing associations, the CNA (2005a) developed an evaluation framework to determine the impact of nursing staff mix decisions and the utilization of health human resources in the health sector (CNA, 2005c). The CNA commissioned Harris and McGillis Hall (2012) to undertake a focused literature review "to guide revisions to the evaluation framework with

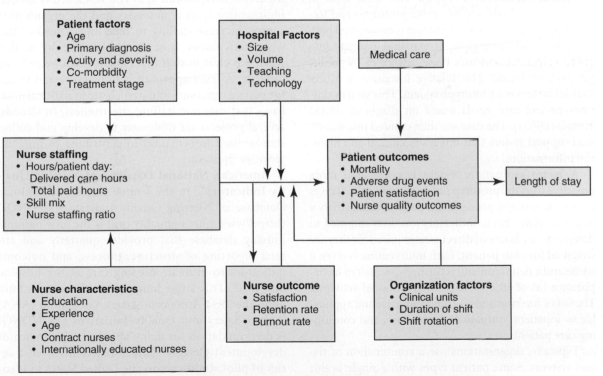

FIGURE 15-1 Conceptual framework of nurse staffing and patient outcomes.

the goal of supporting evidence-informed decision-making regarding staff mix in today's healthcare system" (p. 2). In terms of nurse staffing and outcomes, Harris and McGillis Hall (2012) concluded that "no gold standard for the measurement of nurse staffing exists" (pp. 2–3).

Patient Factors. The acuity or severity of patients' conditions, which is influenced by age, primary diagnosis, co-morbidity, and treatment stage, is a key component in determining staffing required for safe care. However, the dynamic nature of patient care often makes it difficult to quantify the care needs of patients at any given time.

Patient classification systems have been developed in an effort to give nurse managers the tools and language to describe the acuity of patients. "Sicker" patients receive higher classification scores, indicating that more nursing resources are required to provide patient care. Nurse managers may use the classification data to adjust the unit's staffing plan for a given time or to quantify acuity trends over longer periods in order to forecast staffing requirements for strategic, workforce, or budget planning processes.

Patient Classification Types. Two basic types of patient classification systems exist: prototype and factor. A prototype evaluation system is considered both subjective and descriptive. It classifies patients into broad categories and uses these categories to predict patient-care needs. The relative intensity measures (RIMs) system is a prototype system. This system classifies patient-care needs based on diagnosis-related groups (DRGs). The data are then entered into a decision support system that integrates clinical and financial information.

A factor evaluation system is considered more objective than the prototype evaluation system. It gives each task, thought process, and patient-care activity a time or rating. These indicators are then summed to determine the hours of direct care required, or they are weighted for each patient. Each intervention is given a name and a definition and is further specified to incorporate a list of all associated interventional activities. The list of interventions is comprehensive and applicable to inpatient, outpatient, home care, and continuing care patients.

Typically, organizations use a combination of the two systems. Some patient types with a single health care focus, such as maternal deliveries or outpatient surgical patients, would be appropriately classified with a prototype system. Patients with more complex care needs and a less predictable disease course, such as those with pneumonia or stroke, are more appropriately evaluated with a factor system.

Numerous potential problems exist with patient classification systems. The issue most often raised by administrators relates to the questionable reliability and validity of the data collected through a self-reporting mechanism. Another concern with patient classification data relates to the inability of the organization to meet the prescribed staffing levels outlined by the patient classification system. If the patient classification data indicate that six caregivers are needed for the upcoming shift but the organization can provide only five caregivers, what are the potential consequences for the patient and the organization if an untoward event occurs?

Concern over the accuracy of biased data and the inability to meet predicted staffing levels outlined by patient classification systems has caused many health care organizations to abandon patient classification as a mechanism for determining appropriate staffing levels. Staff morale is at risk when acuity models indicate one level is necessary and the organization cannot increase staffing to meet those needs. Likewise, staff morale is at risk without acuity models when it is clear to staff that patient needs exceed care capacity. A truer approach is to measure and monitor patient outcomes and participate in national databases that monitor staffing effectiveness. In Canada, several projects are underway to develop and collect standardized information to contribute to nursing-sensitive indicators.

American National Database of Nursing Quality Indicators®. In the United States, the National Database of Nursing Quality Indicators (NDNQI) (http://www.nursingquality.org) is the only national nursing database that provides quarterly and annual reporting of structure, process, and outcome indicators to evaluate nursing care at the hospital unit level. This large, longitudinal database is built upon the 1994 American Nurses Association (ANA) Patient Safety and Quality Initiative. The NDNQI is the foundation for many approaches to indicator development globally. This initiative involved a series of pilot studies across the United States to identify nursing-sensitive indicators to use in evaluating quality of patient care. These nursing-sensitive indicators include both structures of care and care processes, which in turn influence care outcomes. Nursing-sensitive indicators are distinct and specific to nursing and different from medical indicators of care quality (Montalvo, 2009).

Data for the NDNQI database are collected for eight types of units: critical care, step-down, medical, surgical, combined medical–surgical, rehabilitation, pediatric, and psychiatric. RN survey data are collected for all hospital unit types, including outpatient and interventional units (Dunton, Gajewski, Klaus, et al., 2007). Hospitals may join the NDNQI project, submitting data regarding nursing-sensitive indicators. Hospitals can benchmark (or compare) their own data against other similar hospitals and participate in ongoing research on nursing-sensitive data. Table 15-1

outlines the nursing-sensitive indicators included in the NDNQI project.

A component of the NDNQI database is the hours per patient day (HPPD) required to provide the necessary care for patients on the unit. This figure may include the HPPD of total nursing care provided or the HPPD of RN care provided. The NDNQI project reports a number of findings related to the HPPD required by patients. For example, in their review of nursing outcomes research, Dunton et al. (2007) suggested the following:

- Lower falls rates were related to higher total nursing hours (including RN, licensed practical nurse, and unlicensed nursing assistants) per patient day and a higher percentage of nursing hours supplied by RNs.
- For every increase of 1 hour in total nursing HPPD, fall rates were 1.9% lower.

TABLE 15-1 NURSING-SENSITIVE INDICATORS INCLUDED IN THE NDNQI® PROJECT

INDICATOR	SUBINDICATORS		MEASURE(S)
1. Nursing hours per patient day (HPPD)*†	a.	Registered nurses (RNs)	Structure
	b.	Licensed practical (LPNs)	
	c.	Unregulated care providers (UCPs)	
2. Patient falls*†			Process and outcome
3. Patient falls with injury*†	a.	Injury level	Process and outcome
4. Pediatric pain assessment, intervention, reassessment (AIR) cycle			Process
5. Pediatric peripheral intravenous infiltration rate			Outcome
6. Pressure ulcer prevalence*	a.	Community acquired	Process and outcome
	b.	Hospital acquired	
	c.	Unit acquired	
7. Psychiatric physical/sexual assault rate			Outcome
8. Restraint prevalence†			Outcome
9. RN education/certification			Structure
10. RN satisfaction survey options*‡	a.	Job satisfaction scales	Process and outcome
	b.	Job satisfaction scales—short form	
	c.	Practice environment scale (PES)†	
11. Skill mix: percent of total nursing hours supplied by agency staff*†	a.	RNs	Structure
	b.	LPNs	
	c.	UCPs	
12. Voluntary nurse turnover†			Structure
13. Nurse vacancy rate			Structure
14. Health care-associated infection			Outcome
a. Urinary catheter–associated urinary tract infection (UTI)†			
b. Central line catheter–associated bloodstream infection (CABSI)*†			
c. Ventilator-associated pneumonia (VAP)†			

*Original American Nurses Association (ANA) nursing-sensitive indicator.
†National Quality Forum (NQF)–endorsed nursing-sensitive indicator "NQF-15."
‡The RN survey is annual, whereas the other indicators are quarterly.

From Montalvo, I. (2007, September). The National Database of Nursing Quality Indicators™ (NDNQI®). *OJIN: The Online Journal of Issues in Nursing, 12*(3), 2.

- For every increase of 1 percentage point in the nursing hours supplied by RNs, the fall rate was 0.7% lower (Dunton et al., 2007).
- Nurse managers may also use clinical or human resources indicators other than those identified by NDNQI to evaluate the effectiveness of the staffing and quality of patient care. Box 15-1 identifies some of these indicators.

In Canada, three initiatives have been undertaken in recent years to develop and advance Canadian-specific nursing-sensitive indicators. In 2010, the CNA and the Academy of Canadian Executive Nurses (ACEN) joined forces to create the Canadian National Nursing Quality Report, or NNQR (C). The NNQR (C) is a benchmark of structural and contextual indicators such as nursing hours per patient day, RNs to total nursing staff, absenteeism, satisfaction; process indicators such as hand hygiene, pressure ulcer risks, fall risks, restraint use, medication incidents; and outcome indicators such as pressure ulcers, falls, therapeutic self-care, pain, and functional status (VanDeVelde-Coke, Doran, Grinspun, et al., 2012). The Canadian Health Outcomes for Better Information and Care (C-HOBIC) program in Ontario and the Nursing Quality Indicators for Reporting and Evaluation (NQuiRE) database led by the Registered Nurses Association of Ontario are two other examples of work on nursing-sensitive indicators in Canada (VanDeVelde-Coke et al., 2012).

Nurse Staffing. The growth in evidence on nursing-sensitive indicators has been accompanied by significant controversy regarding the level of nurse staffing required for various groups of patients, primarily in acute care hospitals. Spence Laschinger, Sabiston, Finegan, et al. (2001) surveyed nurses in Ontario about working conditions and the effect of these conditions on patient safety outcomes. They noted four major areas of concern: quality of work life, quality of patient care, relations with management, and cumulative impact of work conditions. In 2008, the American Nurses Association (ANA) polled more than 10 000 nurses nationally to determine their perceptions of the impact of staffing levels on their work environment. In all, 73% of respondents did not believe the staffing on their unit or shift was sufficient, and 59.8% said they knew of someone who left direct care because of concerns about safe staffing. Of the 51.9% of respondents who were considering leaving their current position, 46% cited inadequate staffing as the reason. Almost 52% of respondents said that they thought the quality of nursing care on their unit had declined in the past year, and 48.2% would not feel confident having someone close to them receiving care in the facility where they work (American Nurses Association [ANA], 2008).

The recognition that the number of nurses providing care to patients is associated with patient outcomes in some areas of acute care leads to a discussion regarding the best model to ensure sufficient staffing. Two major approaches to sufficient staffing have been put forward. The first requires a specific number of patients to be cared for by one nurse per shift (mandated nurse–patient ratios). Legislation to mandate specific nurse–patient ratios was implemented in California in 1999 (Keepnews, 2007). No such legislation exists in Canada. However, frameworks that guide managers when making staff mix decisions do exist in Canada. One example appears in Table 15-2.

The second major approach requires the development of a staffing plan that projects the nursing needs on each unit for a period of time, typically coinciding with budget cycles, for 6 months, or for a year. A **staffing plan** is the conceptual approach of

---

BOX 15-1 OTHER INDICATORS OF STAFFING EFFECTIVENESS

Clinical or Service Indicators
- Family complaints
- Patient complaints
- Adverse drug events
- Injuries to patients
- Postoperative infections
- Upper gastrointestinal bleeding
- Shock/cardiac arrest
- Length of stay

Human Resource Indicators
- Overtime
- Staff vacancy rate
- Staff turnover rate
- Understaffing as compared with the hospital's staffing plan
- Nursing care hours per patient day
- Staff injuries on the job
- On-call or per diem use
- Sick time

TABLE 15-2	NURSING STAFF MIX DECISION-MAKING FRAMEWORK

COMPONENT	SELECTED CRITERIA
Patient factors	Complexity of care needs Predictability of outcomes Risk of negative outcomes
Care provider competencies	Education Experience Expertise
Practice environments	Availability of and access to resources including support for nurses, policies, procedures, care pathways and protocols to guide clinical decision-making

From Canadian Nurses Association. (2005). Nursing staff mix: A key link to patient safety. *Nursing Now—Issues and Trends in Canadian Nursing.* *19*(1):1-6. © Canadian Nurses Association. Reprinted with permission. Further reproduction prohibited.

accomplishing the work to be done on a given unit. Hospitals are also responsible for monitoring the extent to which actual staffing matches staffing plans and making revisions as necessary. These plans often require that direct care nurses be part of the nurse staffing committee to ensure that safe nurse-to-patient ratios are based on patient needs and other related criteria. The first legislation mandating such a committee was passed by the Texas state legislature in 2002. As of October 2008, seven states had some sort of legislation requiring a nursing staffing plan in acute care hospitals (Haebler, 2008). Again, no such legislation exists in Canada. However, some collective agreements do include provisions for joint staffing committees. *Joint*, in this instance, refers to combined union, staff, and leadership staffing committees whose purpose is to review issues of staffing and workload and make recommendations to address these issues.

Those who support a specified nurse–patient ratio based on the type of unit (e.g., critical care unit, medical–surgical unit) believe that this approach will ultimately require hospitals to either find sufficient numbers of nurses to meet the ratio or shut down units. Those who prefer the nurse staffing plan approach believe that use of a staffing plan is built on nursing judgement that will allow staffing to be flexible, depending on patient acuity, nurse experience, team composition, configuration of the unit, and other factors.

The CNA (2005a) developed a comprehensive template for institutions to use when planning nurse staffing at the macro level (Figure 15-2). The following principles guide this framework for evaluating the impact of nursing staff mix decisions:

1. Patient, nurse, and system outcomes are central to the evaluation of nursing staff mix decisions.
2. Evaluation of the impact of nursing staff mix decisions is complex and requires a systematic and comprehensive approach using all of the components of this framework.
3. This evaluation framework recognizes and respects the value and contribution of each regulated nursing group.
4. This evaluation framework applies to all sectors and patient populations.

The CNA has a number of documents on its website that can help nurse managers and staff make staffing decisions, including the following:

- "Position Statement: Staffing Decisions for the Delivery of Safe Patient Care" (2003): http://www.cna-aiic.ca/~/media/cna/page%20content/pdf%20en/2013/09/04/16/27/9%20-%20ps67_staffing_decisions_delivery_safe_nursing_care_june_2003_e.pdf.
- "Nursing Staff Mix: A Key Link to Patient Safety" (2005): https://www.cna-aiic.ca/~/media/cna/page%20content/pdf%20en/2013/07/26/10/40/nn_nursing_staff_mix_05_e.pdf.
- "Position Statement: National Planning for Human Resources in the Health Sector" (2005): https://www.cna-aiic.ca/~/media/cna/page%20content/pdf%20fr/2013/09/05/19/16/ps81_national_planning_e.pdf.

24-Hour Staffing. Most of the research on safe staffing has been done in acute care hospitals or long-term care facilities. As a result, these findings must be applied to other health care settings with some caution. In addition, little research exists on the differences in staffing in any clinical environment during off-peak hours (nights and weekends). Despite the fact that hospital activity is at its peak from 7:00 to 19:00 weekdays, when maximum resources are available in the nurse's work environment, this time represents only 36% of the time that nurses work in acute care or long-term care. During the remaining 64% of the time, nurses work in off-peak environments with (1) scaled back ancillary personnel, (2) fewer (often less-experienced) staff,

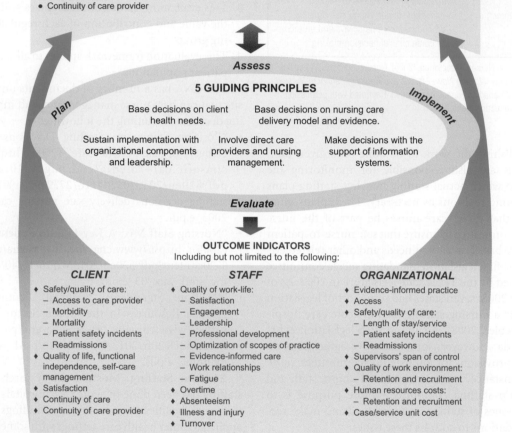

FACTORS TO CONSIDER
Including but not limited to the following:

CLIENT	STAFF	ORGANIZATIONAL
• Health-care needs	• RNs, LPNs, RPNs, UCPs:	• Nursing care delivery model
• Acuity, complexity, predictability, stability, variability, dependency	– Numbers	• Physical environment
	– Availability	• Resources and support services
• Type:	– Education	• Practice setting
– Individual	– Competencies	• Legislation and regulations
– Family	– Experience	• Workplace health and safety
– Group	• Teamwork and collaboration	• Policies
– Community/population	• Clinical support and consultation	• Collective agreements
• Cohort:	• Continuity of assignment	• Vision, mission and nursing philosophy
– Numbers	• Continuity of care	
– Range of conditions		• Culture
– Fluctuations in mix		• Leadership support
• Continuity of care provider		

Assess

5 GUIDING PRINCIPLES

Plan

Implement

Base decisions on client health needs.

Base decisions on nursing care delivery model and evidence.

Sustain implementation with organizational components and leadership.

Involve direct care providers and nursing management.

Make decisions with the support of information systems.

Evaluate

OUTCOME INDICATORS
Including but not limited to the following:

CLIENT	STAFF	ORGANIZATIONAL
◆ Safety/quality of care:	◆ Quality of work-life:	◆ Evidence-informed practice
– Access to care provider	– Satisfaction	◆ Access
– Morbidity	– Engagement	◆ Safety/quality of care:
– Mortality	– Leadership	– Length of stay/service
– Patient safety incidents	– Professional development	– Patient safety incidents
– Readmissions	– Optimization of scopes of practice	– Readmissions
◆ Quality of life, functional independence, self-care management	– Evidence-informed care	◆ Supervisors' span of control
	– Work relationships	◆ Quality of work environment:
	– Fatigue	– Retention and recruitment
◆ Satisfaction	◆ Overtime	◆ Human resources costs:
◆ Continuity of care	◆ Absenteeism	– Retention and recruitment
◆ Continuity of care provider	◆ Illness and injury	◆ Case/service unit cost
	◆ Turnover	

FIGURE 15-2 Evaluation framework to determine the impact of nursing staff mix decisions.

(3) less supervision and support, and (4) strained communication with on-call health care providers (Hamilton, Eschiti, Hernandez, et al., 2007). In a study to determine the organizational effects of off-peak (weekend and night shift) environments on the work that critical care nurses do, Eschiti and Hamilton (2011) learned that support services and numbers

of non-nurse staff are greatly diminished on off-peak shifts.

The problems identified by Hamilton et al. (2007) are corroborated in other studies. Researchers have associated weekends and nights with increased mortality in hospitals for more than 25 diagnoses/patient groups. For example, Becker (2007) found acute myocardial infarction more likely to result in death among Medicaid (a US government health insurance plan) patients admitted on weekends, and Cram, Hillis, Barnett, et al. (2004) found that major teaching hospitals had a larger weekend effect than did nonteaching hospitals. Peberdy, Ornato, Larkin, et al. (2008) found lower survival rates from inpatient cardiology units at nights and on weekends, even after adjusting for potentially confounding factors. Although the reasons for the differences in risk in off-peak hours are under investigation, managers must be cognizant of these differences and staff during off-peak times in a prudent manner to minimize patient risk.

Overtime. Overtime may affect staffing plans and patient outcomes. Kane et al. (2007) reviewed seven descriptive studies that used survey methodology to find that nurses are working long hours. Because more nurses are choosing to work 12-hour shifts, the risk of working more than 12 hours is high, given that nurses on occasion cannot finish their work by the end of their scheduled shift. Preliminary evidence shows that working more than 12 hours and rotating shifts can lead to errors that compromise patient safety. This finding suggests that as many nurses and other staff are required to work rotating shifts, nurse managers need to carefully consider these effects. Nurses should be educated about the effect of fatigue on the quality of their practice (Kane et al., 2007).

Rogers (2008) reported that working overtime at the end of a shift or exceeding regular weekly work hours was associated with a statistically significant increase in making an error. The most significant elevations in risk of making an error were associated with working a consecutive 12.5 hours or longer. It should be noted that the risk did not change based on whether the nurse had volunteered to work longer, was scheduled to work longer, or was mandated to work overtime.

Requiring staff to stay on duty after their shift ends to fill staffing vacancies is called **mandatory overtime**. Professional nursing associations, unions, and regulatory bodies across the country continue to debate the issue of mandatory overtime. Regular and mandatory overtime have become a major negotiating point for nurses in unionized settings. Nursing associations tend to oppose mandatory overtime because it is seen as a risk to both patients and nurses. The Canadian Federation of Nurses Unions (2009) rejected the practice of officially mandating nurses to work overtime as well as the practice of coercing or pressuring a nurse into accepting overtime.

In contrast, *requesting* staff to stay on duty after their shift ends to fill staffing vacancies is called **overtime**. This differs from mandatory overtime because there are no employment consequences to the staff response to the request. In addition, in a given week, nurses may work in more than one employment setting as a means of increasing their income. Although this practice is an individual decision, tired and overworked nurses are more likely to have compromised decision-making abilities and technical skills because of fatigue.

EXERCISE 15-1

Review a health care organization's policies on overtime. Is mandatory overtime covered in the policy? Are the consequences for failing to work mandatory overtime when requested to do so by a supervisor outlined in the policy?

How would you respond to a manager who required you to stay on the job after your shift was over? Develop a list of questions you might ask during a job interview relating to use of overtime in the organization.

What does the professional nursing association or regulatory body in your province or territory allow regarding mandatory overtime? As a nurse manager, how would you respond to a nursing staff shortage without mandatory overtime as an option? Develop a list of strategies for eliminating mandatory overtime, if it exists. Refer back to the applicable sections of Chapter 5 and reflect upon your findings.

Float Pools and Agency Staff. Some nurses may choose to work for staffing agencies. They may be hired by a hospital or the nursing unit as an independent contractor for a shift, a week, or longer. There may be advantages to the nurse to work for an agency, such as higher hourly rates of pay, diversity in work assignments, exposure to a variety of work teams, and the ability to travel.

Organizations may use supplemental (contract or agency) staff to fill temporary staff vacancies. Although they must respond to unexpected vacancies, nurse managers must consider the potential negative aspects of depending on supplemental staff to fulfill staffing plans. Patients should be unable to distinguish agency staff from unit staff. However, the ability to provide that level of orientation to agency or contract staff is often difficult.

The evidence regarding the impact of the use of contract nurses on patient outcomes is mixed. Cho (2002), as cited in Kane et al. (2007), showed no association between hours worked by a contract nurse and the rates of urinary tract infection, pneumonia, pressure ulcers, surgical wound infections, and bloodstream infections. In contrast, Kane et al. (2007) reviewed research by Cho (2002) and Donaldson, Bolton, Aydin, et al. (2005), which found that an increase in rates of patient falls corresponded to the use of additional contract hours.

Another strategy that may be used to deal with unanticipated staff vacancies involves "floating" nurses from one clinical unit to another to fill the vacancies. Two studies included in Kane et al. (2007) indicated that the use of "float" nurses was associated with an increased risk of nosocomial infections and rate of bloodstream infections; however, further research is necessary to validate this finding. In practice, the use of float nurses may be effective if the nurses are deployed from a centralized flexible staffing pool and they have the competencies to work on the unit to which they are assigned. Nurses willing to work as float nurses may be generally experienced nurses who maintain a broad range of clinical competencies. However, they may also be fairly inexperienced newly graduated nurses who require ongoing education, orientation, and support.

When an organization does not have the flexibility of a staffing pool, the organization may expect nurses to float across clinical units to fill vacancies. To ensure patient safety and nurse satisfaction, the organization must develop a policy regarding the reassignment of the staff to clinically similar units. If staff nurses are asked to be reassigned to an area outside of their sphere of clinical competence, they should be given appropriate orientation and asked to support only basic care needs and nursing care they feel comfortable they can provide within their competence and not assume a complete and independent assignment. This practice should be used only on an emergency basis or with the nurse's agreement, because being required to float is often a "dissatisfier" for nurses.

External Factors Influencing Staffing. Provincial and territorial professional nursing associations and regulatory bodies along with some provincial governments offer recommendations that can guide projections of staffing requirements. Staffing requirements can relate to the minimum number of regulated nurses on an acute or critical care unit at a given time or to the amount of minimum staffing in an ambulatory care program, a continuing care facility, or a correctional facility. For example, some provincial governments set out the minimum staffing required to license long-term care facilities.

However, it is important to note that licensing standards and staffing recommendations by provincial and territorial governments, professional associations, and regulatory bodies are not the only mechanisms that affect staffing plans. A number of national organizations have missions related to continuous improvement in the areas of patient safety and quality care. Accreditation Canada is an example of such an organization. Accreditation Canada supports performance improvements in health care organizations by establishing standards and by monitoring accreditation processes. For example, to comply with Accreditation Canada's (2010) leadership standards, an organization must promote a healthy and safe work environment, support a positive quality of work life, and design and organize services to meet the needs of the community. Accreditation Canada is not prescriptive as to what constitutes "adequate" staffing. However, for contracted services, Accreditation Canada (2010) has set out standards for investing in health care services, engaging prepared and proactive staff, providing safe and appropriate services, monitoring quality, and achieving positive outcomes. During the Accreditation Canada process, external reviewers (surveyors) follow patients (tracing) through the care continuum. It is possible that staffing concerns may arise during these surveys. The surveyor also interviews staff outside of the presence of managers to inquire about staff perceptions of the units' staffing adequacy, among other factors. Additional agencies that provide review services or carry out comparative benchmarking similar to those provided by Accreditation Canada include Health Facilities Review Committees, Health Quality Councils, the Trauma Association of Canada, Canadian Association for Laboratory Accreditation, and the Canadian Institutes of Health Research.

Patient and family expectations may also play a role in the development and implementation of staffing plans. Patient expectations and patient satisfaction reports frequently cite staffing levels and other staffing factors as important. Recognizing that patients expect to receive high-quality nursing care that is delivered promptly and efficiently by nurses who are capably managing their workload has a significant influence on the development of a staffing plan.

Organizational policies and clear expectations communicated to staff are essential to managing high and low volume as well as changes in acuity. Proposed human resources budgets and staffing plans that cannot flex up or down when patient acuity or volumes change put the manager in a position in which patient safety may not be maintained and financial obligations may not be met. In addition, mechanisms that allow staff to ask for additional help as needed must be in place and internally publicized. Patient, staff, and physician satisfaction; service and care improvement; and patient safety improvement are all outcomes of a solid staffing plan. Nurse managers are obligated to consider these variables when preparing the human resources budget.

Nurse Characteristics. Estabrooks et al. (2011) define *nurse characteristics* as including age, education, skill mix (RN to total nurse staff), employment status, nurse work satisfaction, autonomy, nurse–physician relationships, and experience. In addition, the local supply of nurses and the use of supplemental (e.g., contract) nurses are variables that influence nurse staffing.

Ridley (2008) undertook a review of literature from 1986 to 2006 regarding the relationship between patient safety and nurse education level. She found that when studies discriminated between RNs and other types of nursing personnel (e.g., licensed practical nurses, registered psychiatric nurses) or unregulated care providers (UCPs), they showed that an increased number of RNs and a larger percentage of RNs relative to other nursing personnel decreased adverse patient outcomes sensitive to nursing care. In 2003, Aiken, Clarke, Cheung, et al. found that hospitals with a higher proportion of RNs educated at the baccalaureate level or above had a lower 30-day mortality and failure-to-rescue rate; interest in this idea has

persisted. Further research is necessary to validate this claim (Ridley, 2008). However, Dunton et al. (2007) found that for every increase of a year in average RN experience, the fall rate was 1% lower and the number of hospital-acquired pressure ulcers was reduced by 0.7%. Cho, Hwang, and Kim (2008) found that in secondary hospitals, every additional patient per RN was associated with a 9% increase in the odds of dying. However, these authors did not find a significant relationship between nurse experience and mortality. Aiken, Cimiotti, Sloane, et al. (2011) concluded that the positive effect on patient outcomes of increased nurse education is consistent across all hospitals, as is the lowering of patient-to-nurse ratios. Kendall-Gallagher, Aiken, Sloan, et al. (2011) indicated that nurse specialty certification is associated with better patient outcomes.

Hospital Factors. According to Tourangeau, Doran, McGillis Hall, et al. (2006) hospital factors include the size of the hospital, the type of hospital (e.g., major teaching or nonteaching), and location (e.g., urban or rural). Other hospital factors include the volume and acuity of patients seen, and the extent to which technology is used in the hospital. A number of studies have found that the type of unit affected hospital RN staffing. Critical care, pediatric, and oncology units had significantly higher RN staffing than medical–surgical or maternity units. Controlling for size, rural hospitals also had higher RN staffing (Kane et al., 2007). Studies exploring the relationship between increased RN-to-patient ratio found that the effect of increasing the number of RNs to patients was greater in surgical patients and in critical care units. The evidence of the effect of increased RN-to-patient ratios in medical units is less consistent and needs further investigation (Kane et al., 2007). The nurse surveillance capacity of a hospital (those factors that strengthen or weaken the nurses' ability to observe patients for signs of difficulty) also affects the quality of care given. Nurse surveillance capacity is composed of nurse staffing, education, expertise, and experience, as well as nurse practice environment characteristics. Kutney-Lee, Lake, and Aiken (2009) found that greater nurse surveillance capacity was significantly associated with better quality of care and fewer adverse effects. (See the following Literature Perspective.)

LITERATURE PERSPECTIVE

Resource: Kutney-Lee, A., Lake, E. T., & Aiken, L. H. (2009). Development of the hospital nurse surveillance capacity profile. *Research in Nursing & Health, 32*(2), 217–228. doi:10.1002/nur.20316

Surveillance by nurses is a key component of improved patient care. This article defines, operationalizes, measures, and evaluates nurse surveillance capacity, which includes organizational features that enhance or weaken nurse surveillance. Nurse surveillance capacity is composed of nurse staffing, education, expertise, and experience, as well as nurse practice environment characteristics. This study found that greater nurse surveillance capacity was significantly associated with better quality of care and fewer adverse effects.

Implications for Practice

Evaluating the nurse surveillance capacity in a particular nursing work environment may help the nurse manager improve nurse surveillance and patient outcomes on his or her unit.

Regardless of the characteristics of the hospital, nurse managers must be concerned with the financial health of the institution. As a result, hospital financial officers are often reluctant to increase the number of RN staff because of fear of escalating costs. However, Dall, Chen, Seifert, et al. (2009) found that for each additional patient care RN employed at 7.8 hours per patient day, over $60 000 annually will be saved from reduced medical costs and improved productivity (accounting for 72% of labour costs). This finding is only a partial estimate of the economic value of nursing because the estimate omits the intangible benefits of reduced pain and suffering by patients and family members, the reduced risk of rehospitalization, benefits to the hospital such as improved reputation and reduced patient concerns or legal issues, and other indirect costs.

Nurse Outcomes. Nurse outcomes are the results of nursing work, including staff vacancy rate, nurse satisfaction, staff turnover rate, retention rate, and nurse burnout rate. Kane et al. (2007) noted that while patient outcomes are the ultimate concern, nurse outcomes can interact with nurse staffing to affect patient outcomes. In addition, patient outcomes will, in turn, affect length of stay (LOS), and greater complication rates may increase the LOS for patients.

Spence Laschinger and Leiter (2006) tested a theoretical model for professional nurse work environments, linking conditions for professional nursing practice to burnout and subsequent patient safety outcomes. The results suggested that nurses who feel that the environment they work in is supportive of professional practice are more likely to engage in the work leading to safer patient care. The results also reinforced the key role of strong nursing leadership in creating conditions for staff engagement and safe, quality care for patients. These results were also supported by the findings of Stone, Mooney-Kane, Larson, et al. (2007), who carried out an observational study of nurse working conditions related to outcomes for older adult patients in intensive care environments and determined that system approaches and improving nurse working conditions improved patient safety.

Organizational Factors That Affect Staffing Plans. Other organizational factors that affect staffing plans include the type of clinical unit and the duration of the shift nurses work, as well as the extent to which shifts are rotated. These factors are typically addressed in the structure and philosophy of the unit, program, service, department, hospital, or health organization staffing policies, organizational supports, and services offered. Chapter 14 also discusses care delivery strategies that may influence staffing plans.

Structure and Philosophy of the Nursing Services Department. A nursing philosophy statement outlines the vision, values, and beliefs about the practice of nursing and the provision of patient care within an organization (see also Chapter 9). The philosophy statement is used to guide the practice of nursing in various nursing units on a daily basis. Nurse managers should propose a staffing plan and a human resources budget that allow consistency between the written philosophy statement and the observable practice of nursing on the units. It is demoralizing for nurses to feel that they cannot comply with their nursing philosophy statement or professional values because of problems associated with consistently inadequate staffing.

The philosophy statements may exist for an organization as a whole and for various parts of the organization. These statements also guide the establishment of the overall structure of the clinical service departments and the staffing models that are used within the organization. Staffing models adopted by organizations play a major role in determining the mix of regulated and unregulated health care staff needed to provide patient care.

Organizational Staffing Policies. An organization's staffing policies guide nurse managers in the development of unit human resources budgets. For example, an organization develops a policy or follows one or more collective agreements that identify the rate at which an employee earns overtime and other benefit time. Nurse managers will be in compliance with these requirements if they adhere to organizational staffing policies.

Organizational Support Systems. A critical variable that affects the development of the human resources budget is the presence, or absence, of organizational systems that support clinical staff in providing care. If an organization has recognized the need to keep the registered nurse at the bedside, support systems will be in place to allow that to happen. Examples of support systems that enhance the nurse's ability to remain on the unit and provide direct care to patients include patient and material transport services, clerical support services, and hospitality services.

However, registered nurses often work in organizations that require them to function in the role of a multi-purpose worker, particularly in acute or long-term care. Because nurses in these settings are generally scheduled to work 24 hours a day, 7 days a week, they may be required to offer services to other health care providers who deliver more limited hours of care to patients. It is wise for nurse managers to identify what costs are being incurred in the unit as a result of the absence of organizational support systems and to develop strategies to put those systems in place or justify the budget accordingly. For example, introducing a supply clerk role on weekends and evenings may prevent nursing staff from seeking supplies, and reduce overall nursing requirements, which could give nurses more time with patients and be a more effective utilization of budget dollars. Important to this consideration is the study by Upenieks, Akhavan, and Kotlerman (2008), which found that a number of activities that were not actual direct care activities performed at the patient's bedside were considered value-added activities because they represented a direct benefit to the patient. (See the Research Perspective.)

🔍 RESEARCH PERSPECTIVE

Resource: Upenieks, V., Akhavan, J., & Kotlerman, J. (2008). Value-added care: A paradigm shift in patient care delivery. *Nursing Economic$, 26*(5), 294–300.

The purpose of the study was to (1) gain an understanding of how much time front-line RNs spent in value-added care and (2) determine whether increasing the combined level of RNs and UCPs increased the amount of time spent in value-added care compared with time spent in necessary tasks and waste. The study found that a number of activities that were not actual direct care activities performed at the patient's bedside—including collaborating with team members, reviewing charts, preparing medications, teaching activities, and communicating with family members—were considered value-added activities since they represented a direct benefit to the patient.

Implications for Practice
This study validated the work done by Robert Wood Johnson Foundation's initiative Transforming Care at the Bedside, which was designed to increase the amount of time nurses spend in value-added activities and to reduce time spent in nonvalue-added activities to improve workflow efficiency, encourage care processes free of waste, and promote continuous flow of patient activities through the appropriate use of nurses and UCPs.

Services Offered on the Unit. When developing a staffing budget, nurse managers must consider the services offered on the unit, as well as organizational plans to provide new or expanded clinical services. For example, a nurse manager of an inpatient surgical unit must consider the potential effect of offering a new surgical procedure to the community. What projections have been made for this service need? What is the expected length of stay for patients undergoing this new procedure? What are the provincial or territorial and national standards for care for this type of patient? Has another organization developed the best "benchmarked" way to deliver this service in an accessible, quality, sustainable way? A nurse manager will use this information to project additional staff requirements to manage these changes in service.

Conversely, nurse managers must also be aware of any organizational plans to adjust or delete an existing service that their unit supports. For example, if a nurse manager in a home care setting knows that service pressures exist related to the distribution of existing home care resources, services may need to be rationed to allow for structuring staffing resources in any fiscal period. Decisions about service rationing should be based on clinical decision making related to individual patient needs.

FORECASTING UNIT STAFFING REQUIREMENTS

Recognizing elements, including related research, that influence staffing is essential to the development of a staffing plan. However, additional factors must be considered when determining the appropriate staffing level for a specific unit. The staffing plan for a unit is initiated in concert with the development of the human resources budget. The person(s) responsible for projecting the staffing needs of the unit should consider a number of factors when forecasting the unit's workload for the upcoming year, including the following:

1. Projected units of service—productivity target; e.g., hours per visit for emergency departments
2. Projected population needs
3. Historical staffing requirements
4. Effectiveness of the current staffing plan
5. Trends in acuity on the unit
6. Anticipated skill mix or other human resource changes
7. Experience and education of staff
8. New physicians, programs, services, or technology anticipated to affect staffing
9. Patient outcomes
10. Need for educational updates driven by changes in patient-care guidelines
11. Enablers such as technology, new knowledge

Various mathematical formulations are used to create human resources budgets and staffing patterns. However, these formulas were developed when the average length of stay and funding mechanisms were much different than they are today. The current difficulties related to staffing in health care suggest that current methods used to predict human resources budgets and staffing patterns have become increasingly complex and ineffective. Fitzpatrick and Brooks (2010) suggest the use of optimization models that rely on computer and logistical sciences to identify the best solution to particular staffing problems. (See the following Literature Perspective.)

LITERATURE PERSPECTIVE

Resource: Fitzpatrick, T., & Brooks, B. (2010). The nurse leader as logistician: Optimizing human capital. *Journal of Nursing Administration, 40*(2), 69–74.

Ten-day hospital length of stays, cost-based reimbursements, and unlegislated staffing ratios were common when the mathematical formulas currently used to create human resources budgets and staffing patterns were developed. However, health care delivery has become much more dynamic and complex in the twenty-first century and the old formulas, based on averages, are no longer adequate. Because these formulas use a single number, usually an average, to represent uncertain outcomes, the "flaw of averages" tends to promote zero-sum solutions. For example, if the solutions meet financial goals, staff satisfaction may be sacrificed. Conversely, if staff satisfaction is achieved, financial targets may not be met.

The authors suggest that optimization models, using the power of computer science and logistics science, can simulate solutions for complex staffing problems. These solutions consider myriad constraints and variables and arrange them in such a way as to produce the optimal answer solution. For example, real-world problems are defined as a set of mathematical equations, addressing objectives (minimize cost, maximize preferences, and perfect coverage), variables (skill and staff mix, demand fluctuation, and cost differentials), and constraints (staff availability, union rules) to determine the best solution.

Implications for Practice
Although these modelling tools and techniques have not yet been widely used in health care, they are available. The authors suggest that executive teams should include experts with these modelling and analytical skills. In addition, nurse executives also may want to gain these skills.

Units of Service

A **unit of service** is a measure of the work being produced by the organization; for example, patient days, clinic or home visits, hours of service, admissions, deliveries, or treatments. The units of service multiplied by the volume for a clinical area determine the number of staff needed in a given time period. The formula can be adjusted for total paid staff or just for those required for the delivery of direct patient care.

When developing an adequate human resources budget, the amount of work performed by a **cost centre** (an organizational unit for which costs can be identified and managed) is referred to as its workload. **Workload** is measured in terms of the units of service defined by the cost centre. Nurse managers must understand the nature of the work in their area of responsibility to define the units of service that will be used as the workload statistic and to forecast, or project based on multiple sources of data, the volume of work that will be performed by a cost centre during the upcoming year.

Calculation of Full-Time Equivalents

Nurse managers use the unit's forecasted workload to calculate the number of full-time equivalents (FTEs) that will be needed to construct the unit's overall staffing plan. An FTE is an employee who works full-time, typically 37.5 hours per week (1950 hours per year). It is important to remember that an employee in a staff position and an FTE are distinct. Chapter 13 describes FTEs and how they are calculated. To achieve a balanced staffing plan, managers must determine the correct combination of full-time and part-time positions that will be needed.

Nurse managers must also consider the effect of productive and nonproductive hours when projecting the FTE needs of the unit. Productive hours are paid time that is actually worked. Productive hours can be further defined as direct care hours and indirect care hours. Direct care hours are paid time used for the care of patients. Indirect care hours are paid time used for other required unit activities, such as staff meetings or continuing education.

Nonproductive hours are paid time that is not worked, such as vacation, statutory holidays, orientation, education, and sick time (see Chapter 13). In most practice settings, nurses and other staff must be replaced when they are off duty and accessing their paid benefit time off. Nurse managers must be aware of the average benefit hours required for the unit, or FTE needs may be understated. Thus, nurse managers must carefully consider how to allocate budgeted FTEs into full-time and part-time positions to meet the staffing requirements for the unit when a portion of the staff is taking paid time off. In addition, looking at the number of employees being paid for any specific day may not reflect the number actually providing care. So, the nurse manager must have competencies in finances, information technology, and automated staffing and scheduling programs.

> **EXERCISE 15-2**
>
> Select a hospital-based unit and determine the hours of operation (e.g., 24-hour/7-days-a-week inpatient or 7.5 hour/day outpatient). Assess the master scheduling plan and determine how many RNs are needed to ensure that each shift has one RN present. Assuming that a 37.5-hour work week will equal one FTE, convert the required number of RN positions to FTEs. Compare your findings with those for an inpatient unit where 12-hour shifts and 8-hour shifts are scheduled.

Distribution of Full-Time Equivalents

Managers must consider a number of variables when they begin the process of distributing FTEs in the unit staffing plan. The staffing plan, which is based on the unit's approved human resources budget and the projected staffing needs to ensure patient safety, serves as a guide for creating unit schedules for the upcoming year. Variables that must be considered by managers when creating master staffing plans include the following:

1. The hours of operation of the unit
2. The basic shift length for the unit
3. Known activity patterns for the unit at various times of day
4. Maximum work stretch for each employee
5. Shift rotation requirements
6. Weekend requirements
7. Personal and professional requirements and requests for time off (e.g., school schedule, meetings for professional development, and support for models of staff involvement in organizational initiative planning and implementation).

Each of these variables interrelates with the others, so few "absolutes" are possible. For example, initially one might think that a 24/7 unit might require more staff than a unit that operates from 7:00 to 18:00. However, if the 24/7 unit provides basic care all day and few activities at night (e.g., a long-term care facility), fewer staff might be needed than for the 7:00 to 18:00 unit if that were, for example, a day surgery unit.

The master staffing plan must consider the distribution of fixed FTEs in the plan. Fixed FTEs are full-time equivalent positions that do not fluctuate based on patient-care demands. Fixed FTEs are scheduled to work, no matter what the volume of activity. These employees generally hold a fully funded salaried position, meaning that their compensation does not depend on the unit's workload. Employees who typically hold a fixed FTE include nurse managers, regular staff, and support staff such as clinical nurse specialists and education staff.

The nurse manager then distributes the variable FTEs in the staffing plan. Variable FTEs are full-time equivalent positions that depend on the demand for care, and are typically staff positions. Variable FTEs are scheduled to work based on changes in the workload of the unit or replacement needs. These employees are considered hourly wage or casual employees, meaning that their compensation depends on the actual number of hours worked in a given pay period. Employees who typically hold a variable FTE position include casual staff nurses, casual clerical staff, and other casual ancillary support staff assigned to the unit.

SCHEDULING

Scheduling, as indicated earlier, is the implementation of the staffing plan by assigning unit personnel to work specific hours and days of the week. The nurse manager is often challenged to take the FTEs that are allotted through the human resources budget, distribute them appropriately, and create a master schedule for the unit that also meets each employee's personal and professional needs. Although completely satisfying each individual staff member is not always possible, a schedule can usually be created that is both fair and balanced from the employee's perspective while still meeting patient-care needs. Creating a flexible schedule with a variety of scheduling options that leads to work schedule stability for each employee is one mechanism likely to retain staff, which is within the control of nurse managers.

Constructing the Schedule

Mechanisms are typically in place within an organization for staff to request days off and to know when the final schedule will be posted. In addition, most organizations have written policies and procedures that must be followed by managers to ensure compliance with provincial or territorial and federal labour laws or contractual requirements relative to scheduling. These policies also help nurse managers make scheduling decisions that will be perceived as fair and equitable by all employees.

Schedules are usually constructed for a predetermined block of time based on organizational policy or contractual requirements—for example, weekly, biweekly, monthly, or quarterly. The unit schedule may be prepared in a decentralized fashion by managers or by unit staff through a self-scheduling method. In some organizations, centralized staffing coordinators may oversee all of the schedules prepared for the patient-care units. Each method of schedule preparation has pros and cons.

Decentralized Scheduling—Nurse Manager. One decentralized method for preparing the schedule involves nurse managers developing the schedule in isolation from all other units. In this model, the nurse manager approves all schedule changes and spends time on a regular basis drafting the staff schedule, considering only the staffing needs of the unit. In other decentralized models, nurse managers do the preliminary work on schedules and then submit them to a centralized staffing office for review and for the addition of any needed supplemental staff. The advantage of this decentralized method is that the accountability for submitting a schedule in alignment with the established staffing plan rests with nurse managers. Ultimately, nurse managers are responsible for maintaining unit productivity in line with the human resources budget, so the incentive to manage the schedule tightly is strong. The disadvantage of this decentralized method relates to the inability of any individual nurse manager to know the "big picture" related to staffing across multiple patient-care units. Requests for time off are approved in isolation from all other units, and a real potential exists that each nurse manager will make a decision at the unit level that will be felt in aggregate as a "staffing shortage" across multiple units.

Staff Self-Scheduling. A self-scheduling process has the potential to promote staff autonomy and to increase staff accountability. In addition, team communication, problem-solving, and negotiating skills can be enhanced through the self-scheduling process. Successful self-scheduling is achieved when each individual's personal schedule is balanced with the unit's patient-care needs.

Self-scheduling has become more complicated in the wake of care delivery changes and the decentralization of many activities to the individual patient-care units. The professional nursing staff cannot work in isolation from other care team members when creating a schedule. Assessing the readiness of support staff to participate in this type of initiative is critical as resource utilization and cost containment continue to be major areas of concern.

Self-scheduling needs to be properly managed. Although it is important to meet the personal needs of staff, patient-care needs on the unit are the most important focus for building a schedule. Unit standards for a staffing plan are usually established by the staff, typically based on criteria set out in collective agreements. A negotiated schedule that meets the needs of staff and patients is the expected and ultimate outcome.

Centralized Scheduling. One benefit to centralized scheduling is that the staffing coordinator is usually aware of the abilities, qualifications, and availability of supplemental personnel who may be needed to complete the schedule. In many organizations, the centralized staffing coordinator is also aware of each unit's human resources budget and any constraints the budget may impose on the schedule. On the other hand, a disadvantage to centralized staffing is the limited knowledge of the coordinator relative to changing patient acuity needs or other patient-related activities on the unit. Developing a mechanism for the centralized staffing coordinator to share unit-specific knowledge with the respective manager can resolve this disadvantage satisfactorily.

Many organizations have invested in computer software designed to create optimal schedules based on the approved staffing plans for individual units. The centralized staffing coordinator maintains the integrity of the computerized databank for each unit; enters schedule variances daily; generates planning sheets, drafts, and final schedules; and runs any specialized productivity reports requested by nurse managers. Nurse managers review the initial schedule created by the computer, make necessary modifications, and approve the final schedule.

Variables That Affect Staffing Schedules

Nurse managers must consider many variables to create a fair and balanced schedule. Examples of variables nurse managers can anticipate and must consider as they prepare a unit schedule appear in Box 15-2. Other unanticipated variables can complicate the best-prepared schedule. When faced with calls related

---

BOX 15-2	ANTICIPATED SCHEDULING VARIABLES

- Hours of operation
- Shift rotations
- Weekend rotations
- Approved benefit time for the schedule period—for example, vacations and holidays
- Approved leaves of absence/short-term disability
- Approved orientation, seminar, and continuing education time
- Scheduled meetings for the schedule period
- Current filled positions and current staffing vacancies
- Number of part-time employees

---

to illness, bereavement leaves, jury duty, or an emergent need for a leave of absence (LOA), nurse managers must attempt to fill a shift vacancy on short notice. Requesting staff to add hours over their planned commitment, floating staff from another unit, securing someone from a staffing pool, contracting with agency nursing staff, and seeking overtime are examples of strategies that nurse managers may be compelled to use to ensure safe staffing. However, as discussed, potentially negative consequences are associated with using these strategies.

EXERCISE 15-3

Assume that you are going to a job interview. Considering your personal preferred work schedule, what scheduling practices would be most satisfying to you and might lead you to accept employment with the organization? What scheduling practices might cause you to look elsewhere for a job? Develop a list of questions to ask your potential employer regarding scheduling practices in his or her organization.

EVALUATING UNIT STAFFING AND PRODUCTIVITY

Nurse managers are increasingly pressed to justify staffing decisions to staff, senior management, and occasionally external agencies such as unions, professional associations, or review committees. Unit activity and production reports, which provide a variety of measures of unit workload, can be helpful in such justification. In addition, a review of the extent to which the actual staffing over a specific time period matches the staffing plan, particularly coupled with various outcomes over the same period, gives a picture of the productivity and effectiveness of the unit. Although the format of these reports may vary, the kinds of information typically available to nurse managers in an activity report appear in Box 15-3.

In the inpatient setting, the average daily census (ADC) is a measure considered by nurse managers to project the potential workload of the unit. The ADC is a simple measure of the average number of patients being cared for per day in the unit during a reporting period. The formula for calculating the ADC appears in Box 15-3. If a unit's ADC is trending upward, the nurse manager may propose additional personnel to manage this increase in patient volume. If the ADC is trending downward, the nurse manager may propose the need for fewer resources to manage this downward

patient census trend. In an acute care setting, the ADC of a unit can be extremely volatile based on patterns of admissions, transfers, and discharges in the unit. Therefore, nurse managers may need the ability to make short-term adjustments to resources; for example, by making changes to the skill mix or floating a staff member out in response to short-term volatility. In a long-term care setting, however, the ADC of the unit may be very stable over prolonged periods. Nurse managers may note patient census trends based on a particular shift, the day of the week, or the season of the year. The addition of new physicians, the creation of new programs or services, and many other variables may also affect a unit's average daily census. Admissions and discharges increase staffing demands. Nurse managers must maintain a strong grasp on these workload measures to prepare an adequate staffing plan for the unit.

BOX 15-3   TYPICAL UNIT ACTIVITIES PRODUCTIVITY REPORT INDICATORS

- Volume statistic: number of units of service for the reporting period
- Capacity statistic: number of beds or blocks of time available for providing services
- Percentage of occupancy: number of occupied beds for the reporting period
- Average daily census (ADC): average number of patients cared for per day in the unit for the reporting period
- Average length of stay (ALOS): average number of days that a patient remained in an occupied bed

Formulas for Calculating Volume Statistics

Assume that a 20-bed medical–surgical unit (i.e., capacity statistic) accrued 566 patient days in June (i.e., volume statistic). Ninety-eight of these patients were discharged during the month.

Average daily census on this unit is 18.9:

Formula: patient days for a given time period divided by the number of days in the time period

    a. 30 days in June
    b. 566 patient days/30 days = ADC of 18.9

Percentage of occupancy for June is 95%:

Formula: daily patient census (rounded) divided by the number of beds in the unit

19 patients in a 20-bed unit =
19 patients/20 beds = 95% occupancy

Average length of stay for June is 5.8:

Formula: number of patient days divided by the number of discharges

566 patient days/98 patient discharges = 5.8 (rounded)

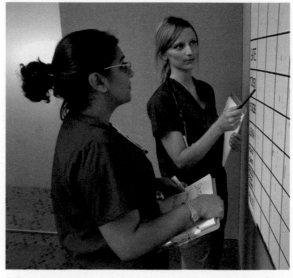

Calculating the percentage of occupancy is essential when developing a unit's staffing plan.

Another way of assessing a unit's activity level is to calculate the percentage of occupancy, or the patient census divided by the number of beds in the unit. The unit's occupancy rate can be calculated for a specific shift, on a daily basis, or as a monthly or annual statistic. The formula for calculating the percentage of occupancy appears in Box 15-3. Managers use the percentage of occupancy to develop the unit's staffing plan. Optimal occupancy rates may vary by practice setting. In a long-term care facility, the organization would desire 100% occupancy rates. However, in an acute care facility, 85% occupancy rates would ensure the best potential for patient throughput.

Another measure of a unit's activity level is the average length of stay (ALOS), or the average number of days that a patient remained in an occupied bed. As dollars have decreased, so have lengths of stay. However, the cost of treating the patient has not decreased as dramatically because patient acuity is greater; essentially, hospitals need to provide more care in less time for fewer dollars with the same, if not better, outcomes. For this reason, as a unit's ALOS trends downward, the need for staffing resources may not change substantially or may actually climb. The formula for calculating the average length of stay appears in Box 15-3.

The measures just mentioned provide the nurse manager with an understanding of the number of patients who have been admitted to the unit over a period of time. The nurse manager is then charged with matching the needs of these patients with the appropriate number of staff members. The positions and subsequent budgeted nursing salary dollars in the human resources budget are based on the estimated units of service that will be provided in the patient-care unit. If nurse managers can provide more care to more patients while spending the same or fewer salary dollars, they have increased unit productivity. Conversely, if the same or more salary dollars are spent to provide less care to fewer patients, nurse managers have decreased unit productivity.

Nursing productivity is a formula-driven calculation that represents the ratio of required staff hours to actual provided staff hours. Unit of service (UOS) multiplied by volume (patient days or emergency department visits) equals hours available to create direct productive staffing plans. Those hours multiplied by a nonproductive factor (e.g., 1.12) to account for paid time off equals the total hours available for the staffing plan. To complete the calculation, it is essential to set a ratio of patients to RNs. This ratio is then applied to the total hours available, and the support structure (e.g., health care aides or unit clerks) can then be built accordingly. Patient type, scope of service, patient acuity, and classification of the patient are all factors correlated with patient outcomes that drive staffing decisions. Meeting these productivity standards is important to ensure

the financial well-being of an organization. However, if the safety needs of patients are put at risk to achieve a productivity level, the consequences are harmful to patients, staff, and the organization as a whole.

Calculating nursing productivity is challenging for nurse managers because it is difficult to quantify the efficiency and effectiveness of individual nurses providing care to patients. Individual nurses can vary greatly in their critical-thinking abilities, skill levels, and ability to make timely and accurate decisions that affect patient outcomes.

Variance Between Projected and Actual Staff

Organizations can use labour costs or a straight FTE model to compare actual versus projected staff. Labour cost per unit of service is a simple measure that compares budgeted salary costs per budgeted volume of service (productivity target) with actual salary costs per actual volume of service (productivity performance). This measure requires nurse managers to staff according to their staffing plan because the plan reflects the approved human resources budget. Box 15-4 shows an analysis of labour costs per unit of service.

Typically, nurse managers must evaluate and explain changes in productivity resulting in a difference between the projected staffing plan and the actual schedule using a variance report. If nurse managers compare the two numbers and the actual productivity performance number is higher than the target, they have spent more money for care than budgeted. A number of variables may cause the labour costs to be higher than anticipated, such as increased overtime or sick time, using costly agency resources, or a higher-than-anticipated amount of indirect education or orientation time.

If nurse managers compare the two numbers, and the actual productivity performance number is lower than the target, they have spent less money for care than budgeted. Managers must also explain this high degree of productivity. One variable that may cause the labour costs to be lower than anticipated is an increased UCP skill mix or the consistent understaffing of the unit.

Having a productivity performance number that is either higher or lower than that planned does not represent effective management. Assuming that staffing plans were an accurate reflection of the

BOX 15-4   ANALYSIS OF LABOUR COSTS PER UNIT OF SERVICE

1. A manager of a cardiac telemetry unit proposes the following in the human resources budget. These are the unit's productivity targets.
   Total patient days: 5840
   - ADC = 16
   - Staffing plan for ADC of 16:
     - Day shift: 3 RNs and 3 UCPs (50% RN skill mix)
     - Evening shift: 3 RNs and 3 UCPs (50% RN skill mix)
     - Night shift: 3 RNs and 1 UCP (75% RN skill mix)
   - Direct care labour costs are also projected by the manager based on the average RN and UCP salaries for this unit.
   - Target = $139.32 per patient, or $2229.12 per day
2. The manager actually staffs as follows:
   - ADC = 16
   - Actual staffing for ADC of 16:
     - Day shift: 4 RNs and 2 UCPs (66% RN skill mix)
     - Evening shift: 4 RNs and 2 UCPs (66% RN skill mix)
     - Night shift: 3 RNs (100% RN skill mix)
   - Direct labour costs for this day = $145.44 per patient, or $2327.04 per day
3. The manager has incurred a variance:
   - Exceed target by $6.12 per patient, or $97.92 for the day

ADC, average daily census; *RN*, registered nurse; *UCP*, unregulated care provider.

conditions on the specific units, if the nurse manager compares the actual productivity performance with the productivity target and the two numbers match, the nurse manager has probably managed effectively. However, given the dynamic nature of patient care, an ongoing evaluation of the conditions on the unit as well as the extent to which proposed staffing levels are reached or exceeded should be monitored on an ongoing basis. Variance reports provide an opportunity for such evaluation.

EXERCISE 15-4
Assume that you are working as a charge nurse in a hospital. One of the nursing staff assigned to work with you becomes ill and must go home suddenly, leaving his designated patient assignment to be assumed by someone else. As a charge nurse, what factors would you consider as you determine how to reassign this work to other nurses? If you were a co-worker on the shift, instead of the charge nurse, what effective follower behaviours might you demonstrate to support the charge nurse in this situation? Can you identify behaviours of co-workers that would complicate the staffing situation further?

Impact of Leadership on Productivity

Nurse managers must possess staffing and scheduling skills to prepare a staffing plan that balances organizational directives with unit needs for care and services. They must spend time each month evaluating the unit's productivity performance. Yet it is also important that nurse managers improve unit productivity by spending more of their work time coaching and mentoring staff and providing clear information and direction related to meeting unit productivity goals. Nurse managers are the chief retention officers and need to perform their duties accordingly.

CONCLUSION

Staffing and scheduling are two of the greatest challenges for a nurse manager. When these functions are performed well, the resulting satisfaction of the unit staff contributes to positive patient outcomes. If these functions are not performed well, low morale and discontent may result. The nurse manager has various data available to help in planning the staffing patterns for the unit. Success, however, depends on the unit staff and the nurse manager working collaboratively to meet the needs for care.

A SOLUTION

Samantha called staff meetings on an ongoing basis at the regional hospital to discuss the impact of the new NICU at the local children's hospital. Staff were informed about the size of the new neonatal unit and the methods for staffing the new unit. Staff members were assured that their jobs would not be lost and that appropriate training would be provided to current staff to ensure that they know new procedures in relation to collaboration with and patient transfers to the new NICU. Samantha also informed staff that eight neonatal intensive care beds would be incorporated into the existing PICU, and other local hospitals would help with capacity over the 3 years until the new NICU opened. She involved staff members in the design of the space and the selection of the in-room supplies and equipment they would need.

Samantha established a staffing plan for the new neonatal intensive care beds; that entailed consulting with the union to incorporate its feedback and respond to concerns, and proposing that staff members

A SOLUTION—cont'd

of the existing NICU and PICU at the regional hospital be first to be offered positions at the new NICU. The new unit's staffing plan was filled with staff members from the existing NICU as well as a related staffing pool. Samantha also developed staff orientation programs. The existing NICU and PICU nursing staff members were open and welcoming when the new staff rotated and partnered with the staff in the two critical care environments. The new unit's nursing staff also provided backup to the regional hospital's NICU and PICU nurses when needed.

Samantha held continuous discussions with the medical staff involved through an idea champion who was identified within the department of pediatric critical care. She distributed talking points to the medical staff and other hospital staff to keep everyone current with the progress. The interdisciplinary teams that were developed around the care models are now engaged in daily patient-care conferences to monitor the progress of patients.

The unit has been open for 5 months and is a success. It has no vacant positions, the number of neonatal intensive care beds available have helped alleviate capacity constraints, the medical staff are pleased with the care delivered, patient and family satisfaction is very good, and the staff feel accomplished and proud of their contribution to the overall capacity challenge!

Would this be a suitable approach for you? Why or why not?

THE EVIDENCE

Kane et al. (2007), in a meta-analysis of 94 observational studies done between 1990 and 2006, found consistent evidence that suggested an increase in the number of RNs relative to the number of patients in a unit was associated with a reduction in hospital-related mortality, failure to rescue, and other nursing-sensitive outcomes. The increased number of nurses also influenced a reduced length of stay after adjustment for patient characteristics was considered. However, none of these studies demonstrated a causal relationship. Kane et al. (2007) noted that hospitals with an overall commitment to high-quality care through sufficient staffing may also invest in other actions that improve quality.

NEED TO KNOW NOW

- Know what your provincial or territorial practice regulations and related rules such as collective agreements say about staffing requirements.
- Know how staffing is determined for the unit where you work or are considering working.

- Know to ask for help if your assignment is limiting your ability to provide safe patient care.

CHAPTER CHECKLIST

This chapter addresses the managerial functions of staffing and scheduling and asserts that skills in both functions are needed by the nurse manager to maintain unit productivity and patient and staff satisfaction.

- The nurse manager must consider the impact of patient and hospital factors, nurse staffing, nurse characteristics, nurse outcomes, and organizational factors on staffing and patient outcomes.
- The nurse manager must also consider the following external factors when preparing the budget and the unit staffing plan:
  - Staffing requirements

- Patient and family expectations
- Organizational policies
- When forecasting the staffing needs for the unit, the nurse manager must consider the following:
  - The staffing model of the unit
  - The skill mix of the nursing and other staff
  - The number of positions and FTEs needed to meet the anticipated units of service
  - The amount of nonproductive paid-benefit time allotted to each staff member
  - Patient outcomes
  - Availability of resources

- When constructing the unit schedule, the nurse manager must consider the following:
  - Unit hours of operation
  - Shift or weekend rotations required in the unit
  - Approved paid time off for vacations, holidays, and other benefit hours
  - Staffing vacancies
  - Availability of automation
- Organizational policies on overtime and use of agency personnel
- When evaluating unit staffing and productivity, the nurse manager should consider the following:
  - Acuity trends identified through patient classification systems and/or staff input
  - Labour cost per unit of service
  - Periodic unit activity reports

TIPS FOR STAFFING AND SCHEDULING

- Know provincial regulations and acts and voluntary accreditation (professional association and institutional) standards for staffing.
- Integrate ongoing research regarding the impact of various factors on patient outcomes into staffing plans.
- Identify current demands for staff and anticipate externally imposed changes such as services offered

and the availability of RNs, licensed practical nurses, registered psychiatric nurses, and UCPs.
- Value the various responses to short staffing from the manager, staff, and patient perspectives.
- Recognize the complexity of staffing issues and how they relate to staff satisfaction, community perception, budget, and accreditation standards.

evolve WEBSITE

Visit the Evolve website for Suggested Readings, Internet Resources, and additional resources related to the content in this chapter: http://evolve.elsevier.com/Canada/Yoder-Wise/leading/.

REFERENCES

Accreditation Canada. (2010). *Qmentum program standards: Health care staffing services (Version 4)*. Ottawa, ON: Author. Retrieved from http://www.accreditation.ca/health-care-staffing-services.

Aiken, L. H., Cimiotti, J. P., Sloane, D. M., et al. (2011). Effects of nurse staffing and nurse education on patient deaths in hospitals with different nurse work environments. *Medical Care, 49*(12), 1047–1053. doi:10.1097/MLR.0b013e3182330b6e

Aiken, L. H., Clarke, S. P., Cheung, R. B., et al. (2003). Educational levels of hospital nurses and surgical patient mortality. *Journal of the American Medical Association, 290*(12), 1617–1623. doi:10.1001/jama.290.12.1617

American Nurses Association. (2008). *Principles for nurse staffing*. Washington, DC: American Nurses. Retrieved from http://www.nursingworld.org/principles.

Becker, D. J. (2007). Do hospitals provide lower quality care on weekends? *Health Services Research, 42*(4), 1589–1612. doi:10.1111/j.1475-6773.2006.00663.x

Canadian Federation of Nurses Unions. (2009). The national voice for nurses: A position statement on mandatory overtime. Retrieved from http://nursesunions.ca/sites/default/files/Mandatory_Overtime_Position_Statement.pdf.

Canadian Nurses Association.(2003, June). *Position statement: Staffing decisions for the delivery of safe nursing care*. Ottawa, ON: Author. Retrieved from http://www.cna-aiic.ca/~/media/cna/page%20content/pdf%20en/2013/09/04/16/27/9%20-%20ps67_staffing_decisions_delivery_safe_nursing_care_june_2003_e.pdf.

Canadian Nurses Association. (2005a). *Evaluation framework to determine the impact of nursing staff mix decisions*. Ottawa, ON: Author. Retrieved from http://www.cna-aiic.ca/.../2013/09/05/19/21/Evaluation_Framework_2005_e/en/1.

Canadian Nurses Association. (2005b). Nursing staff mix: A key link to patient safety. *Nursing Now—Issues and Trends in Canadian Nursing, 19*(1), 1–6. Retrieved from http://www.cna-aiic.ca/.../2013/09/05/19/20/NN_Nursing_Staff_Mix_05_e/en/1.

Canadian Nurses Association. (2005c). Position statement: National planning for human resources in the health sector. Ottawa, ON: Author. Retrieved from http://www.cna-aiic.ca/.../PDF FR/2013/09/05/19/16/PS81_National_Planning_e/en/1.

Cho, S. H. (2002). Nurse staffing and adverse patient outcomes: A systems approach. *Nursing Outlook, 49*(2), 78–81. Retrieved from http://www.nursingoutlook.org.

Cho, S. H., Hwang, J. H., & Kim, J. (2008). Nurse staffing and patient mortality in critical care units. *Nursing Research, 57*(5), 322–330. doi:10.1097/01.NNR.0000313498.17777.71

Cram, P., Hillis, S., Barnett, M., et al. (2004). Effects of weekend admission and hospital teaching status on in-hospital mortality. *The American Journal of Medicine, 117*, 151–157. doi:10.1016/j.amjmed.2004.02.035

Dall, T., Chen, Y., Seifert, R., et al. (2009). The economic value of professional nursing. *Medical Care, 47*(1), 97–104. doi:10.1097/MLR.0b013e3181844da8

Donaldson, N., Bolton, L. B., Aydin, C., et al. (2005). Impact of California's licensed nurse-patient ratios on unit-level nurse staffing and patient outcomes. *Policy, Politics & Nursing Practice, 6*(3), 198–210. doi:10.1177/1527154405280107

Dunton, N., Gajewski, B., Klaus, S., et al. (2007). The relationship of nursing workforce characteristics to patient outcomes. *Online Journal of Issues in Nursing, 12*(3). doi:10.3912/OJIN.Vol12No03Man03

Eschiti, V., & Hamilton, P. (2011). Off-peak nurse staffing. *Dimensions of Critical Care Nursing, 30*(1), 62–69. doi:10.1097/DCC.0b013e3181fd03cd

Estabrooks, C. A., Midodzi, W. K., Cummings, G. G., et al. (2011). The impact of hospital nursing characteristics on 30-day mortality. *Journal of Nursing Administration, 41*(7/8), S58–S68. doi:10.1097/NNA.0b013e318221c260

Fitzpatrick, T., & Brooks, B. (2010). The nurse leader as logistician: Optimizing human capital. *Journal of Nursing Administration, 40*(2), 69–74. doi:10.1097/NNA.0b013e3181cb9f3b

Haebler, J. (2008, August 1). Safe staffing legislation: Win-win for Ohio and others. *Nevada RNformation.* Retrieved from http://www.highbeam.com/doc/1G1-183554756.html.

Hamilton, P., Eschiti, V. S., Hernandez, K., et al. (2007). Differences between weekend and weekday nurse work environments and patient outcomes: A focus group approach to model testing. *Journal of Perinatal Neonatal Nursing, 21*(4), 331–341. doi:10.1097/01.JPN.0000299791.54785.7b

Harris, A., & McGillis Hall, L. (2012). Evidence to inform staff mix decision-making: A focused literature review. Ottawa, ON: Canadian Nurses Association. Retrieved from http://www.nurseone.ca/docs/NurseOne/KnowledgeFeature/StaffMix/Staff_Mix_Literature_Review_e.pdf.

Hyun, S., Bakken, S., Douglas, K., et al. (2008). Evidence-based staffing: Potential roles for informatics. *Nursing Economic$, 26*(3), 151–173. Retrieved from http://www.nursingeconomics.net/cgi-bin/WebObjects/NECJournal.woa.

Kane, R. L., Shamliyan, T., Mueller, C., et al. (March 2007). *Nursing staffing and quality of patient care: Evidence report/technology assessment no. 151.* (Prepared by the Minnesota Evidence-based Practice Center under Contract No. 290-02-0009.) AHRQ Publication No. 07-E0005. Rockville, MD: Employer for Healthcare Research and Quality. Retrieved from http://archive.ahrq.gov/downloads/pub/evidence/pdf/nursestaff/nursestaff.pdf.

Keepnews, D. (2007). Evaluating nurse staffing regulations. *Policy, Politics, and Nursing Practice, 8*(4), 235–236. doi:10.1177/1527154408315641

Kendall-Gallagher, D., Aiken, L. H., Sloane, D. M., et al. (2011). Nurse specialty certification, inpatient mortality, and failure to rescue. *Journal of Nursing Scholarship, 43*(2), 188–194. doi:10.1111/j.1547-5069.2011.01391.x

Kutney-Lee, A., Lake, E. T., & Aiken, L. H. (2009). Development of the hospital nurse surveillance capacity profile. *Research in Nursing & Health, 32*(2), 217–228. doi:10.1002/nur.20316

Montalvo, I. (2007, September). The National Database of Nursing Quality Indicators™ (NDNQI®). OJIN: *The Online Journal of Issues in Nursing, 12*(3), 2.

Montalvo, I. (2009). The national database of nursing quality indicators® (NDNQI®). OJIN: *The Online Journal of Issues in Nursing, 12*(3), Manuscript 3. Retrieved from http://www.nursingworld.org/MainMenuCategories/ANAMarketplace/ANAPeriodicals/OJIN/TableofContents/Volume122007/No3Sept07/NursingQualityIndicators.html.

Peberdy, M. A., Ornato, J. P., Larkin, G. L., et al. (2008). Survival from in-hospital cardiac arrest during nights and weekends. *Journal of the American Medical Association, 299*(7), 785–792. doi:10.1001/jama.299.7.785

Ridley, R. T. (2008). The relationship between nurse education level and patient safety: An integrative review. *Journal of Nursing Education, 47*(4), 149–156. doi:10.3928/01484834-20080401-06

Rogers, A. E. (2008). The effects of fatigue and sleepiness on nurse performance and patient safety. In R. G. Hughes (Ed.), *Patient safety and quality: An evidence-based handbook for nurses* (pp. 2-509–2-545). Rockville, MD: Agency for Healthcare Research and Quality.

Spence Laschinger, H. K., & Leiter, M. P. (2006). The impact of nursing work environments on patient safety outcomes. The mediating role of burnout/engagement. *Journal of Nursing Administration, 36*(5), 259–267. Retrieved from http://journals.lww.com/jonajournal/pages/default.aspx.

Spence Laschinger, H. K., Sabiston, J. A., Finegan, J., et al. (2001). Voices from the trenches: Nurses' experiences of hospital restructuring in Ontario. *Canadian Journal of Nursing Leadership, 14*(2), 6–13. doi:10.12927/cjnl.2001.16305

Stone, P. W., Mooney-Kane, C., Larson, E. L., et al. (2007). Nurse working conditions and patient safety outcomes. *Medical Care, 45*(6), 571–578. Retrieved from http://journals.lww.com/lww-medicalcare/pages/default.aspx.

Tourangeau, A. E. (2008). Choices and tradeoffs: Decreasing costs of improving hospital mortality rates. *Healthcare Quarterly, 11*(1), 23–24. doi:10.12927/hcq.2013.19493

Tourangeau, A. E., Doran, D. M., McGillis Hall, L., et al. (2006). Impact of hospital nursing care on 30-day mortality for acute medical patients. *Journal of Advanced Nursing, 57*(1), 32–44. doi:10.1111/j.1365-2648.2006.04084.x

Upenieks, V., Akhavan, J., & Kotlerman, J. (2008). Value-added care: A paradigm shift in patient care delivery. *Nursing Economic$, 26*(5), 294–300. Retrieved from http://www.nursingeconomics.net/cgi-bin/WebObjects/NECJournal.woa.

VanDeVelde-Coke, S., Doran, D., Grinspun, D., et al. (2012). Measuring outcomes of nursing care, improving the health of Canadians: NNQR (C), C-HOBIC and NQuiRE. *Canadian Journal of Nursing Leadership, 25*(2), 26–37.

CHAPTER 16

Selecting, Developing, and Evaluating Staff

Diane M. Twedell
Adapted by Arden Krystal

Two of the most important functions of a nurse manager are interviewing and hiring employees for an organization. Once hired, it is essential that individuals understand the expectations associated with their role. Role clarity can improve performance, increase job satisfaction, and improve the quality of care delivered. Role theory is a useful organizing framework for the nurse manager and the employee to follow throughout the process of role development. This chapter also explores the process and tools of performance appraisal as well as the role of the nurse manager as coach who empowers employees to grow as followers and develop their leadership skills in a learning environment.

OBJECTIVES

- Understand role concepts and role theory.
- Define *position description*.
- Know how to approach the interview process when hiring a new employee.
- Describe the guidelines for performance appraisal.
- Describe the various performance appraisal tools.
- Understand how collective agreements affect hiring decisions and performance appraisals.

TERMS TO KNOW

coaching	performance appraisal	role conflict
empowerment	position description	role theory
halo effect	role ambiguity	

? A CHALLENGE

Marie-Claude, an experienced nurse manager, offers education sessions to patient care managers (PCMs) to help them run highly effective and efficient teams. The biggest challenge for PCMs is nurse turnover, vacancies, and a very junior staff composition. The balanced experience levels of old are long gone; now many PCMs are faced with having a majority of staff with 5 years or less of experience.

How can Marie-Claude help the PCMs address nurse turnover, develop staff, and increase retention?

INTRODUCTION

Health care delivery systems in Canada, though largely not-for-profit, have a strong "value for money" imperative. Whether the setting is inpatient or outpatient, the emphasis is on providing the highest quality of care at an affordable cost. The nurse manager is a key individual whose leadership can directly influence many environmental functions. Nurse managers must have a specific set of competencies to ensure the delivery of effective clinical services (Pangman & Pangman, 2009). Nurse managers are increasingly being held accountable for nurse retention. They begin with the selection of the right person for the right position. As a coach, the nurse manager can support and encourage employees to perform at their highest levels in an empowered and self-directed manner. The nurse manager also clarifies the organization's mission and expectations, and teaches the necessary followership skills to student nurses. A strong patient-care unit has both effective leadership and team members who understand their roles in meeting the goal of quality patient care. Health care providers must clearly understand what is expected of their performance, including the ramifications of not meeting those expectations. Effective organizational performance can be achieved only when all members of the organization have clearly defined roles and overall objectives. Ambiguous roles are more detrimental to role performance and employee work satisfaction than is role conflict.

ROLE CONCEPTS AND THE POSITION DESCRIPTION

The acquisition of a role requires an individual to assume the personal as well as the formal expectations of that specified role or position. Many individuals function within multiple roles. As discussed in the Theory Box below, role theory—a framework used to understand how individuals perform within organizations—provides an appreciable framework for the development and evaluation of staff. Today's nurse is often a parent, spouse, and community volunteer and maintains full-time employment outside the home. Many skills are necessary for each role. In addition, the role-taker (i.e., the individual actually performing the role) has specific performance objectives within the social context in which the role is enacted. The social context includes the physical and social environment.

? THEORY BOX

Role Theory

THEORY/CONTRIBUTOR	KEY IDEAS	APPLICATION TO PRACTICE
Role theory and role dynamics in organizations (Kahn, Wolfe, Quinn, et al., 1964)	Roles within organizations affect an individual's interactions with others. Acquisition of these roles is time-dependent and varies based on individual experiences and value systems. For effective communication to take place, role expectations for performance must be understood by all individuals involved.	The role of the nurse is complex. Role acquisition, role clarity, and role performance are enhanced by the use of clear position descriptions and evaluation standards.

From Kahn, R. L., Wolfe, D. M., Quinn, R. P., et al. (1964). *Occupational stress: Studies in role conflict and ambiguity.* New York, NY: Wiley.

Role ambiguity in the workplace creates an environment for misunderstanding and hinders effective communication. When employees have ambiguous roles, they do not have a clear understanding of what is expected of their performance or how they will be evaluated. **Role conflict** is easier to recognize: employees know what is expected of them, but they are either unable or unwilling to meet those expectations.

Employees must have clear role expectations and perceive that their contributions are valued. Employee empowerment and control over certain aspects of the environment can lead to increased personal health, job satisfaction, and individual performance. Valued employees with clear roles are more likely to be committed to the organization and provide a higher level of patient care. These principles are applicable to both nurse managers and staff members. An organization that consistently focuses on developing staff creates a learning environment directed toward excellence. Landmark studies reiterate that nurses want to be appreciated and respected by physicians and the administrative team; they want to be recognized for their expertise, and they want to take responsibility and participate in the decision-making processes concerning patient care (Aiken, 1984; Johnson, 2000; Trossman, 2002).

Acquisition of a role is time-dependent; that is, the more complex the role, the longer it will take to assimilate that role. Individuals bring their life experiences to each role and interpret the role within their own value system. Nursing graduates enter the profession with various levels of education and life experiences. The nurse manager plays an integral role in helping these individuals develop and acquire the complex role of the nurse. It is important to remember that an individual's role evolves over time at a pace that is specific to the individual. Moreover, nurses may acquire new roles numerous times during their career. For example, the registered nurse (RN) who completes additional education and becomes an advanced practice registered nurse takes on a new role. The staff nurse who moves to a new or different specialty takes on a new role. Coaching is a technique that nurse managers can use to facilitate individual development; this technique is discussed in "Performance Appraisals," later in the chapter.

The **position description** is a statement of the roles and responsibilities of a specific position in an organization. It describes the scope and duties of the work assignment, as well as to whom the individual reports. It also serves as a contract between the manager and employee.

The position description should reflect current provincial or territorial practice guidelines and may include competency-based requirements. Most collective agreements contain provisions that pertain to the approval of job descriptions as well as clauses that govern job postings and selecting applicants. As nursing delivery systems shift to the home and community, nurses must have a clear understanding of the performance that is expected of them. The nurse is also responsible for clearly understanding the position descriptions of the paraprofessionals to whom care is delegated. Clear and concise position descriptions for all employees are extremely important because they provide the basis for roles within the organization. Sample statements from a position description for a staff nurse in a medical–surgical patient-care unit appear in Box 16-1.

EXERCISE 16-1

Obtain a position description for a nursing role from a health care setting such as a home health care agency or a hospital. Compare them. Analyze the general categories (e.g., communication, responsibilities) and the specific behaviours associated with the role. What competencies do you already have? How will you develop other competencies? What are the common competencies for the nursing role in both contexts?

BOX 16-1 **EXCERPTS FROM A STAFF POSITION DESCRIPTION FOR A REGISTERED NURSE**

- Accountable for the coordination of nursing care, including direct patient care, patient/family education, and discharge planning
- Maintains basic cardiac life support (BCLS) competency
- Required to accurately assess and prioritize patient-care needs and delegate care appropriately to licensed practical nurses and patient care aides
- Works collaboratively with multidisciplinary team members

SELECTING STAFF

The selection of staff would seem to be a relatively simple process. The nurse manager just needs to choose the most qualified individual for a position. However, choosing the right individual can be a challenge! Moreover, the cost of recruiting and orienting a new nurse "drives home the necessity of carefully selecting nurses who'll work well within your hospital's culture" (Brooke, 2008, p. 50). Health care is centred on caring for people, and nurses with appropriate people skills are essential for ensuring satisfied patients and families. For example, if an applicant values that the needs of the patient come first and this view is also valued by the organization, he or she has similar values related to the work of the organization. The applicant and the nurse manager must also agree on what defines quality care and the manner in which it should be delivered. As well, the nurse manager must decide whether members of the existing staff should be included in the screening and interview process for new employees. The guidelines for selecting staff that follow are suggestions for nurse managers and staff as well as prospective employees.

Guidelines for Selecting Staff

The nurse manager must be prepared for the interview and have well-thought-out questions. Questions must be based on the key elements of the role as per the position description—essentially, they should accurately reflect the job for which the nurse manager is hiring. Developing a standardized interview tool, including objective criteria for ranking applicants, is highly recommended. This tool allows the nurse manager to determine who is the best applicant and allows for a legitimate defence of a hire in the case of a dispute by an unsuccessful applicant. Many collective agreements require that the employer use an objective process for hiring, and some may also require the applicant's seniority to be factored into the hiring equation. Nurse managers should always ensure that they are well aware of any constraints around interviewing and hiring, and should seek advice on these areas from human resources professionals in their organization.

The interviewing environment should be comfortable and provide privacy without interruptions. It is important to remember that the nurse manager's attitude sets the tone of the interview (Parrish, 2006). The interview questions should be related to the applicant's experience and geared to evaluating the applicant's values and critical-thinking skills. These objectives can be met by asking the applicant to describe his or her reactions to challenging situations previously experienced. Behavioural interviewing is considered the most effective way to predict a future employee's success in the job (Graham, 2011). Behavioural interviewing involves asking the applicant to use past experiences and actions to answer applied questions. A question related to teamwork in an interview could be, *Tell me about a time when you were working in a group and there were problems with other individuals who were not pulling their weight. What did you do to maintain a team environment?*

Technical skills, such as specific certificates, are also important for the work environment and, therefore, must be discussed and verified. The applicant may be given a case study to read and discuss with the interviewer. The case study could describe a situation for the work area in which the applicant is being interviewed; the content of the case study may require the applicant to prioritize the care of one patient or a group of patients. Questions from the applicant should be answered honestly. The nurse manager should also provide an overview of the organization, the job, required work hours, any benefits package, and any other related information (Parrish, 2006). A tour of the unit and a review of the position description are helpful to give the applicant information about the expectations of the role. If staff members are included in the interview, they can provide information to the applicant as appropriate. At the conclusion of the interview, it is important for the nurse manager to clarify concrete issues and offer closure beyond a "don't call us, we'll call you" (McConnell, 2008). Applicants should know the time line of when they can expect to hear about their interview result, who will contact them, and how they will be contacted. The nurse manager should thank each applicant for attending the interview, and end each interview on a positive note.

The applicant also has responsibilities in preparation for the employment interview (see also Chapter 29). It is important to be on time and appropriately dressed. Conservative dress is always acceptable. A uniform is not necessary and usually not even preferable. First impressions may be lasting impressions. Reviewing in advance the organization's goals and mission statement as well as the position description for which the interview is being conducted is appropriate. The applicant should be prepared to answer each question honestly and thoughtfully. It is as important to the prospective employee to make the right decision as it is to the employer. The nurse manager and the applicant must have a clear understanding of the organization's values and goals for nursing care to ensure that the applicant is well-suited for the role. The applicant should focus on the topic and avoid irrelevant conversations. He or she must prepare for any questions that might be discussed. In addition to describing previous situations and how they were handled, the applicant may be asked to describe personal strengths and weaknesses. At the end of the interview, the applicant should thank the nurse manager and any other interviewers for their time and verify when the selection will be made and how it will be communicated. It is also appropriate to send the nurse manager a brief note of appreciation for the interview.

DEVELOPING STAFF

Once the interview and offer are completed and an applicant has accepted the position, strategies are used to help the individual acclimatize to the new organization, new role, or both. Some health regions and provinces use residency-type programs for new graduates that may last for several months after the initial hire. These programs are often very successful in enhancing the transition from student to professional nurse. Other staff development strategies in organizations may last a short time or for several weeks, focusing on orientation to the role and the organization. Orientation to an organization is usually a structured program that is generally applicable to all new employees. It may include outlining the mission, benefits, safety programs, and other specific topics. Orientation to the work area usually depends on the specialty area involved, the skills that need to be verified, and the environment itself. Every individual brings various experiences and skills to a new position. A nurse manager assists new employees by advising them about educational programs and experiences that will aid in their entry to the organization. It is imperative that the orientation period be used efficiently for both the employee and the organization. Retention of new nursing personnel begins on the day of their hire. Consider that replacing just one medical–surgical nurse costs $92 442 (Robert Wood Johnson Foundation, 2006). This dollar figure includes human resources expenses, temporary replacement costs, lost productivity, training, and any severance pay. Although the amount depends on the employee's role and the organization, there is no question that the cost of replacement is high.

Orientation can accomplish a variety of goals. It offers new employees the opportunity to learn about the work environment and meet the staff. Most organizations have preceptors, who are expert clinicians and mentors that help new graduates, younger staff, and nurses moving into a new role (preceptees) learn new skills and knowledge and integrate both into practice, thereby helping nursing departments achieve their health care goals (Moore, 2008). Preceptors teach in the clinical setting. Clinical nurse educators can help develop a range of strategies that cover a variety of learning styles of preceptees. Doing so helps the preceptor ensure the uptake and retention of information in preceptees.

Nurse managers are responsible for the continued development of staff. It is a challenge to merge a group of individuals with varying levels of expertise and experience. If the focus is centred on professional socialization and development, a common thread will "weave" itself throughout all employees. That common thread may be a particular philosophy of care delivery, further development of critical-thinking skills for a specific specialty, or advocacy activities in which various employees are involved. Some units encourage a monthly journal club or a brief presentation by employees to summarize information learned from a conference. One nursing unit could send a staff member to monthly open meetings of the provincial nursing association or regulatory body. This staff member then could summarize the report of the meeting for the rest of the staff to keep them informed on current issues in professional nursing.

Empowerment strategies are useful for individual professional development as well as for overall staff development. *Empowerment* is the process of exercising one's own power; it is also the process by which we facilitate the participation of others in decision making and taking action so they are free to exercise power. In the A Challenge and A Solution sections in this chapter, employee self-development and professional empowerment are a couple of the strategies managers have used to create more effective work teams.

For individuals to feel empowered, the organizational environment must be open and individuals must feel safe to explore and develop their own potential. The organizational environment must also encourage individuals to employ the freedom of making decisions while retaining accountability for the consequences of those decisions. Management must relinquish some control to followers so that the followers might work more effectively as individuals and as part of a team. It is important that the student nurse develop good "followership" skills or styles, as ineffective followership can be detrimental to an organization (Kelley, 1992). Followership styles fall on a continuum ranging from those who are passive to active followers, along with those with uncritical to critical thinking styles. Those individuals who actively participate and are critical thinkers are the most valuable to an organization (Kelley, 1992). Several provinces in Canada have implemented initiatives such as Care Delivery Model Redesign (CDMR) and Releasing Time to Care™, which are aimed at developing problem-solving skills and professional accountability in nurses. A key element of these initiatives is the use of Plan-Do-Study-Act (PDSA) cycles (Langley, Nolan, Nolan, et al., 2009), where staff groups identify a problem on their unit and test possible solutions in a rapid cycle. These initiatives also help nursing unit groups learn to function better as cohesive teams and have been shown to improve quality, reduce sick time, and improve job satisfaction (Stevenson, Joyce, Eastman et al., 2011).

Specific work environment challenges and situations (e.g., working short staffed, adapting to new care models) can influence employee attitudes, feelings of empowerment, and performance. These challenges can affect commitment to the organization and individual work satisfaction. Positive feedback or coaching, achievement recognition, and support for new ideas may enhance employees' feelings of empowerment and their ability to perform effectively.

One strategy for empowering staff is to provide timely feedback for performance contributions, not simply one annual performance appraisal. Supporting the implementation of innovative ideas and providing opportunities for mentoring relationships are also valuable approaches for nurse managers who wish to empower staff. Many organizations use shared governance as a guide for accountability. A premise of shared governance is that power, control, and decision making can empower staff and enhance individual and group accountability.

PERFORMANCE APPRAISALS

Feedback to employees regarding their performance is one of the strongest rewards an organization can provide. Performance appraisals are individual evaluations of work performance. Ideally, evaluations are conducted on an ongoing basis, not just at the conclusion of a predetermined period. Evaluations, however, are usually done annually and also may be required after a scheduled orientation period for new employees. Chandra (2006) outlined the purpose of performance appraisals:

> Administrators may conduct performance appraisals to monitor performance quality and quantity, evaluate job standards and expectations, provide a basis for personnel decisions (e.g., promotions, transfers, releases, staffing needs), and provide other information that may signal potential problems or successes of daily operations. (p. 34)

The process of providing feedback for either an above-average or a below-average performance is best received at a time closest to the incidents being evaluated. Nurse managers might consider the actual appraisal as a negative and time-consuming process of endless paperwork. Instead, nurse managers should embrace the appraisal process as a key time to engage in staff development. The actual appraisal session should be productive (Chandra, 2006). At the same time, appraisals should be designed so that they can be supported in grievances and legal actions if the need arises. Labour relations decisions can be made based on the evidence, or lack of evidence, presented in a performance appraisal. Consider, for example, the individual who has been terminated for reasons of poor work performance. Depending on the province, territory, and relevant collective agreement, a progressive series of notifications must occur to the employee to communicate clearly that performance is unsatisfactory, and that notice must specify what the employee must accomplish to achieve satisfactory performance. Often this process begins as a verbal warning, progressing to a more formal written notice. Good documentation of performance issues can make the difference for either the employee or the employer to justify the fairness for termination.

Performance appraisals can be either formal or informal. Performance appraisals may also include personal and peer evaluations, as well as managerial components. A formal performance appraisal involves written or online documentation according to specific organization guidelines. An informal appraisal might be as simple as immediate praise and recognition of the individual for performance. A compliment from a family member or patient might be conveyed. Some units have a specific bulletin board for thank-you notes from patients and their families. Some organizations have developed significant appreciation programs that recognize both individuals and teams for their outstanding contributions, which can include e-mail "thank-you" templates, thank-you cards, and employee-of-the-month awards. Sometimes a simple "Thank you for all your hard work today!" can be extended from the nurse manager to staff. In addition, staff members have a responsibility to show the nurse manager their appreciation and give positive and negative feedback. Whether the evaluation is formal or informal, it does not preclude interim evaluations. The primary reason for an interim evaluation is so that praise or corrections are made as close to an episode as possible.

Keeping brief anecdotal notes on a regular basis about an employee's performance is important. These anecdotal notes, when accumulated over time, provide a more accurate cumulative appraisal. The anecdotal note describes an occurrence, either favourable or unfavourable, in a brief and concise manner. The purpose is to help the nurse manager have information for an entire rating period. When the nurse manager gives feedback to an employee, making a quick note about the interaction can help trigger memory to ensure both positive and constructive content makes its way into the performance appraisal.

Example of an Anecdotal Note: Nurse "Banister"

2/14/14: Patient (Jacqueline Allard) and family described the wonderful care that she received from Ms. Banister during this hospitalization. All members of the family noted that when Ms. Banister was in the room, "we felt like we were the most important people in the world." She made the patient feel "special and not just like another number." Compliment relayed to employee on 2/15/14. (Note in employee's anecdotal record with a signature and date by nurse manager.)

EXERCISE 16-2
Select a partner. Observe some clinical or classroom behaviour and prepare an anecdotal note. Ask your partner for feedback about the content.

Additional methods may be incorporated into the performance appraisal in the form of competency assessment tools as specified by the position description. Competency assessment tools can focus on "observable clinical performances and behaviours, such as accurate cardiac rhythm interpretation, safe blood product administration, and appropriate laboratory value

interpretation" (Kollman, Liedl, Johnson, et al., 2007, p. 422). Integration of relevant competency assessment data into the evaluation process further enhances the individual employee's sense of empowerment, as well as the accountability of the evaluation process.

Coaching

The overall evaluative process can be enhanced if the nurse manager employs the technique of coaching. Coaching is a process in which a manager helps others learn, think critically, and grow through communications about performance. This coaching process is a personal approach in which the manager and the employee interact on a frequent and regular basis with the ultimate outcome that the employee performs at an optimal level. Coaching can be individual or may involve a team approach; when implemented in a planned and organized manner, it can promote team building and the optimal performance of employees. Coaching is a learned behaviour that takes nurse managers time and effort to develop. The rewards for both the employee and the nurse manager are significant; communication is enhanced, and the performance appraisal process is an active one between the employee and the nurse manager. Another related element in enhancing individuals is mentoring. This is an important approach in developing staff and is addressed in detail in Chapter 27.

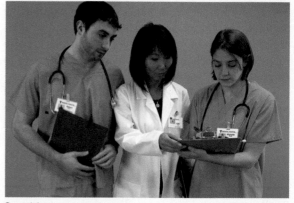

Coaching can promote team building and the optimal performance of employees.

The formal performance appraisal, a useful tool for coaching, usually involves some type of predetermined evaluation tool or instrument. The tool may be a simple one or may involve the integration of a variety of measuring methods. The instruments should reflect the philosophy of the organization and be as objective and specific as possible regarding the employee's performance. Numerous instruments and a variety of simple to complex scoring methods for each exist. New employees must have a clear understanding of the timing and content of appraisals at the onset of employment. The example in Box 16-2 illustrates a type of peer performance appraisal method in which a staff nurse could evaluate another staff nurse within the area-specific context of assessment documentation. It is important to note that some collective agreements stipulate the circumstances under which peers may engage in the assessment of others; it is always advisable to consult with a human resources professional before undertaking such an approach.

EXERCISE 16-3

Think back to your last performance appraisal, either in the clinical situation as a nurse or in the role of nursing student. Did you feel you were fairly and adequately evaluated? Were the comments reflective of your current practice and made by someone who had directly observed the care that you provided? What was the environment like for the interview? Were you comfortable with the evaluator? Was feedback given, both positive and negative? How did you feel at the conclusion of the interview? Taking the time to think about the answers to these questions might provide you with insight and direction before your next performance appraisal interview.

BOX 16-2	PEER PERFORMANCE APPRAISAL, STAFF NURSE

Area of Responsibility

Assessment/Diagnosis: Provides continuous holistic assessment to include physical, psychosocial, spiritual, and educational needs. Directs outcome criteria so that discharge plans are timely and optimal quality care is delivered.

a. Completes database (history/physical assessment) within 12 hours of admission (Score 4)

b. Illustrates documentation reflective of continuous assessment per unit guidelines (e.g., neurovascular assessment of extremity after cardiac catheterization) (Score 3)

c. Initiates plan of care according to critical path guidelines within 12 hours of admission (Score 4)

d. Provides for safe environment (Score 4)

The scoring procedures for evaluations can be as simple as *satisfactory/unsatisfactory*. A more complex scoring system that includes a numerical rating scheme (using a range of 1 to 4, with *1* meaning "rarely meets standards," to *4* meaning "always exceeds standards") also appears in Box 16-2. The results from the peer-review process are then summarized and incorporated into the manager's formal performance appraisal.

PERFORMANCE APPRAISAL TOOLS

The type of appraisal tool used is not as important as how it is used, and, as the Research Perspective below shows, little consistency exists across organizations in terms of the appraisal tools use. A formal written or electronic tool may have specific guidelines or a more open-ended format. General topics may be addressed in an anecdotal or "incident" type of format. The tool or evaluation form should facilitate accurate appraisal of the individual's performance and provide an opportunity to identify personal goals of the individual and goals of the organization. The Literature Perspective below discusses the importance of developing objective performance metrics that align with overall strategic initiatives and organizational goals.

🔍 **RESEARCH PERSPECTIVE**

Resource: Hamilton, K. E., Coates, V., Kelly, B., et al. (2007). Performance assessment in healthcare providers: A critical review of evidence and current practice. *Journal of Nursing Management, 15,* 773–791.

The authors evaluated methods of performance assessment through an international literature review and a survey of current practice. In terms of methodology, the authors completed a comprehensive literature review. They also asked all Northern Ireland health care organizations to submit their performance appraisal tools. The results indicated that performance was not universally defined; a range of assessments were in use; and each method had advantages and disadvantages. The conclusion noted that no single method of performance appraisal is appropriate for assessing clinical performance. Multiple strategies are needed to capture employee performance accurately.

Implications for Practice

When organizations link performance appraisal tools to their mission, adopting a wide variety of assessment tools is logical because doing so ensures that all attributes necessary for nursing are assessed. Knowing the advantages and disadvantages of each performance appraisal tool is important.

LITERATURE PERSPECTIVE

Resource: Topjian, D. F., Buck, T. F., & Kozlowski, R. (2009). Employee performance for the good of all. *Nursing Management, 40*(4), 24–29.

The authors called for the development of objective performance metrics for all nursing personnel that align with overall strategic initiatives and organizational goals. A task force was formed to (1) develop a model of evaluation that was understandable and easily used by staff nurses and managers; (2) align staff with achievement of success at both unit and individual levels; (3) provide clear criteria to distinguish meeting from exceeding expectations; and (4) develop a tool that would avoid bias.

The authors provided concrete examples of how a peer or manager could evaluate a nurse's performance. A specific number of criteria must be successfully met to hit the threshold that exceeds expectations. The methodology used could be very helpful in assisting nurses and managers assess performance.

Implications for Practice
Reviewing examples of other performance appraisal tools can help organizations develop their own tools. Having a specific number of criteria to assess clarifies for everyone what the expected behaviours are.

BOX 16-3   EXAMPLES OF STRUCTURED AND FLEXIBLE PERFORMANCE APPRAISAL TOOLS

Structured (Traditional Method)
• Graphic rating scales

Flexible (Collaborative Method)
• Behaviourally anchored rating scales (BARS)
• Management by objectives (MBO)
• Self-review

Performance appraisal tools are either structured or flexible. Box 16-3 summarizes examples of structured and flexible performance appraisal tools.

Structured Performance Appraisal Tools

Graphic Rating Scales. Graphic rating scales are examples of structured approaches to evaluation. They comprise numbering systems that indicate high and low values for evaluating performance (Figure 16-1). The rating scale is popular because it is easy to construct and use. Problems with these types of scales are that they lack specificity and may promote a halo effect. The halo effect is "a type of cognitive bias where our perception of one personality trait influences how we view a person's entire personality" (Cherry, 2013). According to Chandra (2006), "managers may give higher ratings to individuals they like (a positive halo effect) and lower ratings to individuals they do not like (a negative halo effect)" (p. 36).

When undertaking a structured performance appraisal, it is important to include information about employee performance gathered over the entire evaluation period. Evaluations should not be reflections of isolated incidents (Chandra, 2006). It is human nature to remember incidents that are recent or sensational because those that deviate from the norm make a greater impression. However, these are usually a poor basis for overall evaluations.

Flexible Performance Appraisal Tools

Evaluation can also be conducted collaboratively. Flexible performance appraisal tools focus on how the nurse manager can help the individual nurse develop professionally.

Behaviourally Anchored Rating Scales. Behaviourally anchored rating scales (BARS) can be implemented as a collaborative or flexible approach. The focus is on behaviour and should include employees in the development. BARS combine ratings with critical incidents (specific examples that have occurred) or criterion references (examples usually based on standards of practice or competency-based standards). The criteria used for this scale are specific to the specialty of nursing delivered and pre-established outcomes. This scale is also considered more advantageous in the case of potential grievances or litigation. BARS describe the employee's performance both quantitatively and qualitatively. Staff who are involved in the development of these instruments are more likely to understand the importance of evaluation for each criterion selected and to have an understanding of their performance expectations. This scale is another method for clarifying roles and role expectations within the organization. The primary drawback of this scale is that it is expensive to develop and time consuming to implement; it must be designed for each specific position description

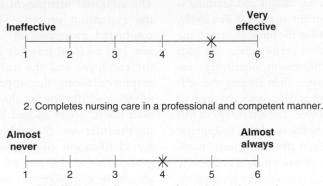

1. Effectiveness of patient teaching.

Ineffective				Very effective	
1	2	3	4	X 5	6

2. Completes nursing care in a professional and competent manner.

Almost never				Almost always	
1	2	3	X 4	5	6

FIGURE 16-1 Examples of graphic rating scales.

or standard of practice. However, it provides the nurse manager with concrete information regarding an employee's performance, with minimal subjective interference. Box 16-4 provides an example of how established nursing standards of practice, or protocols for practice, can be incorporated into the appraisal process using peer review. The data might also be used in an outcome review process as a component of a continuous quality-improvement program. The final result would be summarized by the nurse manager and incorporated into the employee's performance appraisal.

Management by Objectives. Management by objectives (MBO), which was popularized by Peter Drucker (1954), has been used for many years as a method of participative goal setting. In the MBO approach, performance goals are established jointly

between the nurse manager and the employee for the upcoming evaluation period. Progress regarding the accomplishment of these goals is documented throughout the rating period. An MBO approach requires that the employee establish clear and measurable objectives at the beginning of each rating period. Then, during the performance appraisal evaluation, both the employee and the manager address these objectives individually and in writing. In effect, the employee has created a "performance contract," as well as defined goals for future professional performance. For the nurse manager, MBO focuses on results and value and is therefore logically connected to managing the business of nursing (Pollok, 1983). Box 16-5 illustrates performance goals and accomplishments that could be part of an MBO method of performance appraisal.

BOX 16-4   EXAMPLE OF A BEHAVIOURALLY ANCHORED RATING SCALE

Emergency department (ED) staff nurse responsibilities for patient admitted with chest pain: (ED records evaluated per protocol; minimum 10/rating period). Met/Unmet

1. Vital signs recorded within 5 min of admission _____
2. Cardiac monitor, IV, lab tests, and ECG done within 15 min _____
3. If sublingual nitroglycerin given, vital signs recorded every 5 min for 30 min _____
   a. Chest pain changes evaluated per protocol _____
   b. Post–chest pain 12-lead ECG documented _____

BOX 16-5   LEARNING GOALS AND ACCOMPLISHMENTS

Learning Goals

1. Prepare for and take advanced cardiac life support (ACLS) certification examination
2. Participate in shared governance committee as unit representative

Accomplishments (12 Months Later—Summary)

1. Successfully passed ACLS certification
2. Participated in monthly meetings; chaired task force for development and implementation of new delivery system; presented in-service class to staff on several units

Self-Review. A common strategy used in Canadian contexts to encourage personal insight and learning is the self-review, or self-assessment, process (Kilty, 2005). Using the same appraisal tool as the nurse manager, the employee rates his or her own performance and adds multiple examples of goal achievement, identifying areas for growth. The nurse manager then reviews the self-appraisal to ensure alignment and discusses any areas of disagreement with the employee. The advantage of this approach is that it encourages the employee to appraise his or her own work critically, it affords the nurse manager a perspective on the employee's insight and ability to improve performance, and it avoids any favouritism or union concerns that might arise with peer review.

Summary of Appraisal Instruments

Which instrument or method of appraisal is best? The missions and goals of the organization determine the tools used. A combination of several tools is probably superior to any one method. The primary success of any performance appraisal lies in the skills and communication abilities of the nurse manager. It is also the nurse manager's responsibility to educate employees about the process and tools for performance appraisal. Role ambiguity and uncertainty of standards of practice and methods for evaluation are significant contributors to decreased work satisfaction. The best-designed instrument will fail if the nurse manager is ineffective and cannot communicate with the employee. Although nurse manager workloads in many jurisdictions have been cited as a deterrent to providing regular performance appraisals for staff, finding time-efficient ways of giving regular feedback is essential to creating and sustaining a high-performing team.

EXERCISE 16-4

Which performance appraisal tool is used by the local health care organization from which you obtained a position description (see Exercise 16-1)? How would you characterize the tool? Is it structured or flexible? Is it quantitatively based, qualitatively based, or both? Indicate whether the tool is well suited to appraising the performance of an individual in the position you described in Exercise 16-1.

Appraisal Interview Environment

The appraisal instrument is not the only factor in the evaluation process. The interview should be conducted professionally and in a positive manner. It is an ideal time for communication between the employee and the nurse manager. Advise the employee about the appraisal interview well in advance so that he or she has the opportunity to plan for it. There should be no interruptions during the interview, if possible. This time is important for clarification of employee and organizational goals. The evaluation of employee performance should be objective and unemotional. The evaluation instruments should be clearly completed, and time should be allowed for discussion. Goals may be established. The nurse manager and the employee should sign the appraisal forms, and each should be provided a copy. The effectiveness of the entire appraisal method relies on the manner in which the nurse manager uses the tools and the feedback that the employee receives. Effective communication between the nurse manager and employees can prevent potential performance problems on a unit. Specific behaviours by the nurse manager enhance the appraisal interview (Box 16-6).

BOX 16-6   KEY BEHAVIOURS FOR THE PERFORMANCE APPRAISAL INTERVIEW

- Provide a quiet, controlled environment, without interruptions.
- Maintain a relaxed but professional atmosphere.
- Put the employee at ease; the overall objective is for the best job to be done.
- Review specific examples for both positive and negative behaviour (keep an anecdotal file for each employee).
- Allow the employee to express opinions, orally and in writing.
- Write future plans and goals, training needs, and such (a "performance contract" for the future).
- Set a follow-up date as necessary to monitor improvements, if cited.
- Show the employee confidence in his or her performance.
- Be sincere and constructive in both praise and criticism.

A SOLUTION

Marie-Claude asked patient care managers (PCMs) attending the education session to share successful strategies for developing and retaining staff. These strategies included regular staff development sessions, journal clubs, and active engagement in quality improvement projects through either Plan-Do-Study-Act (PDSA) cycles or Lean-type initiatives (i.e., initiatives that look for ways to reduce spending and streamline processes). A number of PCMs explained that they actively mentored existing employees and coached new employees, which helped create a welcoming and supportive environment in their units. A few PCMs also noted that conducting annual performance appraisals could be challenging due to their large portfolios. Marie-Claude suggested integrating self-appraisal tools, online forms, and plenty of just-in-time feedback. She also suggested that PCMs obtain sponsorship from their organizations to support staff nurses in specialty certifications and other educational endeavours as a retention technique. Despite the many pressures facing nurse managers in Canada, it is clear that energy spent on developing and engaging staff, mentoring and coaching staff, and evaluating performance is beneficial and results in more effective and efficient clinical environments.

Would these approaches be suitable in your context? Why or why not?

THE EVIDENCE

The first year of a nurse's career can be a very difficult time for retention in the acute care setting. Recruiting, orienting, and providing ongoing education to a newly hired nurse is costly. Thus, it is important to use best practices in the acute care environment. Funderbunk (2008) identified the benefits of mentoring in acute care settings. She also suggested how to establish a mentoring program and provided information about mentoring of leadership and developing goals for a mentoring program. A comprehensive view of how to establish a mentoring program and what supports are necessary is outlined.

NEED TO KNOW NOW

- Consider how well job applicants fit with the position and the organization.
- Know what professional development opportunities are available to staff.

- Review position descriptions and performance appraisals with staff.

CHAPTER CHECKLIST

The nurse manager plays a key role in the selection and development of staff. As a role model, the nurse manager is also key in the establishment of the type of work environment that exists. Nurse managers must be supportive and develop their staff to their highest potential. They must have accurate position descriptions and tools for the evaluation of employee performance. These are integral to role development and professional socialization. Nurse managers must also use various communication methods to empower their employees. Coaching and the implementation of empowerment strategies positively contribute to overall staff performance as well.

- When seeking to fill a position, the interviewer should do the following:
  - Prescreen applicants.
  - Prepare questions in advance, based on the position description.
  - Ensure that the interview environment is comfortable and private.
  - Provide role clarification.
  - Be a good listener.
  - Answer questions honestly.
  - Provide closure.
  - Inform the applicant when he or she will be notified.

- The applicant should do the following:
  - Be on time and dress appropriately.
  - Review the organization's mission and goals.
  - Prepare questions in advance.
  - Answer questions honestly and completely.
  - Note appreciation for the interview.
- Staff development includes the following:
  - Organized and efficient orientation and residency
  - Plans for education, team building, and professional socialization
  - Active coaching
  - Implementation of empowerment strategies
- Development of accurate position descriptions and tools for evaluation of employees is integral to role development and professional socialization. Nurse managers should use various communication methods, including coaching techniques.
  - Role theory describes how individuals perceive their position in an organization.

- Distinction and clarity among the various positions are imperative if partnerships in quality patient care are to exist.
- The position description serves several purposes:
  - Provides a statement that describes roles and responsibilities
  - Reflects the position's scope and duties
  - Reflects current practice guidelines for the role
  - Serves as a contract between the manager and employee
- Performance appraisals are a method of providing feedback to the employee in relation to individual performance.
  - Types of structured (traditional) performance appraisals include the following:
    - Graphic rating scale
  - Types of flexible (collaborative) performance appraisals include the following:
    - Behaviourally anchored rating scales (BARS)
    - Management by objectives (MBO)
    - Self-review

TIPS FOR CONDUCTING A JOB INTERVIEW

- Prescreen the applicants and schedule a time for each interview.
- Prepare questions in advance. Be concise but thorough.
- Control the environment for noise and interruptions.

- Explain and clarify the role for which the applicant is interviewing.
- Be a good listener.
- Answer questions honestly.
- Inform the applicant when he or she will be informed of the decision.

evolve WEBSITE

Visit the Evolve website for Suggested Readings, Internet Resources, and additional resources related to the content in this chapter: http://evolve.elsevier.com/Canada/Yoder-Wise/leading/.

REFERENCES

Aiken, L. (1984, December). A new game plan for the doctor nurse team. *The New Physician.*

Brooke, P. (2008). Hiring and firing: Know the consequences. *Nursing Management, 39*(9), 50–52. doi:10.1097/01.NUMA.0000335260.31344.58

Chandra, A. (2006). Employee evaluation strategies for healthcare organizations: A general guide. *Hospital Topics, 84*(2), 34–38.

Cherry, K. (2013, May 31). Halo effect—Psychology definition of the week. Retrieved from http://psychology.about.com/b/2013/05/31/halo-effect-psychology-definition-of-the-week.htm.

Drucker, P. F. (1954). *The practice of management.* New York, NY: Harper.

Funderbunk, A. (2008). Mentoring: The retention factor in the acute care setting. *Journal for Nurses in Staff Development, 24*(3), E1–E5. doi:10.1097/01.NND.0000320652.80178.40

Graham, S. (2011). Prepare to win the behavioural interview. Retrieved from http://www.higherbracket.ca.

Hamilton, K. E., Coates, V., Kelly, B., et al. (2007). Performance assessment in healthcare providers: A critical review of evidence and current practice. *Journal of Nursing Management, 15,* 773–791.

Johnson, J. E. (2000). The nursing shortage: From warning to watershed. *Applied Nursing Research, 13*(3), 162–163.

Kahn, R. L., Wolfe, D. M., Quinn, R. P., et al. (1964). *Occupational stress: Studies in role conflict and ambiguity.* New York, NY: Wiley.

Kelley, R. E. (1992). *The power of followership.* New York, NY: Doubleday.

Kilty, H. L. (2005). *Nursing leadership development in Canada.* Retrieved from http://www.cna-aiic.ca/CNA/documents/pdf/publications/Nursing_Leadership_Development_Canada_e.pdf.

Kollman, S., Liedl, C., Johnson, L., et al. (2007). Rookies of the year: Successfully orienting new graduate registered nurses to the cardiovascular surgical intensive care unit. *Critical Care Nursing Clinics of North America, 19,* 417–426. doi:10.1016/j.ccell.2007.07.007

Langley, G. L., Nolan, K. M., Nolan, T. W., et al. (2009). *The improvement guide: A practical approach to enhancing organizational performance* (2nd ed.). San Francisco, CA: Jossey-Bass.

McConnell, C. R. (2008). Conducting the employee selection interview: How to do it effectively while avoiding legal obstacles. *JONA's Healthcare Law, Ethics and Regulation, 10*(2), 48–56. doi:10.1097/01.NHL.0000300781.72981.40

Moore, M. L. (2008). Preceptorships: Hidden benefits to the organization. *Journal for Nurses in Staff Development, 24*(1), E9–E15.

Pangman, V. C., & Pangman, C. (2009) *Nursing leadership from a Canadian perspective.* Philadelphia, PA: Lippincott.

Parrish, F. (2006). How to recruit, interview and retain employees. *Dermatology Nursing, 18*(2), 179–180.

Pollok, C. S. (1983). Adapting management by objectives to nursing. *The Nursing Clinics of North America, 18*(3), 481–490.

Robert Wood Johnson Foundation. (2006). Wisdom at work: The importance of the older and experienced nurse in the workplace. Retrieved from http://www.rwjf.org/content/dam/supplementary-assets/2006/06/wisdomatwork.pdf.

Stevenson, L., Joyce, S., Eastman, N., et al. (2011, June). *Finding a "new right way": Collaborating on care delivery model redesign.* Panel presented at the CCHL Rising to the Challenge: Relationships, Resources and Realities, Whistler, BC.

Topjian, D. F., Buck, T. F., & Kozlowski, R. (2009). Employee performance for the good of all. *Nursing Management, 40*(4), 24–29. doi:10.1097/01.NUMA.0000349686.01295.b5

Trossman, S. (2002). Nursing magnets: Attracting talent and making it stick. *The American Journal of Nursing, 102*(2), 87, 89.

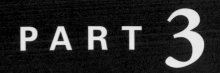

Changing the Status Quo

PART 3

Changing the
Status Quo

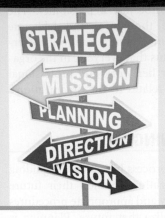

Strategic Planning and Goal Setting

Mary Ellen Clyne
Adapted by Sandra Regan

This chapter discusses how organizations plan for the future, with a focus on the strategic planning process and goal setting. It also presents specific examples of strategic planning in health care organizations.

OBJECTIVES

- Understand the phases of the strategic planning process.
- Articulate the value and importance of conducting an assessment of external and internal environments.
- Review the purpose of an organization's mission statement, philosophy, goals, and objectives.
- Describe the four key steps in implementing a goal-setting program.
- Know the guidelines for developing S.M.A.R.T. objectives.

TERMS TO KNOW

environmental assessment
goal setting
S.M.A.R.T. objectives

strategic planning
SWOT analysis

❓ A CHALLENGE

In an effort to ensure patient safety, Ray, a registered nurse, and other staff nurses identified concerns with the interruptions they faced administering medications. Specifically, they were interrupted from medication administration to answer phone calls and random questions, redirect visitors, and check medications with nurses of other patients. Ray and the staff nurses wanted to bring their vision of patient safety to the process of medication administration on their unit. However, Ray and the staff nurses faced challenges in bringing this vision to reality because they lacked a clear plan. Ray agreed to take the lead on the matter and considered what he might do.

What do you think you would do if you were Ray?

INTRODUCTION

Given the rising costs of health care and our society's aging population, now, more than ever, health care organizations are under enormous pressure to deliver services while reducing expenses and containing costs. Major reforms are required, and the health care system has responded by the following initiatives:

- Empowering patients
- Ensuring care across the continuum that is both coordinated and comprehensive
- Ensuring appropriate utilization of resources, advanced technology, and the workforce
- Focusing on health promotion and prevention

Nurses are instrumental in developing, planning, and executing new strategies for the future, and thus are a major influence in the direction of health care. In the twenty-first century, technology has a strong influence on care delivery, nurse leaders, and organizations (Mayo & Nohria, 2005). Health technologies, defined as "the application of organized knowledge and skills in the form of devices, medicines, vaccines, procedures and systems developed to solve a health problem and improve quality of lives" (World Health Organization, 2007, p. 1) are rapidly advancing, and it is paramount for nurses to be at the forefront of influencing the implementation of new technologies. Doing so will require nurses to embrace the use of new technologies and evaluate their effectiveness. Across health care settings, new models of care will increasingly utilize and depend on new technologies. For example, mobile information technologies, such as hand-held devices, are increasingly being used at the point-of-care by nurses to document patient care (Doran, Mylopoulos, Kushniruk, et al., 2007). By adopting and regularly using new technology, nurses will not only enhance their nursing expertise but also earn the credibility to serve as advisors, directors, and influencers of technology. Nurses should be proactive and ensure that new technologies are used to meet nursing's information needs, to advance nursing practice, and to ensure nursing's continued viability.

The operational definition of *proactive* is simply "aggressive planning." It provides direction for one's efforts and toward which others must then react.

Thus, greater control is possible so that one's vision becomes a probability, not just a possibility. The importance of proactive, thoughtful, and deliberate planning in the face of uncertainties cannot be overestimated. *Proactive* means that everyone in the organization manages his or her work and professional life and how he or she relates to the organization's goals and missions.

STRATEGIC PLANNING

Strategic planning is a process by which the guiding members of the organization envision their future and develop the necessary and appropriate procedures and operations to actualize that future. Planning is designed to encompass the organization's emphasis on mission statements, strategic action plans, changes in policies and procedures, environmental factors affecting the organization, and the development and execution of new services.

The strategic planning process shown in Figure 17-1 consists of the following key phases:

1. Assess the internal and external environments to determine those forces or changes that may affect the work of the organization or that may be crucial to its survival. These assessments entail analyzing the *S*trengths, *W*eaknesses, *O*pportunities, and *T*hreats (SWOT analysis) facing the organization and the organization's ability to deal with change (SWOT analysis is also discussed in Chapter 7).
2. Review the organization's mission, philosophy, goals, and objectives.
3. Determine major strategies, establish goals, and develop a plan of action to respond to the identified opportunities and threats. The best strategic option balances the organization's potential with the challenges of changing conditions, taking into account the values of its management and its social responsibilities.
4. Implement the plan of action.
5. Evaluate the strategic plan on a regular basis to determine its effectiveness and whether adjustments need to be made.

Reasons for Strategic Planning

In today's health care environment, which is marked by turbulence and complexity, strategic planning is imperative for health care organizations to remain

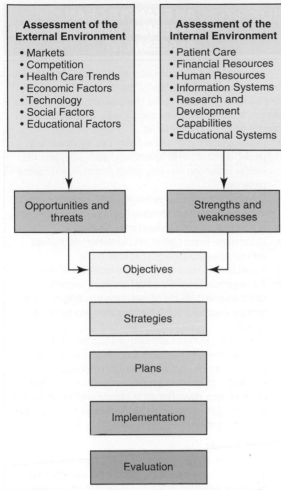

Assessment of the External Environment
- Markets
- Competition
- Health Care Trends
- Economic Factors
- Technology
- Social Factors
- Educational Factors

Assessment of the Internal Environment
- Patient Care
- Financial Resources
- Human Resources
- Information Systems
- Research and Development Capabilities
- Educational Systems

Opportunities and threats

Strengths and weaknesses

Objectives

Strategies

Plans

Implementation

Evaluation

FIGURE 17-1 Key phases in the strategic planning process.

responsive to internal and external forces. Therefore, to survive the ongoing change and restructuring of the health care system, the strategic plan becomes the fundamental tool for creating and sustaining the organizational vision for the future. The strategic planning process leads to the achievement of goals and objectives, gives meaning to work life, and provides direction and improvement for the operational activities of the organization. Furthermore, a strong and dynamic strategic plan, if used, results in the efficient and effective use of resources and reflects the organizational culture and patient focus. Strategic planning occurs in large and small health care organizations and across sectors from hospitals to long-term care facilities to home health care agencies. Nurse leaders plan in a proactive, systematic manner because (1) knowledge regarding philosophy, goals, and external and internal operations of the organization is necessary to lead change; and (2) an understanding of the planning process is paramount to managing decisions.

Phases of the Strategic Planning Process

The strategic planning process is proactive, vision-directed, action-oriented, creative, innovative, and oriented toward positive change. For a strategic plan to succeed, a system must be developed that creates a plan for each approved initiative; this plan is integrated with a financial plan so that resources can be allocated and the time for implementation and the required capital resources can be determined (Ruder & O'Connor, 2007).

The *strategic planning process* involves developing a plan of action that covers 3 to 5 years. The initial phase—assessing the external and internal environments—is the most difficult. An **environmental assessment** is carried out to understand the specific internal and external forces that influence the health care setting (e.g., a hospital or community agency). Figure 17-1 presents some of the key forces in an external and internal environmental assessment.

Visionary leaders ensure that those around them understand the direction the organization is taking (Ibarra & Obodaru, 2009). These visionaries search for a new path through a vigorous dialogue with various constituents, both internally and externally, because great visions will not actualize from solitary analysis (Ibarra & Obodaru, 2009). It is also important that visionaries test their ideas practically based on current resources from the following perspectives: financial, human resources, and overall organizational capabilities (Ibarra & Obodaru, 2009). True strategists provide an organization with more than a vision statement, "they articulate a clear point of view about what will transpire and position their organizations to respond to it" (Ibarra & Obodaru, 2009, p. 66). Although strategic planning often takes place at the executive level of an organization, nurse managers and staff nurses can provide a valuable perspective through established processes such as committees. In addition, nurse managers and staff nurses often engage in clinical strategic planning processes.

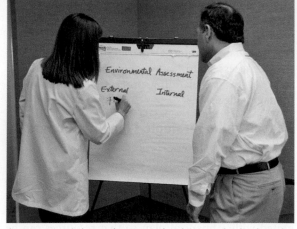

A strong and dynamic strategic plan results in the efficient and effective use of resources.

Phase 1: Assessment of the External and Internal Environments

External Environmental Assessment. An external environmental assessment takes place first in the strategic-planning process. The legal–political forces, economic forces, sociocultural forces, accreditation, technology, professional associations and unions, and regulatory bodies are assessed according to a SWOT analysis. By assessing and monitoring external forces, health care leaders can make effective plans for their organization and develop creative and visionary programs that respond to external changes within the framework of their institutional mission and goals. An example of an external environmental assessment appears in Box 17-1.

EXERCISE 17-1

Research the demographics of the city you work in. Specifically, find information on age, socioeconomic factors (income, education, employment, and housing), and the ethnic origin of the population. What is the gap between the actual health care needs of the population and the services provided to patients in your organization?

Internal Environmental Assessment. Internal environmental assessment involves a SWOT analysis of the health care organization's structure, size, programs, financial resources, human resources, information systems, and research and development capabilities. It also includes a review of the education

---

BOX 17-1 AN EXAMPLE OF AN EXTERNAL ENVIRONMENTAL ASSESSMENT

A community-based acute care hospital is undertaking a study to examine accessibility, availability, quality, and effectiveness of developing an orthopedic centre of excellence. One of the initial steps is to conduct an environmental scan. The hospital considered the following external forces:

- Legal–political forces such as health care legislation and provincial and territorial government health policy priorities such as addressing wait lists, health promotion, and disease prevention
- Economic forces such as escalating health care costs and shifts in provincial and territorial funding as well as the cost of orthopedic care from admission to discharge
- Sociocultural forces such as the community organizations with volunteer groups supporting older adults
- Accreditation Canada standards and accreditation processes
- The diagnostic services available, including magnetic resonance imaging (MRI) and nuclear diagnostic imaging, along with the availability of rehabilitative and home health care services
- The numbers and types of health care providers, including certified orthopedic physicians specialized in innovative joint replacement, operating room (OR) orthopedic nurses, orthopedic staff nurses (specialty certified), case managers, social workers, physiotherapists, occupational therapists, and pain management specialists and their respective unions and regulatory bodies

Patient Trends

- Demographic and population trends (e.g., age, size, and distribution of the population, employment, socioeconomic indicators, education, ethnicity, and lifestyle issues, with particular emphasis on priority populations)
- Trends in health care (increased emphasis on wellness programs and enhanced technologies)
- Prospective users' input about current and future services

---

and training needs of staff and patient demands or needs. The management team involves all levels of staff in this assessment and focuses on the purpose of the organization; its mission and goals; the capabilities, skills, and relationships of various health care providers and related staff; and the weaknesses and strengths of staff in areas such as leadership, planning, coordination, research, and staff development. Also, the organizational climate must be assessed because it can shape the strategic direction of the organization.

Phase 2: Review of the Mission Statement, Philosophy, Goals, and Objectives

Mission Statement and Philosophy. A mission statement reflects the purpose and direction of the health care organization or a department within it. A statement of philosophy provides direction for the organization and/or department. The content usually specifies organizational beliefs regarding the patient, health and nursing, the expectations of practitioners, and the commitment of the organization to professionalism, education, evaluation, and research. The importance of the mission statement cannot be overstated, yet it is questionable how many individuals in an organization, when asked, can articulate their organization's mission statement or its philosophy.

Covey (1990) considered that the mission statement is vital to the success of an organization and believed that everyone should participate in its development: "The involvement process is as important as the written product and is the key to its use" (p. 139). "An organizational mission statement, one that truly reflects the deep shared vision and values of everyone within that organization, creates a unity and tremendous commitment" (p. 143). Chapter 9 further discusses organizational mission statements.

> **EXERCISE 17-2**
> Select a health care organization with which you have been affiliated. How effective is the organizational structure (i.e., is the organization operating effectively and efficiently?)? What human resources are present (refer to the organizational chart, note the various titles, and find out the number of employees)? Where are nurse leaders in the organizational chart? What information systems are used in the organization?

Building on the example in Box 17-1, an example of a mission statement for a newly developed total joint replacement program within the orthopedic centre might be as follows: to provide quality care, to be integrated with the community, and to support a patient-centred approach to care.

Goal Setting. Goal setting is the process of developing, negotiating, and formalizing the targets of an organization. If goals are not appropriate to the organization, frustration and poor performance could result (Hader, 2008).

The new joint replacement program might have five goals:

1. Provide comprehensive patient and family education across the continuum of care.
2. Develop protocols for standardized patient-care programs in terms of activities of daily living, physiotherapy, occupational therapy, recreational exercise, and pain management.
3. Incorporate an interdisciplinary approach to patient care through a team consisting of physicians, nurse practitioners, nurses, case managers, social workers, physiotherapists, occupational therapists, nutritionists/dietitians, home support workers, and clergy or other spiritual support roles.
4. Enhance community support programs for arthritic patients.
5. Ensure that the Web site is current, with information and services available to patients.

> **EXERCISE 17-3**
> Obtain and review a health care organization's mission statement. Based on what it says and means to you, create a goal statement that fits.

Specific goals are more likely to lead to higher performance than are vague or very general goals, such as "try to do your best." Feedback, or knowledge of results, is more likely to motivate individuals toward higher performance levels and commitment to goal achievements. For example, as organizations have become more focused on patient outcomes, they have been able to focus on specific goals and behaviours that result in better care.

Four key steps in the goal-setting process are as follows:

1. Set goals that are specific, and adhere to a deadline.
2. Promote goal commitment by providing instructions and support to employees and managers.
3. Support the achievement of goals with appropriate feedback as soon as possible.
4. Monitor performance at appropriate intervals.

Objectives. Objectives are an important way to set out specific actions for goal achievement. Objectives tend to be short- or medium-term statements that support people's efforts to attain stated goals. The ability to write clear and concise objectives is an important aspect of nursing leadership. Effective objectives are known as S.M.A.R.T. objectives. The acronym *S.M.A.R.T.* refers to key attributes of effective objectives. Namely, that objectives are *Specific, Measurable,*

Agreed on (or some use the word *Achievable*), *Realistic*, and *Time* bound. Consider the following guidelines when developing S.M.A.R.T. objectives:

Specific The objective statement must be properly constructed and describe exactly what is to be accomplished.

- It begins with the word *to,* followed by an action verb.
- It specifies a single result to be achieved.
- It specifies a target date for its attainment.

Measurable The objectives must be measurable.

- They provide the level of accomplishment of the end result.
- They leave no question as to what is expected.

Agreed On The objectives must be agreed on by all parties.

- There is mutual agreement by all parties on who will be responsible for execution and monitoring.

Realistic The objectives must be created within the realm of possibility and a challenge.

- They should not be unrealistic or unattainable.
- They must be written in the span of control for the specific team working toward the goals.
- The team has to be accountable for follow-through.

Time Bound The objectives should establish a time frame for which the activity or improvement must be achieved.

- The timeline and deadlines are adhered to.
- The timeline must be well-defined, avoiding statements such as "in the future."

Examples of S.M.A.R.T objectives appear in Box 17-2.

Phase 3: Identification of Strategies. The third phase of the strategic planning process involves identifying major issues, establishing goals, and developing strategies to meet the goals. The term *strategy* can be defined as an organized and innovative plan that

---

BOX 17-2   EXAMPLES OF S.M.A.R.T. OBJECTIVES

1. To provide training for 20 registered nurses in the use of the new electronic health record by June 1, of the current year.
2. To increase by four the number of medical–surgical units in the ABC hospital to implement electronic health records by August 31, of the current year.
3. To deliver ten additional smoking cessation clinics per month in the local public health unit starting January 1, of the current year.

---

assists an organization to achieve its objectives. All departmental managers are involved in this process and are responsible for preparing a detailed plan of action, which may include the following: development of short-term and long-term objectives, formulation of annual department objectives, allocation of resources, and preparation of the budget. Table 17-1 identifies a plan of action for developing, implementing, and evaluating an orthopedic centre of excellence based on the internal and external environmental assessment in Box 17-1 on page 322.

EXERCISE 17-4

You are a staff nurse working in home care within a Regional Health Authority (RHA). The chair of the Professional Practice Council has assigned you to work on a planning committee with staff nurses and nurse managers from across the RHA in acute care, community, long-term care, and home care. The purpose of the committee is to devise long-term and short-term goals for nursing within the RHA.

The population of the community served by a local hospital is 55 000, and the population is aging. The older adult population will increase over the next 5 years. Many patients in the community are seeking assistance for arthritis complications such as building better bones and exercise programs, physiotherapy opportunities, and access to education.

The hospital has both an inpatient and an outpatient rehabilitation program with a specialized orthopedic unit; the inpatient orthopedic unit is staffed with nurses who are Canadian Nurses Association–certified in orthopedics and world-renowned Royal College of Physician and Surgeons of Canada–certified orthopedic surgeons. The hospital has implemented an early discharge program for patients who have had knee or hip replacement surgery. Nurses in home care are increasingly providing postoperative orthopedic care to these patients.

Considering the parameters of this strategic planning situation, in what direction should nursing in the hospital consider moving during the next 5 years to meet the needs of the community? How will you determine short-term and long-term plans? What additional information will your committee need to plan, realistically, for the next 5 months and the next 5 years?

Phase 4: Implementation. In the fourth phase of the strategic planning process, the specific plan of action is executed in order of priority. Implementation requires open communication with staff (this is paramount) regarding the priorities for the next year and subsequent periods; the development of revised policies and procedures regarding the changes; and the creation of area and individual objectives related to the plan. The specific plan needs to be focused on communications, programs, operations, a budget, and human resources.

TABLE 17-1	**STRATEGIC PLAN OF ACTION FOR THE DEVELOPMENT, IMPLEMENTATION, AND EVALUATION OF AN ORTHOPEDIC CENTRE OF EXCELLENCE**		
GOAL	**ACTIVITIES**	**RESPONSIBLE COUNCIL**	**TIME FRAME**
1. To develop an orthopedic centre of excellence	1.1 To conduct an internal and external environmental assessment • Primary and secondary service area • Demographic review • Out migration	Director of nursing Orthopedic manager Strategic planning director	January 2016
	1.2 To conduct a literature review related to each of these topics: • Orthopedic product lines • Innovative orthopedic joint replacement procedures • Programs related to orthopedics evidenced-informed practices for joint replacement	Orthopedic manager Operating room (OR) director Vice-president of medical affairs Director of rehabilitative services Nurse practitioner Staff nurse	January 2016
	1.3 To form an advisory committee comprising community representatives to oversee the development and implementation of the centre	Quality assurance director Physician champion Vice-president of patient-care services Orthopedic staff across the continuum of care Director of rehabilitation services Vice-president of medical affairs	February 2016
	1.4 To develop the organizational structure, mission statement, philosophy, and objectives, and revise accordingly	All parties	March 2016
	1.5 To develop policy and procedure manuals for staff in all areas	Orthopedic staff across the continuum of care Medical staff Standards staff Nurse practitioners Director of education Staff nurses	Ongoing
	1.6 To determine the business structure of the organization (i.e., legalities regarding partnerships, corporations, and proprietorship)	Nurse practitioners Medical staff Vice-president of medical affairs Orthopedic manager Vice-president of patient-care services Assistant vice-president of patient-care services Office of general counsel	Ongoing
	1.7 To develop a budget	Assistant vice-president of patient-care services Orthopedic manager/nurse manager	March 2016 Ongoing
	1.8 To develop a business site for the organization: • All renovations • Equipment • Supplies	Consultants and orthopedic manager	April 2016

Continued

TABLE 17-1	STRATEGIC PLAN OF ACTION FOR THE DEVELOPMENT, IMPLEMENTATION, AND EVALUATION OF AN ORTHOPEDIC CENTRE OF EXCELLENCE —cont'd		
GOAL	**ACTIVITIES**	**RESPONSIBLE COUNCIL**	**TIME FRAME**
	1.9 To develop a communications program (internal and external communications)	Communications office Patient engagement office Nurse practitioners Orthopedic manager Director of strategic planning Medical staff Staff nurses	February 2016 Ongoing
2. To implement and evaluate the effectiveness and efficiency of these programs	2.1 To develop patient questionnaires related to satisfaction regarding care provided	Nurse practitioners Orthopedic managers Quality assurance director Orthopedic front-line staff across the continuum Staff nurses	April 2016
	2.2 To develop cost-effective analysis studies to evaluate each of the programs being provided	Orthopedic manager	Ongoing
	2.3 To collect and collate data related to utilization of services by orthopedic patients	Nurse practitioners Staff across the continuum of care Pharmacists Medical staff Orthopedic manager Quality and patient safety director	Ongoing

Phase 5: Evaluation. The strategic plan is reviewed on a regular basis at all levels to determine whether the goals, objectives, and activities are on target. It is important to keep in mind that objectives may need to change in response to legislation, government funding, organizational budget constraints, restructuring, and other environmental factors. Therefore, alternative activities may need to be used to adapt to respond to new situations. For example, imagine that an employer is informed that the budget must be decreased by $250 000 over the next 3 months. Management involves the staff in developing creative alternative methods for ensuring that the necessary changes will occur. Three months later, savings have been realized through restructuring, reducing expenses, and, when appropriate, using oral (PO) rather than intravenous (IV) medication administration.

The strategic planning process is similar in nature to the nursing process, as Figure 17-2 shows.

> **EXERCISE 17-5**
> Obtain a copy of a health care organization's strategic plan. You can often go to the Web site for a particular regional health authority, hospital, long-term care facility, primary health care centre, home health agency, public health unit, or other health care related organization and type in "strategic plan" in the search box. Keep in mind that not all organizations will have their strategic plan on their Web site. How does the strategic plan you obtained compare with what you have learned in this chapter about the key phases in the strategic planning process? Can you find information that illustrates most of the phases of the planning process?

The strategic planning process can also be useful to develop programs within organizations. The Literature Perspective on page 328 illustrates how one Canadian hospital applied the strategic planning process to develop a nursing strategic plan. Box 17-3 outlines key elements of a strategic plan to reduce breast cancer deaths in the workplace. Notice the goal setting and use of S.M.A.R.T objectives.

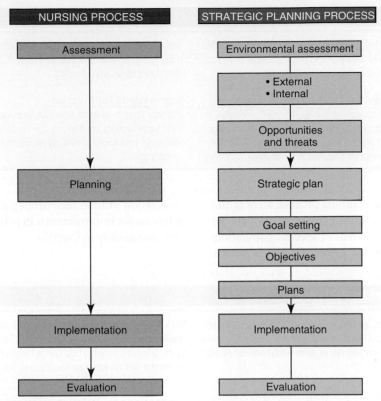

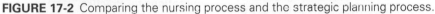

FIGURE 17-2 Comparing the nursing process and the strategic planning process.

BOX 17-3 MISSION STATEMENT, GOALS, AND OBJECTIVES OF A BREAST CANCER SCREENING PROGRAM

Mission Statement

To reduce the leading cause of cancer deaths in women by delivering a comprehensive, organized, and evaluated breast cancer screening program for female health care workers in an acute care setting. The Breast Cancer Screening Program is committed to deliver a program that is sensitive to women's needs, builds on health-promoting behaviours, and fosters partnerships with interest groups in the health care community.

Overall Goals

To integrate health promotion strategies and medical practice to reduce mortality from breast cancer by having 100% of eligible female health care workers participate in annual mammography screening and conduct self-breast examinations.

Objectives

- To detect breast cancer earlier than would occur if organized screening were not available
- To develop and implement a hospital mobilization plan for the program
- To develop and implement a social marketing plan, including a health education component for the program
- To articulate protocols and standards for health care providers associated with the program
- To establish protocols for the interaction of the target population with the program
- To develop and implement training and technical assistance for those associated with the delivery of the program
- To develop a partnership with health care providers that will facilitate program delivery
- To establish a regional breast screening service so that all women in the target population have equal access to breast screening
- To document the follow-up of all women in whom an abnormality has been detected
- To provide screening that is sensitive and acceptable to the target population
- To evaluate the program on a continual basis, including needs assessment and measurement of process, economic, and outcome variables

📖 LITERATURE PERSPECTIVE

Resource: Jeffs, L., Merkley, J., Jeffrey, J., et al. (2006). Case study: Reconciling the quality and safety gap through strategic planning. *Canadian Journal of Nursing Leadership, 19*(2), 32–40.

A strategic planning process was applied to enhance the nursing professional practice environment at St. Michael's Hospital in Toronto, Ontario. The authors reported on the steps of the strategic planning process used to develop a nursing strategic plan (NSP). They concluded with several key lessons learned in the process, including the importance of linking a change agenda, such as enhancing the nursing professional practice environment, to an external strategic direction such as patient safety.

Implications for Practice

The key lessons learned from the strategic planning process can help nurse leaders undertaking similar processes achieve success and avoid challenges commonly encountered in strategic planning processes.

During the strategic planning process, an organization may identify significant gaps in health care services or the health care needs of specific populations. The Research Perspective below illustrates how an association utilized their strategic planning process to advocate for improvements in primary care delivery in one community in Ontario.

🔍 RESEARCH PERSPECTIVE

Resource: Doey, T., Hines, P., Myslik, B., et al. (2008). Creating primary care access for mental health care clients in a community mental health setting. *Canadian Journal of Community Mental Health, 27*(2), 129–138.

The authors described how a strategic planning exercise conducted by Canadian Mental Health Association was used as a point of advocacy to address the unique primary care needs of people with mental illness in Windsor-Essex County in Ontario. A Primary Care Working Group was established to explore options to provide mental health care within a primary care model. The working group reports on the process that led to City Centre Health Centre, an interdisciplinary mental and primary care facility, and the patient-focused evaluation of the services provided.

Implications for Practice

Strategic planning processes can be used to identify gaps in service delivery and to advocate for patient-focused strategies.

💡 A SOLUTION

The first step in addressing any problem is to define the problem and identify its root causes. Ray talked to the staff nurses on his floor. Their concerns about the disruptions during medication administration were also shared by nurses on other units. Given that the hospital had recently implemented a Professional Practice Council (PPC), Ray proposed and the staff nurses agreed that bringing their concerns forward to the PPC would be a first step in addressing the problem. Most hospitals and other health care settings have implemented PPCs or something similar as a forum for nurses, other staff, and nurse managers to discuss issues arising in practice, identify evidence-informed solutions, and make decisions. At the PPC, it was agreed that the goals of supporting nurses to meet medication administration standards and ensuring patient safety were shared among the staff nurses and nurse managers. To address these concerns, the PPC undertook the following:

1. It conducted an assessment of the internal environment, gathered information about medication errors, and interviewed staff nurses and nurse managers to gain their perspectives on the problem. The PPC also consulted with key people responsible for patient safety in the organization.

2. It obtained and reviewed provincial nursing regulatory body's standards for medication administration. It also reviewed and summarized research on medication administration and patient safety, identifying solutions that had been implemented in other health care settings to address similar concerns.

3. It established the following goal: to ensure that staff nurses were able to meet medication administration standards, minimize disruptions during medication administration, and ensure patient safety. In order to understand the resources required to support staff nurses, the PPC conducted an assessment of the process of "typical" medication administration on a unit, which included shadowing some staff nurses to identify the full nature of the problem.

4. It involved nursing staff and nurse managers in all aspects of planning to address the problem. During this process, the nursing staff felt a strong sense of ownership of the issue and the potential solutions. Nurse managers communicated the concerns to other key executives in the hospital, including the patient safety officer and the director of nursing.

A SOLUTION—cont'd

5. After examining the standards, reviewing the research, and understanding the work processes that nurses enact to administer medication, the PPC identified solutions that could be implemented to minimize interruptions during medication administration. It reported its recommendations to the vice-president, Patient Care Services.

PPCs provide staff nurses with a strong professional voice within their organization. They are also an avenue for bringing professional and patient safety issues to the attention of managers, identifying a shared vision or goal, reviewing evidence, working on solutions, and developing actions that can make a difference for nursing practice and address patient safety issues.

Would this be a suitable approach for you? Why or why not?

THE EVIDENCE

Connelly (2005) explored how six departmental nursing leaders dealt with high nurse turnover rates in their organization. The goal of the nursing leaders was to not have any new nurses leave the organization unless they were asked to leave.

The nursing leaders conducted a SWOT analysis through a focus group of staff nurses who had recently resigned from the organization. Based on feedback from the former staff nurses, a new strategic plan for nurse retention was developed, and the resulting new Welcoming Process transformed the nursing department as a whole.

The Welcoming Process incorporated six elements: establishing connections, greeting new staff, individualizing orientation, acceptance into the workgroup, checking in periodically, and supporting new staff. In addition to decreasing the nurse turnover rate, the organization realized significant cost savings by retaining the new nursing staff and improved nurse satisfaction of both the new nursing staff and the nursing leaders.

NEED TO KNOW NOW

- Consider how a health care organization's vision and mission statement would affect your practice.
- Know the strengths, weaknesses, opportunities, and threats facing your health care organization.
- Listen for ideas about needs from your patients.

CHAPTER CHECKLIST

The operational effectiveness of any organization depends on its strategic planning. Nurse managers and leaders must be knowledgeable of the critical elements to facilitate the process.

- The strategic planning process leads to attainment of goals and objectives and provides meaning to work life and direction for the organizational activities.
- Strategic planning is similar in nature to the nursing process and involves the following:
  - Assessment of the environment (internal and external) based on SWOT analysis
- Review of the organization's mission statement, philosophy, goals, and objectives
- Identification and development of strategies to respond to opportunities and threats
- Implementation of the plan of action
- Evaluation of the strategic plan
- Nurses can play a pivotal leadership role in the development of visionary programs and services that meet the needs of patients by participating in planning processes at all levels of the organization.

TIPS FOR PLANNING AND GOAL SETTING

- Be clear about the organization's mission and vision, ensuring that they meet the needs of those you serve, and stay true to them.
- Read and listen to wide sources of information to determine what is happening and what trends could

affect you and your organization, and be flexible if changes are imminent.
- Be clear about your role in the organization and its success. Actively participate in the process.

℮volve WEBSITE

Visit the Evolve website for Suggested Readings, Internet Resources, and additional resources related to the content in this chapter: http://evolve.elsevier.com/Canada/Yoder-Wise/leading/.

REFERENCES

Connelly, L. (2005). Welcoming new employees. *Journal of Nursing Scholarship, 37,* 163–164. doi:10.1111/j.1547–5069.2005.00029.x

Covey, S. (1990). *The seven habits of highly effective people.* Toronto, ON: Simon & Schuster.

Doey, T., Hines, P., Myslik, B., et al. (2008). Creating primary care access for mental health care clients in a community mental health setting. *Canadian Journal of Community Mental Health, 27*(2), 129–138.

Doran, D. M., Mylopoulos, J., Kushniruk, A., et al. (2007). Evidence in the palm of your hand: Development of an outcomes-focused knowledge translation intervention. *Worldviews on Evidence-Based Nursing, 4*(2), 69–77. doi:10.1111/j.1741-6787.2007.00084.x

Hader, R. (2008). Know your targets, then align your goals. *Nursing Management, 39*(1), 6. doi:10.1097/01. NUMA.0000305982.90946.5a

Ibarra, H., & Obodaru, O. (2009). Women and the vision thing. *Harvard Business Review, 87*(1), 62–70.

Jeffs, L., Merkley, J., Jeffrey, J., et al. (2006). Case study: Reconciling the quality and safety gap through strategic planning. *Canadian Journal of Nursing Leadership, 19*(2), 32–40. doi:10.12927/cjnl.2006.18171

Mayo, A., & Nohria, N. (2005). Zeitgeist leadership. *Harvard Business Review, 83*(10), 45–60.

Ruder, S. M., & O'Connor, D. J. (2007). Strategic planning: What's your role? *Nursing Management, 38*(12), 54–56. doi:10.1097/01. NUMA.0000303874.18693.84

World Health Organization. (2007). Health technologies: Report by the secretariat. Geneva, Switzerland: Author. Retrieved from http://apps.who.int/gb/ebwha/pdf_files/EB121/B121_11-en.pdf.

Leading Change

Mary Ann T. Donohue
Adapted by Suzanne Johnston

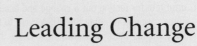

This chapter describes the general nature of change in health care organizations. It presents the theories, models, processes, responses, principles, and strategies typically involved in creating and leading change. The nurse manager's and leader's primary role is that of change agent. This role includes anticipating, acting on, and managing the dynamic forces of change to achieve desired change outcomes. Nurse managers face change on a regular basis, and leading proactively offers multiple opportunities to enhance patient outcomes. Moreover, as effective change agents, nurse managers ensure that staff are empowered to participate in and achieve change outcomes.

OBJECTIVES

- Analyze the general characteristics of change in open-systems organizations.
- Understand the models of planned change, and describe linear and nonlinear approaches for managing change.
- Describe the major change management functions.
- Understand how people respond to change.
- Evaluate the use of strategies, functions, and principles for initiating and managing change.
- Describe the qualities of effective change agents.

TERMS TO KNOW

barriers	chaos theory	nonlinear change
change agent	cybernetic theory	Plan-Do-Study-Act (PDSA) cycle
change fatigue	facilitator	planned change
change management	high-complexity change	strategies
change process	learning organization	
change situations	low-complexity change	

? A CHALLENGE

As a nurse manager on a rehabilitation unit, Tarryn often noticed that nurses did a lot of running around in and out of patients' rooms. They often answered call bells for the same things, repeatedly, all day long. Tarryn attended a quality improvement conference and learned about the Plan-Do-Study-Act (PDSA) cycle, which is a powerful tool for testing out a change and accelerating improvement. Tarryn decided to apply the PDSA cycle to help nurses undertake their rounds more efficiently. She knew that the evidence suggested that implementing comfort rounds on nursing units could improve patient care, reduce call bell demand, and increase patient and staff satisfaction. Before she began the PDSA cycle, Tarryn asked herself the following questions: *How can I integrate the evidence of comfort rounds and build on that idea to engage the multidisciplinary team on our unit to provide care in a different way to patients? How can I do that without resistance? Would our patient and staff satisfaction increase? How would the staff adjust to the change?*

What would you do if you were Tarryn?

INTRODUCTION

Change is a natural social process of individuals, groups, organizations, and society. The forces of change in health care organizations may have external or internal origins or both. We do know that change is constant, inevitable, and varies in rate and intensity. Change influences individuals, technology, and systems at all levels of every organization. Even if we did not want to change, the fast pace and the staggering amount of change affecting the health care environment leads us to embrace the future. If we do not accept change, we risk becoming frustrated and dissatisfied and, perhaps, may end up expending more energy obstructing growth than promoting opportunities for success.

Because most health care organizations operate as open systems, they are especially receptive to a wide variety of influences. Health care organizations do not exist in a stable state. Instead, they exist in the context within which they operate and interact with forces both inside and outside of the organization, such as government funding, governance boards, technological advances, and patient needs. The impact of organization-wide change depends on the organization's particular stage of development, degree of flexibility, and experience with change. The role of change agents is to lead change within the organization. *Change agents* are individuals with formal or informal legitimate power whose purpose is to initiate, champion, and direct or guide change. Their activities are rooted in thinking that is systems and theory based. They are tolerant of ambiguity and mindful of the bigger picture. Managing change in organizations requires moving easily back and forth from an emphasis on long-range planning and established goals to a greater focus on managing competing, dynamic forces in change situations (the field comprising various factors and dynamics within which change is occurring). The successful manager of change constantly moves the group toward a set of predetermined, achievable outcomes. Balancing change in the long and short term is always a key challenge in any given situation, and the capacity to manage change is one of the marks of a true leader.

CONTEXT OF THE CHANGE ENVIRONMENT

In the increasingly uncertain world of health care, nurse managers and leaders must be skilled in using change theory, being change agents, and supporting staff during times of change. According to the Canadian Nurses Association (2014), leadership is a critical requirement in moving change forward within organizations. Leadership as a stand-alone concept evokes a wide variety of reactions and questions when introduced to nursing students. For example, "not everyone wants to be a supervisor," or "I don't want to be a leader, I just want to be a nurse." Leadership is inextricably linked to the role of nurse. Nurses may be formal leaders or informal leaders. Informal leaders are those nurses that step up and get the job done. Each of us can point to nursing leaders we admire (and some we do not). Nurses, whether they be new graduates or experienced practitioners, are expected to be leaders.

Health care in Canada is in the midst of unprecedented change. Shrinking health care dollars, the increasing demand for services, human resources shortages, health care reform, and a growing body of research on the need for innovation mean that the health care system is evolving. Nurses are called upon to implement change and innovation that will ensure a sustainable health care system. Using planned linear change was useful when cycles in society and health care were somewhat stable (low-complexity change). However, the highly complex, accelerated, and unpredictable change situations of today still require planning, and a purposeful approach to change remains effective (Burnes, 2004; Mitchell, 2013). True leaders are able to integrate the proven principles of planned linear change with those of more complex nonlinear change theories, resulting in techniques that move change forward.

Context is a key variable in change. Paying attention to the context within which the change is to be implemented will influence the degree of success that will be achieved. For example, the change leader who is going to implement a new technology in a large urban centre must know whether technology use is already a part of the organizational culture. The same knowledge would be required for a rural community hospital. Differences in context will inform the implementation process for a particular change.

Nurses are key players in health care delivery. They are partners with multiple care providers and pivotal players in open-systems organizations. In their classic work, "Altering Nursing's Dominant Logic: Guidelines from Complex Adaptive Systems Theory," Begun and White (1995) said that it was important for nursing to consider its dominant logic as a source of structural inertia. Using chaos theory components, they suggested that nursing in certain organizations is "stuck" and thus unresponsive and unable to adapt

to rapid change. Today, nurse managers and leaders can lead change by putting into place structures and processes that capitalize on rapid change and thus improve patient safety and nurses' work environment to achieve quality outcomes. One way nurse leaders can alter the dominant logic is shown in Box 18-1. Using this methodology, the nurse manager or leader can become adept at planning and managing change over time rather than reacting to change sporadically or from one episode to another (Shanley, 2007). Scenario planning (i.e., raising multiple "what if" questions with many possible alternative answers) is an example of the flexibility and creativity urgently needed in nursing today.

The two common approaches to change in organizations are linear and nonlinear. Planned change models, or linear approaches, can be used to guide directional, incremental, low-level, less-complex changes. Examples are a plan to reorganize the storage of unit supplies and a plan to publish staff development courses for nurses monthly. Changes that represent higher-level thinking, on the other hand, are characteristically more fluid and complex because of the number of interacting factors and the activities of multiple players across the organization. There are tools that help facilitate change that support moving from linear change

BOX 18-1 GUIDELINES FOR ALTERING THE DOMINANT LOGIC

DECREASE	INCREASE
• Long-term forecasting	• Short-term forecasting
• Preplanned strategies	• Emergent strategies
• Emphasis on past successes	• Search for new opportunities
• One future vision	• Multiple scenarios
• Rigid, permanent structures	• Self-organizing, temporary structures
• Structural isolation in the workplace	• Structural interdependence in the workplace
• Stability of leadership	• Leadership turnover
• Standardization	• Innovation, experimentation, diversity
• Insulation from other professions and marketplace	• Cooperation and competition
• Marketplace "passivity"	• Marketplace "aggression"
• Expectation of job security	• Self-learning

From Begun, J.W., & White, K.R. (1995). Altering nursing's dominant logic: Guidelines from complex adaptive systems theory. *Complexity and Chaos in Nursing, 2*(1), 10.

to more complex change. For example, applying the principles of Lean (see Chapter 13) to a change model helps the leader move forward through a change plan. Usually, nonlinear change (change occurring from self-organizing patterns, not human-induced ones, in complex, open-systems organizations) is inherent in chaos theory (sometimes referred to as *complexity theory*), and learning organization theory. Change agents who engage in planned linear changes focus on specific goals and the incremental steps needed to attain those goals. Change agents who engage in nonlinear changes serve as monitors of the environment, negotiators of influences on a change, and precise forecasters of possible scenarios and their anticipated outcomes. One methodology that can bring both approaches together effectively is project management, which is a framework for implementing changes (Schifalacqua, Costello, & Demnan, 2009). While traditionally used for a singular change process, project management can help leaders deliver large-scale complex organizational change by using a variety of proven principles and tools to run multi-parallel processes.

PLANNED CHANGE USING LINEAR APPROACHES

Most models of planned change (change expected and deliberately prepared in advance using systematic processes) advocate that change can occur in a sequential and directional fashion when guided by effective change agents. The early planned change models, such as those of Lewin (1951), Lippitt, Watson, and Westley (1958), and Havelock (1973), explain the nature of change processes (ongoing efforts applied to managing a change) and offer systematic problem-solving methods designed to achieve change. A model of change is necessary to achieve desired results (Mitchell, 2013).

Flexibility in the implementation of the plan and moderating the situational factors (which are advocated by nonlinear approaches) can improve overall outcomes. However, to make change happen, the group has to progress through it. The group cannot let only a few make the changes. Inevitably, people will develop a positive attitude toward change when involved in the change from the beginning (Stichler, 2011). Sticking with and advancing the change is daily work that requires the commitment of all team members.

Lewin's Change Theory

According to Lewin (1951), an analysis of change situations, which he called *force field analysis*, includes early and ongoing assessment of barriers and facilitators. In change situations, barriers are factors that can hinder the change process; facilitators are factors that can expedite the change process. These factors may originate from people, technology, organizational structure, or values. For change to be effective, the force of facilitators must exceed the force of barriers; thus, the work of change agents is to reduce the barriers in the situation and support or enhance the facilitators. Figure 18-1 presents an example of how to diagram forces that visually portrays the facilitators and barriers of any change. In this case, the facilitators outweigh the barriers.

Lewin (1951) asserted that change in organizations should follow three stages: unfreezing, experiencing the change, and refreezing.

Unfreezing refers to the awareness of an opportunity, need, or problem for which some action is necessary; it also requires subsequent mental readiness to approach the issue. This phase may occur naturally as a progressive development, or it may result from a deliberate activity as a first step in planning a change. For example, when the current way of communicating shift-to-shift reports is ineffective, as evidenced by a lack of hand-off communication, the staff becomes aware of the problem and the need for change. As the Challenge described at the start of this chapter, changes to how patients' needs were anticipated on a regular round schedule, with formal processes introduced to the staff on one unit, brought about unfreezing.

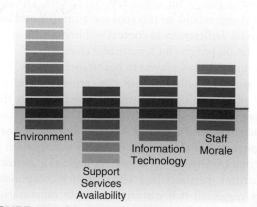

FIGURE 18-1 Examples of forces of change: facilitators and barriers.

Identify the facilitators and barriers in the following situation. Rate the potential strength of each in hindering or expediting attainment of the change. Use "+5" for the highest positive strength toward change occurring and "−5" for the greatest negative strength against the change:

The inpatient psychiatric unit is about to convert 12 of its 20 voluntary beds into short-term care facility (STCF) beds for patients who are involuntarily committed. These beds would coexist with the voluntary beds that are already on the unit. The involuntary beds were transferred from a nearby facility as a result of a capital expansion project. The talent and the expertise of the former facility were highly desirable to help with the transition to a unit with a higher acuity with sicker patients; therefore, 12 of the former facility's nursing staff members were hired; others were placed into available positions within the broader facility. So far, the staff's reaction to the merger has been mixed. Individuals from the former facility, while welcomed enthusiastically by the staff from the present unit, were less than enthusiastic. Added to the change was the news that the former employees' seniority would not be transferable to the new facility as it was a different bargaining unit certification.

observations, or other data-collection methods can be conducted at various points after the implementation of a specific change to measure the effectiveness of the new approach. Analysis of these data can help evaluate the degree of implementation and identify additional alterations needed to ensure an effective change outcome.

Havelock's Model for Planning Change

Although Havelock's (1973) six-stage model for planning change had particular application to education (see the Theory Box below), its elements are similar to those of the directional phases recommended by other planned-change models. Two adjuncts to Havelock's model advocate development of the effective change agent and use of his model as a rational problem-solving process. The rational problem-solving process is "how change agents can organize their work so that successful innovation will take place" (p. 3).

Lippitt, Watson, and Westley's Model for Planning Change

Lippitt, Watson, and Westley's (1958) model suggests seven sequential phases to use to plan change (see the Theory Box below). Inherent in this model is the change agent's appraisal of the "change and resistance forces which are present in the client system at the beginning of the change process as well as others which may be revealed as the process advances. Being continuously sensitive to the constellation of change forces and resistance forces is one of the most creative parts of the change agent's job" (p. 92).

Experiencing the change or solution leads to the incorporation of what is new or different into work and interpersonal processes (Lewin, 1951). Deciding to begin to adopt the change or being unexpectedly thrust into the change can result in the potential integration of the new way of thinking or doing.

Refreezing occurs when the participants in the change situation accept and adopt the new attitude or behaviour (Lewin, 1951). Acceptance is assumed once most staff members integrate the change into their work processes. Surveys, structured or unstructured

THEORY BOX

Theories for Planned Change

KEY CONTRIBUTORS	KEY IDEAS	APPLICATION TO PRACTICE
Six phases of planned change* Havelock (1973) is credited with this planned change model.	Change can be planned, implemented, and evaluated in six sequential stages. The model is advocated for the development of effective change agents and used as a rational problem-solving process. The six stages are as follows: 1. Building a relationship 2. Diagnosing the problem 3. Acquiring relevant resources 4. Choosing the solution 5. Gaining acceptance 6. Stabilizing the innovation and generating self-renewal	Useful for low-level, low-complexity change.

Continued

Theories for Planned Change

KEY CONTRIBUTORS	KEY IDEAS	APPLICATION TO PRACTICE
Seven phases of planned change[†] Lippitt, Watson, and Westley (1958) are credited with this planned change model.	Change can be planned, implemented, and evaluated in seven sequential phases. Ongoing sensitivity to forces in the change process is essential. The seven phases are as follows: 1. The patient system becomes aware of the need for change. 2. A relationship is developed between the patient system and change agent. 3. The change problem is defined. 4. The change goals are set, and options for achievement are explored. 5. The plan for change is implemented. 6. The change is accepted and stabilized. 7. The change entities redefine their relationships.	Useful for low-level, low-complexity change.

*Adapted from Havelock, R. G. (1973). *The change agent's guide to innovation in education.* Englewood Cliffs, NJ: Educational Technology.
[†]Adapted from Lippitt, R., Watson, J., & Westley, B. (1958). *The dynamics of planned change.* New York, NY: Harcourt Brace.

Kotter's Strategies for Implementing Complex Change

Another popular change theorist, Kotter (1995), recommended a strategy for implementing complex change: establish a sense of urgency for the change by creating a compelling reason for the change; form a powerful coalition of people who will lead the change; create and communicate the vision; empower others to act on the vision; celebrate accomplishments; and incorporate the change into the organizational culture.

NONLINEAR CHANGE: CHAOS THEORY AND LEARNING ORGANIZATION THEORY

Chaos Theory

Organizations can no longer rely on rules, policies, and hierarchies to enforce change and achieve outcomes. According to chaos theory, the rapidly changing nature of human and world factors underscores how an emphasis on rules and policies is short-sighted, wastes time, and fails to accomplish goals in the long run. Chaos theory is a theoretical construct defining the random-appearing yet deterministic characteristics of complex organizations. Organizations are open systems operating in complex, fast-changing environments. The term *open* by itself suggests that such systems (health care organizations and health

care services) are affected by and simultaneously affect their environment. These systems are similar to semipermeable membranes, allowing some exchanges between the internal and external environments. Non-human-induced responses are characterized by random-appearing yet self-organizing patterns. Constant adaptation and the mere anticipation of change force organizations to remain relevant in their environment. Traditionally, the cycle of change allowed for periods of stability interrupted by periods of intense transformation, thus demonstrating "spurts" of change rather than continuously steady, incremental change. Although not immediately predictable in the long run, small changes in the internal or external environment can certainly result in significant consequences to organizational work processes and outcomes. Chaos theory further explains that the conditions present in a particular organizational change will not occur again in the same form (Vicenzi, White, & Begun, 1997). Figure 18-2 illustrates the contrasting patterns of linear and nonlinear change.

Learning Organization Theory

Learning organizations continually expand their capacity to create their future and provide opportunities and incentives for their members to learn continuously. Specifically, they are complex organizations that are responsive to internal and external influences, trying to survive in an unpredictable

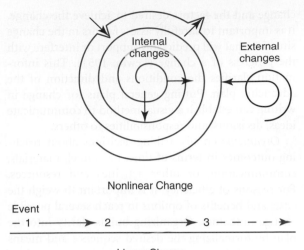

Nonlinear Change

Event

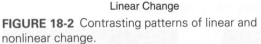

Linear Change

FIGURE 18-2 Contrasting patterns of linear and nonlinear change.

environment (such as the health care environment). They can best respond and adapt when members of the organization work with others using the results of learning to achieve better results. Senge (1990) identified five disciplines (or components) that converge to support innovation in learning organizations. The disciplines are five interrelated components that function effectively only when all elements are present, linked, and interacting. For example, an automobile with a working engine and other essential operational features but no tires could not be driven as designed.

Senge's (1990) five disciplines of learning organizations are as follows:

1. Systems thinking
2. Personal mastery
3. Mental models
4. Shared vision
5. Team learning

Communication promotes individual, group, and organizational learning processes. *Systems thinking* refers to the need for organizations to view the world as a set of multiple visible and invisible parts that interact constantly. When the organization values and facilitates development of the deeper aspirations of its members in addition to professional proficiency, it successfully matches organizational learning and personal growth, or *personal mastery*. Each individual

and each organization base their activities on a set of assumptions, beliefs, and mental pictures about the way the world should work. When these invisible *mental models* are uncovered and consciously evaluated, it is possible to begin to determine their influence on work accomplishment. Building a *shared vision* occurs when leaders involve all members in moving personal visions of the future into a consolidated yet ongoing vision common to members and leaders. *Team learning* refers to the need for a cohesive group to learn together to benefit from the abilities of each member, thereby enhancing the overall outcomes of the team's efforts. Organizations value employees who learn continuously, interact and communicate effectively as team members, and seek to meet their potential as team members.

An example of the application of chaos and learning organization theories is a community hospital that has been sensitive to and has adapted to external and internal environmental forces, such as the need to make changes when governments reorganize health care delivery systems and move to form large regional health care organizations. The process of adaptation involves times of fluctuation interrupted with times of stability. The implications of regionalization may not be predictable, but they have significant consequences for the leaders in community hospitals. These regional structures have created the need for community hospitals to come together under one umbrella organization. Accelerated change of such magnitude has created change that, at times, appears chaotic. However, the result is that all hospitals are transformed and we can observe that some degree of order exists in the middle of perceived general chaos. It is likely that these exact conditions will not occur again for these hospitals. Yet, hospital administrators and other employees have shown resilience and assumed a "learning" philosophy to seek overall organizational adaptation and, when able to do so, have been able to integrate nicely into the regional structures.

MAJOR CHANGE MANAGEMENT FUNCTIONS

Change management is the coordination of processes and strategies used to transition from situation A to situation B and achieve lasting results. Change agents selectively use change management functions and activities to help create and manage change to reach specific outcomes. The functions may or may not be used sequentially; they may also be applied simultaneously, depending on the nature of the change process. Flexibility and appropriateness of use are essential. The six change management functions are as follows:

1. Planning (includes assessment)
2. Organizing
3. Implementing
4. Evaluating
5. Seeking feedback
6. Communication

Feedback works in conjunction with the first four management functions as a way to assess the ongoing status of the change process and movement toward desired change outcomes.

Planning is simply the activity of looking ahead to decide how to achieve some result, goal, or outcome. For any plan to be effective, both those who will implement the plan and those who will be affected by the changes must participate in the change-planning process from the beginning. Planning ideally occurs before implementation. Part of the initial and ongoing planning activity includes assessing the "who, what, when, where, how, and why" of the situation needing

change and the factors desired to achieve the change. It is important to carefully assess factors in the change situation that will predictably support or interfere with the progress of a change (Lewin, 1951). This information clarifies the conditions and direction of the advancing plan. Putting general plans for change in writing can establish a visual method to communicate ideas, decisions, and responsibilities to others.

Organizing entails making decisions about reaching outcomes in terms of time, personnel, materials, communication, or other activities and resources. For reasons of efficiency, it is important to weigh the costs and benefits of options to reach several possible change outcomes. Organizing builds clarity into the plan by formalizing the desired sequence and means of accomplishing the change.

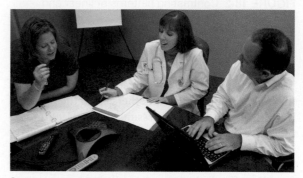

Converting to an electronic health record must involve an inclusive process to be successful.

Implementing ideally occurs after a plan is established. However, unexpected change may sometimes require immediate action. Plans made quickly after the change can facilitate handling the effects of the change. Successful implementation, or putting the plan into action, depends on the appropriateness of the change and the involvement of those who are part of the change. An important aspect of change is that change in one part of a system can affect the function of other, related systems. Understanding the context within which the change will occur is critical to the success of the change being undertaken.

Evaluating entails continually judging the degree to which the change process is moving toward desired outcomes or goals and whether or when outcomes are met. Monitoring, or ongoing data collection, assists the change agent to course correct as required. Judging whether an outcome has been fully or partially met occurs in the final stage of the change process.

EXERCISE 18-3

From the perspective of a manager applying these functions to a change process, consider the manager's and clinical educator's responsibility to orient two nurses to staff a new infusion centre for a rural community hospital, and identify the appropriate functions.

Both nurses were long-term employees; one was from the medical–surgical unit, and the other was the discharge planner whose position was eliminated because of budget reductions. Ideally, the manager and the clinical educator will map out the following in writing: (1) the goals of the program, (2) the activities for meeting orientation goals, and (3) a schedule for accomplishing the goals. The manager and the clinical educator agree to "check in" with each other daily, as well as to meet weekly for a more formal review of the team's progress. Part of this plan includes the option to alter the plan based on unexpected changes. The two nurses will begin the position in four weeks and put the prearranged outline of activities into action. The nurse manager's responsibility will be to guide and support the education of the nurses. Unexpected occurrences, such as the nurse manager extending her medical leave of absence by a few days, will create the need to modify the goal, activities, or time frame of the orientation plan (dynamic quality of process). New information (feedback) guides the overall process.

Effective change agents *seek feedback* by continuously gathering accurate, comprehensive, and timely information about the progress of the change process from a variety of sources. According to classic references (Ashby, 1957; Cadwallader, 1959), cybernetic theory (the regulation of systems by managing communication and feedback mechanisms) purports that access to negative feedback establishes communication networks that act as monitors of specific types of information. Analysis of this negative feedback, or information indicating a correction must occur within the system, informs the change agent where problems exist: whether the course of the accelerated change process has veered away from its progress toward desired outcomes or some action is needed to facilitate continued progress toward a particular goal. Although some typical organizational feedback mechanisms include computerized data findings, town hall–style meeting discussions, and informal or formal observations such as in "round-the-clock" chief nursing officer (CNO) meetings or scheduled staff meetings, negative feedback sources are found specifically in the reports of exceptions, such as risk management incident reports, variances in budget expenditures, or new clinical policies. Multiple sources of feedback produce information to build a picture of the success of the change process.

Alternatively, Hirschhorn (2002) described the major change management functions in terms of campaigns. He proposed that effecting change requires a multifaceted approach that entails three campaigns: political, marketing, and military. The key is that all three campaigns must take place simultaneously for the change to be successful. Table 18-1 illustrates the key concepts of the campaigns and provides an example of each.

Furthermore, when making a change it is critical to use emotional intelligence rather than knowledge intelligence. This means that a change agent has to have the knowledge of both the nature of the change and the nature of the people with whom he or she is working to effect the change. Lakoff (2004) suggested that we think in frames and that if the knowledge we are given does not fit our frame about a topic or event, we should dismiss the information. It is a challenge to help a co-worker adjust his or her frames. Consider what it might be like to work with a group of people who have multiple frames and trying to help them exchange well-entrenched frames for something new. The critical issues are to help people change their behaviour and to realize that communication more likely involves people's emotions and feelings rather than their intellect. Therefore, to bring about change, a leader of change must be equally skilled at knowing the various elements of the change and how to affect

TABLE 18-1 EXAMPLES OF THE THREE CAMPAIGNS FOR CHANGE

TYPE OF CHANGE	DESCRIPTION	EXAMPLE
Political	Coalition-building to create more influence Changes in structures	Working with pharmacy to effect a change in the delivery of medications to patients Creating new communication approaches to enhance patient-safety outcomes
Marketing	Listening to what is important to team members Working with key groups such as physicians who typically admit patients to a given unit Creating a theme	Explaining to patients' families why certain approaches are taken Determining what motivates others to change Creating huddles to map out the plan for the day Using messages to convey a full set of values around a change (e.g., nothing about me without me . . . a theme for patient safety)
Military	Engaging with resistance by providing attention, testing beachheads, and creating a war room	Paying attention (asking questions about, seeking reports about) to the change outcomes Determining the tough choices that need to be made and going after them strategically Creating a space for resources and meetings about the change that symbolizes to others that the change is moving ahead

Adapted from Hirschhorn, L. (2002). Campaigning for change. *Harvard Business Review, 80*(7), 98–104.

them and understanding how to "read" people and their relationship with the change at hand.

RESPONSES TO CHANGE

Change affects people, technology, and systems. Change can be influenced by external mandates, or it can originate within a department or unit or at the level of care delivery. Often, those in senior leadership create a change for managerial staff to integrate new practices into their work areas. Therefore, it follows that the responses that arise across the organization will depend on how change is perceived. Effective change agents anticipate possible responses and apply strategies to deal with them for the best possible change outcomes.

Organizational culture and staff readiness influence responses to change. Knowing the values and beliefs of work groups (staff and their managers and administrators—all part of organizational culture) is critical to identifying responses to change. Readiness can be viewed as individuals' current attitudes or willingness, as well as their nursing abilities. An assessment of organizational culture and the readiness of staff and others to engage in making or participating in a change, whether minor or extensive, sets the stage for the selection and use of strategies. For example, in Exercise 18-3, the willingness of the two nurses to learn new skills and the combined talents of the nursing, clinical education, and administrative managerial staff to work together successfully helped achieve the very different nursing and organizational skills required by the new infusion centre. Answering the self-assessment questions in Table 18-2 can help determine how receptive one is to change and innovation.

> **EXERCISE 18-4**
> Answer the self-assessment questions in Table 18-2.

Human Side of Change

The *human side* of managing change refers to staff responses to change that either facilitate or interfere with change processes. Responses to all or part of the change process by individuals and groups may vary from full acceptance and willing participation to outright rejection or even rebellion. Some nurses may manifest their dissatisfactions visibly; others may quietly undermine the change. There are individuals, in all of our professional careers, who may consistently reject any new thinking or ways of doing things, just to disagree. Furthermore, in today's tumultuous health care environment, multiple change initiatives are often underway simultaneously. These initiatives vary in complexity and intensity however; sustained change that is occurring in many organizations today can result in what is known as change fatigue. **Change fatigue** occurs when key leaders and staff get tired of new initiatives and the way they are implemented (MacIntosh, Beech, McQueen, et al., 2007).

TABLE 18-2   SELF-ASSESSMENT: HOW RECEPTIVE ARE YOU TO CHANGE AND INNOVATION?

Read the following items. Circle the answer that most closely matches your attitude toward creating and accepting new or different ways.

1. I enjoy learning about new ideas and approaches.	Yes	Depends	No
2. Once I learn about a new idea or approach, I begin to try it right away.	Yes	Depends	No
3. I like to discuss different ways of accomplishing a goal or end result.	Yes	Depends	No
4. I continually seek better ways to improve what I do.	Yes	Depends	No
5. I commonly recognize improved ways of doing things.	Yes	Depends	No
6. I talk over my ideas for change with my peers.	Yes	Depends	No
7. I communicate my ideas for change with my manager.	Yes	Depends	No
8. I discuss my ideas for change with my family.	Yes	Depends	No
9. I volunteer to be at meetings when changes are being discussed.	Yes	Depends	No
10. I encourage others to try new ideas and approaches.	Yes	Depends	No

If you answered "yes" to 8 to 10 of the items, you are probably receptive to creating and experiencing new and different ways of doing things. If you answered "depends" to 5 to 10 of the items, you are probably receptive to change conditionally based on the fit of the change with your preferred ways of doing things. If you answered "no" to 4 to 10 of the items, you are probably not receptive, at least initially, to new ways of doing things. If you answered "yes," "no," and "depends" an approximately equal number of times, you are probably mixed in your receptivity to change based on individual situations.

The initial responses to change may be, but are not always, reluctance and resistance. Reluctance and resistance are common when the change threatens personal security. For example, changes in the structure of an organization can result in changes of position for employees. Eliminating a critical care nurse position and displacing the nurse to the only open position, perhaps that of home health nurse, can certainly result in the nurse feeling angry, and even temporarily incompetent and isolated.

The change agent's recognition of the ideal and common patterns of individuals' behavioural responses to change can facilitate an effective change (Rogers, 1995). These responses and brief descriptions are as follows:

- *Innovators* thrive on change, which may be disruptive to the unit stability.
- *Early adopters* are respected by their peers and thus are sought out for advice and information about innovations and changes.
- *Early majority* prefer doing what has been done in the past but eventually will accept new ideas.
- *Late majority* are openly negative and agree to the change only after most others have accepted the change.
- *Laggards* prefer keeping traditions and openly express their resistance to new ideas.
- *Rejectors* oppose change actively, even use sabotage, which can interfere with the overall success of a change process.

The change agent's challenge is to deal with individuals' responses to behaviour by providing opportunities to channel those responses into those supportive of the change process. Helping innovators "test" new ideas might be accomplished in a contained manner so that they are not disruptive yet feel supported. The work of the Institute for Healthcare Improvement (IHI) has been beneficial to organizations in this area. The focus of IHI is to accelerate rapid small tests of change, often at the point of care (http://www.ihi.org/ihi). For example, there may be times when you have a hunch that what you are doing could be done differently, be improved, or be a better way to practice. The idea may be no more than a fleeting thought or a brief "what if" moment. Leading authors suggest that those fleeting ideas can be tested (Gillam & Siriwardena, 2013; Langley, Nolan, Nolan, et al., 2009). Based on the work of Walter Shewhart and W. E. Deming, the **Plan-Do-Study-Act (PDSA)** cycle is an effective way to test and measure incremental changes in a safe and innovative manner for patients and point-of-care providers (Langley et al., 2009). PDSA is shorthand for testing a change in the real-work setting—it involves *planning* the change to be implemented, *doing* (carrying out) the plan, *studying* the results, and then *acting* on what is learned to plan full implementation. Testing a change before a full-scale implementation presents the opportunity for staff involvement, which leads to less resistance to change. The testing cycles are time and cost effective because change is made on one process, patient, or clinic at a time. The PDSA cycle provides an opportunity to immediately understand and evaluate the effect of a change, test expansion (spread of change) and collect data during testing, and identify barriers and possibilities for continuous evaluation and improvement.

Unit-based decisions to change processes and policies revolve around the staff members working on the unit and depend highly on their ongoing adaptation to evolving realities. For example, a staff nurse champion of change may report to her unit colleagues that she is frustrated with many interruptions while preparing and administering medications, which can increase the likelihood for error. Discussing the problem may lead to the trial of a solution to the interruptions, such as wearing a prominently coloured vest that says, "Do not disturb: Medication administration in process." We do know that the more rapidly change can be incorporated, the more effective the organization is at remaining relevant. Connecting early adopters, such as unit-based champions, to new ideas and innovators (e.g., the Canadian Patient Safety Institute's online Communities of Practice; http://tools.patientsafetyinstitute.ca/Pages/welcome.aspx) keeps those early adopters at the cutting edge. When innovators and early adopters are supported, an early majority can occur. The challenge of working with the laggards is to make them feel comfortable enough to transition to new practices. Thus, an equal challenge is to help them feel sufficiently uncomfortable that remaining where they are is no longer the place of comfort. Finally, the goal of working with the rejectors is to minimize their effects and to encourage them to find work that is more satisfying. The change agent's challenges are to be sensitive to employees' stages of loss and to promote transition by responding with appropriate interventions.

Systems and Technological Side of Managing Change

The *systems and technological side of managing change* refers to responses that influence the efficiency and effectiveness of work processes and outcomes. The change agent's challenge is to monitor, recognize, and implement appropriate strategies to minimize responses that are destructive and maximize those that support the dynamics of an ongoing change.

Organizational systems and technology can both influence and be influenced by change. System responses to change may emerge as signs of more or less efficiency or effectiveness. Changes in the type of staff or technology used to deliver care may lead to initial responses of confusion followed by a period of adaptation by the staff and other systems. The quality of care and the morale of staff may change. Productivity and safety outcomes may be different. Reparation of the breakdowns in the affected work processes can restore efficient and effective functioning. Managing uncertainty is critical.

STRATEGIES

The change agent uses various strategies to facilitate both planned and nonlinear change processes. **Strategies** are approaches designed to achieve a particular purpose based on anticipation and consideration of myriad human, technological, and system responses. In addition, the change agent assesses the organizational readiness for change (Weiner, 2009). The following strategies can help support the successful implementation of change (Devereaux, Drynan, Lowry, et al., 2006):

- Consider the demographic variables, such as age and years of experience.
- Establish and promote constant feedback communication loops.
- Support training that is convenient and just in time.
- Involve the early adopters from the beginning.
- Include change implementation in annual performance appraisals.
- Create project priorities so staff are not unduly pressured or overwhelmed.
- Promote prioritization and accountability throughout the entire process.

Lehman (2008) identified strategies that can help avoid pitfalls that stand in the way of successful change:

- Identify what process will be replaced, affected, or created.
- Create a description of the current state of the process being changed or affected.
- Determine how this change is aligned with the organization's key mission statements.
- Evaluate the deriving and restraining forces.
- Identify stakeholders potentially affected by this change.

As supported by chaos and learning organization theories, the change agent also uses vision development, relationship building, information management strategies, and people skills to achieve change.

Figure 18-3 provides an example of a chart that can be used to ensure that the strategy fits the situation. *Communication* and *education* refer to interchanges among the change agent, the change participants, and others for the purpose of integrating the elements of the change process. Staff meetings, focus groups, town hall meetings, and other informal discussion groups inform staff and clarify change activities. One effective strategy is the Leadership Rounding Tool developed by the Studer Group. The following are examples of actions that leaders are encouraged to practise weekly (Studer, 2009):

- Establish and maintain a human rapport with their staff (*How are your children, your vacation?*).
- Ask what is working well for the staff as they perform their daily functions (*Can you tell me something that is working well for you today?*).
- Ask what is not working well (*Can you tell me something that is a barrier for you today?*).
- Ask if they would like to especially recognize someone as a contributor to outstanding patient care.
- Answer any tough questions (*Is there anything you've been thinking about asking me that you'd like to know?*).

Active and empathetic listening is always essential. However, staff members need much more than listeners—they need energetic, accountable "do-ers." Feeding information back to the staff creates trust and a belief that leaders are there to help them meet patients' needs. An effective strategy is "walking a mile in my shoes," when a leader periodically shadows a staff member for a defined period (e.g., 4 to 12 hours) to experience first-hand what it is like to work on any particular unit. Early discussions of problems, especially with the

Situation	Education	Support	Facilitation	Communication	Participation	Negotiation	Manipulation	Cooptation	Coercion	Learning	Visioning	Relationships	Information
Staff is not sure of the next best step in the change process	√	√	√	√						√	√	√	√
Two staff members reluctantly try change	√	√	√	√	√	√				√		√	√
Staff has heard rumours about new program	√			√						√	√		√
Several staff members propose a different method		√	√		√					√	√	√	√
One nurse consistently lags behind in accepting a change	√		√		√					√	√	√	√
A group of staff expresses loss of previous roles		√	√	√						√		√	√
Three staff members challenge the need for a change	√		√	√	√	√				√	√		√
Staff member avoids change in task force membership				√		√		√		√		√	√
Four staff members have become change agents with manager	√	√	√	√	√					√	√	√	√
A group of staff verbalizes satisfaction with status quo	√		√	√	√	√	√			√	√	√	√
One nurse disrupts the change process with other ideas	√			√	√	√	√	√		√	√	√	√
Two nurses try to get others to oppose change	√			√		√	√	√	√				

FIGURE 18-3 Matching strategies to situations.

unit's informal leaders, can facilitate change in a positive environment and lead to better outcomes such as staff satisfaction and decreased turnover (Mohrman, 2008). Leadership is one of the most important elements of planned change (Schifalacqua et al., 2009).

Empowerment of staff through *participation* and *involvement* promotes ownership of both the process and the decisions made during the process. It is important to include staff at all levels at the beginning or as early as possible and then throughout the change process.

Facilitation and *support* strategies typically are used to reassure and assist those in the change situation who do not accept a change because of anxiety and fear. When personal security is threatened or when loss and grief are experienced, people tend to want to continue doing what they have always done. A staff member with financial problems may believe that a new benefit plan or implementation of a no-mandatory-overtime policy will result in less take-home pay. The change agent can reassure that person by providing the actual calculation to show that the fear is unfounded if, in fact, that is true. On the other hand, it would be important to deal directly and answer the tough questions and admit when fears have a foundation in reality.

Individuals or groups in a change situation may have the power or resources to adversely affect the success of a particular change. *Negotiation* and *agreement* strategies can revise the terms of the change to accommodate the involved parties and embrace diversity.

Cooptation usually entails manipulated involvement through an appointed or assigned role. An example of this strategy is appointing a highly resistant individual to a change task force that necessitates that the individual be more involved in the change process. *Manipulation* appeals to the motivational needs of others and influences them to participate in change when they might not do so on their own initiative. Expecting staff to be cooperative by participating in a pilot project of the proposed change on a 3-month basis can identify and help reduce barriers whenever possible.

Coercion involves the use of power to force others to make a change, particularly when time is critical to implementation. An example of coercion would be offering to retain a staff member's position during staff reductions if that individual accepts certain conditions.

The ongoing creation of goals and visions (*visioning*) by all the change participants or change teams shows overt responsiveness to the dynamic nature of change (Senge, 1990). This required dialogue continually redefines the future, whether for the organization or for a project. Development of a set of possible outcomes rather than the rigid pursuit of one outcome opens the possibilities to respond to unpredictable environmental influences (Begun & White, 1995). Change agents build work environments that support the time needed to create a shared vision and accept varied beliefs of staff (Senge, 1990).

Information management by the change agent focuses on delivery of the right information to the right place at the right time. Information may produce decisions that are relevant and flexible!

Relationship management involves how individual capabilities and potential can facilitate creative solutions to projected organizational outcomes and is essential to change management. Formal position titles become irrelevant. Matching a staff member who has the needed abilities and attitudes with the demands of an appropriate project, for example, can lead to more creative outcomes. Peers can become coaches and teachers to help develop others' competencies.

The strategies discussed are useful when used appropriately. Moreover, typically, combinations of strategies are applied simultaneously rather than one at a time. It is important to recognize cognitive responses or concerns that can be met with education, information, or other forms of communication. Participation, facilitation, and support can be choices to address the emotional components of accepting change, such as fear, anxiety, or grief. When the issue is sustained lack of motivation or unwillingness to cooperate, the more effective strategies may be manipulation, cooptation, or coercion. Effective change agents develop work environments that support continuous individual and group learning. Because of the dynamic nature of accelerated change environments, effective change agents stay focused on the dynamics of change by consistently managing information, relationships, and vision.

Diffusion theory (Rogers, 2003) describes how, why, and at what rate new ideas spread through a culture or group. Diffusion is the process through which the new idea is communicated. It may be planned, as with the introduction of the newest generation of iPod, or unplanned, as in the immediate response of governments to shut down the airline industry immediately after the events of September 11, 2001. In both cases, the idea is new and is accompanied by a degree of uncertainty (Should we believe/buy it? What is it all about? Is danger involved?). Diffusion also introduces a new social order because consequences can occur that influence the choice. For example, the peak in the epidemiological occurrence of SARS led to policy changes across Canada that impacted care at the bedside. For many health care providers, great uncertainty existed regarding whether or not these changes would be enough to protect them.

ROLES AND FUNCTIONS OF CHANGE AGENTS

Initiating change and managing its dynamics using linear and nonlinear approaches are the key roles of change agents. The appropriate application of related functions, principles, and strategies can assist in meeting the challenges of any kind of change on the change continuum from low-complexity change to high-complexity change. *Low-complexity change* is an uncomplicated change situation characterized by the interactions of the limited influences of people, technology, and systems. By contrast, *high-complexity change* is a complicated change situation characterized by the interactions of multiple variables of people, technology, and systems. The ultimate goal is a unified movement toward the adoption of something new or different. For example, the Research Perspective below describes a case study on leading a multi-site change initiative to implement a new documentation system at two hospitals in Vancouver, British Columbia.

RESEARCH PERSPECTIVE

Resource: Walker, A. R. (2006). Case study: Leading change across two sites: Introduction of a new documentation system. *Nursing Leadership, 19*(4), 34–40.

The project task was to implement a new documentation system across 18 medical–surgical units at the different sites of two large hospitals in Vancouver, British Columbia. Recognizing the complexity of the change project, the nurse leaders used a number of strategies suggested by Kotter's theory for implementing change, including communicating the vision for the change, forming a coalition with other powerful leaders, helping others to be involved in the change, finding opportunities to celebrate the successes, and making the change part of the organization's culture. This case study illustrates how nursing leaders can use a transformational change approach and implement wide-scale change.

Implications for Practice
Implementing a wide-scale change requires a well-designed plan and effective leadership. Drawing on early adopters and harnessing the willingness of nurses to serve as coaches to the change process can have a significant impact on the success of a change initiative.

Lencioni (2002) suggested that the key dysfunction of a team is lack of trust. Building trust, therefore, is a critical success factor. Change agents use their personal, professional, and managerial knowledge and skills to lead or influence change and to build trust in the team. Staff members who are not officially in charge—possessing only informal power—can also fulfill important change agent functions. Through their early interest and expertise (early majority), informal leaders can model

the new way of doing or thinking for others to emulate. Their positive attitudes toward integrating the change can favourably influence staff participation and unity. The informal leader's close interaction with the formal change agent can lead to reinforcement with other staff members about changes in direction.

Brafman and Beckstrom, in *The Starfish and the Spider* (2006), made the case that organizations that do not have a rigid, authoritarian leader actually have an advantage when they are confronted with the need for change. Their premise is that there are two types of leadership styles: one is exemplified by the starfish and the other by the spider. The spider is a creature with one central head and eight legs and serves as the metaphor for a centralized organization. The starfish, on the other hand, is a creature with redundancy throughout each arm and is a "neural network of cells" (p. 35). Therefore it exemplifies a decentralized system because it has no head and no central command. The authors illustrated these concepts through the examples of the Aztecs and the Apaches. When Spain attempted to raid the Aztec nation, it only took approximately 2 years for a society that had been in existence before the birth of Christ to collapse in ruins. Theirs was a culture that had one single decision maker who ruled by coercive power with many complex rules and regulations. They were the spiders. In contrast, the Apache tribe distributed political power throughout its complex network of individuals and had very little centralized leadership structure. Yet, for two centuries, the Apache nation was able to deter the strength of the Spanish invaders while the Aztecs were not. The reason lies in the characteristics of the starfish, of a decentralized organization in which there is flexibility, shared power, and ambiguity and in which there was truly no vocabulary word for the phrase, "you should." Individuals were free to follow the leader or to choose not to. When struck in battle, the Aztecs had nowhere to go but to collapse and die. When the Apaches were attacked, they simply abandoned their former homes and villages and moved on, taking their culture and their society with them. Seemingly, the starfish model means that power lies not in any central figure but, rather, in each one of the members.

Similarities may be drawn by examining the success of worldwide organizations such as Alcoholics Anonymous (AA), most definitely a starfish organization, which has no centralized leadership yet is nearly always mutating and changing to address people's needs. For example, the 12-step program has transcended the combat of alcoholism as its focus. As our society has arrived at new definitions of addictions, such as gambling, food, and even shopping, AA members have created specific 12-step programs to address these needs. In nursing, we have often bemoaned our lack of singularity and vision, perhaps believing that we should mimic the prevailing worldview and seek to become a spiderlike organization. The authors of *The Starfish and the Spider* endorse a different approach, suggesting that we need to develop and endorse more starfish as well as spider qualities. Nursing leadership, when it embodies a starfish, might mean that we celebrate more innovation and diversity, decide to "break the rules" whenever possible, and embrace the contributions of everyone. Developing a shared understanding of the changes of which individuals are a part, understanding the business logic of the change, having the freedom to be part of adapting the change to the local level, and learning from failure and from the experiences of others are also critical to the achievement of change outcomes (Mohrman, 2008). Staff who share the creation of change that affects them directly and who trust the change agent usually are more receptive to change and integrate change more willingly. Giving and receiving information that includes clear explanations also encourages receptivity. Assertive communication projects self-confidence and a belief that the change will have some perceived benefit to both the individual and to the group at large. Persistence and persuasion can communicate the change agent's commitment to the change outcome.

Rewarding and recognizing change agents makes good business sense. According to a study published in the *Harvard Business Review* (Gunn, 2008), executives who embraced change and developed change leaders met or exceeded leadership's expectation, and 62% of the executives were promoted. The fate of executives who did not embrace change and developing change leaders had serious consequences. In such companies, a quarter of the leaders most comfortable with taking risks and leading during times of uncertainty left the organization.

Having credibility, often as a result of their expertise and legitimate power, allows leaders to sometimes make independent decisions without negative responses. Leaders can role-model the change by actively participating in the change situation, which can translate into expectations for others to follow.

For example, a manager who uses the new computerized medication dispenser may be more likely to earn the respect of the change participants.

EXERCISE 18-5

Recall a work or personal situation in which a particular individual tried to get you or a group to do something. What rationale supported the decision to cooperate or not? Was the idea worthwhile from your perception? Was the person making the suggestions known, understood, and trusted? Was the person making the suggestions aware of the real situation, an essential part of carrying out the idea, or had he or she not received official sanctioning to influence activities? Can you see that change agents need specific qualities and abilities to be trusted by others?

PRINCIPLES

Principles are assumptions and general rules that guide behaviour and processes. Principles are useful for creating and leading change. Classic principles that characterize effective change implementation appear in Box 18-2.

BOX 18-2   CLASSIC PRINCIPLES CHARACTERIZING EFFECTIVE CHANGE IMPLEMENTATION

- Change agents within health care organizations use personal, professional, and managerial knowledge and skills to lead change.
- Change agents have high emotional intelligence.
- The recipients of change believe they own the change.
- Administrators and other key personnel support the proposed change.
- The recipients of change anticipate benefit from the change.
- The recipients of change participate in identifying the problem warranting a change.
- The change holds interest for the change recipients and other participants.
- Agreement exists within the work group about the benefit of the change.
- The change agents and recipients of change perceive a compatibility of values.
- Trust and empathy exist among the participants of the change process.
- Revision of the change goal and process is negotiable.
- The change process is designed to provide regular feedback to its participants.

Adapted from Harper, C. L. (2007). *Exploring social change* (5th ed.). Englewood Cliffs, NJ: Prentice Hall.

EXERCISE 18-6

Prepare an actual or hypothetical change that is meaningful to you in your personal, work, or school life. Select a change that provides an opportunity to apply the linear (planned) and nonlinear principles of change. Draft a hypothetical or an actual plan for change, drawing on the chapter content and paying particular attention to the array of change principles discussed. Share your plan and the rationale used with peers or a small group of other health care providers. Ask for their comments and suggestions. If you need a hypothetical change to work with, consider this one: You are the case manager for a home health care agency. The agency administrator just informed you by memorandum that in 1 month, because of new policies, the agency will change criteria for assessing whether clients qualify for home care services. How will you prepare for this change?

CONCLUSION

Change is inevitable. Some change is formally planned, but much is not. Change involves specific steps as well as a positive attitude to embrace the concept of change. Leaders are accountable for facilitating change that contributes to the vision and mission of the organization and working closely with employees to bring about proposed changes. It is the combined strength of these two groups that can effect powerful improvements in patient care and the workplace.

💡 A SOLUTION

The practice and benefits of trying out comfort rounds were introduced to the staff on the rehabilitation unit. Tarryn presented the evidence to the staff and explained that a Plan-Do-Study-Act (PDSA) cycle would be used to try out the change. All members of the unit's multidisciplinary team were asked to participate in the process. They gathered baseline data on current rounds, including the number of call bells experienced by the staff, and asked patients and nurses to complete a satisfaction survey. Once the data were collected and analyzed, comfort rounds began to be carried out every 2 hours. A member of the multidisciplinary team would visit each patient's room and ask the patient if he or she was comfortable. The team member conversed with the patient and asked if he or she needed anything, such as a glass of water, pain medication, or repositioning. Once the patient's needs were satisfied, the team member announced to the patient that someone would be back in 2 hours. Each time a comfort round was completed, the team member initialled a chart on the door indicating that a comfort round was completed on the even hour. Comfort rounds were supported by ongoing education sessions and an instructional video for nursing and allied health team members. After the first week of implementing comfort rounds, data on the number of call bells as well as nurse and patient satisfaction were collected. The number of call bells had decreased significantly, and nurse and patient satisfaction results improved. Implementing comfort rounds produced the predicted results. Team members found that comfort rounds helped them anticipate patients' needs rather than be in a reactive mode. The practice of comfort rounds has been implemented in the rehabilitation unit, and other units in the hospital are considering making the change.

Would this be a suitable approach for you? Why or why not?

■ THE EVIDENCE

Dickson, Lindstrom, Black, et al. (2012) developed an evidence-informed approach to supporting change in health care organizations. The four steps in the approach are as follows:

1. *Getting ready for change:* understanding the context of the change and assessing the readiness and capacity for change
2. *Implementing change:* setting the direction in terms of the expected improvement or goals (e.g., effectiveness, efficiency, accountability)
3. *Spreading change:* applying strategies and tactics that will move the change across an organization or system
4. *Sustaining change:* evaluating and monitoring the change process and how the change has met stated goals

NEED TO KNOW NOW

- Know how to recognize when change is needed and how to retrieve literature related to the change process.

- Understand how to be proactive and prepared for change, regardless of how and when it occurs.

- Role-play with a friend or colleague some scenarios related to change so you know how you react.

- Expect people to respond differently to change, which may either keep movement toward the outcome on course or slow it down.

CHAPTER CHECKLIST

Change is an unavoidable constant in the rapidly evolving health care delivery system. As a result, uncertainty is an element in most workplaces. Creating and leading change rather than merely reacting to it can promote overall organizational effectiveness.

The nature of accelerated change demands flexibility and prompt response to sometimes unpredictable environmental pressures as opposed to inflexible thinking and acting. Although planned change has a linear approach, it can be used to implement both low-level, less-complex change and change that requires more sophisticated approaches. Linked together, linear and nonlinear approaches to change can produce remarkable results in sustaining change.

- The characteristics of change include the following:
  - Is a natural social process
  - Involves individuals, groups, organizations, and society
  - Is constant and accelerates at various rates and intensities
  - Is inevitable and complicated
  - Varies from high complexity to low complexity
- Planned change can occur in sequence:
  - Lewin:
    - Unfreezing
    - Experiencing the change
    - Refreezing
  - Havelock:
    - Building a relationship
    - Diagnosing the problem
    - Acquiring relevant resources
    - Choosing the solution
    - Gaining acceptance
    - Stabilizing the innovation and generating self-renewal

- Lippitt, Watson, and Westley:
  - The patient system becomes aware of the need for change.
  - A relationship is developed between the patient system and change agent.
  - The change problem is defined.
  - The change goals are set, and options for achievement are explored.
  - The plan for change is implemented.
  - The change is accepted and stabilized.
  - The change entities redefine their relationships.
- Kotter:
  - A sense of urgency for the change is established by creating a compelling reason for the change.
  - A powerful coalition of people is formed who will lead the change.
  - The vision is created and communicated.
  - Others are empowered to act on the vision.
  - Accomplishments are celebrated.
  - The change is incorporated into the organizational culture.
- Nonlinear change is more complex, according to nonlinear change theories:
  - Chaos theory:
    - Organizations as open systems
    - Nonhuman-induced, self-organizing patterns
    - Periods of stability interrupted with intense transformation
    - Small changes resulting in significant consequences
    - Conditions in one situation not recurring in the same pattern
  - Learning organization theory:
    - Emphasis on flexibility, responsiveness, and learning

- Five disciplines interrelated by dialogue
  - Systems thinking
  - Personal mastery
  - Mental models
  - Shared vision
  - Team learning
- Major change management functions:
  - Planning
  - Organizing
  - Implementing
  - Evaluating
  - Seeking feedback
  - Communication
- The human responses to change manifest in various behavioural patterns that may help or hinder movement toward achievement of the change outcome:
  - Innovators
  - Early adopters
  - Early majority
  - Late majority
  - Laggards
  - Rejectors
- Multiple strategies are used selectively to promote involvement by the participants of change and to facilitate the overall change process:
  - Education and communication
  - Participation and involvement
  - Facilitation and support
  - Negotiation and agreement
- Cooptation and Manipulation
- Coercion
- Visioning
- Information management
- Relationship management
- Effective change agents, both formal and informal, exhibit the following characteristics in the change situation:
  - Leadership skills
  - Excellent communication skills
  - Observation skills
  - Knowledge of how groups work
  - Understanding of political issues
  - Trustworthiness
  - Ability to establish positive relationships
  - Ability to empower others
  - Flexibility
  - Conflict management skills
  - Active participation in change
  - Credibility and respect in the eyes of members of the organization or community
  - Expert and legitimate power
  - Understanding of the change process
  - Appropriate timing
- Principles guide change:
  - Ownership of change
  - Anticipated benefits as change consequence
  - Negotiation skills
  - Benefits of feedback to change process

TIPS FOR LEADING CHANGE

- Create a list of outcome and goal scenarios with prospective actions.
- Assume the role of continuous learner during accelerated change.
- Be open to who will assume the leader role in a change process. People involved in change may assume the role of leader and may emerge from both informal and formal roles.
- Be flexible. Creating a detailed plan using a project management approach and rigidly adhering to it reduces opportunities to moderate the inevitable and changing aspects of implementing change, especially in an accelerated change environment.
- Build ambiguity and flexibility into a plan and how it is managed to promote responsiveness and movement toward desired outcomes.

evolve WEBSITE

Visit the Evolve website for Suggested Readings, Internet Resources, and additional resources related to the content in this chapter: http://evolve.elsevier.com/Canada/Yoder-Wise/leading/.

REFERENCES

Ashby, W. R. (1957). *An introduction to cybernetics*. New York, NY: John Wiley & Sons.

Begun, J. W., & White, K. R. (1995). Altering nursing's dominant logic: Guidelines from complex adaptive systems theory. *Complexity and Chaos in Nursing, 2*(1), 5–15.

Brafman, O., & Beckstrom, R. A. (2006). *The starfish and the spider*. New York, NY: Penguin.

Burnes, B. (2004). Kurt Lewin and the planned approach to change: A reappraisal. *Journal of Management Studies, 41*(6), 977–1002. doi:10.1111/j.1467-6486.2004.00463.x

Cadwallader, M. L. (1959). The cybernetic analysis of change in complex social organizations. *The American Journal of Sociology, 65*, 154–157. doi:10.1086/222655

Canadian Nurses Association. (2014). Leadership. Retrieved from https://www.cna-aiic.ca/en/on-the-issues/best-nursing/leadership.

Devereaux, M. W., Drynan, A. K., Lowry, S., et al. (2006). Evaluating organizational readiness for change: A preliminary mixed-model assessment of an interprofessional rehabilitation hospital. *Healthcare Quarterly, 9*(4), 66–74. doi:10.12927/hcq..18418

Dickson, G., Lindstrom, R., Black, C., et al. (2012). *Evidence-informed change management in Canadian healthcare organizations*. Ottawa, ON: Canadian Health Services Research Foundation.

Gillam, S., & Siriwardena, A. N. (2013). Frameworks for improvement: Clinical audit, the plan-do-study-act cycle and significant event audit. *Quality in Primary Care, 21*(4), 253–259.

Gunn, R. W. (2008). The rewards of rewarding change. *Harvard Business Review*. Retrieved from http://hbr.org/2008/04/the-rewards-of-rewarding-change/ar/1.

Harper, C. L. (2007). *Exploring social change* (5th ed.). Englewood Cliffs, NJ: Prentice Hall.

Havelock, R. G. (1973). *The change agent's guide to innovation in education*. Englewood Cliffs, NJ: Educational Technology.

Hirschhorn, L. (2002). Campaigning for change. *Harvard Business Review, 80*(7), 98–104.

Kotter, J. P. (1995). Leading change: Why transformation efforts fail. *Harvard Business Review, 73*(2), 59–65.

Lakoff, G. (2004). *Don't think of an elephant! Know your values and frame the debate*. White River Junction, VT: Chelsea Green.

Langley, G. L., Nolan, K. M., Nolan, T. W., et al. (2009). *The improvement guide: A practical approach to enhancing organizational performance* (2nd ed.). San Francisco, CA: Jossey Bass.

Lehman, K. L. (2008). Change management: magic or mayhem? *Journal for Nurses in Staff Development, 24*(4), 176–184. doi:10.1097/01.NND.0000320661.03050.cb

Lencioni, P. (2002). *The five dysfunctions of a team: A leadership fable*. San Francisco, CA: Jossey-Bass.

Lewin, K. (1951). *Field theory in social science*. London, UK: Tavistock.

Lippitt, R., Watson, J., & Westley, B. (1958). *The dynamics of planned change*. New York, NY: Harcourt Brace.

MacIntosh, R., Beech, N., McQueen, J., et al. (2007). Overcoming change fatigue: Lessons from Glasgow's National Health Service. *Journal of Business Strategy, 28*(6), 18–24. doi:10.1108/02756660710835879

Mitchell, G. (2013). Selecting the best theory to implement planned change. *Nursing Management, 20*(1), 32–37.

Mohrman, S. A. (2008). Leading change: Do it with conversation. *Leadership Excellence, 25*(10), 5.

Rogers, E. M. (1995). *Diffusion of innovations* (4th ed.). New York, NY: Free Press.

Rogers, E. M. (2003). *Diffusion of innovations* (5th ed.). New York, NY: Free Press.

Schifalacqua, M., Costello, C., & Demnan, W. (2009). Roadmap for planned change, part 1: Change leadership and project management. *Nurse Leader, 7*(2), 26–29. doi:10.1016/j.mnl/2009.01.003

Senge, P. M. (1990) *The fifth discipline: The art and practice of the learning organization*. New York, NY: Doubleday.

Shanley, C. (2007). Management of change for nurses: Lessons from the discipline of organizational studies. *Journal of Nursing Management, 15*(5), 538–546.

Stichler, J. F. (2011). Leading change: One of the leader's most important roles. *Nursing for Women's Health, 15*(2), 166–170. doi:10.1111/j.1751-486X.2011.01625.x

Studer, Q. (2009). *Hardwiring excellence*. Gulf Breeze, FL: Fire Starter.

Vicenzi, A. E., White, K. R., & Begun, J. W. (1997). Chaos in nursing: Make it work for you. *American Journal of Nursing, 97*(10), 26–31.

Walker, A. R. (2006). Case study: Leading change across two sites: Introduction of a new documentation system. *Canadian Journal of Nursing Leadership, 19*(4), 34–40. doi:10.12927/cjnl.2006.18598

Weiner, B. J., (2009) A theory of organizational readiness for change. *Implementation Science, 4*(67). doi:10.1186/1748-5908-4-67

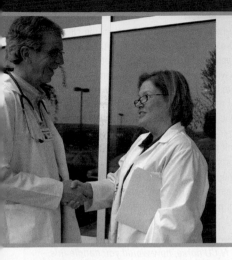

CHAPTER

19

Building Teams Through Communication and Partnerships

Karren Kowalski
Adapted by Colleen A. McKey

This chapter presents major concepts and tools important to creating and maintaining effective teams. To ensure safety for patients and co-workers, health care providers must work together collaboratively and respectfully, communicate effectively, and develop productive partnerships. Research has demonstrated that teams are critical to quality care and patient safety because they encourage frequent and ongoing communication and inform a system in which safeguards and support are part of health care delivery. This chapter also provides an overview of the different types of teams, the qualities of team members, the importance of communication and conflict management in teams, the characteristics of effective teams, and the role of leadership in team success.

OBJECTIVES

- Describe the differences between a group and a team.
- Compare and contrast types of teams.
- Describe the qualities of a team member.
- Critique a team that functions synergistically, including the team's outcomes.
- Understand how generational differences can affect teams.
- Describe the value of team building.
- Explore the role of conflict in teams.
- Apply the guidelines for acknowledgement to a situation in your workplace.
- Know the guidelines for effective communication.
- Explain why it is important for individuals to manage their emotions.
- Describe the process of reflective practice and why it is important.
- Understand the concepts of interdisciplinary and interprofessional teams.
- Explain how the role of leadership can contribute to team success.

TERMS TO KNOW

active listening	group	synergy
conflict	interdisciplinary team	team
dualism	interprofessional team	

351

A CHALLENGE

A large team provides care to neonates and their families in a neonatal intensive care unit (NICU) in a large academic teaching hospital. The team members include physicians, registered nurses, licensed practical nurses, respiratory therapists, physiotherapists, social workers, neonatal nurse practitioners, and ancillary staff. Occasionally, specialists are consulted on specific cardiac, neurological, or gastrointestinal problems; they are intermittent team members who play a crucial role in neonates' care.

Recently, a new group of specialists joined the team. These specialists are known for their expertise and reputation. The existing team was excited to have the specialists join the NICU, particularly because they expected that there would be an increase in the number of referrals to the hospital. However, the integration of the new team members did not go smoothly. Clinical disagreements, communication breakdowns, and interpersonal conflicts arose. The experience evolved into a state of mutual distrust and perceived issues of control over clinical practice decisions.

As disagreements, insults, and complaints escalated on both sides, the situation came to a defining moment when one of the specialists said, "I'm never bringing any patients here. I'm sending them to another teaching hospital." The response from the NICU team was "Fine with us; we don't need you, your patients, or the hassle." It seemed unreasonable to continue to work "together" because, in fact, the two groups worked separately and sometimes against each other. This inability to work together was in direct conflict with the belief that the NICU team provided a valuable service and made a difference for both the babies and their families. This conflict posed a dilemma for the staff, but everyone felt the situation was hopeless.

Team members felt that they could no longer function effectively and that further efforts to work together would be futile. All parties believed they had tried and failed. The new mantra was "Let's just cut our losses and move on." How does one create a team when no one believes it is possible and some believe that it is not even necessary?

If you were an NICU nurse, how would you handle this situation? What help would you need from your nurse manager?

INTRODUCTION

Teamwork has become critical to quality care and safety. We are in an era in which teams are accountable for patient outcomes. Health care organizations focus not only on quality care and safety but also on linkages with the public, consumer groups, other provider organizations, and government in the forms of accountability agreements and funding models. Team communication is the bedrock of safe quality care. It will be increasingly important as teams negotiate with internal and external key stakeholders.

In our society, emphasis is often placed on individual achievement. However, we still need individuals to work together to achieve goals that one person alone would not be able to achieve. Teams often function with the yin and yang of cooperation and competition. They do so in many forums, from health care to sports. Sports teams are premier models of cooperation and competition. They are the model for teamwork in business today, and they represent a group following their respective leader or "coach" (Parcells, 2000). In order to create and sustain teams that are able to function effectively in complex health care environments, it is important to understand what a team is, the different types of teams, when it is appropriate to create a team, and how to best utilize teams in the delivery of quality care.

GROUPS AND TEAMS

A **group** is a number of individuals assembled together or who have some unifying relationship. Groups could be all the parents in an elementary school, all the members of a specific church, or all the students in a school of nursing because the members of these various groups are related in some way to one another by definition of their involvement in a certain endeavour. A **team**, on the other hand, is a number of individuals who work closely together toward a common purpose and are accountable to one another. Not every group is a team, and not every team is effective.

A group of people does not constitute a team. A team is a group of interdependent individuals who seek out opportunities to combine their expertise to achieve common goals (Thompson, 2011). It has a high degree of interdependence geared toward the achievement of a goal or a task. Often, we can recognize intuitively when the so-called team is not functioning effectively. We say things such as "We need to be more like a team" or "I'd like to see more team players around here."

Consequently, in the process of defining *team*, effective versus ineffective teams should be considered. Teams have defined objectives, ongoing relationships, and a supportive environment and are focused on accomplishing specific goals. Teams are essential in providing cost-effective, high-quality care. As resources are expended more prudently, teams must develop clearly defined goals, use creative problem solving, and demonstrate mutual respect and support.

Types of Teams

A number of types of teams exist, each fulfilling a distinct purpose. As a first step, it is important to decide whether a team is required to reach a specific goal or address a specific issue. Often we create teams without a clear mandate or specific goals or team roles. As a result, an effective team of individuals—no matter how knowledgeable, creative, and productive—can fail.

Understanding the different types of teams can be helpful in deciding which team approach is appropriate.

- *Manager-led team:* The manager is the team leader and controls the agenda, decisions, direction, and outputs of the team.
- *Self-managing team:* The manager sets the overall direction and defines the goal and outcome for the team. The members of the team determine the direction, strategies, and focus of the team to achieve the goal.
- *Self-directed team:* The manager identifies the outcome, and the team members determine the direction, strategies, methods, and focus to achieve the outcome. Often, these teams function in quality improvement initiatives to address quality challenges and opportunities.
- *Self-governing team:* This team is a collection of individuals who come together to create something new or address an opportunity or challenge. The team determines appropriate membership, sets its own direction, defines the outcomes, and then manages team performance and outcomes (Thompson, 2011).

Each of these types of teams is appropriate for and often used in health care organizations. They assist in the achievement of organizational goals and address issues of competition (both internal and external) to the organization.

Interdisciplinary and Interprofessional Teams

Teams are essential to quality patient care. Nurses, physicians, dietitians, social workers, case managers, pharmacists, and physiotherapists, to name but a few, must work together to achieve cost-effective care while providing the highest quality of care for patients. This means that health care providers must understand the various roles and educational backgrounds of each discipline. Two types of teams, interdisciplinary teams and interprofessional teams, are common to health care.

An interdisciplinary team comprises members from different clinical disciplines who have specialized knowledge, skills, and abilities. They often work alongside one another and may or may not collaborate closely on patient care. Much of the care in hospitals is delivered through interdisciplinary teams. For example, nurses, surgeons, and physiotherapists work together to address the needs of a patient receiving postoperative care after orthopedic surgery. Each health care provider on the team has a specific role in patient care, often has his or her own approach to patient documentation, and may or may not meet together with other team members to discuss a patient's plan of care.

In the last decade or so, a body of literature has emerged that has highlighted the importance of interprofessional collaboration. An interprofessional team comprises "different healthcare disciplines working together towards common goals to meet the needs of a patient population. Team members divide the work based on their scope of practice; they share information to support one another's work and coordinate processes and interventions to provide a number of services and programs" (Virani, 2012, p. 3). This type of team implies a deep degree of collaboration among team members. Studies of interprofessional teams have identified positive outcomes for clients (e.g., lower readmission rates, improved self-care), health care providers (e.g., higher rates of job satisfaction, retention in the workplace), and the health care system (e.g., cost savings associated with improved patient and health care provider outcomes) (Barrett, Curran, Glynn, et al., 2007; Suter, Deutschlander, Mickelson, et al., 2012).

The Canadian Interprofessional Health Collaborative has developed the National Interprofessional

Competency Framework. This framework addresses interpersonal and communication skills, patient-centred and family-focused care, collaborative practice, and team functioning (Canadian Interprofessional Health Collaborative, 2010). In addition to focusing on collaborative teams in the health care setting, health professional educational programs, such as those in nursing and medicine, have included opportunities for interprofessional education. That is, students from different disciplines are encouraged to take courses or participate in educational initiatives together to learn about one another's role, share knowledge and skills, and learn how to collaborate (World Health Organization, 2010).

EXERCISE 19-1

Think of a team or group of which you were a part. How did the team function? Use the "Team Assessment Exercise" in Table 19-1 to assess aspects of the team more specifically. Address each of the identified areas and discover how well the team functioned. Think about roles, activities, relationships, and the general environment. Consider examples of shared decision making, shared leadership, shared accountability, and shared problem solving. These concepts can be used to evaluate the functioning of almost any team.

Key Concepts Related to Teams

In rare instances, a group of individuals may work as a team spontaneously, like kids in a schoolyard at recess. However, most management teams learn about teamwork because they need and want to work together. Working together requires that individuals observe how they function in a group and that they unlearn ingrained self-limiting assumptions about the exclusive value of individual effort and authority that are contrary to cooperation and teamwork. Ineffective teams are often dominated by a few members, leaving others bored, resentful, or uninvolved. Leadership tends to be autocratic and rigid, and the team's communication style may be overly stiff, formal, and not focused on the team goal. Members tend to be uncomfortable with conflict or disagreement, avoiding and suppressing it rather than using it as a catalyst for change. When criticism is offered, it may be destructive, personal, and hurtful rather than constructive and problem-centred. Team members may begin to hide their feelings of resentment or disagreement, sensing that they are inappropriate. Doing so

---

TABLE 19-1   TEAM ASSESSMENT EXERCISE

ARE WE A TEAM?

Directions: Select a team with which you work or in your educational program. Place a checkmark beside each item that is true of your team. If the statement is not true, place no mark beside the item.

1. The language we use focuses on "we" rather than "you" or "I."
2. When one of us is busy, others try to help.
3. I know I can ask for help from others.
4. Most of us on the team could say what we are trying to accomplish.
5. What we are trying to accomplish on any given work day relates to the mission and vision of nursing and the organization.
6. We treat each other fairly, not necessarily the same.
7. We capitalize on people's strengths to meet the goals of our work.
8. The process for changing policies, procedures, equipment is clear.
9. Meetings are focused on the goals we are focused on.
10. Our outcomes reflect our attention to goals and efforts.
11. Acknowledgment is individual and goal-oriented.
12. Innovation is supported by the team and management.
13. The group makes commitments to each other to ensure goal attainment.
14. Promises are kept.
15. Kindness in communication is evident, especially when bad news is delivered.
16. Individuals can describe their role in the overall work of the group.
17. Other members of the team are seen as trustworthy and valued.
18. The group is cost-effective and time-effective in attaining goals.
19. No member is excluded from the process of decision-making.
20. Individuals can speak highly of their team members.

Tally the number of checkmarks and multiply that number by 5. The resultant number is an assessment of how well your team is functioning. The higher the score, the better the functioning.

©The Wise Group, 2007, Lubbock, Texas.

---

creates the potential for later eruptions and discord. Similarly, the team avoids examining its own team dynamics, or members may wait until after meetings to voice their thoughts and feelings about what went wrong and why.

In contrast, the effective team is characterized by its clarity of purpose, informality, congeniality, commitment, and high level of participation. It is also characterized by members' ability to listen respectfully to one another and communicate openly, which helps them handle disagreements in a professional manner and work through them rather than suppress them. Through goal-focused discussions of issues, the team reaches decisions by consensus or other predetermined ways. Roles and work assignments are clear, and members share the leadership role, recognizing that each person brings his or her own unique strengths to the effort. This diversity of styles helps the team adapt to changes and challenges, as does the team's ability and willingness to assess its own strengths and weaknesses and respond to them appropriately. Signs that a team is functioning effectively include the following: discussions progress productively, team members have a good understanding of team-specific goals and tasks, team members listen to one another, the team is able to handle disagreements, decisions are usually made by consensus, and feedback is given and received respectfully. MacGregor (1960), whose work is still relevant today, identified the characteristics of effective and ineffective teams (Table 19-2).

In today's health care system, complex patient safety, quality, and cost-effective care issues are at the forefront. Ongoing rounds of restructuring, realignment, budget cuts, declining patient days, ever-changing funding models and incentives, and staff adjustment abound. Effective teams need to engage in effective problem solving and increased creativity in order to improve patient outcomes and health care. The impact of effective teams on patient safety and quality care is critically important.

TEAM DEVELOPMENT

When individuals come together in a group, they spend considerable time in group processes or social dynamics, which allows the group to advance toward becoming a team and achieving its goal. Each member of the team often struggles with three key questions that must continually be re-evaluated and renegotiated (Weisbord, 1988). These questions are as follows:

1. Am I in or out?
2. Do I have any power or control?
3. Can I use, develop, and be appreciated for my skills and resources?

TABLE 19-2	CHARACTERISTICS OF EFFECTIVE AND INEFFECTIVE TEAMS	
CHARACTERISTIC	**EFFECTIVE TEAM**	**INEFFECTIVE TEAM**
Working environment	Informal, comfortable, relaxed	Indifferent, bored, tense, stiff
Discussion	Focused	Frequently unfocused
	Shared by almost everyone	Dominated by a few
Objectives	Well understood and accepted	Unclear, or many personal agendas
Listening	Respectful—encourages participation	Judgemental—much interruption and "grandstanding"
Ability to handle conflict	Comfortable with disagreement	Uncomfortable with disagreement
	Open to discussion of conflicts	Disagreement usually suppressed, or one group aggressively dominates
Decision making	Usually reached by consensus	Decisions often occur prematurely
	Formal voting kept to a minimum	Formal voting occurs frequently
	General agreement is necessary for action; dissenters are free to voice opinions	Simple majority is sufficient for action; minority is expected to go along with opinion
Criticism	Frequent, frank, relatively comfortable, constructive	Embarrassing and tension-producing; destructive
	Directed at removing obstacle	Directed personally at others
Leadership	Shared; shifts from time to time	Autocratic; remains clearly with committee chairperson
Assignments	Clearly stated	Unclear
	Accepted by all despite disagreements	Resented by dissenting members
Feelings	Freely expressed; open for discussion	Hidden; considered "explosive" and inappropriate for discussion
Self-regulation	Frequent and ongoing; focused on solutions	Infrequent, or occurs outside meetings

Adapted from MacGregor, D. (1960). *The human side of enterprise*. New York, NY: McGraw-Hill.

Moreover, when a team begins to develop, it is essential to establish ground rules for the team as well as build trust in the team, both of which are essential to collaboration, creativity, and achieving the desired goals.

"In" Groups and "Out" Groups

Most of us want to be valued and recognized by others as a member of the team, one who "knows" or understands. Most people want to be at the core of decision making, power, and influence. In other words, they want to be part of the "in" group, and researchers have demonstrated that those who feel "in" cooperate more, work harder and more effectively, and bring enthusiasm to the team. The more people feel they are not a part of the key group, the more "out" they feel and the more they withdraw, work alone, daydream, and engage in self-defeating behaviours. Often, intergroup conflict results when individuals who feel they are "out" and want to be "in" create a schism or a division that prohibits the team from accomplishing its goals.

Team members need to get to know one another to feel part of the team. Therefore, it is important to take the time at the beginning of a new team to introduce all team members and their role on the team.

Power and Control

Everyone needs to feel that they have some control over their work environment. A component of that control is a sense of power. When faced with changes that individuals feel they cannot influence, they experience a loss of that sense of power and influence. Consequently, everyone wants to feel in control of his or her immediate environment and be able to exert the power and influence to make valued contributions in the workplace.

EXERCISE 19-2

Think about a time when you were a member of a team in your workplace that was not able to successfully make a change in a patient-care practice. How did you, as a member of the team, feel? What was the response from other members of the team? Did team members engage in gossip to make others appear wrong? Using the content in this section, and reflecting on the preceding questions, answer the following:

- Do you believe issues related to "power and control" were impacting the team? If so, what were they? If not, how did you come to this conclusion?
- What were the warning signs that the team was becoming ineffective? How might these have been managed differently?

Using, Developing, and Being Appreciated for Skills and Resources

Each member of the team has unique skills and resources to bring to the goals and tasks to be accomplished. In its evaluation of the work environment, Gallup research is clear that one of the most powerful indicators of a successful, supportive work environment is the score from the question "At work, do you have the opportunity to do what you do best every day?" (Buckingham & Clifton, 2001). When the score is low in this area, team members clearly do not feel their skills are recognized, well utilized, or appreciated. An effective and knowledgeable team leader is key to ensure that each team member feels recognized, encouraged, and utilized to the fullest potential. Fewer than 20% of employees feel their strengths are used every day (Wagner & Harter, 2006). When team members do not feel their skills are used, they are more prone to be in the "out group," which can lead them to feel disengaged from the team and the workplace.

Ground Rules

One of the most helpful tools in team development is to have team members come to an agreement about the ground rules concerning their relationships with one another (Leggat, 2007). Ground rules are the foundation "rules of the game" that focus on both team dynamics and processes. Multiple types of guidelines or rules can be used to set the context for how team members work together. An example of a set of guidelines appears in Box 19-1. A team's ground rules may go through multiple transitions and redesign over time, but the basic tenets essentially remain the same. People must agree on the goals and mission with which they are involved. They have to reach some understanding of how they will work together. Tenets or rules such as "We will speak supportively" go a long way to avoid gossiping, backbiting, bickering, and misinterpreting others. An essential success factor for these team agreements is the willingness of members to be accountable for upholding the agreements and to give feedback when the agreements have been violated. Without rules, people have implicit permission to behave in any manner they choose toward one another, including angry, hostile, hurtful, and acting-out behaviour.

BOX 19-1	GROUND RULES

- Only one person speaks at a time.
- Team meetings begin and end on time.
- An agenda is sent prior to the team meeting.
- Team decisions are made by consensus.
- If the team cannot make decisions by consensus, then majority plus one is employed.
- Team members complete assigned work between team meetings.

Adapted from Leggat, S. (2007). Effective healthcare teams require effective team members: Defining teamwork competencies. *BMC Health Services Research, 7,* 17–27. doi:10.1186/1472-6963-7-17

Trust

Trust can be a major issue among team members, and one of the first questions to come up in the team often concerns who one can trust and not trust. In the early days of organizational development, MacGregor (1967) defined *trust* in the following way:

> Trust means: "I know that you will not—deliberately or accidentally, consciously or unconsciously—take unfair advantage of me." It means, "I can put my situation at the moment, my status and self-esteem in this group, relationship, my job, my career, even my life, in your hands with complete confidence." (p. 163)

The *Canadian Oxford Dictionary* (2004) defines *trust* as "faith or confidence in the loyalty, veracity, reliability, strength, etc., of a person or thing." Trust is fundamental to well-functioning teams. Leaders model trust through behaviours such as setting the ground rules and agreements by which the team will function and holding themselves and the team members accountable. Trust is probably the most delicate aspect within relationships and is influenced far more by actions than by words. What people do is often more powerful than what they say. Trust is a fragile thread that can be severed by one act. Once destroyed, trust is more difficult to re-establish than its initial creation. When speaking of trust, we often hear the adage "years to create and moments to destroy."

Trust is the basis on which each team member assumes a role in the activities and the progress of the team. Kouzes and Posner (2007) conducted research on personal best leadership practices that mobilize others to get extraordinary things done. They focused on how leaders build high-performance teams through five key behaviours: modelling the way, inspiring a shared vision, challenging the process, enabling others to act, and encouraging the heart. Poorly performing teams show little evidence of these relational behaviours and, consequently, trust is low for the leader and among team members.

QUALITIES OF A TEAM MEMBER

Most people have participated in teams that did not work and in those that worked very well. Maxwell (2002) identified 17 characteristics that make a good team member:

1. *Adaptable:* Inflexibility does not work in teams. Being rigid in thinking or behaviour is destructive to both the individual and to the team.
2. *Collaborative:* Collaboration is more than cooperation. It means each person brings something to the project that adds value to the team and supports the creation of synergy.
3. *Committed:* Commitment is a passion in the face of adversity to take action and make things happen. It is the passion to do whatever it takes to accomplish the team objectives.
4. *Communicative:* Communication should happen early and often. Frequency of interaction with other team members, talking with them and sharing thoughts, ideas, and experiences: these are the activities that support teamwork.
5. *Competent:* Competence translates as someone who is quite capable and highly qualified and does the job well.
6. *Dependable:* Team members who are dependable follow through and do what they have agreed to do well, without prodding or delay.
7. *Disciplined:* Discipline is doing what you really do not want to do so you can accomplish the goals you really want and includes paying attention to the details in thinking, in emotions, and in the actions you take.
8. *Enlarging:* Helping a teammate advance or grow into a better person or a good team member; helping teammates advance the team; believing in your teammates before they believe in themselves are examples of value-added.

9. *Enthusiastic:* Enthusiasm focuses on becoming a highly energetic team member who has a positive attitude and believes that the team, together, can be better than anyone dreamed they could.

10. *Intentional:* The team and its members have a purpose for themselves and for the team. Every action counts and is meaningful. The focus is on doing the right things in each moment and following through with these actions to their logical conclusion.

11. *Mission conscious:* Each team member has a sense of purpose and mission that drives all thoughts, ideas, and actions to do what is best for the team and the cause.

12. *Prepared:* Being prepared translates into preparation for every meeting and event and begins with a thorough assessment of what is needed, aligning the appropriate work with the appropriate effort, addressing the mental aspects of the right attitude, and being ready to take action.

13. *Relational:* The ability to be connected to other members of the team, to be in a relationship with them, is the core of being relationship-oriented. These relationships and the mutual respect upon which they are built create cohesiveness on the team.

14. *Self-improving:* As a team member, you strive to continually grow and reflect, both routinely and periodically, on how well each venture of assignment went and what you could have done better. This is a process of self-reflection.

15. *Selfless:* Putting others on the team ahead of yourself through being generous to team members, avoiding "playing politics," showing loyalty toward team members, and valuing interdependence among team members over the value of being independent are all examples of selflessness.

16. *Solution-oriented:* Do not be consumed with all of the problems associated with the endeavour; rather, focus on finding the solutions; think about what is possible.

17. *Tenacious:* Being tenacious means giving your all, with determination, and refusing to stop until the goal has been accomplished.

> **EXERCISE 19-3**
> Think about the last team project in which you participated. What worked about the team? What did not work about the team? Was there a member who did not carry his or her share of the work? Was there a team member who was a "know it all"? How did you handle the situation? Was there a person on the team who took the lead? How many of the qualities of a good team member do you possess? Be honest. What are areas in which you could improve? What are your strengths; that is, where do you shine?

CREATING SYNERGY

Teams function with varying levels of effectiveness. The interesting part is that effectiveness can be created systematically. Effective teams are ones in which people work together to produce results and achieve a common goal that could not have been achieved by any one individual. This phenomenon is often described as synergy. In the physical sciences, synergy is found in metal alloys. Bronze, the first alloy, was a combination of copper and tin and was found to be much harder and stronger than either copper or tin separately; the tensile strength of bronze cannot be predicted by merely adding the tensile strength of tin to that of copper. It is far greater than simple addition.

We see the same properties of synergy in human endeavours. Consider the gold-medal win of the women's hockey team in the 2014 Winter Olympics in Sochi, Russia, for example. The success of the women's hockey team was the result of grit and hard work by all team members. No individuals took credit for winning. The women's ice hockey team won gold because its members knew how to work together to produce extraordinary results. Working cooperatively, an effective team produces results that no one team member could have achieved alone. Creating synergy requires a clear purpose. Each member of the team must understand the reason the team is together, determine what he or she wishes to accomplish (as delineated by defined goals and objectives), and express his or her belief in both the value and feasibility of the goals and tasks. Teams function best when the members cannot only tell others about their purpose but also define and operationalize succinctly the meaning and value of this purpose.

Synergy cannot occur when one team member becomes a self-proclaimed expert who has the "right" answer. Nor can synergy occur when people refuse to communicate. Each team member has good ideas, and these need to be shared. They are not shared, however, when someone feels uncomfortable in the team. It is difficult to speak up and appear wrong or inadequate. The challenge each person faces is to push through discomfort and become a full participant in problem identification and resolution for the overall benefit of the team.

Our society tends to be dualistic in nature. Dualism means that most situations are viewed in terms of two opposing sides or parts (right or wrong, yes or no), limiting the broad spectrum of possibilities that exists between. Exercising creativity and exploring numerous possibilities are important. Doing so allows the team to operate at its optimal level.

We have all known people who were self-proclaimed experts, to whom it was critically important that they be right and acknowledged as right and who become judgemental of others whose perspectives and opinions differ from theirs. Consequently, being able to tell the truth to one's team and to encourage team members to stretch and look at different ways of functioning is vital. This ability requires strong skills in negotiation and conflict resolution, something for which few teams have been trained. If self-proclaimed experts think we are judging them, they will not hear the questions, the observations, or the "truth" because the message seems to be making them wrong rather than originating from compassion. The most valuable contribution a team can make to an organization is the creation of synergistic teams.

GENERATIONAL DIFFERENCES AMONG TEAM MEMBERS

Most workplaces have a mix of team members from different generations: Baby Boomers, Generation X, and Generation Y. Each generation, traditionally interpreted as a span of 20 years, grew up in a different era and was influenced by different historical events and cultural developments (Weingarten, 2009). For example, Baby Boomers lived through the Cold War and Post–World War II social change. Generation X-ers are accustomed to working independently, having grown up as part of the "latch key" generation where both parents worked outside the home. Once they entered the workforce, job stability was no longer guaranteed. Generation Y-ers are technology-savvy and grew up

with massive amounts of information. They are culturally diverse and view education as the key to success.

Efforts to understand and bridge these generational differences can be the difference between a dysfunctional and an effective team. Chapter 3 provides more details about these generations. Understanding and capitalizing on their unique attributes can strengthen the team.

Understanding the diversity of team members is crucial at all stages of team development but in particular during the formation of the team and when the team encounters challenges and difficulties. Team building, discussed next, can help teams overcome any challenges and achieve their goals. Team building can be the cornerstone to effective teams.

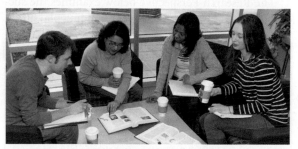

Teams can form strong relationships outside the work environment.

THE VALUE OF TEAM BUILDING

Team building can enhance functioning in any one or all of the following processes (Mackin, 2007):
- The establishment of goals and objectives
- The allocation of the work to be performed
- The manner in which teams make decisions
- The relationships among the people doing the work
- Clearly define performance expectations and team outcomes

When things are not going well in an organization and problems need to be resolved, the first intervention people think of is "team building." Naturally, for teams to be effective, they must function cohesively in a culture of learning (Mackin, 2007). The difficulty is that when organizations are under pressure and facing difficulties, they generally do not have teams whose members function well together. Team building can address any one of the aforementioned activities, depending on the available time and other resources. A team-building exercise can teach a team how to set goals and priorities; help a team analyze the distribution of the workload using various team members' strengths; examine a team's process, norms, decision-making processes, and communication patterns; and promote the resolution of interpersonal conflicts or problems within the team.

Regardless of which areas are problematic, appropriate assessment of the team is essential. The problems may be in priority or goal setting, allocation of the work, team decision making, or interpersonal relationships among the members. Box 19-2 presents guidelines you can use to determine areas in which your team would benefit from team building.

The Research Perspective below examines the success of the team and the role team building plays.

RESEARCH PERSPECTIVE

Resource: Klein, C., Granados, D., Salas, E., et al. (2009). Does team building work? *Small Group Research, 40*, 191–222. doi:10.1177/1046496408328821

The authors undertook an extensive meta-analysis of team-building research that focused on four specific components of teams: goal setting, interpersonal relationships, problem solving, and role clarification. The meta-analysis included 103 articles published between 1950 and 2007 and expanded the original work conducted in 1999. The outcomes measured were cognitive, affective, process, and performance based. The results suggested that team-building activities have a moderately positive effect across all team outcomes, whereas the strongest effect existed for goal setting and role clarification. The size of the team can also be important, and teams of 10 or fewer members seem to have more success.

These findings indicated that most work teams need to be limited in size (with 10 or fewer members per group) and that the focus when forming the team is on clarifying the goals of the team and the role of each team member.

Implications for Practice
The implications of this meta-analysis are important for nursing practice. How often do we find ourselves in teams of more than 10 individuals? Is this really a team or a group of individuals who have come together to address or provide input on an issue? Often, when a team is formed, we look to people we like to work with, who think the same way we do, and who have a similar set of skills that we do. A team should be formed based on the knowledge and skills required to address the issue. When a team has varying skills and backgrounds, it is very helpful to take the time to clarify roles, set team goals, and use tools that help with problem solving. Try these strategies (or suggest to the leader to try these strategies) the next time you are asked to be part of a team.

BOX 19-2   QUESTIONS TO ASSESS THE NEED FOR TEAM BUILDING

1. What do you see as the issues currently facing your team?
2. What are the current strengths of your work group? What are you currently doing well?
3. Do other members of the team affect your ability to be as effective as you would like to be?
4. Does the leader of the team engage in activities or behaviours that prevent you from being as effective as you would like to be?
5. What would you like to accomplish at your upcoming team-building session? What changes would you be willing to make that would facilitate a more effective team and accomplishment of the team goals?

CONFLICT AND TEAMS

Conflict Management

When thinking about conflict, it is helpful to realize that conflict is fundamental to the human experience and is an integral part of all human interaction (Porter-O'Grady & Malloch, 2011). **Conflict** is defined as two or more competing responses to a single event. It is a problem to be solved when differences exist between and among individuals or groups (Cahn & Abigail, 2007). Challenges arise when a breakdown in communication processes occurs that requires an appropriate response to preserve working relationships (Porter-O'Grady & Malloch, 2011). Conflicts are usually based on attempts to protect a person's self-esteem or to alter perceived inequities in power because most human beings believe that other people have greater power, and they are unlikely to achieve their objectives (Sportsman, 2005). When a team leader recognizes conflict between two team members, the following steps can be helpful (Sportsman, 2005):

• Identify the triggering event.
• Discover the historical context for each person.
• Assess how interdependent they are on each other.
• Identify the issues, goals, and resources involved in the situation.
• Uncover any previously considered solutions.

Assessing the level of working relationship between the conflicted parties is essential, particularly if they work together on a regular basis.

Working together requires that team members understand how to conduct interpersonal relationships and communicate with their peers in thoughtful, supportive, and meaningful ways. It requires that team members be able to resolve conflicts among themselves and do so in ways that enhance rather than inhibit their working relationship. In addition, team members must be able to trust that they will receive what they need while being able to count on one another to complete tasks related to team outcomes. To communicate effectively, people must be willing to confront issues and to openly express their ideas and feelings—to use interactive skills to accomplish tasks. In nursing, constructive confrontation has not been a well-used skill. Consequently, if communication patterns are to improve, the onus is on each individual to change communication patterns. In essence, for things to change, each of us must change. In order to create an environment that allows for conflict management, a number of contextual factors must be in place. These include a focus on the mission, a willingness to cooperate, a commitment to the team, and a commitment to resolve issues that arise in the team.

Singleness of Mission

Every team must have a purpose—that is, a plan, an aim, or an intention. However, the most successful teams have a mission—some special work or service to which the team is 100% committed. The mission and purpose of the team must be clearly understood and agreed to by all (Thompson, 2011). The more powerful and visionary the mission, the more energizing it will be to the team. The more energy and excitement on the team, the more motivated all members will be to do the necessary work.

Willingness to Cooperate

Just because a group of people has a regular reporting relationship within an organization does not mean that the members are a team. The boxes and arrows of an organizational chart are not in any way related to the technical and interpersonal coordination or the emotional investment required of a true team. In effective teams, members are required to work together in a respectful manner. Most of us have been involved in organizations in which people could accomplish assigned tasks but were not successful in their interpersonal relationships. In essence, these employees received a salary for not getting along with a certain person or persons. Some of these employees have not worked cooperatively for years! Organizations can no longer afford to pay people to not work together. Personal friendship or socialization is not required, but cooperation is a necessity. Traditionally, these interpersonal skills were considered "soft" skills and difficult to coach people on or to hold people accountable for. That is no longer the case. In most organizations, employees can now be terminated for a lack of willingness to work cooperatively with team members.

Commitment to the Project

Commitment is a state of being emotionally impelled and is demonstrated by one's passion for and dedication to a project or event—a mission. In other words, people go the extra mile because of their commitment. They do whatever it takes to accomplish the goal or see the project through to completion. Charles Garfield, an expert on team management, described what it was like to be a part of the team that created the lunar landing module for the first trip to the moon (Albrecht, 2003). People did all kinds of things that looked crazy, including working extended hours and shifts, calling in to see how the project was progressing, and sleeping over at their workstation so as not to be separated from the project—all because everybody knew that he or she was a part of something that was much bigger than himself or herself. They were all a part of sending a man to the moon, something that human beings had been dreaming about for many years. It was a historical moment, and people were intensely committed to making it happen.

Many people go through their entire lives hating every single day of work. Needless to say, most of them are not committed. Because we spend an extensive amount of time in the work setting, it is critically important to both physical and mental well-being that we are engaged in it. If this is not the case for you, then try to find a different job or profession—one you might love. Life is too short to do something that you hate doing every day. While you are moving into whatever you decide you love doing, commit to yourself to do your best at whatever you are now doing. Be 100% present wherever you are. Do the best work you are capable of doing. This honours you as a human being, and it honours your co-workers and patients.

Commitment to the Resolution

Being committed to a resolution means that you are dedicated to finding a workable response to a problem. It means that you are willing to hear and listen to others' perspectives, identify similarities and differences, and creatively seek solutions to resolve the areas of difference to reach a common ground. The parties need to then agree that they feel heard and agree to the resolution. This approach differs greatly from the compromise and majority vote that are part of the democratic process. When compromise exists, there is acquiescence or relinquishing of a significant portion of what was desired. Compromise generally leaves both parties feeling negative about themselves or the agreement. Consequently, most compromises must be reworked at some future date. Conflict can either be constructive or destructive (Table 19-3), but it is essential to effectively functioning teams (Cahn & Abigail, 2007).

Commitment to the resolution is integral to the needs of the team. One team member may disagree with another team member, but the successful work of the team is at stake in this conflict. Without commitment to the resolution for the sake of the team, individuals often have less impetus to seek a common ground or to agree to disagree.

COMMUNICATION

The only thing humans do more often than communicate is breathe. Communication is the most important component of daily activities. It is essential to clinical practice, to building teams, and to leadership.

A person cannot be without communication. Cahn and Abigail (2007) define *communication* as the sending and receiving of messages that leads to a process of creating meaning in our interactions and relationships. It is the exchange of a message between two or more individuals. Communication can occur as a verbal or nonverbal exchange. Because communication consists of both verbal and nonverbal signals, individuals are continuously expressing thoughts, ideas, opinions as well as emotions. Once the message is sent, it cannot be retracted; it can be amended, but the first impression of the communication usually is lasting. However, as important as this initial impression is, it is often an unconscious response or reaction.

Communication is learned from watching others. A host of poor examples can be seen in movies and television. Poor communication leads to relationship breakdowns, misunderstandings, high levels of emotion, judgement, and an excess of drama. Nursing programs teach therapeutic communications with patients and their families. However, little focus is placed on effective communication in the workplace, even though communication is essential to building and maintaining smoothly functioning teams.

A basic model of communication patterns between the sender and the receiver appears in Figure 19-1. Effective communication develops a rhythm in which messages are sent and received in a productive, respectful, and supportive manner (Nemeth, 2008). Communication begins to break down as the rhythm is disrupted. The sender–receiver pattern disintegrates into a nonrhythmic

---

TABLE 19-3   ASPECTS OF CONFLICT

DESTRUCTIVE	CONSTRUCTIVE
• Diverts energy from more important activities and issues • Destroys the morale of people or reinforces poor self-concepts • Creates differences in a group that cannot be addressed and leads to team paralysis • Deepens differences in values • Leads to actions and behaviours such as anger, anxiety, withdrawal, or combative communication	• Opens up dialogue regarding issues of importance, resulting in their clarification • Results in a focus on finding the solution to issues • Increases the involvement and commitment of individuals in issues • Supports authentic communication with expression of individual needs • Serves as an opportunity for mutual respect • Helps build cohesiveness among team members engaged in the conflict • Provides opportunities for professional growth

Adapted from Cahn, D., & Abigail, R. (2007). *Managing conflict through communication* (3rd ed.). New York, NY: Pearson.

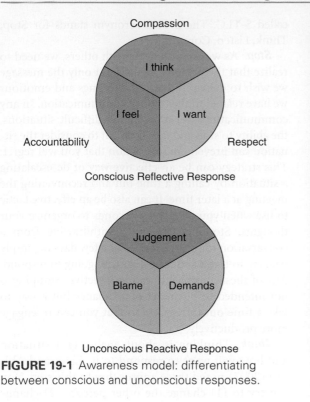

FIGURE 19-1 Awareness model: differentiating between conscious and unconscious responses.

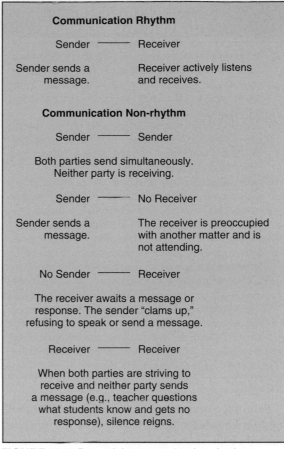

FIGURE 19-2 Potential communication rhythms.

event, as described in Figure 19-1. When non-rhythmic patterns develop, the participants may feel disrespected, upset, and even fearful.

Positive Communication Model

Whenever human beings are in distress, unengaged, disengaged, or have an emotional reaction to a situation or the actions of another, a conditioned response is to move into one or all of the following: *blame*, *judgement*, or *demand*. These ideas are depicted in the awareness model that appears in Figure 19-2. With effort and practice, it is possible to create a positive communication interaction that produces a significantly improved outcome.

When an individual is reacting at the feeling level, he or she tends to move unconsciously to blame. By taking accountability for these feelings, one can move out of blame and own one's feelings by stating, "I feel . . ."

Likewise, when an individual is trapped in distress or reaction at the thinking level, he or she most often turns to judgement. By thinking compassionately, one can dismantle the judgement and state what one thinks in a compassionate way: "I think . . ."

Finally, when in distress, we make demands that are often unreasonable. By calming oneself, one can find respect for the other human being and make a request: "I want . . ."

Most broken relationships are stuck in blame, judgement, and demand. Being accountable, compassionate, and respectful helps clarify what goes on inside each of us.

Everyone needs to feel as though his or her skills, tools, and contributions are needed and valued and that he or she is respected for what personal contributions are offered to the workplace, team, or group. Everyone has weaknesses, but rather than emphasize them, focus should be placed on people's strengths; specifically, acknowledging and emphasizing what people do well.

BOX 19-3   GUIDELINES FOR ACKNOWLEDGEMENT

1. Acknowledgement must be specific. The specific behaviour or action that is appreciated must be identified in the acknowledgement; for example, "Thank you for taking notes for me when I had to go to the dentist. You identified three key points that appeared on the test."
2. Acknowledgement must be "eye to eye," or personal. Look the person in the eye when you thank him or her. Do not run down the hall and say "Thanks" over your shoulder. Written appreciation also qualifies as "eye to eye."
3. Acknowledgement must be sincere, that is, from the heart. Each of us recognizes insincerity. If you do not truly appreciate a behaviour or an action, do not say anything. Insincerity often makes people angry or upset, thus defeating the goal.
4. Acknowledgement is more powerful when it is given in public. Most people receive pleasure from public acknowledgement and remember these occasions for a long time. For people who are shy and may prefer no public acknowledgement, this is an opportunity to work on a personal growth issue with them. Public acknowledgement is an opportunity to communicate what is valued.
5. Acknowledgement needs to be timely. The less time that elapses between the event and the acknowledgement, the more powerful and effective it is and the more the acknowledgement is appreciated by the recipient.

Part of focusing on people's strengths is being willing to acknowledge peers, faculty, and the other significant people in one's life (Roman, 2001). We do not always give acknowledgement in a way that it can be received and valued. Box 19-3 provides guidelines for giving acknowledgement.

To deal with the three personal issues discussed in this section, team members must learn how to state openly what is on their minds and be responsive and respectful as other members of the team do the same. In other words, team members must give and receive feedback constructively.

EXERCISE 19-4

Within the next three days, find three opportunities to acknowledge a peer (e.g., a student) or acquaintance using the five guidelines for acknowledgement shown in Box 19-3. In addition, use the guidelines to accept at least one self-acknowledgement.

Communicating During Conflict

Cahn and Abigail (2007) proposed a framework to help guide effective communication during conflict called S-TLC. The S-TLC acronym stands for Stop, Think, Listen, Communicate.

Stop. As we communicate with others, we need to realize that the primary focus is not only the message we wish to deliver but also the feelings and emotions we have related to the topic of communication. In any communication, but especially in difficult situations, the ability to stop and take time out to consider the situation can prevent an interaction that you will regret. This strategy can be an effective way of de-escalating a situation by calling a time out and reconvening the meeting at a later time. It can also be an effective tactic to use when you need a few seconds to organize your thoughts. Stopping can mean withdrawing from a conversation for a few minutes or a few days or simply pausing to think about how you are going to respond. Any of these approaches can be effective. Stopping is not intended to be an act of avoidance but a way to take a time out to regroup so that you can re-engage more productively.

Think. Thinking is about analyzing a situation and how you want to respond to it. Cahn and Abigail (2007) noted three approaches to this step. You can try to (1) change the other person, (2) change the situation, or (3) change yourself. Knowing the communication goals you wish to reach is fundamental to this stage of the framework. Identifying those goals will help you choose which of the steps to engage in.

Listen. This step is the most challenging. As another person begins to speak, we automatically begin to mentally prepare our response; in doing so, we miss vital pieces of the other person's message. True listening is a learned skill and provides a means for connecting with the other person. Giving your complete attention to the conversation and the other individual(s) engaged in the conversation is critical. Eye contact, positive nonverbal messages, and remaining open to understanding the other person's perspective are important activities that support listening.

Communicate. Cahn and Abigail (2007) offered two approaches to communication: linear and transactional. In the linear approach, the focus is on goals, purpose, and intention of the message. In the transactional approach, the focus is on the process of communication; that is, what and how we communicate with one another. The transactional approach can be very effective in resolving conflict because it considers that the conflict is not one-sided but a result of the behaviours of each person. Cahn & Abigail (2007) suggested that communication is like a dance; individuals need to engage and partner with each other in order to achieve a goal.

Factors That Hinder Effective Communication

Stress. In her classic work, Satir (1988) identified the connection between stress and self-worth that can evolve as a result of a breakdown in communication. She defined *stress* as a threat to positive self-worth. Individuals tend to feel stress or anxiety whenever there is an unconscious linking of feelings, behaviours, or comments from others to a lowering of self-esteem or an attack on self-worth. A conscious effort ought to be made to relieve stress through activities such as ensuring specific or scheduled quiet time, requesting peer support, keeping a journal, treating yourself to something special, or going for a walk (Weiss, 2001).

Stress Response Model. When a threat is identified, the receiver often reacts using one of five communication patterns: attribution of blame, placation, constrained cool-headedness, immaterial irrelevance, or congruence (Bradley & Edinberg, 1990; Satir, 1988). The communication patterns, types of interaction, sources of the interaction, and related examples appear in

Table 19-4. The pattern that produces effective communication—the one to strive for—is congruence. Congruent communication occurs when both the verbal and nonverbal actions fit the inner feelings of the sender and are appropriate to the context of the message. This communication pattern creates the kind of connection between the sender and the receiver that fosters respect, support, and the creation of relationship. Further discussion on stress appears in Chapter 28.

Communication Barriers. A number of communication barriers can interfere with clear, focused, and effective communication. Olen (1993) identified potential problems to allow both the sender and receiver to be prepared to minimize them.

- *Distractions:* Distractions most commonly come through sensory perceptions, such as poor lighting or background noise. Electronic communication, reports, and heavy workloads can also be distracting.
- *Inadequate knowledge:* The sender and receiver may be at different levels of knowledge, particularly in this time of highly specialized and technical knowledge bases. For multiple reasons, one person may not seek clarity from the other.
- *Poor planning:* The process of organizing, planning, and clearly thinking through what needs to be communicated is very helpful. If the interaction

TABLE 19-4   COMMUNICATION PATTERNS DURING STRESS

PATTERN	INTERACTION	SOURCE	EXAMPLE
Attribution of blame	Sender blames receiver	Fault-finder dictator acts superior as camouflage for fear and low self-esteem	Mostly "you" messages; for example, "You made a mistake."
Placation	Sender placates receiver	Sender's low self-worth: puts herself/himself down	"I was wrong. I'm sorry. It's all my fault."
Constrained cool-headedness	Sender is correct and very reasonable without feeling or emotion	Feelings of vulnerability covered by cool analytical thinking	"I decided to use research data in coming to a solution."
Irrelevant	Sender is avoiding the issue, ignoring own feelings and feelings of the receiver	Fear, loneliness, and purposelessness	"Wait a minute. Let me tell you about . . ." (changes the subject)
Congruence	Sender's words and actions are congruent; inner feelings match the message	Any tension is decreased, and self-worth is at a high level	"For now, I feel concerned about the anger and hostility exhibited by Nurse X. I'm wondering what approach would de-escalate the situation."

Adapted from Satir, V. (1988). *The new peoplemaking.* Mountain View, CA: Science & Behavior Books; and Bradley, J., & Edinberg, M. (1990). *Communication in the nursing context* (3rd ed.). Norwalk, CT: Appleton & Lange.

is more spontaneous, it can more easily fall into a nonrhythmic pattern.

- *Differences in perception:* Both the sender and the receiver have their individual mental filters—the way in which they see the world. Because of this individuality, no two filters are the same. Thus, the same message is interpreted differently. Add to this, for example, sociocultural, ethnic, and educational differences, and it is easy to see how differences in perception can occur.

- *Emotions and personality:* Someone who is experiencing distress may not be able to receive another message or may have difficulty keeping his or her emotions out of an unrelated message. Most individuals, at some point, bring distress or problems from home to the workplace. If these remain unconscious, they can influence the work setting in a negative or nonproductive way.

Communication Pitfalls. Effective communication suggests that the interaction is a rhythmic pattern that is respectful and clear, promotes trust, and encourages the expression of feelings and viewpoints. On the other hand, pitfalls in communication comprise actions, behaviours, and words that create distrust, are dishonouring, and decrease the feelings of self-worth in the receiver. Box 19-4 lists the major pitfalls of communication. These pitfalls lead to communication breakdowns that affect not only the team but also the quality of care to patients (Jason, 2000).

Guidelines for Effective Communication

A number of communication tools can help individuals communicate effectively. For example, Situation-Background-Assessment-Recommendation (SBAR) is a standardized approach to communication often used in health care settings to convey clinical information from one caregiver to another (Box 19-5). The purpose of communication tools is to create an environment in which the communicator can achieve the desired outcome. Box 19-6 lists some basic guidelines on how to

---

BOX 19-4   COMMUNICATION PITFALLS

1. Giving advice

It is so tempting to give advice when a co-worker comes with an issue or problem. Do not! Most often what the person wants is to work through the issue by talking out loud. Just listen.

2. Making others wrong

When telling others "our" story of distress, the adversary is always "wrong." The telling of the story to a third party only reinforces how right "I" am and how wrong, bad, or terrible the other person is. If you have an issue or problem, take the problem to the person with whom you have the issue.

3. Being defensive

Defensiveness occurs when you do not listen, are hostile or aggressive, or respond as if attacked when there was no attack. Look for a physiological signal in your body so that you can identify your own distress. Stop. Breathe. Acknowledge that the message did not come out the way you intended, and begin again.

Also, defensiveness can occur when met with hostile, aggressive behaviour from another. Rather than choose an emotional response or react to the attack, know that the other person's behaviour has nothing to do with you personally but is the response chosen by that person in a moment of stress. Any one of a dozen other responses could have been chosen. Understand that the person may be motivated by fear or hurt.

4. Judging the other person

Evaluating another person as "good" or "bad," as someone you like or do not like, or judging the person's actions or behaviour as "stupid," "crazy," or "inappropriate" is a reflection of how you judge yourself. Who is the hardest person on you? Of course, you are. Know that you can have feelings about situations or behaviours without judging the other person in a negative way. Rather, you can feel compassion for his or her stress and fear, which often drives behaviour.

5. Being patronizing

Speaking to others as though they are less than human or are not equal to you as a person fails to honour them as human beings. You do not have to be condescending or seek to humiliate in an overly sweet voice. These are merely other versions of judging or making the person wrong. Another approach is to question what is at issue for them in the moment.

6. Giving false reassurance

One of the great temptations is to "fix" things and make them better, to rescue the situation or the person involved. To accomplish this goal, sometimes we reassure inappropriately. Know that you do not have to fix every situation. You can support people to work through situations themselves.

7. Asking "why" questions

When working in the team, refrain from asking "why" questions. These tend to create a defensive response in the other person. Instead, ask "What makes you think . . . ?"

8. Blaming others

Saying things such as "You make me so angry" is blaming the other person for your feelings, which you choose at any given time. In nearly every situation, the responsibility for communication breakdown is a joint responsibility. You can always choose your response, even if that response is to say, "I can't discuss this with you now. I would like to talk about this later when I am calmer."

BOX 19-5 SBAR COMMUNICATION

Miscommunication is the most commonly occurring cause of sentinel events and "near misses" in patient care. Situation-Background-Assessment-Recommendation (SBAR) is one of the most popular structured communication techniques used in health care and was created by health care providers at Kaiser Permanente of Colorado. It is used throughout North America and focuses on providing information to health care providers that can be easily applied to decision-making trees. SBAR honours the structured transfer of information.

Situation. The health care provider identifies the patient, the physician, the diagnosis, and the location of the patient. The health care provider describes the patient situation that has led to this SBAR communication.

Background. Next, the health care provider provides background information, which could include information relevant to the current situation, mental status, current vital signs (all of them), chief complaint, pain level, and physical assessment of the patient.

Assessment. The health care provider offers an assessment of the chief problem and describes the seriousness of the situation. Any specific changes in the patient's condition should be described.

Recommendation. The health care provider can make a request of the health team members.

Adapted from NHS Institution for Innovation and Quality. (2014, February 20). SBAR. Retrieved from http://www.institute.nhs.uk.

BOX 19-6 GUIDELINES FOR EFFECTIVE COMMUNICATION

- Approach each interaction as though the other person has no knowledge of effective communication. Assume responsibility for creating the sender-receiver rhythm.
- Share your thoughts and feelings. Be self-revealing.
- Use casual conversation or "small talk": It can be important to relationships, particularly when it is light and humorous. It balances deep, meaningful talk.
- Acknowledge, praise, and encourage the other person; doing so is supportive and brings life and energy to the relationship.
- Present messages in a way that the other person can receive them.
- Take responsibility for any problem or issue you have with another, and speak about it as your problem or issue also.
- Use language of equality even when position titles are not of the same level.

Adapted from Olen, D. (1993). *Communicating: Speaking and listening to end misunderstanding and promote friendship.* Germantown, WI: JODA Communications.

communicate effectively and avoid misunderstandings. It is important to keep in mind that active listening, being compassionate, telling the truth, and being flexible are essential to the process of communicating effectively.

EXERCISE 19-5

In pairs or small groups, compare the effective guidelines for communication with the communication pitfalls. Give examples of each from your own recent personal experience. Hypothesize how you could have changed the pitfalls into a positive interaction.

Use Active Listening. Active listening means completely focusing on the individual who is speaking. It means listening without judgement. It means listening to the essence of the conversation so that you can actually repeat to the speaker most of the speaker's intended meaning. It means being 100% present in the communication. Box 19-7 presents guidelines for active listening.

Active listening means avoiding developing a defensive response or argument in your head while the other person is still speaking. To listen actively, a person must be absorbing words, posture, tone of voice, and all the clues accompanying the message so that the

BOX 19-7 GUIDELINES FOR ACTIVE LISTENING

1. Slow down your internal processes and seek data. Do not interrupt the speaker.
2. The more information you acquire through listening, the less interpretation you do (making up the missing pieces or motivations). The less information you have, the more interpretation you do.
3. Realize that the first words from the other person are not necessarily representative of inner thoughts and feelings. Be patient.
4. When listening, suspend your own beliefs, views, and judgements, at least temporarily. Attempt to understand the perspective of the other person, particularly if it is different from yours.
5. Realize that any judgements or "labels" strongly influence the manner in which you listen to the other person.
6. Appreciate the difference between understanding other people's perspective and agreeing with them. First strive to understand. Then you may agree or disagree.
7. Effective listening is based on an inner desire to learn about another's unique experience of the world.

Adapted from Olen, D. (1993). *Communicating: Speaking and listening to end misunderstanding and promote friendship.* Germantown, WI: JODA Communications.

TABLE 19-5   ACTIVE LISTENING

USE OF ACTIVE LISTENING	EXAMPLES
To convey interest in what the other person is saying	I see! I get it. I hear what you're saying.
To encourage the individual to expand further on his or her thinking	Yes, go on. Tell us more.
To help the individual clarify and understand the issue	Then the issue as you see it is . . .
To get the individual to hear what he or she has said in the way it sounded to others	This is your decision, then, and the reasons are . . . If I understand you correctly, you are saying that . . .
To pull out the key ideas from a long statement or discussion	Your major point is . . . You feel that . . .
To respond to a person's feelings more than to his or her words	I hear you say you feel strongly that . . . You don't believe that . . .
To summarize specific points of agreement and disagreement as a basis for further discussion	We seem to be agreed on the following points . . . But we seem to need further clarification on these points . . .
To express a consensus of group feeling	As a result of this discussion, we as a group have decided to . . .

intent of the communication can be received. Specific purposes used in active listening, including examples, appear in Table 19-5.

Be Compassionate. Being compassionate means having a sympathetic consciousness of another's position. Consequently, it is appropriate to focus time and energy on the other person's perspective. It means listening from a caring perspective—one that is focused on understanding the viewpoint of the other person rather than insisting on the "rightness" of one's own point of view.

Tell the Truth. Telling the truth means speaking clearly to personal points and perspectives while acknowledging that they are, merely, personal perspectives. If an observation is made about the tone or behaviour of a speaker that affects the ability of others to hear the message, feedback can be provided in a way that does not make the speaker wrong. This is accomplished in an objective rather than subjective manner using neither a cynical nor a critical tone of voice. To be effective, one must own—be responsible for—personal opinions and attitudes.

Be Flexible. Being flexible reflects a willingness to hear another team member's point of view rather than being committed to the "rightness" of a personal point of view. This flexibility is critical for a team to work well together. No single person has all the right answers. Therefore, acknowledging that each person has something to contribute is important.

MANAGING EMOTIONS

Because people spend such a large percentage of their time in the work setting, it would be unrealistic to

believe that they continually appear in an unemotional and controlled state. People simply do not function that way. What is observed are people's aspirations, their achievements, their hopes, and their social consciousness; they are observed being excited, sad, fearful, and anxious. Consequently, these "feelings" are important components of organizational life. Most of us know of situations in which, because of an emotional disagreement, two individuals have avoided each other for years. Because of the power of emotions and the inevitability of their presence, their effect on interpersonal relationships, and their influence on productivity, the quality of work, and the safety of patients, they should be a high priority when examining the functioning of the team. Fortunately, research addresses the importance of emphasizing the "emotional intelligence" of individuals and team members (Cahn & Abigail, 2007). Those teams that address these issues are much more successful and create a positive work environment.

According to Bocialetti (1988), people are sensitive to what happens when emotions are revealed. When people yell or get angry or upset and when goals, objectives, and tasks are disputed, employees see the following:

- Unprofessional behaviours including intimidation and bullying
- A member overstating or exaggerating another's view to appear right
- Defensive and hostile responses by one or more members of the team
- Concern for oneself to the point of self-absorption
- Gossip
- Attempts to stop or subvert the "real work" of the team

- Conflict in the team that becomes unproductive and distracts the team from its purpose

These behaviours can destroy the team. What are needed are behaviours that support team members in growing, learning, and achieving goals. On the other hand, the cost of suppressing emotions or "feelings" includes the following:

- Physical and psychological stress
- Withdrawal from participation
- Loss of energy and direction of the team
- Lost opportunities for team learning
- Hidden agendas
- Prevention of others from being acknowledged
- Decreased motivation
- Weakening of the ability to receive constructive feedback
- The loss of one's influence

These types of outcomes indicate that suppressing emotions at work is neither healthy nor constructive for team members.

When emotions are handled appropriately within the team, there are several positive outcomes for the work setting. One creates a sense of internal comfort with the workings of the team and the organization. When stress is lowered, problems are much more easily resolved. This phenomenon is similar to releasing steam slowly with a steam valve rather than having the gasket blow. Interpersonal relationships on the team are more stable, and people have a sense of closer ties and collegiality when emotions are addressed. Fewer negative relationships or interactions develop, which results in more effective and pleasant working relationships all around.

Work group effectiveness improves when the team is functioning smoothly and emotions and "feelings" are addressed as a part of normal team functioning rather than waiting for a volcanic eruption. The skills and tools previously discussed (e.g., speaking supportively) are the basic tools one needs to handle the emotional aspects of the team. Choosing to cope with emotional aspects of team interactions must be a conscious choice, one that requires practice to improve the skill.

REFLECTIVE PRACTICE

The process of reflective practice consists of the active, careful consideration of a belief or knowledge and can derive from "learning from experience." It is an internal learning process in which an issue of concern is closely examined (Freshwater, Taylor, & Sherwood, 2008). Through this reflective process, the team member may come to see the world differently and, as a result of these new insights, see the work world differently, which can translate into acting differently. Thus, upon reflection of how an interaction progressed within the team, the team member can examine how this event unfolded compared with how he or she might have wanted the event to occur. This is an opportunity to learn experientially from what works and what does not work as well. Many of us think about what happened during our day as we travel home. The major area for growth is when we identify specific behaviours to enact differently and make a commitment to actually enact them differently. Bringing issues to the conscious level is the first step in personal and professional growth.

THE ROLE OF LEADERSHIP IN TEAM SUCCESS

The team leader plays a key role in the success of a team. Kouzes and Posner (2007) have identified five practices of exemplary leaders in their Leadership Practices Framework, which are presented in the Literature Perspective.

Teams usually have a formal leader as well as informal leaders (team members who by virtue of their knowledge and experience are seen by their peers as leaders). These leaders often have followers who learn from them, act on their behalf, and are inspired by them. In addition, teams function within large organizations that have leaders. Without the approval and the support of the leader, team building, which can be a costly endeavour in terms of consultation fees as well as work time and the resources of the team, is difficult to undertake and of questionable effectiveness. Although very strong teams may be able to educate themselves regarding some of the issues, such as establishing goals and priorities or clarifying their own team process, addressing any kind of relationship issue among team members without a more objective party facilitating the process is exceedingly difficult.

Because leadership is such a pivotal part of smoothly functioning teams, it is illuminating to examine leaders more carefully. Effective leaders need to create opportunities for teams to be innovative and be willing to give up the old way of doing things. Porter-O'Grady

📖 LITERATURE PERSPECTIVE

Resource: Kouzes, J. M., & Posner, B. Z. (2007). *The leadership challenge* (4th ed.). San Francisco, CA: Jossey-Bass, John Wiley & Sons.

Kouzes and Posner's (2007) Leadership Practices Framework focuses on how leaders—whether formal or informal—can mobilize people to get extraordinary things done. For example, informal leaders such as novice nurses can guide others along pioneering journeys to phenomenal accomplishments. The research and work that Kouzes and Posner have done establish relationships as the core of leading any change or initiative. Five key aspects of establishing and maintaining relationships constitute the heart of this leadership model:

- **Model the way:** Credibility is the foundation of leadership. It is established by consistently *doing what you say you will do* or by *setting the example* for the other team members.
- **Inspire a shared vision:** Imagine exciting and ennobling possibilities, and enlist others in these dreams through positive attitude, excitement, and hard work.
- **Challenge the process:** Seek innovative ways to change, grow, and improve—experiment and take risks.

- **Enable others to act:** Foster collaboration by promoting cooperation and building trust. Create a sense of reciprocity or give and take. Establish a sense of "We're all in this together."
- **Encourage the heart:** Novice leaders encourage their constituents to carry on. They keep hope and determination alive, recognize contributions, and celebrate victories.

When nurses use this model to approach leadership, they can strengthen their skills. Each of the examples above provides a way for new, emerging, and established leaders to remain committed to the team with which they work.

Implications for Practice

Each of us has leadership qualities that we bring to every encounter. Think about using the strategies for each of the practices in dealing with patients, families, peers, co-workers, and the team. If each of us consciously engages in "doing what we say we will do" and "setting examples," imagine the positive impact this would have on ourselves and others. The five leadership practices speak to the core of the profession of nursing.

and Malloch (2011) call this the work of the contemporary leader. The leader must do more than talk about innovation. He or she must behave in an inspirational way. The leader must be willing to take risks and allow team members to take risks. Teams led by contemporary leaders make informed decisions and identify their successes and failures in a way that promotes more innovation (Porter-O'Grady & Malloch, 2011). For the contemporary leader, team building is a natural process. This type of leader understands that the best in a person is tied intimately to the individual's deepest sense of himself or herself—to his or her spirit. Warren Bennis (2009), a pioneer in the field of leadership, once said that leaders simply care about people. Consequently, this caring manifests itself in doing whatever it takes to improve team functioning. This may imply involving oneself in team building with the team. The risk in such an endeavour is that the team leader is open to being vulnerable, to being judged by others, and to being wrong. However, if the leader has been a role model for the "rules of the game" and has held people to these rules, the team-building exercise will not degenerate into judging and placing blame.

If true leadership is about character development as much as anything, then character development is also beneficial for followers—that is, members of the team. The areas of character development often addressed

include communication, particularly those aspects of speaking supportively that avoid placing blame and justifying and enhance understanding the other person's message.

Leaders understand the multiple aspects of the issue of control. They take control of their lives rather than put themselves at the mercy of others. They have clarity regarding opportunities and areas for improvement. They focus time and energy primarily and almost exclusively on those issues, events, and behaviours over which they have control. Their activities are thus focused primarily on areas relating directly to them—not on world events or other happenings over which they have neither influence nor control.

Confidence, which loosely translates as faith or belief that one will act in a correct and effective way, is a key aspect of character. Thus, it follows that confidence in oneself can be closely tied to self-esteem, which is satisfaction with oneself. The greatest deterrent to self-esteem and self-confidence is fear. Fear is described by some as "false evidence appearing real." Jeffers (2006) believes the core fear—the one that rules our lives—is one of "I can't handle it." So, the core of our fears is "I can't handle it," and it is exactly the opposite of being confident or holding oneself in high esteem. Working on self-confidence requires an attitude of belief, of confidence, of I "CAN DO" whatever is required.

A SOLUTION

The Challenge presented at the beginning of the chapter is a very complex one. It includes a number of issues: conflict that impacts individual nurses and other health care providers; patient and family outcomes; and the functioning of the neonatal intensive care unit (NICU) as a whole. No easy responses exist to these issues. The common theme that affects each individual in the Challenge scenario is communication. Communication strategies for the NICU nurse and the nurse manager are explored here.

The NICU nurse must focus on recognizing the communication patterns that are occurring. Understanding the aspects of conflict and how these are impacting the nursing role is very important. As the nurse works with team members, it would be important not to use language that blames or judges others. Staying focused on the patient and family care issue and not the conflict can be difficult but achievable. Using the S-TLC framework would be especially helpful. Also, using SBAR principles can make both verbal and written

communication more effective. The nurse can also reflect on the communication pitfalls and identify areas for growth. The nurse can seek feedback from peers and the nurse manager on his or her communication strategies. Managing emotions and using the strategies identified in this chapter can help prevent an escalation of the conflict.

The nurse manager is in a challenging position. He or she must bring team members together to focus on the issues and not individual team members. The nurse manager should also utilize the communication strategies identified in the preceding paragraph. The nurse manager can draw on the organization's vision, mission, values, and goals to drive the work of the team. Support from the senior administration team would be essential to success. It is also important to ensure that the individuals who are on the team will help achieve a positive outcome.

THE EVIDENCE

The Canadian Interprofessional Health Collaborative (CIHC) is made up of health organizations, health educators, researchers, health care providers, and students from across Canada. The CIHC holds that interprofessional education and collaborative patient-centred practice are key to building effective health care teams. In 2008, the CIHC established a working group to review the existing literature on competency frameworks in interprofessional education and interprofessional practice. From this work, the CIHC developed the National Interprofessional Competency Framework. This framework provides an integrative approach to describing the competencies required for effective interprofessional collaboration. The framework comprises six competency

domains that are essential for interprofessional collaborative practice. The six competency domains are as follows:

1. Interprofessional communication
2. Patient/family/community-centred care
3. Role clarification
4. Team functioning
5. Collaborative leadership
6. Interprofessional conflict resolution (Canadian Interprofessional Health Collaborative, 2010, p. 9)

This framework is used by health care educators, students, regulators, practitioners, employers, and accreditors. The framework is reproduced in Chapter 26 on page 490.

NEED TO KNOW NOW

- Remember that team members are your colleagues.
- Apply effective communication techniques, such as SBAR.

- View all members of the team as colleagues and team members who want only the best possible care for patients.

CHAPTER CHECKLIST

Nurse managers must help build teams. Although a nurse manager may not be the team leader, he or she must ensure that the team can function effectively. The team members must be able to communicate with one another effectively, share a single mission, be willing to cooperate with one another, and be committed to achieving their objectives. Successful teamwork requires leadership, trust, and willingness to take risks.

- A team is an interdependent group of people that has the following characteristics:
  - It has defined goals and objectives.
  - It communicates effectively with one another.
  - It has an ongoing relationship.
  - It is focused on accomplishing a task.
- An effective team is characterized by the following:
  - Clarity of purpose
  - Informality
  - Congeniality
  - Commitment
  - High level of participation
  - Listening
  - Effective communication
  - Civilized disagreement
  - Consensus decisions
  - Clear roles and work assignments
  - Shared leadership
  - Diversity of styles
  - Self-assessment and self-regulation
- Each team member deals continually with the following three questions:
  - Am I in or out?
  - Do I have any power or control?
  - Can I use, develop, and be appreciated for my skills and resources?
- One of the most helpful tools in team development is to have team members come to an agreement about the ground rules concerning their relationships with one another.
- Trust among team members is essential for successful teamwork.
- A team member is adaptable, collaborative, committed, communicative, competent, dependable, disciplined, enlarging, enthusiastic, intentional, mission conscious, prepared, relational, self-improving, selfless, solution-oriented, and tenacious.
- Synergy allows a team to produce results that could not have been achieved by any one individual.
- Efforts to understand and bridge generational differences can be the difference between a dysfunctional and an effective team.
- Focusing on team members' strengths and acknowledging what they do well are key to team building.
- To be effective, acknowledgement must be specific, personal, sincere, timely, and public.
- Conflict can either be constructive or destructive, but it is essential to effectively functioning teams.
- When communicating during a conflict with another person, try the S-TLC approach to arrive at a productive outcome.
- Managing emotions is a key to successful team building.
- Leadership is a pivotal part of a smoothly functioning team.
  - Leadership relies on personal character development as much as on education.
  - Confidence is a key aspect of the leader's character. A "can-do" attitude is one of the most important confidence-building strategies a leader can adopt.
  - The leader must be willing to take risks and allow team members to take risks.

TIPS FOR TEAM BUILDING

- Commit to the purpose of the team.
- Develop team relationships of mutual respect.
- Communicate effectively and use active listening.
- Create and adhere to team agreements concerning function and process.
- Build trust.

℮volve WEBSITE

Visit the Evolve website for Suggested Readings, Internet Resources, and additional resources related to the content in this chapter: http://evolve.elsevier.com/Canada/Yoder-Wise/leading/.

REFERENCES

Albrecht, K. (2003). The power of minds at work: Organizational intelligence in action. New York, NY: AMACOM.

Barrett, J., Curran, V., Glynn, L., et al. (2007). CHSRF synthesis: Interprofessional collaboration and quality primary healthcare. Ottawa, ON: Canadian Health Services Research Foundation. Retrieved from http://www.cfhi-fcass.ca/Migrated/PDF/SynthesisReport_E_rev4_FINAL.pdf.

Bennis, W. (2009). On becoming a leader. Reading, MA: Addison-Wesley.

Bocialetti, G. (1988). Teams and management of emotion. In W. B. Reddy & K. Jamison (Eds.), Team building blueprints for productivity and satisfaction (pp. 62–71). Alexandria, VA: NTL Institute for Applied Behavioral Sciences.

Bradley, J., & Edinberg, M. (1990). Communication in the nursing context (3rd ed.). Norwalk, CT: Appleton & Lange.

Buckingham, M., & Clifton, D. O. (2001, January 22). The strengths revolution. Gallup Business Journal. Retrieved from http://businessjournal.gallup.com/content/547/the-strengths-revolution.aspx.

Cahn, D., & Abigail, R. (2007). Managing conflict through communication (3rd ed.). New York, NY: Pearson.

Canadian Interprofessional Health Collaborative. (2010). A national interprofessional competency framework. Retrieved from http://www.cihc.ca/files/CIHC_IPCompetencies_Feb1210.pdf.

Canadian Oxford Dictionary. (2004). Trust. Don Mills, ON: Oxford University Press.

Freshwater, D., Taylor, B., & Sherwood, G. (2008). Reflective practice in nursing. Chichester, UK: Blackwell.

Jason, H. (2000). Communication skills are vital in all we do as educators and clinicians. Education for Health, 13(2), 157–161. doi:10.1080/13576280050074408

Jeffers, S. (2006). Feel the FEAR and DO IT anyway. New York, NY: Ballantine Books.

Klein, C., Granados, D., Salas, E., et al. (2009). Does team building work? Small Group Research, 40, 181–222. doi:10.1177/1046496408328821

Kouzes, J. M., & Posner, B. Z. (2007). The leadership challenge (4th ed.). San Francisco, CA: Jossey-Bass, John Wiley & Sons.

Leggat, S. (2007). Effective healthcare teams require effective team members: Defining teamwork competencies. BMC Health Services Research, 7, 17–27. doi:10.1186/1472-6963-7-17

MacGregor, D. (1960). The human side of enterprise. New York, NY: McGraw-Hill.

MacGregor, D. (1967). The professional manager. New York, NY: McGraw-Hill.

Mackin, D. (2007). The team building tool kit: Tips and tactics for effective workplace teams (2nd ed.). New York, NY: AMACOM.

Maxwell, J. (2002). The 17 essential qualities of a team player. Nashville, TN: Thomas Nelson.

Nemeth, C. P. (2008). Improving healthcare team communication: Building on lessons from aviation and aerospace. Aldershot, UK: Ashgate.

NHS Institution for Innovation and Quality. (2014, February 20). SBAR. Retrieved from http://www.institute.nhs.uk.

Olen, D. (1993). Communicating: Speaking and listening to end misunderstanding and promote friendship. Germantown, WI: JODA Communications.

Parcells, B. (2000). The tough work of turning around a team. Harvard Business Review, 78(6), 179–194. doi:10.1225/R00613

Porter-O'Grady, T., & Malloch, K. (2011). Quantum leadership: A resource for health care innovation (3rd ed.). Sudbury, MA: Jones & Bartlett.

Roman, M. (2001). Teams, teammates, and team building. MedSurg Nursing, 10(4), 161–165.

Satir, V. (1988). The new peoplemaking. Mountain View, CA: Science & Behavior Books.

Sportsman, S. (2005). Build a framework for conflict assessment. Nursing Management, 36(4), 12–40.

Suter, E., Deutschlander, S., Mickelson, G., et al. (2012). Can interprofessional collaboration provide health human resources solutions? A knowledge synthesis. Journal of Interprofessional Care, 26(4), 261.

Thompson, L. (2011). Making the team: A guide for managers (4th ed.). Upper Saddle River, NJ: Pearson Education.

Virani, T. (2012). Interprofessional collaborative teams. Ottawa, ON: Canadian Health Services Research Foundation. Retrieved from http://www.cfhi-fcass.ca/Libraries/Commissioned_Research_Reports/Virani-Interprofessional-EN.sflb.ashx.

Wagner, R., & Harter, J. (2006). 12: The elements of great managing. New York, NY: Gallup Press.

Weingarten, R. (2009). Four generations, one workplace: A Gen X-Y staff nurse's view of team building in the emergency department. Journal of Emergency Nursing, 35, 27–30. doi:10.1016/j.jen.2008.02.017

Weisbord, M. (1988). Team work: Building productive relationships. In W. B. Reddy & K. Jamison (Eds.), Team building blueprints for productivity and satisfaction. Alexandria, VA: NTL Institute for Applied Behavioral Sciences.

Weiss, W. (2001). Attitude: A major managerial challenge. Supervision, 62(6), 3–7. doi:10.1037/a0028893

World Health Organization. (2010). Framework for action on interprofessional education and collaborative practice. Geneva, Switzerland: Author.

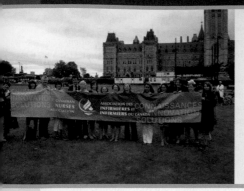

Collective Nursing Advocacy

Susan M. Duncan

In 2006, journalists Buresh and Gordon made a compelling case for ending the silence in nursing and challenged nurses to "envision how things would be if the voice and visibility of nursing were commensurate with the size and importance of the nursing profession" (p. 11). Today, nurses make critical contributions to nursing, health care, and public policy decisions. These decisions involve both the context and the content of their work. Education, knowledge, and experience empower nurses to actively partici-pate in decision making that affects the workplace, health care delivery, and the social determinants of health. Professional nurses are expected to participate in decisions regarding practice. Collective action is one mechanism available to achieve that par-ticipation. Understanding collective action is critical if nurses' efforts to shape practice are to be successful.

OBJECTIVES

- Define what *collective action* means in nursing.
- Identify the three pillars, or program areas, that are essential to the improvement of nursing and health.
- Describe the role of nursing organizations in collective action (e.g., professional associations, labour unions, and regulatory bodies) and how nurses contribute to these organizations.
- Identify evidence on the need for and impact of nurses' collective action initiatives.
- Describe the three strategies nurses use most often to achieve collective action: shared governance, workplace advocacy, and collective bargaining.
- Understand the impact of organizational culture and leadership on nurses' abilities to engage in collective action.
- Evaluate how the participation of staff nurses in decision making affects job satisfaction and patient outcomes.
- Describe how nurses at the beginning of their careers can influence workplace, health care, and public policies.

TERMS TO KNOW

advocacy	nursing professional practice	shared governance
collective action	council	subculture
collective bargaining	organizational culture	union
health equity	professional association	whistle-blowing
nursing governance	role model	workplace advocacy

? A CHALLENGE

Ann, a nurse manager at Seaview Home Health Care, had previously worked in a large urban hospital system as a staff nurse. When Ann moved to Seaview, she took a staff nurse position in home health care and was promoted to nurse manager within the first year. On her team, care provision was disjointed and ineffective, and client and nurse satisfaction levels were low. Moreover, issues were evident in the areas of delegation to and support for health care assistants, and family support and teaching were not consistently a part of nursing practice. After several months of assessing how nurses worked and learning which resources were available to support their practice,

Ann determined that it would be beneficial to redesign how care was delivered. Patient-centred care was a model of care that Ann was familiar with at the large city hospital where she had previously worked, but it was not a model that had been used at Seaview. Ann wondered if she could adapt the model used in the hospital to make positive differences in client outcomes and the delivery of care in home health care nursing.

What do you think you would do if you were Ann?

INTRODUCTION

The excitement of beginning a career in nursing and assuming a leader's role and responsibilities is often balanced by events taking place in health care and society and the effect of these events on nursing, nurses, and the health care system. For instance, the impact of chronic illnesses such as HIV/AIDS and diabetes on families worldwide, public awareness of health inequities, and the promise of health equity are prominent influences on nursing in the twenty-first century. **Health equity**, or *equity in health*, is the absence of unfair or unjust differences in life circumstances and access to resources so that all persons have fair opportunities to achieve their full health potential to the extent possible (Reutter & Kushner, 2010, p. 271). Unfair or unjust differences most often relate to the social determinants of health such as income, housing, access to essential services, and the environment. The knowledge gained in your nursing education provides a background for considering these issues and how you can work with others to make a difference in nursing practice, health care, and health equity.

Nurses are deeply involved in the complex clinical problems of individuals, families, and communities because nursing practice requires the acquisition, synthesis, and retrieval of knowledge to provide competent nursing care. Having the time and resources to engage in high-level preparation for quality, competent care can be achieved through the collective action and advocacy of nurses. Nurses make a difference in various ways and by using various means, which is the main focus of this chapter.

DEFINING COLLECTIVE ACTION AND ADVOCACY

Collective action is defined as activities that are undertaken by a group of people who have common interests or goals. Collective action is a benign phrase; it can be applied to many aspects of daily life. The concept of **advocacy** is normative and involves action to support a cause or an interest; it is often embedded in nursing codes of ethics. For example, the Canadian Nurses Association (CNA, 2008) *Code of Ethics for Registered Nurses* states, "Nurses can advocate for quality work environments that support the delivery of safe, compassionate, competent, and ethical care" (p. 2). Another component of ethical nursing practice is advocacy on behalf of health equity and social justice (CNA, 2008; Reutter & Kushner, 2010). The nature of advocacy has been widely discussed in the literature (Baldwin, 2003; MacDonald, 2007). Gadow's (1990) historic discussion of the manifestations of advocacy is relevant to a discussion of today's workplace advocacy. These manifestations include (1) ensuring that nurses have relevant information to support their practice, (2) enabling nurses to learn about the organization in which they work, (3) encouraging nurses to disclose their personal views on issues in the work environment, (4) providing support to nurses to make and implement decisions, and (5) helping nurses clarify their personal values.

Collective action helps nurses advocate for patients, families, and communities in health care and the political arena. Minarik and Catrambone (1998) suggested that for nurses, collective participation has four main purposes: (1) to promote the practice of professional nursing, (2) to establish and maintain standards of care, (3) to allocate resources effectively and efficiently, and (4) to create satisfaction and support in the practice environment. Collective action helps define and sustain individual nurses in achieving these purposes. Further, the purposes of collective action extend beyond the focus on patient care and practice environments to also focus on health equity and social justice (Spenceley, Reutter, & Allen, 2006).

Individually, nurses can find it challenging to advocate for changes to patient care, the health care system, and societal health. In the absence of collective action, the average individual has limited influence in achieving his or her purpose. Cultivating networks and developing a collective voice require strong leaders; that is, nurses with skill and knowledge in policy and political action. Traditionally, nurses have been able to exert a broad influence on health care by working together through their professional associations and unions. Working collectively requires that nurses understand the purposes and functions of the various nursing organizations, such as professional associations, unions, and regulatory bodies. It also requires that nurses who hold different positions and are at different points in their careers understand how they can participate in advocacy through collective action. Ultimately, it is well documented that to

address systemic problems successfully, it is important for nurses to engage in collective action to create a strong, unified voice that speaks on behalf of the profession (Donovan, Diers, & Carryer, 2012; Mahlin, 2010; Mildon, 2013).

The history, purpose, and functions of key nursing organizations are described in this chapter. So too are examples of their influence. Nursing students need to learn about each of these types of organizations and their functions and consider participation as a professional responsibility in making a difference to nursing, health care, and public policy. Participation in the collective action of nursing organizations is an important aspect of career development, which begins with nursing students in the formative years of their nursing education (Mata, Latham, & Ransome, 2010) (see also Chapter 29).

EXERCISE 20-1

Joshua is a fourth-year nursing student who has just completed a practicum with a street outreach program. During the practicum, he learned that the growing lack of affordable housing in the community has led to serious health risks, including homelessness. Joshua also volunteers at the local shelter and sees that the number of people (including children) in the community who lack access to basic living resources such as shelter and food is growing. Joshua wonders how he can draw on his experiences and work toward positive change in the living conditions of people in his community. He is particularly motivated to engage in advocacy as a nurse after he graduates. He has broached the subject with a few colleagues who have cautioned him that it is not really the nurse's role to take on this issue. If you were Joshua, how would you respond to those who do not consider advocacy to be part of nursing practice?

Doane and Varcoe (2015) asserted that leadership "occur[s] in every moment of practice" provided by nurses in both formal and informal leadership roles (p. 421). Nurses who bring their voice and perspective to the policy arena are providing essential leadership within the profession. Often, nurses (including students) who work directly with patients or populations are in an excellent position to bring their care experiences, "stories," and knowledge to influence a nursing practice, the health care system, or a policy. For example, the Canadian Nursing Students' Association (CNSA) recently lobbied the president of MTV to end the production and airing of the TV show *Scrubbing In*, which presents stereotypes and inaccurate information on nurses. Then-CNSA president Carly Whitmore sent a letter and a petition signed by the membership to MTV to pull the show. After hearing from thousands of individual nurses and nursing students, and receiving letters and petitions from nursing associations including the CNSA and the CNA (Figure 20-1),

the network announced that "it would move the show from 10 pm to midnight, therefore cutting its viewership in half, review three of the remaining episodes to see if more clinical scenes featuring nursing skills could be added, and develop new online features to educate viewers about the real work and challenges that come

The national voice of registered nurses   Porte-parole national des infirmières et infirmiers

CANADIAN NURSES ASSOCIATION   ASSOCIATION DES INFIRMIÈRES ET INFIRMIERS DU CANADA

October 21, 2013

Stephen Friedman
President, MTV
Stephen.Friedman@mtvstaff.com

Dear Mr. Friedman,

Both as president of the Canadian Nurses Association, which represents more than 150,000 registered nurses (RNs), and as an RN of 36 years, I am truly saddened to learn of your network's new program, *Scrubbing In*. First hearing of this show from a young nurse, I am especially concerned about its impact on the new generation of nurses.

RNs provide expert care to their patients, helping them and their families through life's most difficult days. RNs work with people to help them heal and live healthier lives. Between birth and death, the number of interactions RNs have with their patients are among the highest of all health-care providers. *Scrubbing In*'s dramatized account of nurses' lives trivializes the critical work they perform. All of their hard work, from studying and gaining experience to answering nursing's call, will be overshadowed by typical 'reality' show fodder.

Moreover, both the American and Canadian nursing professions are facing real challenges — such as tighter health-care budgets, ever-evolving legislation that governs our practice and increasing demand from growing populations who are living longer lives (often with more complex, chronic illnesses). As we work to fight these real battles that affect our capacity to deliver the best care to patients, it's a shame that we have to add sexual objectification and negative stereotypes to the list because of *Scrubbing In*.

If you respect the nursing profession and the care we provide to millions of people every day, you will cancel *Scrubbing In*.

Regards,

Barbara Mildon

Barbara Mildon, RN, PhD, CHE, CCHN(C)
President

cc.   Jennifer Solari, Vice President of Communications — Jennifer.Solari@mtvstaff.com
Shannon Fitzgerald and David Osper, executive producers for MTV — Shannon.Fitzgerald@mtvstaff.com and David.Osper@mtvstaff.com
Janay Dutton and Nick Predescu, executives in charge of production for *Scrubbing In* — Janay.Dutton@mtvstaff.com and Nick.Predescu@mtvstaff.com
Candice Ashton, senior publicist — Canadice.Ashton@mtvstaff.com

cna-aiic.ca

50 DRIVEWAY OTTAWA ONTARIO K2P 1E2 CANADA
TEL/TÉL 613-237-2133 • 1-800-361-8404 • FAX/TÉLÉC 613-237-3520

FIGURE 20-1 Speaking out on behalf of all nurses: a CNA letter advocating for the cancellation of *Scrubbing In*.

with being a nurse" (Geller, 2014, p. 29). This collective action clearly made an important and real difference to the professional image of nursing.

EXERCISE 20-2
Identify two policy issues for which collective action by nurses has been taken. How did you come to know about these issues, and what was nursing's role in addressing them? Is nursing's collective action in addressing these issues visible to the public? To nurses themselves? What difference did nurses' collective action make on these issues?

NURSING ORGANIZATIONS AND COLLECTIVE ACTION

The International Council of Nurses (ICN, n.d.) identified three pillars, or program areas, that are essential to the improvement of nursing and health:

- Professional practice
- Regulation
- Socioeconomic welfare

Most countries have nursing associations that advance the professional practice of nursing. These associations have regional or national collectives, and they are connected through the ICN, which serves as a unified, global voice for nursing. Regulatory bodies regulate the practice of nursing and license nurses. Nurses' unions advance the socioeconomic welfare of nurses. These three types of organizational functions (represented in the three circles shown in Figure 20-2) appear in some form in most countries, and they may exist in three separate organizations or be combined in one or more organizations.

It is important to understand the mandates of the three pillars because specific types of advocacy and collective action flow from each one. The pillar of professional practice involves advocacy on behalf of the nursing profession to shape health care and public policy and inform decisions on behalf of the profession. Provincial and territorial professional nursing associations have generally held this mandate. Since 1924, registered nurse associations have had membership in the CNA, a national professional nursing association that connects nurses in Canada to the ICN (CNA, 2011a).

The pillar of regulation involves regulatory bodies that ensure nurses provide safe, professional care. The nursing profession is self-regulating and sets standards and monitors professional practice for quality and safety on behalf of the public. Self-regulation is a privilege of the profession: "Through regulation there is the

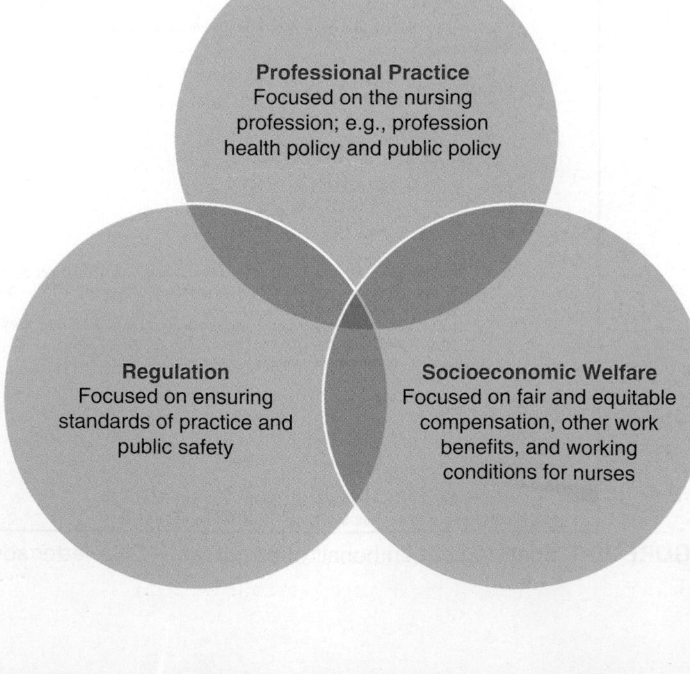

FIGURE 20-2 International Council of Nurses' three pillars.

power to shape nursing. If we, as experts in our field, set our own universal standards of excellence in education and practice, then we can influence what nursing can contribute to health care across the globe" (Affara, 2005, p. 579). Regulatory bodies have been part of the nursing associations in almost every Canadian province, but recent legislation requires that this function be managed separately to avoid perceived conflicts of interest (see also Chapter 5). Nursing regulatory bodies and self-regulation are undergoing change in Canada as a result of new legislation for health care providers as well as greater government oversight. For example, many regulatory bodies are now required to establish mechanisms to ensure health professionals are maintaining their competence to practise. Students must learn about these changes and have in-depth knowledge of professional standards of practice as they relate to the changing landscape of self-regulation.

The pillar of socioeconomic welfare generally involves labour unions. Unions are organizations that undertake collective action on issues such as nurses' working conditions, salaries, and benefits (see also Chapter 5). Nursing unions exist in all Canadian provinces, each with membership in the Canadian Federation of Nurses Unions (CFNU). Nursing unions developed over the last quarter of the twentieth century with a mandate for collective bargaining on behalf of nurses. The first provincial nursing union was established in Saskatchewan in 1973, and others were established in the rest of the provinces over the next 14 years. Nursing unions have made significant gains in nursing salaries, working conditions, and policy for public health care and patient safety. Collective bargaining is a mechanism for negotiating a labour contract between the employer and representatives of the employees. It leads to "an agreement in writing entered into between an employer and a bargaining agent containing provisions respecting terms of conditions of employment and related matters" (*Canada Labour Code*, RSC, 1985, c. L-5, s. 3). Nursing unions enter into collective agreements with employers, such as health care organizations and government ministries. Collective agreements create the mutual obligation for employers and the representatives of the employees to meet at reasonable times to confer in good faith on wages, work hours, and other terms and conditions of employment (and any agreement or question arising from those terms and conditions). The purpose of unionization and collective bargaining by nurses is to secure fair and satisfactory conditions of employment, including the right to participate in decisions regarding nursing practice. As an example, Table 20-1 presents the registered nursing associations, regulatory bodies, and unions of registered nurses in the provinces and territories.

EXERCISE 20-3

If you practise in a setting with a collective agreement, secure a copy. Examine the articles of this agreement. Are they related to practice issues or financial issues? What is the relationship between these two issue areas?

Professional Associations

A professional association is an alliance of practitioners within a profession that provides members with opportunities to meet leaders in the field, hone their own leadership skills, participate in policy formation, continue specialized education, and shape the future of the profession. They carry out a great deal of this work through collective action. The legacy of professional associations in nursing began with the formation of the ICN in 1899, an organization that was initially conceptualized and formed by a group of visionaries including two Canadian nurses—Isabel Hampton Robb and Mary Adelaide Nutting— who were living in the United States at the time (Paul & Ross-Kerr, 2011). In 1908, representatives of 16 organized nursing bodies met in Ottawa to form the Canadian National Association of Trained Nurses (CNATN). By 1924, each of the nine provinces had a professional nursing association with membership in the CNATN, and in that year, the national group changed its name to the Canadian Nurses Association (CNA) (http://www.cna-aiic.ca). Today, the CNA is a federation of provincial and territorial nursing associations and colleges representing over 150 000 registered nurses. The CNA's mission implies advocacy:

CNA is the national professional voice of registered nurses, advancing the practice of nursing and the profession to improve health outcomes in a publicly funded, not-for-profit health system by:

- unifying the voices of registered nurses
- strengthening nursing leadership
- promoting nursing excellence and a vibrant profession
- advocating for healthy public policy and a quality health system
- serving the public interest (CNA, n.d.)

TABLE 20-1 PROVINCIAL AND TERRITORIAL REGISTERED NURSING ASSOCIATIONS, REGULATORY BODIES, AND UNIONS

PROVINCE/ TERRITORY	PROFESSIONAL ASSOCIATION	REGULATORY BODY	PROFESSIONAL ASSOCIATION AND REGULATORY BODY (COMBINED)	UNION
British Columbia	Association of Registered Nurses of British Columbia (ARNBC) http://www.arnbc.ca	College of Registered Nurses of British Columbia (CRNBC) http://www.crnbc.ca		British Columbia Nurses' Union (BCNU) https://www.bcnu.org
Alberta			College and Association of Registered Nurses of Alberta (CARNA) http://www.nurses.ab.ca/Carna/index.aspx	United Nurses of Alberta (UNA) http://www.una.ab.ca
Saskatchewan			Saskatchewan Registered Nurses Association (SRNA) http://www.srna.org	Saskatchewan Union of Nurses (SUN) sun-nurses.sk.ca
Manitoba			College of Registered Nurses of Manitoba (CRNM) http://www.crnm.mb.ca	Manitoba Nurses Union (MNU) http://www.nursesunion.mb.ca
Ontario	Registered Nurses' Association of Ontario (RNAO) http://rnao.ca	College of Nurses of Ontario (CNO) http://www.cno.org		Ontario Nurses' Association (ONA) http://www.ona.org
Quebec			Ordre des infirmières et infirmiers du Québec (OIIQ) http://www.oiiq.org	Fédération interprofessionnelle de la santé du Québec (FIQ) http://www.fiqsante.qc.ca/fr/contents/pages/accueil.html
New Brunswick			Nurses Association of New Brunswick (NANB) http://www.nanb.nb.ca	New Brunswick Nurses Union (NBNU) http://www.nbnu.ca
Nova Scotia			College of Registered Nurses of Nova Scotia (CRNNS) http://www.crnns.ca	Nova Scotia Nurses' Union (NSNU) http://www.nsnu.ca
Prince Edward Island			Association of Registered Nurses of Prince Edward Island (ARNPEI) http://www.arnpei.ca	Prince Edward Island Nurses Union (PEINU) http://www.peinu.com
Newfoundland and Labrador			Association of Registered Nurses Newfoundland and Labrador (ARNNL) http://www.arnnl.ca	Newfoundland and Labrador Nurses' Union (NLNU) http://www.nlnu.ca
Yukon			Yukon Registered Nurses Association (YRNA) http://www.yrna.ca	
Northwest Territories and Nunavut			Registered Nurses Association of Northwest Territories and Nunavut (RNANT/NU) http://www.rnantnu.ca	

The CNA realizes its mission through its ability to speak as the unified voice of Canadian nurses on matters of nursing, health, and public policy. Voice and presence are the essence of political power and influence; they are essential to the mission of professional associations as they advocate on a range of issues, including publicly funded health care, care delivery, nurse staffing models, evidence-informed practice, and the influence of poverty on health. As a nursing student, it is an important part of your education to remain current on the issues of the day and the mandates of your provincial or territorial, national, and international nursing associations. Professional association Web sites and social media make it easier to stay up-to-date on the latest issues and activities in the field.

Professional associations undertake collective action on a variety of topics, including changes to nursing practice, working conditions, care delivery models, public health care, and publicly funded health care. More recently, nurses have been involved in creating healthy public policy in areas such as housing, poverty reduction, and the environment. Many strategies and tools are available to nurses who wish to engage in advocacy initiatives, and many of these have been developed and promoted by professional nursing associations.

Nurses contribute to the work of professional associations by identifying issues and submitting resolutions or motions that can then be voted on by members. Resolutions or motions that are approved by the membership are shared with decision makers or governments on behalf of the nurse membership. It is important to review the kinds of resolutions that have been voted on by the membership of provincial or territorial associations and the CNA at annual general meetings and their outcomes.

Recently, the CNA formed a National Expert Commission on health to influence the government on nurse-led solutions for health care transformation (CNA, 2011b). This initiative and others are clear examples of nurses working together to maximize nursing's voice and influence.

Labour Unions

Today, 80% of nurses in Canada belong to unions, with nurses in managerial positions excluded from membership. Union stewards or regional representatives are elected to represent unionized nurses within regions, practice settings, or both. The CFNU is "the national voice of unionized nurses," with 156 000 nurses represented from unions in nine provinces (Canadian Federation of Nurses Unions, n.d.). Unions' collective bargaining agency is established under various provincial, territorial, and federal labour relations legislation. Although it is possible to bargain collectively without a union, the union model is commonly used.

Union activity in nursing and in health care has grown in the past 30 years and has been stimulated by health care reorganization, work redesign, and changes in patient care delivery models. Some of the major issues that have led to increased union activity in nursing are as follows:

- Lack of professional autonomy and professional practice models in nursing
- Inadequate staffing and increased reliance on unregulated health care providers
- The absence of procedures for the reporting of unsafe work environments and poor quality care
- Mandatory overtime and work overload
- Low wages and poor benefits
- Workplace violence
- The impetus to preserve publicly funded health care
- Social justice issues

As unions evolve to broader mandates of collective influence, they may work in concert with other associations and organizations. It is important that nonunionized nurse managers find ways to work with staff nurses who are union members and union representatives to advance the quality of work environments and patient care, as these interests are not mutually exclusive. In recent years, processes have evolved within unions to address issues of workload, safety, patient care, and other nursing practice issues through a joint problem-solving process between nursing staff and nurse managers.

Nurse who are non-unionized often have supervisory positions that include the authority to act in the interest of the employer in areas such as hiring, terminating, rewarding, and disciplining staff. Many supervisory nurses may think that they are unnecessarily placed in an adversarial relationship with unionized nurses in the hospital. However, supervisory nurses and nonsupervisory nurses both share concern for working conditions, practice standards, and the care delivery environment.

Regulatory Bodies

Self-regulation is a hard-won and essential component of nursing professionalism. Regulatory bodies have the important mandate of establishing professional standards of practice, educational requirements, and scopes of practice. Regulatory bodies exist in an environment of dynamic change and are affected by the evolution of legislation, the inclusion of models of interprofessional practice in health care, and the involvement of nurses in primary health care reform. Regulatory bodies also establish the required competencies for entry-level registered nurse practice, and these competencies are used to guide nursing education program recognition and development. Many provincial regulatory bodies have student representation programs that engage nursing students in learning about professional practice standards, scopes of practice, and ethical issues. Some regulatory bodies have workplace representatives to maintain connection with front-line nurses, and most have practice consultants available to assist registrants with practice questions or practice issues. The regulatory responsibilities of these organizations are discussed in more detail in Chapter 5, but their supportive roles to nurses and their ability to collectively educate and advocate on matters that are in the public interest should not be overlooked.

Inter-organizational Advocacy and Coalitions

At times, associations, regulatory bodies, and unions work together on common issues. For example, an association and a union may decide to work together on policies affecting workplace and care delivery systems. A regulatory body and an association might work together on the matter of expanded nursing practice roles. In addition, nursing associations join with other non-nursing associations to form partnerships in the interest of public policy. Examples include the Canadian Nurses Association, the Canadian Public Health Association, and the Canadian Medical Association, who work in partnership with national patient and consumer advocacy groups in the interests of safeguarding public health care.

The recent partnership of the CFNU, the CNA, the Canadian Healthcare Association, and the Dieticians of Canada produced an initiative entitled "Research to Action: Applied Workplace Solutions for Nurses"

(http://www.thinknursing.ca/rta). This initiative was undertaken as a series of cross-national pilot projects designed to improve working conditions for nurses, and resulted in important lessons learned and recommendations (Box 20-1).

BOX 20-1	"RESEARCH TO ACTION" PROJECT SUMMARY

In recognition of the need to support the practice of new graduates, the CFNU collaborated with the CNA, the Canadian Healthcare Association, and the Dieticians of Canada to initiate the "Research to Action: Applied Workplace Solutions for Nurses" project. Many initiatives across Canada were undertaken as part of Research to Action, all aimed at piloting and evaluating strategies that would improve the quality of working conditions for nurses (Silas, 2012). More details on this project, including lessons learned, appear here: http://www.longwoods.com/content/22815. The project involved staff nurses in research and policy. Through the process of action research, nurses learned about the importance of supporting colleagues, the knowledge and skills required for professional development, mentorship models, and the partnerships and leadership needed to ensure that the initiatives continue to be valued as part of a quality work environment (Silas, 2012).

Collective action requires both leaders and followers. Changes in an initiative or an agenda may mean that today's leader becomes tomorrow's follower. The opposite may also be true: today's follower may become tomorrow's leader. Informed followers are not submissive participants blindly following a cultist personality. They are effective group members, not "groupies." They are skilled in group dynamics and accountable for their actions. They are willing and able to question, debate, compromise, collaborate, and act. Box 20-2 lists the traits of a good follower.

EXERCISE 20-4

Visit the CNA website (http://www.cna-aiic.ca) for the most recent positions and publications on two key issues in nursing: (1) nurse fatigue, and (2) nursing care delivery models and staff mix. Pay particular attention to the recommendations for each of these issues. From your perspective, are these recommendations followed in the health care organizations in your community or areas where you have had clinical practice experiences? What evidence is cited in making these recommendations? Based on your experience, what recommendations for change would you make to your provincial or territorial and national nursing associations?

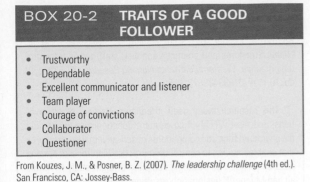

From Kouzes, J. M., & Posner, B. Z. (2007). *The leadership challenge* (4th ed.). San Francisco, CA: Jossey-Bass.

NURSING GOVERNANCE

The governance structure of an organization provides nurses with a framework for participating in decision making regarding their practice to ensure safe, quality care for their patients. Professional nurses are expected to participate in decision making in their health care setting. Doing so provides nurses with greater autonomy and authority over practice decisions regarding care for patients and is a major component of job satisfaction (Kramer, Schmalenberg, Maguire, et al., 2008; Pittman, 2007). Nursing governance is the methodology or system by which a department of nursing controls and directs the formulation and administration of nursing policy. Organizational structure provides a framework for fulfilling the organization's mission. Organizational charts show the relationship among and between roles (see also Chapter 9). The structure of the organization and the relationship among the components of the structure are influenced by the individuals selected to interpret and implement the organization's philosophy. A particular form of governance evolves from the mission and values of the organization and the relationships among and between its components. Thus, nurse managers and leaders who enact their organization's mission and values on a daily basis support nursing more openly. To paraphrase an adage, behaviour speaks louder and has more clout than organizational charts.

The three strategies nurses use most often to achieve collective action are shared governance, workplace advocacy, and collective bargaining. These strategies are not mutually exclusive. Moreover, as noted, governance is influenced by the context within which the organizational culture is embedded. *Organizational culture* is the implicit knowledge or values and beliefs within the organization that reflect the norms and traditions of the organization. Often the culture itself dictates the avenue of collective action.

The culture of the geographical area influences the organizational culture, governance structure, and leadership approaches of a health care setting. Organizational culture comprises value systems and subcultures within organizations. Subcultures differ from the main culture with respect to core values, goals, and relationships, including approaches to issues and conflicts. For example, when a subculture is clearly rooted in the mission of the organization (e.g., delivery of quality care in a cost-effective environment), the possibility of genuine negotiation or problem solving is enhanced. A subculture has its own unique and distinctive features, even as other features overlap with those of the larger culture. Members may adhere to values that are specific to their group while espousing values of the larger society. The presence of congruent subcultures supports healthy relationships. Healthy relationships are an important variable in the development of a strong internal governance structure capable of supporting a professional practice environment that works well for everyone involved.

Too often, nurses and administrators are members of separate subcultures. Several factors may increase the distinct ideologies of the two groups, including the existence of a distant corporate structure and the presence of a union. Both factors may be considered external tensions. Administrators tend to take on greater decision making and be risk averse when faced with economic pressures and the need to maintain a healthy "bottom line." However, history shows that broader input, not less, from nurses is important during these times.

When efforts have been made to address nurses' perceptions about job satisfaction, the relationship between nurses and the top administration of a hospital has been affected. Work environment factors that have a direct impact on nurses' job satisfaction and the ability to influence patient care include supervisory support in patient-care decisions and the provision of adequate staffing to provide quality care, positive working relationships with physicians and nurses, and a clear philosophy of nursing; all of these factors are influenced by the relationship between nurses and administrators (Cummings, Olson, Hayduk et al., 2008; Manojlovich, 2005; Mrayyan, 2004).

EXERCISE 20-5

Identify four factors in your practice (experience) that contribute to job satisfaction. Compare your responses with those of three practising nurses who are not supervisors and three practising nurses who are supervisors. Are your factors similar to the responses of others? Are you surprised by the responses?

Today, nurses expect a motivating, satisfying work environment that includes a role in decision making. Many nurses are and should be unwilling to remain outside the decision-making loop. Work redesign efforts to increase productivity and lower costs have placed a strain on the role of nursing and nurses in decision making. Supporting or creating a system that incorporates others in the decision-making process may be difficult for many in upper-management positions. However, high-performing organizations that provide quality health care have a climate that encourages participation by all stakeholders. Each stakeholder shares responsibility and risk, and that requires optimism and trust.

Shared Governance

Shared governance is described as a democratic, an egalitarian, and a dynamic process resulting from shared decision-making and accountability (Porter-O'Grady, 2009). According to Porter-O'Grady, Hawkins, and Parker (1997), the basic principles of shared governance include partnerships, equity, accountability, and ownership. It is more accurate to say that shared governance *demands* participation in decision making rather than *provides* for participation. Characteristics of self-governance that empower nurses are career ladders, access to power, participation in decision making, recognition of accomplishments, and evidence-informed practice (Kramer et al., 2008) (see the following Research Perspective). In shared governance models, it is important that nurses and others from all levels of the organization participate in making decisions that affect them and the care they are responsible for delivering.

🔍 RESEARCH PERSPECTIVE

Resource: Kramer, M., Schmalenberg, C., Maguire, P., et al. (2008). Structures and practices enabling staff nurses to control their practice. *Western Journal of Nursing Research, 30,* 539–559. doi:10.1177/0193945907310559

This research study used interviews, participant observations, and the CWEQII empowerment questionnaire to examine the characteristics and components of self-governance structures that enabled nurses to control their practice (control over nursing practice [CNP]). The strategic sampling of eight study hospitals all had Magnet™ designation resulting in high CNP scoring. The characteristics that enabled the high CNP scoring, based on both quantitative and qualitative data, were structural components of self-governance and career ladders, as well as the attributes of access to power, participation, recognition, accomplishments, and evidence-based practice initiatives. Findings suggested that self-governance structures are effective in enabling nurses to have control over their practice regarding issues of importance to the nurse, the patient, and the organization.

Implications for Practice
Nurse managers must include nurses in decision making regarding issues that pertain to the role of the nurse and the quality and safety of patients. They should support and encourage nurses to participate actively in unit and department councils and should recognize the accomplishments and achievements of staff.

Some organizations mislabel their governance structures. Although structures may be called "shared governance," they possess few of the characteristics outlined by those who are recognized as experts on the topic. In addition, many organizations have developed thinly veiled mechanisms designed to preclude nurses from participating in collective action. Professional-practice climates recognize individual and team performance. Increasingly, nurses are seeking to work for organizations that provide professional-practice climates—ones that have effective activities, not just effective documents.

Studies demonstrate that health care organizations that provide nurses with authority and autonomy have better patient outcomes, retain nurses at a higher rate, are more cost-effective, and have evidence of greater patient satisfaction than organizations that do not (Aiken, Clarke, Sloane, et al., 2002; Dunton, Gajewski, Klaus, et al., 2007; Kramer & Schmalenberg, 2004). In the United States, Magnet™ hospitals have recognized the benefits of decentralized decision making and its impact on both nursing satisfaction and patient outcomes (see Chapter 9).

Workplace Advocacy

Workplace advocacy is an umbrella term that encompasses advocacy activities within the practice setting. Workplace advocacy includes an array of activities undertaken to address the challenges faced by nurses in their practice settings. These activities include career development, mentorship, participatory decision making, and the promotion of a quality work life for nurses and others with whom they work. The objective of workplace advocacy is to equip nurses to practise in a rapidly changing environment. Advocacy occurs within a context of evidence-informed and participatory decision making.

Participatory Decision Making and Collaboration.

The Registered Nurses' Association of Ontario (RNAO, 2006) recommends that collaborative practice can be achieved by "incorporating non-hierarchal, democratic working practices to validate all contributions from team members" (p. 25). This is the essence of participatory decision making and can be achieved through a variety of means, including the establishment of professional practice councils. Where it is often difficult for individual nurses acting alone to effect change in nursing practice, a nursing professional practice council is a formal committee of nurses in a health care setting that identifies, reviews, and addresses issues that influence nursing professional practice (London Health Sciences, n.d.). Through the NPPC, nurses can advocate for resources and practices needed to maintain and enhance standards and quality of care (Gokenbach, 2007).

A recent research study entitled "Leadership for Ethical Policy and Practice" (LEEP) employed participatory action methods and involved nurses at different levels of practice in various health care sites in British Columbia to identify strategies for action to improve both the ethical climate of health care and the quality of the work environment for nurses (Storch, Rodney, Varcoe, et al., 2009). This three-year study and its findings indicated the need for nurses in senior management to join front-line nurses to understand the need for change and develop approaches and advocacy initiatives. More such initiatives and studies are needed to create the body of knowledge to support the democratization of policy and organizational decision making. The Literature Perspective also illustrates the potential effects of collaborative approaches to everyday ethical situations faced by nurses.

📖 **LITERATURE PERSPECTIVE**

Resource: Scott, S. A., Marck, P., & Barton, S. (2011). Exploring ethics in practice: Creating moral community in healthcare one place at a time. *Nursing Leadership, 24*(4), 78–87. doi:10.12927/cjnl.2012.22736

The authors describe a series of practitioner-led Ethics in Practice (EIP) sessions that provided nurses working in acute care, home health care, and public health with the opportunity to examine their experiences of "everyday ethical situations." For EIP sessions to be successful, they had to explore ethical situations identified by participants. The ethical situations discussed included those that were most relevant to the nurses' daily work, such as handling mistakes in practice, professional boundaries in rural practice, patient autonomy for both adult and pediatric palliative care patients, and vaccine allocation and immunization rollout during disease outbreaks. In the sessions, nurses were able to explore case studies, relevant literature, and hear from nurses who had specific experiences or expertise on the ethical issues. The sessions were highly valued by participants and were easy to arrange and conduct. The authors recommended the sessions as a vital approach to inspiring moral community and moral imagination among clinical colleagues.

Implications for Practice

Nurses experience ethical issues on a daily basis and often lack support for resolving situations or feelings associated with patient-care concerns. The opportunity to come together in a spirit of trust in EIP sessions to explore the often isolating experience of an ethical situation has the great potential to enhance morale and the quality of nursing care. Nurse managers and others in formal leadership positions in health care agencies and hospitals may also learn about the ethical challenges that nurses confront on a daily basis through EIP sessions, which give nurses a forum to present issues. EIP sessions should be considered as a key strategy for enhancing learning and increasing the ability of nurses and others to address everyday ethical situations and concerns, as well as building morale, professional autonomy and accountability, ethical practice through support, and collaboration.

Support for Making and Implementing Decisions.

The support nurses need to make and implement decisions is achieved through role models, mentors, and empowerment. Role models are individuals who enact a role, typically in a positive way, so that others can follow the example. For example, the nurse who has excellent clinical and leadership skills may be a role model. The implementation of a primary mentorship program for nurses may contribute to the development of nurses' leadership and advocacy skills (Crosby & Shields, 2010). Mentoring is a unique dynamic relationship between two individuals, usually in a professional setting (Pinkerton, 2003). A mentoring relationship is an ongoing "hands-on" process. Individuals who have experienced a successful mentorship have identified positive, frequently occurring behaviours that characterized their mentor. These behaviours include trust and the opportunity to make decisions that derive from that trust. The value to the individual is professional growth (Restifo & Yoder, 2004). The value to the organization is in the outcome: the individual will make better decisions that will well serve the organization, the nurse, and the patient.

EXERCISE 20-6

List the characteristics that you would want a mentor to possess. If you have identified a person you would want as a mentor, ask if he or she is willing to mentor you. Identify factors that are contributors and barriers to your seeking a mentorship relationship with the individual. Consider ways that you can address these factors.

Empowerment, or supporting other nurses, is a complex process. Nurses generally want to work hard, continue to learn, perform well, and be involved in the decision-making process. Nurse managers and administrators who support these efforts are empowering nurses and enhancing professionalism and autonomy. An empowered nurse will document an unsafe assignment. Accepting or refusing an unsafe assignment is difficult for nurses—both nurses at the beginning of their careers and those who are experienced. Critical elements to note are date, unit, assignment, staff available, rationale for objections, and documentation of notification of supervisor. Many assignments are classified as unsafe because of a lack of personnel and a lack of training of the existing personnel; therefore, nurses need to be prepared to respond when an assignment is declared unsafe. Accurate, concise, and clear documentation can assist the nurse manager by providing a source of data to support action to address an issue (see the following Research Perspective).

Empowering nurses is important. Powerless nurses feel more depersonalization in the workplace and are less satisfied with their jobs (Laschinger, Finegan, Shamian, et al., 2004; Leiter & Spence Laschinger, 2006). Manojlovich (2007) states that nurses' power develops from an organizational structure that promotes empowerment, a psychological conviction in the ability to be empowered, and the acknowledgement that power is present in the relationships and the caring that nurses provide.

RESEARCH PERSPECTIVE

Resource: Armstrong, K., Laschinger, H., & Wong, C. (2009). Workplace empowerment and Magnet hospital characteristics as predictors of patient safety climate. *Journal of Nursing Care Quality, 24*, 55–62. doi:10.1097/NCQ.0b013e31818f5506

This study was conducted to examine the variables of workplace empowerment and Magnet™ hospital characteristics as predictors of patient safety climate. The framework used to guide the study was Kanter's theoretical model of workplace empowerment in nursing that has linked empowerment in nursing to control over practice, job satisfaction, work productivity, burnout, and organizational commitment. Three hundred randomly selected registered nurses employed in acute care hospitals were surveyed about conditions of work effectiveness, practice environment, and safety climate. Results showed moderate to strong correlations between empowerment and Magnet™ hospital characteristics, empowerment and patient safety climate, and Magnet™ characteristics and patient safety climate. The findings support the Kanter theoretical model of workplace empowerment in nursing and suggest that nurses who feel empowered in their workplace will perceive the patient safety climate as positive.

Implications for Practice

Nurses who feel empowered to make decisions and implement patient-care strategies may feel that the care environment on the unit is safer and more effective and have a higher rating of job satisfaction. Nurse managers should support nurses to make decisions in their practice and include nursing staff in unit-based plans and activities that affect the work and practice environment.

Professional Values. Professional values evolve through education in classroom settings, clinical assignments, and interactions with other nurses. "Professional values are beliefs and attitudes about what is good and right that generally are held in common by members of a profession and that are used to guide professional action" (Chinn & Kramer, 2011, p. 55). Nurses have an opportunity to solidify their own values as skilled mentors guide practice and assist more novice nurses to engage in value clarification. Inherent in professional values are ethical codes, standards of practice, standards for protecting participants, and a willingness to challenge social traditions, cultural mores, and priorities for allocating resources (Chinn & Kramer, 2011).

Organizational patterns may segment the responsibility for the provision of care and the management of resources for that care. It is in the best interest of patients for nurses to participate in decisions regarding the provision of care and resources. The involvement of nurses can vary from none whatsoever to a high degree of input in virtually every decision affecting the conditions of employment and their practice. Nurses must be prepared and willing to participate.

Whistle-blowing. On occasion, individual nurses must act outside of their usual organizational channels of communication to advocate the interests of safety for themselves, colleagues, or patients. Sometimes, one nurse blows the whistle on unsafe actions, practices, and harms. Other times, a group of nurses supported by their professional associations or unions act together as whistle-blowers. Whistle-blowing is defined as "exposing negligence, abuses or dangers, professional misconduct or incompetence, which exists in the organization in which they work" (CNA, 1999, p. 1). A number of prominent cases exist of nurses who have drawn attention to serious breaches of safety and professional conduct in the workplace; for example, in 1994, nurses voiced serious concerns over the preventable deaths of 12 children in the Pediatric Cardiac Surgery Program at the Health Sciences Centre in Winnipeg (Sinclair, 1994). Codes of ethics provide guidance on moral considerations in determining when one should blow the whistle. Nursing associations have also developed guidelines on whistle-blowing (Box 20-3).

BOX 20-3   WHEN SHOULD A NURSE CONSIDER BLOWING THE WHISTLE?

In some situations, nurses have a moral right to disclose harm. The following conditions should be met for a nurse to consider whistle-blowing:

1. The risk exists of actual or potential serious harm to clients, employees, or other persons. The more serious the harm, the more serious the obligation.
2. In most instances, the nurse should have reported the problem to the immediate supervisor or manager.
3. The nurse reported up through the hierarchy of the organization without receiving a satisfactory response or explanation.
4. The nurse consulted the CNA code of ethics for guidance and recognized the moral dimensions of the duty to act.
5. The nurse consulted his or her standards of practice and contacted practice consultants at the regulatory body or professional association for guidance and support in taking action and exposing harm.

Canadian Nurses Association (CNA). (1999). I see and I am silent / I see and speak out: The ethical dilemma of whistleblowing. (1999, November). *Ethics in Practice.* Retrieved from http://www.cna-aiic.ca/cna/documents/pdf/publications/Ethics_Pract_See_Silent_November_1999_e.pdf. © Canadian Nurses Association. Reprinted with permission. Further reproduction prohibited.

CONCLUSION

Nurses deploy a wide range of strategies to challenge the status quo and speak out against inequity and inequality. Nurses can advocate for change and influence public policy in a variety of ways, such as collective action, that will continue to benefit both the nursing profession and patient outcomes.

A SOLUTION

When planning any new change, and particularly a major change, it is important to include all of the stakeholders in the planning process. All Seaview Home Health Care staff, and particularly the nurses, need to have a voice in the decision-making and planning processes for a change in the care delivery system that would affect all of them and the patients. Ann held numerous meetings on the units to discuss the idea of changing to a patient-centred care delivery system and elicited input from all of the nurses and other staff about their feelings, concerns, and thoughts regarding the change. Ann then created a nursing professional practice council to review current evidence on the patient-centred care model and patient outcomes. It was important to identify best practices on a variety of topics, including staff mix, using

decision-making frameworks for quality nursing care when possible. Locating evidence to support best practices would be part of the tasks of the nursing professional practice council, and Ann knew that some nurses would need additional support and education to support these efforts. She arranged for a health region librarian to attend a staff meeting and explain the library support she could offer. Ann believed that the only way to effectively develop and implement any new idea was to engage everyone in the process.

Would this be a suitable approach for you? Why or why not?

THE EVIDENCE

- Nurses who are involved in collective action and who work in organizations where shared governance is practised describe greater job satisfaction and empowerment.

- Nurses who experience a sense of empowerment in the workplace consider that their organization provides a higher quality of care and are more satisfied with the quality of their nursing practice.

NEED TO KNOW NOW

- Validate how the professional practice, regulation, and socioeconomic welfare functions are carried out in your province or territory and by whom.
- Know the collective agreements of the unions active in your workplace as well as the unions' priority issues related to the socioeconomic welfare of nurses.

- Seek clarity from standards of practice and your nursing professional code of ethics about advocacy, whistle-blowing, and the professional practice of nursing.

CHAPTER CHECKLIST

Collectively, nurses possess the knowledge, skills, abilities, and numbers to influence policy and professional practice decisions. Collective action may take many forms. Nursing policy encompasses the three globally recognized functions of professional associations, regulatory bodies, and unions. They are important to nurses, the nursing profession, and the people nurses serve around the world.

Geographical and organizational contexts influence the formal and informal structures in which nurses participate. An organization's structure establishes the parameters for participation in decision making. Nurse managers must employ participatory methods such as nursing professional practice councils and other democratic decision-making processes to engage and empower nurses in all settings of practice.

- The purposes of collective participation by nurses are as follows:
  - To promote standards of practice of professional nursing
    - To establish and maintain standards of care
    - To allocate resources effectively and efficiently
    - To create satisfaction and support in the practice environment
    - To advocate for the social determinants of health, public policy, and health equity in coalition with other organizations and associations
- Collective bargaining is an effective, legal mechanism used by nurses to secure fair and satisfactory conditions of employment and obtain the right to participate in decisions regarding their practice.
- Nursing governance strategies dictate levels of participation. The type and level of participation in decision making influence job satisfaction.
- Shared governance is characterized by partnerships, equity, accountability, and ownership.
- The goal of workplace advocacy is to equip nurses to practice and make ethical decisions in a rapidly changing environment.

TIPS FOR COLLECTIVE ACTION

- Know the issues, positions, and leadership of your province's or territory's nursing associations.
- Be fully aware of what each union active in your workplace brings to the bargaining table and how aware each union may or may not be of workplace issues for nurses.
- Understand that collective action is a professional responsibility of nurses and is most effective when nurses work together to bring an informed perspective to nursing, health, and public policy issues.
- Keep in mind that nurses have the opportunity to bring the experience of patient care and health issues in the community to bear on policy decisions.

℮volve WEBSITE

Visit the Evolve website for Suggested Readings, Internet Resources, and additional resources related to the content in this chapter: http://evolve.elsevier.com/Canada/Yoder-Wise/leading/.

REFERENCES

Statutes

Canada Labour Code, RSC, 1985, c. L-5, s. 3.

Texts

Affara, F. A. (2005). Valuing professional self-regulation. *Journal of Advanced Nursing, 52*(6), 579–579. doi:10.1111/j.1365-2648.2005.03642.x

Aiken, L. H., Clarke, S. P., Sloane, D. M., et al. (2002). Hospital nursing staffing and patient mortality, nurse burnout and job dissatisfaction. *JAMA, 288*, 1987–1993. doi:10.1001/jama.288.16.1987

Armstrong, K., Laschinger, H., & Wong, C. (2009). Workplace empowerment and Magnet hospital characteristics as predictors of patient safety climate. *Journal of Nursing Care Quality, 24*, 55–62. doi:10.1097/NCQ.0b013e31818f5506

Baldwin, M. A. (2003). Patient advocacy: A concept analysis. *Nursing Standard, 17*(21), 33–39. http://dx.doi.org/10.7748/ns2003.02.17.21.33.c3338.

Buresh, B., & Gordon, S. (2006). *From silence to voice: What nurses know and must communicate to the public.* Ithaca, NY: Cornell University Press.

Canadian Federation of Nurses Unions. (n.d.). Why unions. Retrieved from https://nursesunions.ca/why-unions.

Canadian Nurses Association (n.d.). Vision and mission. Retrieved from https://www.cna-aiic.ca/en/about-cna/vision-and-mission.

Canadian Nurses Association. (1999, November). I see and I am silent/I see and speak out: The ethical dilemma of whistleblowing. *Ethics in Practice.* Retrieved from http://www.cna-aiic.ca/sitecore%20modules/web/~/media/cna/page-content/pdf-en/ethics_pract_see_silent_november_1999_e.pdf#search=%22whistleblower%22.

Canadian Nurses Association. (2008). *Code of ethics for registered nurses (2008 centennial edition).* Toronto, ON: Author.

Canadian Nurses Association. (2011a). *About CNA.* Retrieved from http://www.cna-aiic.ca/en/about-cna.

Canadian Nurses Association. (2011b). *National Expert Commission: Backgrounder.* Retrieved from http://www.cna-aiic.ca/CNA/documents/pdf/publications/Expert_Commission_2011-2012_Backgrounder_e.pdf.

Chinn, P., & Kramer, M. (2011). *Integrated theory and knowledge development in nursing* (8th ed.). St. Louis, MO: Mosby.

Crosby, F. E., & Shields, C. J. (2010). Preparing the next generation of nurse leaders: An educational needs assessment. *Journal of Continuing Education in Nursing, 41*, 363–368. doi:10.3928/00220124-20100503-09

Cummings, G. G., Olson, K., Hayduk, L., et al. (2008). The relationship between nursing leadership and nurses' job satisfaction in Canadian oncology work environments. *Journal of Nursing Management, 16*, 508–518. doi:10.1111/j.1365-2834.2008.00897.x

Doane, G. H., & Varcoe, C. (2015). *How to nurse: Relational inquiry with individuals and families in changing health and health care contexts.* Philadelphia, PA: Wolters Kluwer Health.

Donovan, D. J., Diers, D., & Carryer, J. (2012). Perceptions of policy and political leadership in nursing in New Zealand. *Nursing Praxis in New Zealand, 28*,15–25.

Dunton, N., Gajewksi, B., Klaus, S., et al. (2007). The relationship of nursing workforce characteristics to patient outcomes. *The Online Journal of Issues in Nursing, 12*(3), Manuscript 3.

Gadow, S. (1990). Existential advocacy: Philosophical foundations of nursing. In T. Pence & J. Cantrell (Eds.), *Ethics in nursing: An anthology.* New York, NY: National League for Nursing.

Geller, L. (2014, January). Feature article: Changing how the world thinks about nursing. *Canadian Nurse, 110*, 26–30.

Gokenbach, V. (2007). Professional nurse councils: A new model to create excitement and improve value and productivity. *Journal of Nursing Administration, 37*, 440–443. doi:10.1097/01.NNA.0000285149.95236.fa

International Council of Nurses. (n.d.). Pillars & programmes. Retrieved from http://www.icn.ch/pillarsprograms/pillars-and-programmes/.

Kouzes, J. M., & Posner, B. Z. (2007). *The leadership challenge* (4th ed.). San Francisco, CA: Jossey-Bass.

Kramer, M., & Schmalenberg, C. (2004). Essentials of a magnetic work environment part 1. *Nursing 2004, 34*(6), 50–54.

Kramer, M., Schmalenberg, C., Maguire, P., et al. (2008). Structures and practices enabling staff nurses to control their practice. *Western Journal of Nursing Research, 30*(5), 539–559. doi:10.1177/0193945907310559

Laschinger, H. K. S., Finegan, J., Shamian, J., et al. (2004). A longitudinal analysis of the impact of workplace empowerment on work satisfaction. *Journal of Organizational Behavior, 25*(1), 527–545. doi:10.1002/job.256

Leiter, M. P., & Spence Laschinger, H. K. (2006). Relationships of work and practice environment to professional burnout. *Nursing Research, 55*(2), 137–146. doi:10.1097/00006199-200603000-00009

London Health Sciences. (n.d.). Nursing professional practice council. Retrieved from http://www.lhsc.on.ca/About_Us/Nursing/Nursing_Professional_Practice/index.htm.

MacDonald, H. (2007). Relational ethics and advocacy in nursing: Literature review. *Journal of Advanced Nursing, 57*(2), 119–126.

Mahlin, M. (2010). Individual patient advocacy, collective responsibility and activism within professional nursing associations. *Nursing Ethics, 17*, 247–254. doi:10.1177/0969733009351949

Manojlovich, M. (2005). The effect of nursing leadership on hospital nurses' professional practice behaviors. *Journal of Nursing Administration, 35*(7), 366–374. doi:10.1097/00005110-200507000-00009

Manojlovich, M. (2007). Power and empowerment in nursing: Looking backward to inform the future. *Online Journal of Issues in Nursing, 12*(1). doi:10.3912/OJIN.Vol12No01Man01

Mata, H., Latham, T. P., & Ransome, Y. (2010). Benefits of professional organization membership and participation in national conferences: Considerations for students and new professionals. *Health Promotion Practice, 11*, 450–454. doi:10.1177/1524839910370427

Mildon, B. (2013). A profession of leaders. *Canadian Nurse, 109*(5), 3.

Minarik, P., & Catrambone, C. (1998). Collective participation in workforce decision-making. In D. Mason, D. Talbot, & J. Leavitt (Eds.), *Policy and politics for nurses: Action and change in the workplace, government, organizations and community* (3rd ed.). Philadelphia, PA: Saunders.

Mrayyan, M. T. (2004). Nurses' autonomy: Influence of nurse managers' actions. *Journal of Advanced Nursing, 45*(3), 326–336. doi:10.1046/j.1365-2648.2003.02893.x

Paul, P., & Ross-Kerr, J. (2011). Nursing in Canada, 1600 to the present: A brief account. In J. C. Ross Kerr and M. J. Wood, (Eds.), *Canadian nursing: Issues and perspectives* (5th ed., pp. 18–41). Toronto, ON: Elsevier Canada.

Pinkerton, S. E. (2003). Mentoring new graduates. *Nursing Economic$, 21*(4), 202–203.

Pittman, J. (2007). Registered nurse job satisfaction and collective bargaining unit membership status. *Journal of Nursing Administration, 37*(10), 471–476. doi:10.1097/01. NNA.0000285148.87612.72

Porter-O'Grady, T. (2009). *Interdisciplinary shared governance: Integrating practice, transforming health care* (2nd ed.). Boston, MA: Jones & Bartlett.

Porter-O'Grady, T., Hawkins, M., & Parker, M. (1997). *Whole systems shared governance: Architecture for integration.* Gaithersburg, MD: Aspen.

Registered Nurses' Association of Ontario. (2006). Healthy work environments best practice guidelines: Collaborative practice among nursing teams. *RNAO Nursing Best Practice Guidelines Program.* Retrieved from http://rnao.ca/sites/rnao-ca/files/Collaborative_Practice_Among_Nursing_Teams.pdf.

Restifo, R., & Yoder, L. (2004). Partnership: Making the most of mentoring. *Nurseweek, 4,* 30–33.

Reutter, L., & Kushner, K. E. (2010). Health equity through action on the social determinants of health: Taking up the challenge in nursing. *Nursing Inquiry, 17*(3), 269–280. doi:10.1111/j.1440-1800.2010.00500.x

Scott, S. A., Marck, P., & Barton, S. (2011). Exploring ethics in practice: Creating moral community in healthcare one place at a time. *Nursing Leadership, 24*(4), 78–87. doi:10.12927/cjnl.2012.22736

Silas, L. (2012, March). The research to action project: Applied workplace solutions for nurses. *Nursing Leadership,* 9–20.

Sinclair, C.M. (1994). Report of the Manitoba pediatric cardiac surgery inquest. Retrieved from www.pediatriccardiacinquest.mb.ca

Spenceley, S., Reutter, L., & Allen, M. (2006). The road less travelled: Nursing advocacy at the policy level. *Policy, Politics and Nursing Practice, 7,* 180–194. doi:10.1177/1527154406293683

Storch, J., Rodney, P., Varcoe, C., et al. (2009). Leadership for ethical policy and practice (LEEP): Participatory action project. *Nursing Leadership, 22*(3), 68–80. doi:10.12927/cjnl.2009.21155

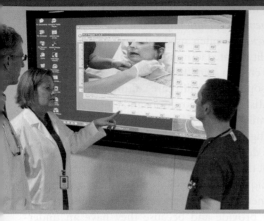

Managing Quality and Risk

Victoria N. Folse
Adapted by Carol A. Wong

This chapter explains key concepts and strategies related to quality and risk management. All health care providers, including nurses, must be actively involved in the continuous improvement of patient care.

OBJECTIVES

- Apply quality management principles to clinical situations.
- Use the six steps of the quality improvement process in practice.
- Understand the roles of leaders, managers, and followers in a culture of quality improvement.
- Describe the value of quality assurance activities at the unit level.
- Apply risk management strategies to a health care organization's quality management program.

TERMS TO KNOW

benchmarking	patient safety	risk management
near miss	performance improvement (PI)	root-cause analysis
never events	quality assurance (QA)	sentinel event
nursing-sensitive outcomes	quality improvement (QI)	
patient outcomes	quality management (QM)	

? A CHALLENGE

Medical errors have become one of the top issues in quality care and risk management and are a source of anxiety for Nadia, a newly graduated registered nurse working in the orthopedic unit of a hospital. Two documents brought the issue of medical errors to the forefront: a landmark report by the US Institute of Medicine (IOM, 2000), *To Err Is Human: Building a Safer Health System* and *The Canadian Adverse Events Study* (Baker, Norton, Flintoff, et al., 2004). However, medical errors have long been a concern before these documents existed and will likely continue to be an issue for years to come. Many policies and procedures, such

as electronic bar coding for medication administration, have been proposed to try to decrease the rate of medical errors in hospitals. Increasing capacity pressures on hospitals and the higher demands placed on nurses mean that it is critical for patient-care units to focus on ways they can advance quality care and prevent errors. Nadia wonders how to ease her anxiety and contribute to patient safety.

What do you think you would do if you were Nadia?

INTRODUCTION

Health care organizations and health care providers strive to provide the highest-quality, safest, most efficient, and cost-effective care possible. The philosophy of quality management and the process of quality improvement need to shape the entire health care culture and provide specific skills for assessment, measurement, and evaluation of patient care. The goal of an organization committed to quality care is a comprehensive, systematic approach that prevents errors or identifies and corrects errors so that adverse events are decreased and safety and quality outcomes are maximized. Leadership must acknowledge safety shortcomings and allocate resources at the patient care and unit levels to identify and reduce risks (Pronovost, Rosenstein, Paine, et al., 2008). Quality management and risk management are focused on optimizing patient outcomes and emphasize the prevention of patient-care problems and the mitigation of adverse events. Hospital leaders, including nurses, must sharpen their expertise in health care quality and patient safety, and staff at all levels must be empowered to act on nursing performance data (Kurtzman & Jennings, 2008).

QUALITY MANAGEMENT IN HEALTH CARE

Health care organizations that demand quality recognize that funding and continued accreditation are directly linked to improved patient outcomes. Success depends on a philosophy that permeates the organization and values a continuous process of improvement. It is essential to integrate patient safety and risk management into broader quality initiatives. Nurses must be prepared to continuously improve the quality and safety of the health care organizations within which they work and must focus on developing the six safety competencies identified by the Canadian Patient Safety Institute (CPSI, 2011): (1) contribute to a culture of patient safety, (2) work in teams for patient safety, (3) communicate effectively for patient safety, (4) manage safety risks, (5) optimize human and environmental factors, and (6) recognize, respond to, and disclose adverse events. Quality necessitates maintaining safety in patient care and a continuous focus on clinical excellence by the entire multidisciplinary team. Patient safety is a key component of quality improvement and clinical governance.

Moreover, the prevention of adverse events is paramount to improved patient outcomes. The terms *quality management*, *quality improvement*, and *performance improvement* are often used interchangeably in health care. Quality-related terminology continues to evolve.

In this chapter, quality management (QM) refers to the philosophy of a health care culture that emphasizes patient satisfaction, innovation, and employee involvement. Similarly, quality improvement (QI) refers to an ongoing process of innovation, error prevention, and staff development that is used by organizations that adopt the quality management philosophy. Nurses have a unique role in quality management and quality improvement because of the amount of direct patient care they provide and because they have an understanding of the day-to-day issues and "real world" nursing involved in the delivery of care. The involvement of nurses in patient-care improvement efforts in a number of areas (e.g., patient flow problems, safe delivery of care during periods of low staffing or high patient census or high acuity, communication problems associated with complex patients, medication safety) not only promotes the quality and safety of patient care but also positively affects job satisfaction and the work environment (Armstrong, Laschinger, & Wong, 2009).

BENEFITS OF QUALITY MANAGEMENT

Health care organizations employing a comprehensive QM program benefit in a number of ways. First, some resource constraints, such as limited government funding and shortages of key staff, may be overcome by greater efficiency and proactive planning. By examining processes, waste in terms of rework and unnecessary steps as well as long wait times can be eliminated and lead to the better use of valuable resources. Second, patient safety can be increased with quality care because QM is based on the philosophy that actions should be right the first time and that improvement is always possible. By standardizing processes, the potential uncertainty and confusion that may lead to errors can be reduced, and patient and clinical outcomes can be improved. Third, job satisfaction could be enhanced because QM involves everyone on the quality improvement team and encourages learning and participation. This participative management approach encourages teamwork and makes employees feel valued as team members who can really make a difference.

PLANNING FOR QUALITY MANAGEMENT

Multidisciplinary planning is integral to the quest for quality. Issues are examined from various perspectives using a systematic process. Planning takes time and money; however, the costs of poor planning can be very expensive. For example, the costs of inadequate planning might involve correcting a patient care error, resulting in an extended length of stay and added procedures. In turn, these errors increase the risk of liability for what was originally done, which can result in a negative public image, employee frustration, and employee turnover. The costs of errors and ineffective nursing actions are avoidable.

EVOLUTION OF QUALITY MANAGEMENT

Non–health care industries have excelled in incorporating process improvement in their core operating strategies. Numerous business management philosophies have been expanded and modified for use in health care organizations. For example, Six Sigma, a data-driven approach targeting a nearly error-free environment, empowers employees to improve processes and outcomes. As health care organizations "go lean," nurses are challenged to eliminate unnecessary steps and reduce wasted processes (saving time and money) to improve the quality of care and the patient

experience (Fine, Golden, Hannam, et al., 2009). Six Sigma uses a five-step methodology known as *DMAIC*, which stands for *d*efine opportunities, *m*easure performance, *a*nalyze opportunity, *i*mprove performance, and *c*ontrol performance, to improve existing processes.

> **D**efine opportunities
> **M**easure performance
> **A**nalyze opportunity
> **I**mprove performance
> **C**ontrol performance

In health care organizations, QI processes are used to assess standards in the following areas: *structure* (e.g., adequacy of staffing, effectiveness of computerized charting, availability of unit-based medication delivery systems), *process* (e.g., timeliness and thoroughness of documentation, adherence to critical pathways or care maps), and *outcome* (e.g., patient falls, hospital-acquired infection rates, patient satisfaction). These three factors are usually considered to be interrelated, and research has been conducted to determine the characteristics of effective structures and processes that would result in better outcomes. The Literature Perspective below expands the classic Donabedian model of the structure, process, and outcome framework in promoting quality in health care organizations.

LITERATURE PERSPECTIVE

Resource: Glickman, S. W., Baggett, K. A., Krubert, C. G., et al. (2007). Promoting quality: The health-care organization from a management perspective. *International Journal for Quality Health Care, 19*(6), 341–348. doi:10.1093/intqhc/mzm047

Although agreement exists about the need for quality improvement in health care, the best approach to measuring and achieving quality has not been identified. Avedis Donabedian developed the structure, process, and outcome framework in 1966 to measure quality initiatives, and the Donabedian model continues to be used today. Structural indicators are based on an assessment of an organization's features or staff characteristics that may affect an organization's performance and quality. Examples might include factors that contribute to accreditation by Accreditation Canada or Magnet™ status designation, such as the leadership climate and staff governance structure. Process standards are based on evidence relating to the quality of the staff's work behaviours and include rates of nosocomial

infections and medication errors. Outcome standards relate to performance measures that can be attributed to the quality of services performed and include patient satisfaction and patient health status.

The focus in most health care arenas has been on process and outcomes, but a need exists to increase the understanding of structure's role in quality initiatives. An updated view of the Donabedian's conceptualization of structure emphasizes five key elements that define structure in today's health care organizations: executive management, culture, organizational design, incentive structures, and information exchange and technology.

Implications for Practice
The updated Donabedian model can be used to enhance organizational performance and quality. Health care leaders must attend to these core structural components to transform quality improvement initiatives and to actively involve direct care providers to improve the quality and safety of the care they deliver to patients.

In Canada, the implementation of the accreditation process for health care organizations was a major influence on the evolution of quality processes. In 1958, the Canadian Council on Hospital Services Accreditation (CCHSA) was established to set standards for Canadian hospitals and monitor their adherence. The CCHSA has acted as a key external stimulus for quality assurance programs in nursing and other professions and organizations. In 2008, CCHSA launched the Qmentum Accreditation Program and changed its name to Accreditation Canada; although its name has changed, its rigorous approach to improving health care through accreditation remains the same. Accreditation Canada's over 1000 clients include Regional Health Authorities, hospitals, and community-based programs and services. A recent study of the accreditation process in Canada confirmed that it is a highly effective tool for introducing QI processes, fostering leadership of QI efforts, and creating links between organizations and stakeholders (Pomey, Lemieux-Charles, Champagne, et al., 2010).

Provincial and territorial professional associations and regulatory bodies in nursing have also been instrumental in the focus on quality processes in nursing by developing guidelines for implementing quality assurance programs, nursing practice standards and guidelines, and resources and tools for nurses to develop QI competencies. The current emphasis in the health care system on improving patient safety has led many hospitals to hire patient safety experts. The findings of the Canadian Adverse Events Study (Baker et al., 2004) were released shortly after the US Institute of Medicine's (IOM, 2000) report *To Err Is Human: Building a Safer Health System*. Baker et al. (2004) reported that in Canada, a 7.5% incidence rate for adverse events (of which 36.9% were highly preventable) accounted for 1.1 million additional hospital days. In 2003, the Canadian Patient Safety Institute (CPSI) was founded to provide a coordinating and leadership role across health care sectors and systems; promote leading practices; and raise awareness by stakeholders, patients, and the general public about patient safety. This not-for-profit organization works with governments, health organizations, health care leaders, and health care providers to inspire improvement in patient safety and quality by developing evidence-informed resources and working to deliver measurable results.

QUALITY MANAGEMENT AND QUALITY IMPROVEMENT PRINCIPLES

The basic principles of both quality management and quality improvement are summarized in Box 21-1 and are developed further below.

Involvement

Senior leaders, nurse managers, and followers must be committed to the QI process. Senior leaders and nurse managers retain ultimate responsibility for QM but must involve the entire organization in the QI process. Although some health care organizations have achieved significant QI results without organization-wide support, total organizational involvement is necessary for cultural transformation. If all members of the health care team are to be actively involved in QI, a clear delineation of roles and responsibilities within a nonthreatening environment must be established (Table 21-1).

To work effectively in a democratic, quality-focused corporate environment, nurses and other health care providers must accept QI as an integral part of their role. Nurses have a direct impact on patient safety and health care outcomes (Kurtzman & Jennings, 2008). Nursing must be empowered to mobilize **performance improvement (PI)** knowledge and practice measures throughout the organization. (*Performance improvement* is the application of QI principles on an ongoing basis.) When a separate department controls quality activities, nurse managers, health care providers, and other workers often relinquish responsibility and commitment for quality control to these quality specialists. Employees working in an organizational

---

BOX 21-1	**PRINCIPLES OF QUALITY MANAGEMENT AND QUALITY IMPROVEMENT**

1. Quality management operates most effectively within a flat, democratic, organization structure.
2. Leaders and followers must be committed to quality improvement.
3. The goal of quality management is to improve systems and processes, not to assign blame.
4. Consumers define quality.
5. Quality improvement focuses on outcomes.
6. Decisions must be based on data.

culture that values quality freely make suggestions for improvement and innovation in patient care. Exercise 21-1 may help nurses make QI suggestions.

EXERCISE 21-1

Think of something that can be improved in your work setting. Define the problem, using as many specific facts as possible. List the advantages to the staff, patients, and employer of addressing this problem. Describe several possible solutions to the problem. Decide whom you would contact about these suggestions.

Goal

The goal of QM is to improve the organization, not to assign blame. Nurse managers strive to provide an environment in which nurses can function effectively. To encourage commitment to QM, nurse managers must clearly articulate the organization's mission and goals. All levels of employees, from nursing assistants to hospital administrators, must be educated about QI strategies.

Communication should flow freely within the organization. When health care providers understand one another's roles and can effectively communicate and work together, patients are more likely to receive safe, quality care. Because QM stresses improving the system, the detection of employees' errors is not stressed; and if errors occur, re-education of staff is emphasized rather than the imposition of punitive measures. When patient safety indicators are used to examine hospital performance, the focus of error analysis shifts from the individual provider to the level of the health care organization (Glance, Li, Osler, et al., 2008).

Consumers

The consumers of a particular product or service define quality. Successful organizations measure the factors that are most important to their consumers and focus their energies on enhancing quality in these areas. As patients (consumers of health care services) become more knowledgeable about their health issues and the health care system, they want input into treatment and care decisions. Although some patients may not be knowledgeable about a specific treatment, they

TABLE 21-1	ROLES AND RESPONSIBILITIES IN QUALITY IMPROVEMENT	
SENIOR LEADER	**NURSE MANAGER**	**FOLLOWER**
• Leads cultural transformation • Sets priorities for house-wide activities, staffing effectiveness, and patient outcomes • Builds infrastructure, provides resources, and removes barriers for improvement • Defines procedures for immediate response to errors involving care, treatment, or services and contains risk • Assesses management and staff knowledge of the QI process regularly, and provides education as needed • Implements and monitors systems for internal and external reporting of information • Defines and provides support system for staff who have been involved in a sentinel event	• Is accountable for quality and safety indicator performance within areas of responsibility • Communicates performance priorities and targets to staff • Meets regularly with staff to monitor progress and help with improvement work • Uses data to measure effectiveness of improvement • Works with staff to develop and implement action plans for improvement of measures that do not meet target • Provides time for unit staff to participate in quality improvement measures • Directly observes staff and coaches as needed • Consults quality management team (e.g., Six Sigma) or risk management team as appropriate • Writes and submits to senior leaders a periodic action plan that includes performance measures and plans for improvement • Shares information and benchmarks with other units and departments to improve organization's performance	• Follows policies, procedures, and protocols to ensure quality and safe patient care • Remains current in the literature on quality and safety specific to nursing; promotes evidence-informed practice standards • Communicates with and educates peers immediately if they are observed not following quality and safety standards • Reports quality and safety issues to supervisor/manager • Invests in the process by continually asking self, "What makes this indicator important to measure?" "What has been done to improve it?" "What can I do to improve it?" • Participates actively in QI activities

know when they are satisfied with their experience with a health care provider.

Every nurse and health care employer has internal and external consumers. Internal consumers are people or units within an organization who receive products or services. A nurse working on a hospital unit could describe patients, nurses on the other shifts, and other hospital departments as *internal consumers. External consumers* are people or groups outside the organization who receive products or services. For nurses, external consumers may include patients' families, physicians, other health service organizations, and the community at large. Some consumers (e.g., physicians, patient families) could be either internal or external consumers, depending on the actual care environment. Nurse managers and staff nurses can use Exercise 21-2 to identify their internal and external consumers.

EXERCISE 21-2

For one week, list every person with whom you interact as a nurse. Internal consumers are those people who work for or receive care in your organization. External consumers come from outside the organization. What is the best method to obtain feedback from each of these groups?

Public reporting of quality and risk data is changing the way consumers make decisions about health care and is intended to improve care through easily accessible information. For example, Health Quality Ontario (n.d.) measures and reports to the public on long-term care, home care, patient safety, and primary care. Topics covered include patient safety and QI indicators such as hospital-associated infections, hand-hygiene compliance, and hospital mortality rates. The public can access a searchable database and yearly reports on Ontario's health care system at the organization's Web site (http://www.hqontario.ca/quality-improvement). The Web site also has a section on quality improvement in health care delivery and is designed to assist the public to become informed users of Ontario's health care system.

Patient satisfaction with health care can be assessed through the use of questionnaires, interviews, focus group discussions, or observation. Patients' perspectives should be a key component of any QI initiative. However, patients cannot always adequately assess the competence of clinical performance, and, therefore, patient feedback and patient satisfaction surveys must serve as only one data source for QI initiatives.

Focus

QI focuses on outcomes. Patient outcomes are statements that describe the results of health care. They are specific and measurable and describe patients' behaviour. Outcome statements may be based on patients' needs, ethical and legal standards of practice, or other standardized data systems. Health care organizations that implement nursing-sensitive performance measures value nurses and have a strong commitment to patients and a goal to continuously improve performance (Doran, 2011; Kurtzman & Jennings, 2008).

Decisions

Decisions must be based on data. The use of statistical tools enables nurse managers to make objective decisions about QI activities. It is imperative that data are not merely collected to support a preconceived idea. Quality information must be gathered and analyzed without bias before improvement suggestions and recommendations are made.

THE QUALITY IMPROVEMENT PROCESS

QI involves the continuous analysis and evaluation of products and services to prevent errors and achieve consumer satisfaction. The QI process is continuous because products and services can always be improved.

In health care, the QI process is a structured series of steps designed to plan, implement, and evaluate changes in care activities. Many models of the QI process exist, but most parallel the nursing process and all contain steps similar to those listed in Box 21-2. The six steps can easily

---

BOX 21-2   STEPS IN THE QUALITY IMPROVEMENT PROCESS

1. Identify the needs most important to the consumer of health care services.
2. Assemble a multidisciplinary team to review the identified consumer needs and services.
3. Collect and analyze data to measure the current status of these services.
4. Establish measurable outcomes and quality indicators.
5. Select and implement a plan to meet the outcomes.
6. Collect data to evaluate the implementation of the plan and the achievement of outcomes.

---

be applied to clinical settings. In the following example, the staff at a community clinic use the QI process to handle patient complaints about excessive wait times.

A community primary care clinic receives a number of complaints from patients about waiting up to 2 hours for scheduled appointments to see a licensed practitioner. The clinic secretary and staff nurses suggest to the clinic manager that scheduling clinic appointments be investigated by the QI committee, which is composed of the clinic secretary, two clinic nurses, one physician, and one nurse practitioner. The clinic manager agrees to the staff's suggestion and assigns the problem to the QI committee. At its next meeting, the QI committee uses a flow chart to describe the scheduling process from the time a patient calls to make an appointment until the patient sees a physician or nurse practitioner in the examining room. Next, the committee members decide to gather and analyze data about the important parts of the process: the number of calls for appointments, the number of patients seen in a day, the number of cancelled or missed appointments, and the average time each patient spends in the waiting room. The committee discovers that too many appointments are scheduled because many patients miss appointments. This overbooking often results in long wait times for the patients who do arrive on time. The QI committee also gathers information on clinic wait times from the literature and through interviews with patients and colleagues.

A measurable outcome is written: "Patients will wait no longer than 30 minutes to be seen by a licensed practitioner." After a discussion of options, the team recommends that appointments be scheduled at more reasonable intervals, that patients receive notification of appointments by phone and by e-mail (where possible), and that all clinic patients be educated about the importance of keeping scheduled appointments. The committee communicates its suggestions for improvement to the manager and staff and monitors the results of the implementation of their improvement suggestions. Within 3 months, the average waiting room time per patient decreased to 90 minutes, and the number of missed patient appointments decreased by 20%. Because the desired outcome has not been met, the QI committee will continue the QI process.

Identify Consumers' Needs

The QI process begins with the selection of a clinical activity for review. Theoretically, any and all aspects of clinical care could be improved through the QI process. However, QI efforts should be concentrated on changes to patient care that will have the greatest effect. To determine which clinical activities are most important, nurse managers or staff nurses may interview or survey patients about their health care experiences or may review unmet quality standards. The results of the research study in the Research Perspective below identified an approach to preventing adverse drug events during hand-off.

RESEARCH PERSPECTIVE

Resource: Berkenstadt, H., Haviv, Y., Tuval, A., et al. (2008). Improving handoff communications in critical care. *Chest, 134*(1), 158–162. doi:10.1378/chest.08-0914

This study was conducted in a medical step-down unit after a patient experienced severe hypoglycemia caused by an infusion of a higher-than-ordered insulin dose. This adverse drug event might have been prevented if the insulin syringe pump had been checked during the nursing shift hand-off. The study included direct observations of nursing shift hand-offs, which led to the development and implementation of a hand-off protocol and the incorporation of hand-off education, including a simulation-based teamwork and communication workshop. The intervention led to an improvement in nurses' communication of crucial information during hand-off, which included the patient's name, events that occurred during the previous shift, and treatment goals for the next shift. However, no change occurred in the incidence of checking and adapting the monitor alarms, checking the mechanical ventilator, or checking medications being administered by continuous infusion.

Implications for Practice
Even minor incidents can reveal safety gaps and needed changes within a health care setting to prevent future occurrences. Reflecting the importance of the hand-off process for safe patient care, the Joint Commission (an American accreditation organization) introduced National Patient Safety Goal (NPSG) 2E. NPSG 2E requires accredited U.S. health care organizations to implement a standardized process to hand off in which information about patient care is communicated in a consistent manner. It also requires that these organizations provide opportunities for nurses to ask clarifying questions and to receive answers in a time frame that is consistent with having complete and accurate information available to the patient's caregivers when they are providing the care. Improving hand-off communication, including when to use certain communication techniques (e.g., Situation-Background-Assessment-Recommendation [SBAR] or repeat-back), is necessary to address time pressures, work overload, and the conflicting demands of nurses.

Assemble a Team

Once an activity is selected for possible improvement, a multidisciplinary team implements the QI process. QI team members should represent a cross-section of workers who are involved with the problem. To maximize success, team members may need to be educated about their roles before starting the QI process.

To develop effective unit-based QI teams, the workplace environment must promote teamwork. Some departments in health care facilities are more open to teamwork than others. Nurse managers and leaders can use Exercise 21-3 to decide whether their clinical unit is ready for a unit-based QI team.

EXERCISE 21-3

Ask yourself the following questions about your department:
1. Is communication between nurses and other health care providers promoted? If so, how?
2. Could the communication process be improved in any way?
3. Does your system encourage nurses to act as a team?
4. Are other disciplines/departments included in team activities?
5. Can the team focus be improved in any way?

Collect and Analyze Data

After the multidisciplinary team forms, the group collects data to measure the current status of the activity, service, or procedure under review. Various data tools may be used to analyze this information. These data tools include flow charts, line graphs, histograms, Pareto charts, and fishbone diagrams. The use of empirical tools to organize QI data is an essential part of the QI process, and although many nurses lack formal training in the use of QI tools, being familiar with those used most frequently in QI work is important (Hughes, 2008).

Flow Charts. A detailed flow chart is used to describe complex tasks. The flow chart is a data tool that uses boxes and directional arrows to diagram all the steps of a process or procedure in the proper sequence. Sometimes, just diagramming a patient-care process in detail reveals gaps and opportunities for improvement. The flow chart in Figure 21-1 depicts the process a home health care agency uses when receiving a new patient referral.

Line Graphs. A line graph presents data by showing the connection among variables. The dependent variable is usually plotted on the vertical scale, and the independent variable is usually plotted on the horizontal scale. In QI, this technique is often used to show the trend of a particular activity over time, and the result may be called a *trend chart*. The line graph in Figure 21-2 illustrates the number of referrals a home health care agency receives during a year.

Histograms. The histogram in Figure 21-3 illustrates the number of home health care referrals that come from five different referral sources during a selected year. A histogram is a bar chart that shows the frequency of events.

Bar Charts. A bar chart that identifies the major causes or components of a particular quality control problem is called a *Pareto chart*. It differs from a regular bar graph in that the highest frequencies of occurrence of a factor are designated in the bar at the left, with the other factors appearing in descending order. Used often in QI, the Pareto chart helps the QI team determine priorities, allowing the most significant problem to be addressed first. The Pareto chart in Figure 21-4 demonstrates that, on a medical–surgical unit over a 1-month period, omission of vital signs was the most common type of documentation error.

Fishbone Diagrams. The fishbone diagram is an effective method of summarizing a brainstorming session. A specific problem or outcome is written on the horizontal line. All possible causes of the problem or strategies to meet the outcome are written in a fishbone pattern. Figure 21-5 uses a fishbone diagram to present possible causes of patients' complaints about extended wait times for clinic appointments.

Although QI teams should be able to use these basic statistical tools, analysis that is more complex is sometimes necessary. In this situation, a statistical expert could be included on the QI team or the team may consult a statistician.

Establish Outcomes

After analyzing the data, the QI team next sets a goal for improvement. This goal can be established in a number of ways but always involves a standard of practice and a measurable nursing-sensitive outcome or patient outcome. **Nursing-sensitive outcomes** are patient outcomes that are sensitive to nursing practice or interventions. Nursing-sensitive indicators reflect the structure, process, and outcomes of nursing care. The structure of nursing care is indicated by the supply of nursing staff, the skill level of the nursing staff,

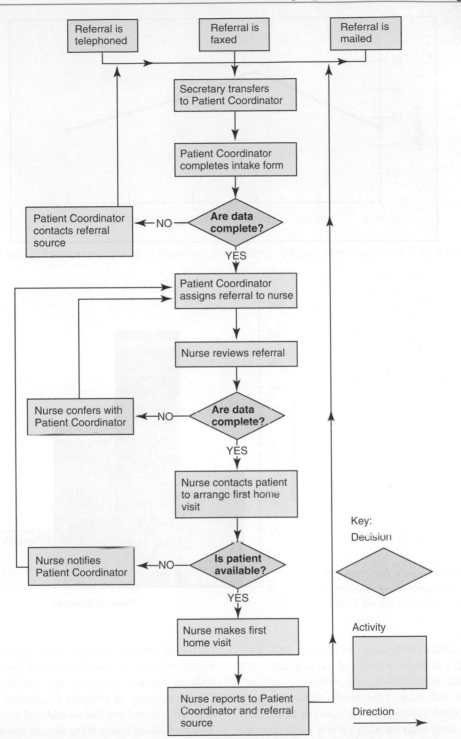

FIGURE 21-1 Steps in a flow chart diagramming process of a new patient referral, starting with the time a home health care referral is made and ending with the first home visit.

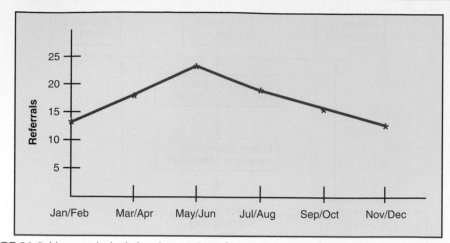

FIGURE 21-2 Line graph depicting the number of home health care referrals received during 1 year.

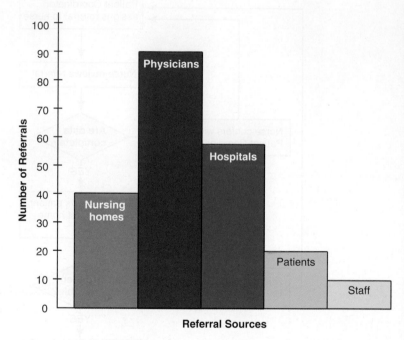

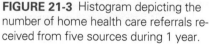

FIGURE 21-3 Histogram depicting the number of home health care referrals received from five sources during 1 year.

and the education/certification of nursing staff. Process indicators measure aspects of nursing care such as assessment, intervention, and nurse job satisfaction. Patient outcomes (the result of patient goals that are achieved through a combination of medical and nursing interventions with patient participation) are determined to be nursing sensitive if they improve with an increase in the quantity or quality of nursing care (e.g., pressure ulcers, falls, and intravenous [IV] infiltrations). Some patient outcomes are more highly related to other aspects of institutional care, such as medical decisions and institutional policies (e.g., frequency of primary Caesarean sections, cardiac failure) and are not considered nursing sensitive. The multidisciplinary team should use accepted standards of care and practice whenever possible. Clinical practice guidelines and standards should reflect evidence-informed practice and should be updated

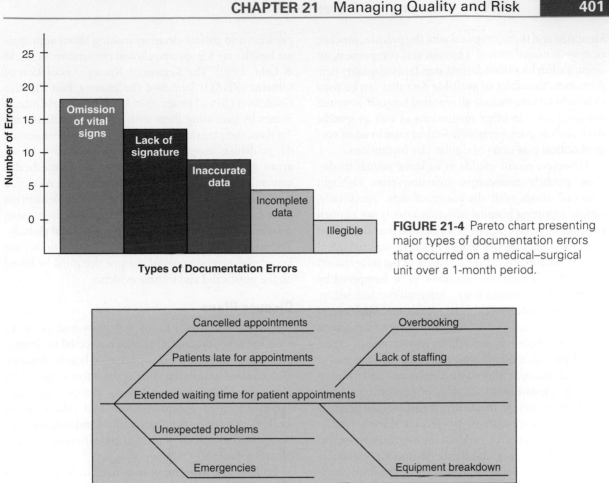

FIGURE 21-4 Pareto chart presenting major types of documentation errors that occurred on a medical–surgical unit over a 1-month period.

FIGURE 21-5 Fishbone diagram showing possible causes of extended wait times for clinic appointments.

as new research emerges. Sources that establish these standards include the following:

1. Provincial or territorial regulatory bodies, nurse practice acts and standards of nursing practice
2. Accrediting bodies such as Accreditation Canada
3. Governmental bodies such as the Canadian Institutes of Health Research (CIHR), Canadian Institute for Health Information (CIHI), and Public Health Agency of Canada (PHAC)
4. Health care advisory groups such as Health Council Canada (HCC), Canadian Patient Safety Institute (CPSI), Institute for Safe Medication Practices (ISMP), National Quality Institute (NQI), Canadian Foundation for Health Improvement (CFHI), and the Canadian Centre for Occupational Health and Safety (CCOHS)

5. Policy statements and reports from nationally recognized professional associations, such as the Canadian Nurses Association (CNA)
6. Nursing evidence-informed Best Practice Guidelines
7. Internal policies and procedures
8. Internal or external performance measurement data such as patient satisfaction surveys, employee opinion surveys, safety assessment surveys, and patient or employee rounds

Although individual health care organizations may have unique patient needs related to their specific population or environment, many targeted outcomes are similar. One way to evaluate the quality of outcomes is to compare one employer's performance with that of similar organizations. In a process called **benchmarking**, best practices, processes, or systems are identified and then compared with the practice, process, or system under review. Through this comparison, an organization identifies desired standards of quality performance. Examples of available data that can be used in benchmarking include all reported hospital-acquired infection rates in other institutions as well as specific data, such as postoperative infection rates in adult surgical critical care units of similar-size institutions.

However, recent mandates in some sectors to disclose publicly nosocomial infection rates highlight potential issues with disclosure of data. Specifically, simply reporting hospital infection rates is not enough to promote hand-hygiene practices and may do little to improve outcomes and reduce hospital-acquired infections. Unfortunately, the usefulness of the information from other institutions continues to be hampered by differences in terminology. Information technology plays a vital role in QI by increasing the efficiency of data entry and analysis. A consistent information system that trends high-risk procedures and systematic errors would provide a useful database regarding outcomes of care and resource allocation. Efforts are underway to develop standardized indicators of performance (such as infection rates) so that true comparisons can be made across health care settings, provinces, and territories.

Nursing has been a leader in the information system field by developing standardized nursing classification systems. The availability of standardized nursing data enables the study of health problems across populations and health care settings, and in relation to caregiving. The consistent use of standardized language enhances the QI process and also makes nursing's contributions clearer to regulators, health care policymakers, and the public. The use of standardized nursing terminology provides a means of collecting and analyzing nursing data and evaluating nursing-sensitive outcomes. In Canada, although there has been limited uptake of specific nursing classification systems in health care organizations, there has been a focus on measuring nursing-sensitive outcomes and implementing evidence-informed practice guidelines in nursing. For more information on nursing-sensitive outcomes, see Chapter 2. For more information on quality indicators in nursing, see Chapter 4.

Evidence-informed Best Practice Guidelines support decision making in the delivery of quality nursing care. Best Practice Guidelines are systematically developed statements based on the best available evidence to assist clinician and patient decision-making about appropriate health care for specific clinical circumstances (Field & Lohr, 1990). The Registered Nurses' Association of Ontario (RNAO) launched the nursing Best Practice Guidelines (BPGs) program in 1999 to support Ontario nurses by providing them with BPGs for patient care. To date, the program has developed and disseminated 41 guidelines covering clinical topics in five broad areas: gerontology, primary health care, home health care, mental health care, and emergency care. As well, a toolkit and an educator's resource kit for implementing these guidelines have been made available to the nursing community in all provinces and territories and globally. The rationale behind the BPG project is that nurses are knowledge professionals whose practice must be based on the most valid and reliable evidence.

Discuss Plans

The team discusses various strategies and plans to meet the new outcome. One plan is selected for implementation, and the process of change begins. Because QM stresses improving the organization rather than assigning blame to employees, change strategies emphasize open communication and education of workers affected by the new standard and outcome. QI is impossible without continual education of all leaders and followers.

Policies and procedures may need to be written or rewritten during the QI process. Policies should be reviewed frequently and updated so that they reflect best practice standards and do not become barriers to innovation. Communication about the change or improvement is essential.

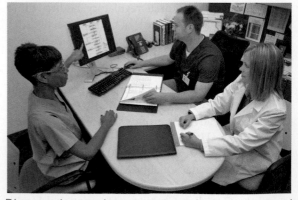

Diagramming a patient-care process in detail can reveal gaps and opportunities for improvement.

Evaluate

As the plan is implemented, the team continues to gather and evaluate data to document that the new outcome is being met. If an outcome is not met, revisions in the implementation plan are needed. Sometimes improvement in one part of a system presents new problems. For example, nurses implemented screening for suicide risk in adolescents and adults presenting to the emergency department. A result of this improvement in care was a greatly increased number of referrals for counselling, which overwhelmed the existing hospital and community resources. The interprofessional team may need to reassemble periodically to handle the inevitable obstacles that develop with the implementation of any new process or procedure. Furthermore, individuals outside the health care centre (external consumers) may need to be included in the process. The example that follows also illustrates this idea.

A hospital is implementing a pneumatic tube system to dispense medications. A multidisciplinary team is assembled to discuss the process from various viewpoints: pharmacy, nursing, pneumatic tube operation managers, aides who take the medications from the pneumatic tube to the patient medication drawers, administrators, and physicians. The tube system is implemented. A nurse on one unit realizes that several patients do not have their morning medications in their medication drawers. The nurse borrows medications from another patient's drawer and orders the rest of the medications "stat" from pharmacy. Other nurses on that unit and other units have the same problem and are taking the same or similar actions. Several problems are occurring—some of the medications are being given late, nurses waste precious time by searching other medication drawers, the pharmacy charges extra for the stat medications and is overwhelmed with stat requests, and the situation increases the nurses' frustration level. In some cases, patients suffer because of late administration of medications. QM principles would encourage the nurses to report the problems to the nurse manager or appropriate team member. The pneumatic tube team could compile data such as frequency of missing medications, timing of medication orders, and nursing units involved. The problems are analyzed with a system perspective to solve the late medication problem effectively.

In some organizations, when a change is implemented successfully, the QI team disbands. One of the crucial tasks of the nurse manager is to publicize and reward the success of each QI team. The nurse manager must also evaluate the work of the team and the ability of individual team members to work together effectively.

Some organizations that have used the QM philosophy for several years establish permanent QI teams or committees. These QI teams do not disband after implementing one project or idea but, rather, may meet regularly to focus on improvements in specific areas of patient care. The use of permanent QI teams or the adoption of a culture driven by QM can provide continuity and prevent duplication of efforts within the quality teams.

QM organizations stress system-level change and the evaluation of outcomes. However, in recent years, the need for process and performance improvement, including individual performance appraisal, has re-emerged within health care organizations. Self-review and peer evaluation are performance-assessment methods that fit within the QM philosophy. Many provincial and territorial regulatory bodies and professional associations have developed self-review tools and resources for performance appraisals.

Any nurse can use the six steps of the QI process in a self-review to improve individual performance. For example, a nurse on a medical unit who wants to improve documentation skills might study past entries on patient records; review current institution policies, professional standards, and literature related to documentation; set specific performance-improvement goals after consultation with the nurse manager and expert colleagues; devise strategies and a timeline for achieving performance goals; and, after implementing the strategies, review documentation entries to see whether self-improvement goals have been met.

QUALITY ASSURANCE

Although QI is a comprehensive process to prevent problems, it is naive to suggest the total abandonment of periodic inspection. Quality assurance (QA) involves regularly monitoring and evaluating services and processes to ensure that they conform to standards of practice. For example, QA focuses on whether an aspect of a provider's care meets the established standard, often in response to an identified problem. QA activities focus on discovering and correcting errors in

TABLE 21-2	COMPARISON OF QUALITY ASSURANCE AND QUALITY IMPROVEMENT PROCESSES	
	QUALITY ASSURANCE (QA) PROCESS	**QUALITY IMPROVEMENT (QI) PROCESS**
Goal	To improve quality	To improve quality
Focus	Discovery and correction of errors	Prevention of errors
Major tasks	Inspection of nursing activities	Review of nursing activities
	Chart audits	Innovation
		Staff development
Quality team	QA personnel or department personnel	Multidisciplinary team
Outcomes	Set by QA team with input from staff	Set by QI team with input from staff and patients

areas such as documentation and adherence to practice standards. An example of a QA question is "Did the nurse document the response to the pain medication within the required time period?" instead of "Did the patient receive adequate pain relief postoperatively?" In contrast, QI activities focus on whether a process, structure, and outcome requires improvement to prevent errors. The similarities and differences between QI and QA are summarized in Table 21-2.

One of the methods most often used in QA is chart review or chart auditing. Chart audits may be conducted using the records of active or discharged patients. Charts are selected randomly and reviewed by qualified health care providers. In an internal audit, staff members from the same hospital or agency that generated the records examine the data. External auditors are qualified professionals from outside the organization who conduct the review. An audit tool containing specific criteria based on standards of care is applied to each chart under review. For example, auditors might compare documentation related to use of restraints for medical–surgical purposes with the criterion "Licensed independent practitioner evaluates patient in person within 4 hours of application." Auditors note adherence or lack of adherence with each audit criterion and report a summary of these findings to the appropriate manager or committee for corrective action.

Because the focus of the chart audit is on detecting errors and determining the person responsible for them, many staff members tend to view QA negatively. The nurse manager must reinforce that QA is not intended to be punitive but, instead, is an opportunity to improve patient care at the unit level. For example, by providing the standard of care for documentation and helping the registered nurse (RN) review several

charts, the nurse manager can reinforce policies and procedures or standards regarding documentation. It is the responsibility of the nurse manager to communicate the importance of daily QA activities and how unit-based monitoring ties into the overall QI program. Moreover, many institutions incorporate both the participation in and the results of QA into annual performance appraisals or clinical ladders.

RISK MANAGEMENT

QM and risk management are related concepts and emphasize the achievement of quality-outcome standards and the prevention of patient-care problems. Risk management is the systematic identification, assessment, and prioritization of risks and the development and implementation of strategies to reduce adverse events and liability associated with these risks. Chapter 5 also discusses risk management. Losses associated with risk include financial loss as a result of malpractice or absorbing the cost of an extended length of stay for the patient, negative public relations, and employee dissatisfaction. The inclusion of patient safety standards in accreditation programs further emphasizes the importance of risk management. For example, Accreditation Canada developed Required Organizational Practices (ROPs) in patient safety, which appear in Box 21-3.

A risk management department has several functions, which include the following:
- Defining situations that place the organization at some financial risk, such as medication errors and patient falls
- Determining the frequency of occurrence of those situations

BOX 21-3 ACCREDITATION CANADA PATIENT SAFETY GOAL AREAS FOR HEALTH CARE ORGANIZATIONS

Culture: Create a culture of safety within the organization

Communication: Improve the effectiveness and coordination of communication among care and service providers and with the recipients of care and service across the continuum

Medication use: Ensure the safe use of high-risk medications

Worklife/workforce: Create a worklife and physical environment that supports the safe delivery of care/service

Infection control: Reduce the risk of health care-associated infections and their impact across the continuum of care/service

Risk assessment: Identify safety risks inherent in the client population

Accreditation Canada. (2013). *Required Organizational Practices Handbook 2014.* Ottawa, ON: Author, p. 2.

- Intervening and investigating identified events
- Identifying potential risks or opportunities to improve care

A major focus of risk management programs in health care organizations is patient safety, which is the absence of preventable harm to a patient during the process of health care. The Canadian Adverse Events Study (Baker et al., 2004) reported the occurrence of 185 000 adverse events per year in Canada, with over one third of these deemed potentially preventable. In a follow-up to the *To Err Is Human* report, the IOM (2004) pointed to the critical role nursing plays in providing safe care and identified health care management practices necessary to create a positive patient safety culture. Those practices included creating and maintaining trust throughout the organization; deploying health care providers in adequate numbers; creating a culture of openness regarding reporting and preventing errors; involving health care providers in decision making regarding work design and work flow; and actively managing the process of change (IOM, 2004). The IOM (2004) emphasized that the quality of patient care is directly affected by the degree to which hospital nurses are active and empowered participants in decisions about their patients' plans of care and by the degree to which they have an active and central role in organizational decision making.

The Canadian Patient Safety Institute (CPSI) created the Safer Healthcare Now! (SHN) program, which is a collaboration of people and organizations committed to improving patient safety. The program is founded on the principle that safe care is a top priority and that all organizations can make a difference when they partner and share information, strategies, and resources. This program is supported by individual clinicians, teams, and health care organizations from across Canada that provide ongoing clinical expertise to SHN's work, including mentorship of health care providers working to implement SHN interventions on the front line. The CPSI has chosen a number of interventions to improve patient safety across Canada through the SHN program, including the prevention of central line-associated bloodstream infections, falls, surgical site infections, ventilator-associated pneumonia, and medication errors. The aim of these interventions is to improve health care delivery by focusing on patients and their safety to reduce the number of injuries and deaths related to adverse events.

"Organizations with a positive safety culture are characterized by communications founded on mutual trust, by shared perceptions of the importance of safety, and by confidence in the efficacy of preventive measures" (Agency for Healthcare Research and Quality [AHRQ], 2004). Singer, Gaba, Geppert, et al. (2003) identified the following elements as integral to a safe culture: leadership commitment to safety, organizational resources for patient safety, priority of safety versus production, effectiveness and openness of communication, transparency about problems and errors, continuous organizational learning, and frequency of unsafe acts.

Each individual nurse is a risk manager and has the responsibility to identify and report unusual occurrences and potential risks. However, active involvement in quality and risk management by direct caregivers can be a challenge complicated by staffing issues and the increased demands on nurses. Increased nursing staff in hospitals is associated with better care outcomes. Consistent evidence shows that an increase in RN-to-patient ratios is associated with a reduction in hospital-related mortality, failure to rescue, and other nursing-sensitive outcomes, as well as reduced length of stay (Kane, Shamliyan, Mueller, et al., 2007). Similarly, favourable patient-care environments are associated with lower rates of serious complications or adverse events (Aiken, Clarke, Sloane, et al., 2008). Findings from the Aiken et al. (2008) and Kane et al. (2007) studies are discussed further in The Evidence section on page 408.

Another barrier to improving patient safety is fear of punishment, which inhibits people from acknowledging, reporting, or discussing errors. One way to minimize errors is to monitor threats to patient safety continually and to recognize that individual errors often reflect organizational and system failures. For example, targeting nurse-to-patient load and work schedules, including 12-hour shifts and overtime, can reduce potential errors from human factors such as fatigue, stress, and distractions. Rotating shifts may have a negative effect on nurses' stress levels and job performance, and working longer hours may have a negative impact on patient outcomes and safety (Kane et al., 2007).

Both risk management and quality management deal with changing behaviour, prevention, focus on the customer, and attention to outcomes. The following clinical examples illustrate how QM and risk management complement each other. First, the implementation of lift teams reduces employee injuries associated with lifting heavy or fully dependent patients and simultaneously, for the patient, decreases adverse events associated with difficult transfers. The implementation of lift teams reflects managing both quality and risk. Second, adherence to the universal safety verification known as "time out" before the beginning of a surgical procedure ensures perioperative safety within a QM framework. Although nurse managers would prefer that all staff intrinsically embrace risk management practices aimed at patient and staff safety, accountability for safety can be one aspect of performance evaluations. Active involvement of staff in risk management activities is key to preventing adverse events. Nurse managers should conduct safety rounds and praise employees for employing safe practices as part of best practice standards. This philosophy reinforces that risk management not only benefits the patient but also works to keep individual employees safe in the workplace.

Adverse-event reduction is a key strategy for reducing health care mortality and morbidity because patients who suffer adverse events are more likely to die or suffer permanent disability. Nurses have always played a pivotal role in the prevention of adverse events and can reduce negative outcomes with a focus on accurate assessment, early identification, and correction of potentially adverse situations. Also, adherence to best practice standards and ensuring quality standards for high-risk/high-volume practices (e.g., restraint use, medication reconciliation) can reduce adverse events. Never events are errors in medical care that are clearly identifiable, preventable, and serious in their consequences for patients and that indicate a real problem in the safety and credibility of a health care facility. Examples of never events include surgery on the wrong body part, a foreign body left in a patient after surgery, mismatched blood transfusion, major medication error, severe pressure ulcer acquired in the hospital, and preventable postoperative deaths. A comprehensive quality and risk program would proactively identify and reduce risks to patient safety by identifying and analyzing select high-risk situations. If an adverse event occurs, nurses should also be able to recognize near misses and sentinel events and participate with a multidisciplinary team in the root-cause analysis. A sentinel event is a serious, unexpected occurrence involving death or physical or psychological harm, such as inpatient suicide, infant abduction, or wrong-site surgery. Similarly, a near miss is a clinical situation that resulted in no harm but highlights an imminent problem that must be corrected; it can provide useful lessons in terms of risk analysis and reduction. After a sentinel event is identified, a root-cause analysis is performed by a team that includes those directly involved in the event and those in leadership positions. A root-cause analysis, while similar to the QI process, involves a deeper review of an incident and the sequence of events that led to it with the goals of identifying and addressing the underlying causes to reduce the likelihood of reoccurence.

Typically, risk or adverse events are communicated through electronic safety reporting systems or through incident reporting. Incident reports are kept separate from the patient's medical record and should serve as a means of communicating an incident that did cause or could have caused harm to patients, family members, visitors, or employees. Aggregated incident reports should be used to improve quality of care and decrease future risk. Trending data can illuminate system issues that need to be modified to reduce risk and achieve quality patient care. Organizations must institute mechanisms to ensure that nurses obtain feedback about the trends identified from analyzing the information gathered from error reporting. They should also establish policies and processes for reporting errors that include clear definitions for what constitute reportable errors. The communication of errors through the appropriate chain of command is essential to improve quality. Nurse managers are encouraged to ensure that the processes used for reporting errors are respectful, the information contained within reports is shared and communicated with discretion, and access to the incident reports is protected (Covell & Ritchie, 2009).

Evaluating Risks

In gathering data about unusual occurrences, the risk management team may involve perspectives from numerous disciplines to discover underlying problems that a single discipline might miss. Risk managers also use multiple data sources, data collection techniques, and perspectives to collect and interpret the data. Quantitative methods such as a questionnaire or records of medication administration can be combined with qualitative methods such as open-ended question interviews. Actionable plans for reducing the incidence of common preventable adverse events such as medication administration errors (wrong patient, time, dose, drug, or mode of delivery) could result from assessment and analysis of both quantitative and qualitative data. Quality and risk management strategies aimed at high-volume and high-risk occurrences are essential. It is important to keep in mind that organizational accountability for quality efforts to provincial and territorial governments as well as public reporting, in which quality data are made available for comparison, have significant implications for nurses. Opportunities to contribute to quality efforts include participation on QI teams, data collection, and involvement in the implementation of quality initiatives.

EXERCISE 21-4

Describe an error that occurred in the health care organization where you practise that resulted in harm to one patient and did not result in harm to another patient. What would you suggest to avoid a reoccurrence? Decide under what circumstances you would inform the patient and family and under what circumstances you would withhold the information.

CONCLUSION

Approaches to quality management and risk management require health care providers to challenge their attitudes that errors are an unfortunate but inevitable part of patient care. Diminished resources and challenges in the work environment have the potential to compromise communication among health care providers and to contribute to an environment in which unsafe practices are overlooked or excused. For example, communication errors between nurses and other health care providers may result from hurried exchanges in crowded hallways or in the midst of a busy nursing station. Poorly designed medication rooms make uninterrupted medication preparation difficult; finding a physical space to take a break can be impossible because the nursing lounge is often used for shift reports and meetings (McGillis-Hall, Peterson, & Fairley, 2010). A team approach to quality and risk management is needed to promote optimal outcomes. Nurses have a responsibility to provide quality care to patients and thus must serve in leadership roles to ensure a culture of integrated quality management and risk management. Moreover, a positive leadership style has been shown to influence the quality of the work environment and safety climate through effective leader–nurse relationships, which in turn have been associated with decreased reported medication errors (Squires, Tourangeau, Laschinger, et al., 2010; Thompson, Hoffman, Sereika, et al. 2011).

A SOLUTION

Nadia decided to participate in the "Safety Huddle" program initiated on her unit to encourage nurses to feel comfortable to openly and honestly discuss safety issues, medical errors, near misses, and good catches. Nurses who have made medical errors are supported to share their experience at the monthly Safety Huddle meeting and discuss the strategies they or the hospital could have taken to prevent the mistake from happening. In addition, nurses review the situations that were "good catches" or "near misses," such as a treatment order that was questioned by a nurse and found to be incorrect or a medication double-checked by another nurse who found a dosage error. These meetings allow nurses to openly discuss their safety problems with co-workers, examine issues from their point of view, foster learning, and influence safety improvement programs and policies. Concise minutes are recorded and provided to anyone unable to attend the meeting so that he or she, too, can learn from others' experiences. Nadia now considers herself part of a team effort to prevent future medical errors from occurring.

Would this be a suitable approach for you? Why or why not?

THE EVIDENCE

A strong correlation has been established between nurse practice environments and patient outcomes. Aiken et al. (2008) analyzed data from 10 184 nurses and 232 342 surgical patients in 168 Pennsylvania hospitals to determine the effects of nurse practice environments on nurse and patient outcomes. Outcomes included nurse job satisfaction, nurse burnout, nurses' intent to leave, quality care, mortality, and failure to rescue patients. This large multi-site study reinforced findings from the systematic review of 94 research studies examining the relationship of nurse staffing to patient outcomes in hospitals for the AHRQ, which was published in 2007 by Kane et al.

Kane et al. (2007) found that increased registered nursing staff was associated with lower patient mortality, failure to rescue, and length of stay. Aiken et al. (2008) found that in better work environments, nurses reported more positive job experiences and fewer concerns about the quality of care and that patients had a significantly lower risk of mortality and failure to rescue. Specifically, surgical mortality rates were more than 60% higher in poorly staffed hospitals with the poorest patient care environments than in hospitals with better care environments, the best nurse staffing levels, and the most highly educated nurses. Approximately 40 000 patient deaths could be avoided annually by improved care environments, nurse staffing, and nurse education. Nurse managers and leaders have several options for improving nurse retention and patient outcomes, including improving RN staffing, moving to a more educated nurse workforce, and improving the care environment. Hospitals (e.g., those with Magnet™ designation) whose practice environment includes investment in staff development, quality management, front-line managerial ability, and good nurse–physician relations are associated with better nurse and patient outcomes.

NEED TO KNOW NOW

- Know how to access clinical practice guidelines and standards for quality and safety using sources such as Accreditation Canada, the Canadian Nurses Association, the Institute of Medicine, Registered Nurses' Association of Ontario Best Practice Guidelines, other provincial or territorial nursing association's guidelines, and Safer Healthcare Now!

- Identify nursing-sensitive outcomes most pertinent to your practice area, and identify evidence-informed practice literature that addresses managing quality and risk.
- Know how to address any patient-care issue using the six steps of the quality improvement process.

CHAPTER CHECKLIST

Many health care organizations are in the process of implementing QM. Greater efficiency with improved quality is the goal of this approach. Effective QI includes identifying consumer expectations, planning, using a multidisciplinary approach, evaluating outcomes, and changing systems to provide an environment in which employees can perform at their best.

- The principles of QM and QI are as follows:
  - QM operates most effectively within a flat, democratic, organizational structure.
  - Leaders and followers must be committed to QI.
  - The goal of QM is to improve systems and processes, not to assign blame.

- Consumers define quality.
- QI focuses on outcomes.
- Decisions must be based on data.
- QM strives to prevent errors. Initial planning requires both time and money, but QM contributes to the bottom line in the long run.
- The steps in the QI process to evaluate and improve patient care are as follows:
  - Identify the needs most important to the consumer of health care services.
  - Assemble a multidisciplinary team to review the identified consumer needs and services.
  - Collect data to measure the current status of these services.

- Establish measurable outcomes and quality indicators.
- Select and implement a plan to meet the outcomes.
- Collect data to evaluate the implementation of the plan and the achievement of outcomes.
- Any process can be improved.

- Risk management focuses on ensuring safety and on minimizing loss after a patient-care error occurs.
- QA involves regularly monitoring and evaluating services and processes; it is the responsibility of all nurses and provides an opportunity to improve patient care at the unit level.

TIPS FOR QUALITY MANAGEMENT

- QM is based on data; anything measured and recorded can be improved.
- Concentrate QI energies on factors that are most important to patient quality and safety.

- Working together to prevent problems is more effective than fixing problems after they occur.

evolve WEBSITE

Visit the Evolve website for Suggested Readings, Internet Resources, and additional resources related to the content in this chapter: http://evolve.elsevier.com/Canada/Yoder-Wise/leading/.

REFERENCES

Accreditation Canada. (2013). *Required Organizational Practices Handbook 2014*. Ottawa, ON: Author.

Agency for Healthcare Research and Quality. (2004). Introduction: User's guide: Hospital survey on patient safety culture. Retrieved from http://www.ahrq.gov/professionals/quality-patient-safety/patientsafetyculture/hospital/userguide/hospcult1.html.

Aiken, L., Clarke, S. P., Sloane, D. M., et al. (2008). Effects of hospital care environment on patient mortality and nurse outcomes. *Journal of Nursing Administration, 38*(5), 223–229. doi:10.1097/01.NNA.0000312773.42352.d7

Armstrong, K., Laschinger, H. K., & Wong, C. A. (2009). Workplace empowerment and magnet hospital characteristics as predictors of patient safety climate. *Journal of Nursing Care Quality, 24*(1), 55–62. doi:10.1097/NCQ.0b013e31818f5506

Baker, G. R., Norton, P. G., Flintoff, V., et al. (2004). The Canadian Adverse Events Study: The incidence of adverse events among hospitals patients in Canada. *Canadian Medical Association Journal, 170*(10), 1678–1686. doi:10.1503/cmaj.1040498

Berkenstadt, H., Haviv, Y., Tuval, A., et al. (2008). Improving handoff communications in critical care. *Chest, 134*(1), 158–162. doi:10.1378/chest.08-0914

Canadian Patient Safety Institute. (2011). The safety competencies. Retrieved from http://www.patientsafetyinstitute.ca/English/toolsResources/safetyCompetencies/Pages/default.aspx.

Covell, C. L., & Ritchie, J. A. (2009). Nurses' responses to medication errors: Suggestions for the development of organizational strategies to improve reporting. *Journal of Nursing Care Quality, 24*(4), 287–297. doi:10.1097/NCQ.0b013e3181a4d506

Field, M. J., & Lohr, K. N. (Eds.). (1990). *Guidelines for clinical practice: Directions for a new program*. Washington, DC: Institute of Medicine, National Academy Press.

Fine, B. A., Golden, B., Hannam, R., et al. (2009). Leading lean: A Canadian healthcare leader's guide. *Healthcare Quarterly, 12*(3), 32–41. doi:10.12927/hcq.2013.20877

Glance, L. G., Li, Y., Osler, T. M., et al. (2008). Impact of date stamping on patient safety measurement in patients undergoing CABG: Experience with AHRQ patient safety indicators. *BMC Health Services Research, 8*, 176. doi:10.1186/1472-6963-8-176

Glickman, S. W., Baggett, K. A., Krubert, C. G., et al. (2007). Promoting quality: The health-care organization from a management perspective. *International Journal for Quality Health Care, 19*(6), 341–348. doi:10.1093/intqhc/mzm047

Health Quality Ontario. (n.d.). Public reporting. Retrieved from http://www.hqontario.ca/public-reporting.

Hughes, R. (2008). Tools and strategies for quality improvement and patient safety. In R. Hughes (Ed.), *Patient safety and quality: An evidence-based handbook for nurses* (Ch. 44). Rockville, MD: Agency for Healthcare Research and Quality.

Institute of Medicine. (2000). *To err is human: Building a safer health system*. Washington, DC: National Academies Press.

Institute of Medicine. (2004). *Keeping patients safe: Transforming the work environment of nurses*. Washington, DC: National Academies Press.

Kane, R. L., Shamliyan, T., Mueller, C., et al. (2007). *Nursing staffing and quality of patient care (Evidence report/technology assessment No. 151)*. Rockville, MD: Agency for Healthcare Research and Quality.

Kurtzman, E. T., & Jennings, B. M. (2008). Capturing the imagination of nurse executives in tracking quality of nursing care. *Nursing Administration Quarterly, 32*(3), 235–246. doi:10.1097/01. NAQ.0000325182.94589.7d

McGillis-Hall, L., Peterson, C., & Fairley, L. (2010). Losing the moment: Understanding interruptions in nurses' work. *Journal of Nursing Administration, 40*(4), 169–176. doi:10.1097/NNA. 0b013e3181d41162

Pomey, M. P., Lemieux-Charles, L., Champagne, F., et al. (2010). Does accreditation stimulate change? A study of the impact of the accreditation process on Canadian healthcare. *Implementation Science, 5*(31). doi:10.1186/1748-5908-5-31

Pronovost, P. J., Rosenstein, B. J., Paine, L., et al. (2008). Paying the piper: Investing in infrastructure for patient safety. *The Joint Commission Journal on Quality and Patient Safety, 34*(6), 342–348.

Singer, S. J., Gaba, D. M., Geppert, A. D., et al. (2003). The culture of safety: Results of an organization-wide survey in 15 California hospitals. *Quality and Safety in Healthcare, 12*, 112–118.

Squires, M., Tourangeau, A., Laschinger. H. K., et al. (2010). The link between leadership and safety outcomes in hospitals. *Journal of Nursing Management, 18*, 914–925. doi:10.1111/j.1365-2834.2010.01181.x

Thompson, D. N., Hoffman, L. A., Sereika, S. M., et al. (2011) A relational leadership perspective on unit-level safety climate. *Journal of Nursing Administration, 41*(11), 479–487. doi:10.1097/ NNA.0b013e3182346e31

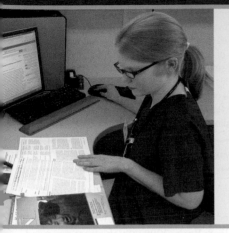

Translating Research into Practice

Margarete Lieb Zalon
Adapted by Barbara Campbell
With contributions from Selvi Roy

Nurses are "vital interpreters at the critical interface of the reality of patient care and the health system" (Pate, 2013, p. 187). This chapter describes the importance of translating and applying research into nursing practice. The role of the nurse as a leader, manager, and team member of a health care organization in applying research to practice is delineated using evidenced-informed data based on the best available research. This chapter also describes the practical aspects of evaluation and utilization of research, the development of evidence-based practice (EBP) in nursing, and the translation of all forms of knowledge into practice. Strategies for translating research into practice that can be used by all nurses in the context of the organization are outlined.

OBJECTIVES

- Value each nurse's obligation to use research in practice.
- Distinguish between research utilization, evidence-based practice, and experiential knowledge.
- Formulate a clinical research question supported by the literature.
- Evaluate resources to access the best available evidence.
- Identify resources for critically appraising evidence.
- Assess organizational barriers to and facilitators of the implementation of research into practice.
- Identify strategies for translating research into practice within the context of an organization.

TERMS TO KNOW

clinical practice guidelines	knowledge translation (KT)	research
diffusion of innovations	meta-analysis	research utilization
evidence-based practice	randomized controlled trial (RCT)	

? A CHALLENGE

Jade, a registered nurse with 7 years of surgical experience, works as a casual nurse on an orthopedic unit. At the beginning of one shift, shortly after midnight, Jade was told that she would receive an admission from the emergency department (ED). Jade prepared for the patient and received the verbal report from the ED nurse. Jade learned that the 58-year-old male patient was being admitted with an open humerus fracture and had a history of schizophrenia. The patient also had a developmental delay and was considered to be a "difficult" patient who was "agitated" and "aggressive." He arrived on Jade's unit in hysterics: he kept trying to climb out of bed, yelled (grunted), and was distraught. The ED nurse failed to tell Jade that the patient was deaf and virtually noncommunicative. The charge nurse immediately intervened with restraints and medication. She administered a large dose of haloperidol (Haldol) and morphine that she thought would surely settle him down. The patient's eyes would continuously roll back in his head. Moreover, he could not hear, could not speak besides the odd grunt, and had been assigned a legal guardian through the province. How was Jade going to communicate and provide ethically responsible care to this patient over the next 12 hours?

What do you think you would do if you were Jade?

INTRODUCTION

The challenge of translating research knowledge for use by practising nurses is a daunting task. Canadian research has lacked innovation in the dissemination of health research information, particularly in clinical nursing practice. **Knowledge translation (KT)** is defined by the Canadian Institutes of Health Research (CIHR, 2009) "as a dynamic and iterative process that includes synthesis, dissemination, exchange and ethically-sound application of knowledge to improve the health of Canadians, provide more effective health services and products and strengthen the health care system" (p. 1). *Canadian Nurse* interviewed leading nurse researchers to identify the importance of nursing research and how to build research capacity through translation and utilization of research to better health care and the profession ("In Conversation," 2010). Nurse researcher Gail Tomblin Murphy suggested that "the current health-care system is challenged by ongoing health professional shortages, increased patient acuity, and an increasing proportion of older workers in the workforce. Therefore it is important to create research utilization strategies that fit within the current context of health care" ("In Conversation," 2010). Nurse researcher Pammla Petrucka stated that "research is important to all nurses in all roles. . . . It augments our effectiveness as clinicians, educators and health-care leaders. It allows us to flourish as health professionals in terms of currency, relevance and evidence for care and quality. It validates our contributions, profiles our achievements and embodies our potential" ("In Conversation," 2010). Although a vast evidence base exists on nursing-related studies,

strategies are needed to adopt this knowledge in nursing practice (Polit & Beck, 2008). Such strategies need to be articulated clearly and in detail.

If you or a loved one required nursing care, you would want that care to be based on the best research evidence available. For example, if a family member needed to be on a ventilator, you would want to be sure that the nurses providing the care were using Best Practice Guidelines to prevent ventilator-associated pneumonia. You would want to know that communication and collaboration are excellent between nurses and physicians on the clinical unit where your family member has been placed. If that family member also had a central venous catheter, you would want to be sure that the nurse who removes that catheter is using an established current practice guideline that minimizes the risk for introducing an air embolism into the circulation. And, when that family member is discharged, you would want to know that the nurses are using evidence-based research and appropriate strategies to help that person transition to home, recover from his or her illness, and manage that illness. As a nurse manager or leader, you should be concerned about incorporating research not only into clinical practices but also into the management of systems of care. You know through research that teamwork and collaboration lead to lower mortality rates and fewer medication administration errors. The challenge, however, is how to (1) find the best research evidence, (2) determine the appropriateness of that research for the practice setting, (3) incorporate the best evidence into practice in a meaningful and timely manner, and (4) motivate clinical nurses and organizational leaders to use research evidence in the midst of all the other challenges facing delivery of high-quality nursing care.

Research is an integral part of professional practice. Research is the "diligent, systematic inquiry or investigation to validate and refine existing knowledge and generate new knowledge" (Burns & Grove, 2009, p. 2). According to nurse researcher Marlene Smadu, "Research answers questions regarding all domains of practice and ensures that practices are current, effective, efficient, patient centred, appropriate etc. The half-life of knowledge is decreasing rapidly, particularly in health care, and nurses must know how to get and create the kind of evidence they need to ensure high-quality practice in all domains" ("In Conversation," 2010). The Canadian Nurses Association (CNA, 2008) states, "Nurses support, use and engage in research and other activities that promote safe, competent, compassionate, and ethical care, and they use guidelines for ethical research that are in keeping with nursing values" (p. 13). Nurses develop and implement research-informed Best Practice Guidelines such as those disseminated through the Registered Nurses' Association of Ontario (RNAO) (http://www.rnao.ca). Best Practice Guidelines allow nurses to assess nursing and health care practices and implement recommendations where needed to enhance the quality of patient care (CNA, 2007). Nurses have the foundational knowledge to identify practice research questions and use research results to provide a scientific rationale for nursing interventions, thereby promoting quality patient care (CNA, 2014; College and Association of Registered Nurses of Alberta, 2005). CNA's latest research is related to nurse fatigue and its impact on patient care and professional health outcomes (Canadian Nurses Association & Registered Nurses Association of Ontario, 2010). Nurses are referred to as "knowledge navigators" who develop and implement research-based Best Practice Guidelines in the CNA (2007) document *Framework for the Practice of Registered Nurses in Canada*. The CNA released a compendium of evidence-based practice (EBP) guidelines in the form of a Primary Care Toolkit, which offers a variety of resources to help registered nurses use evidence in making decisions regarding patient care, including information about theories, clinical judgement, ethics, legislation, and practice environments (CNA, 2014).

As professionals, nurses have an obligation to society that involves rights and responsibilities as well as accountability. The Code of Ethics for Registered Nurses is a "statement of the ethical values of nurses and of nurses' commitments to persons with health-care needs and persons receiving care" (CNA, 2008, p. 3). These values, developed by Canadian nurses for all nurses in any practice environment, are translated through the following CNA statement: "Nurses support, use and engage in research and other activities that promote safe, competent, compassionate, and ethical care, and they use guidelines for ethical research that are in keeping with nursing values" (CNA, 2008, p. 13). Furthermore, an International Council of Nurses' (ICN, 2007) position statement on nursing research indicates that the organization "supports its national nurses associations (NNAs) in their efforts to enhance nursing research, particularly through: improving access to education which prepares nurses to conduct research, critically evaluate research outcomes and promote appropriate application of research findings to nursing practice" (p. 1).

The emphasis of translating research into practice is getting research into the hands of practitioners who can use it to improve patient care. Marlene Smadu suggested that nurse researchers partner with clinicians throughout the "whole research cycle, from working with them to formulate meaningful questions, to choosing appropriate methodologies, to sharing results, and to planning and implementing dissemination, translation and change" ("In Conversation," 2010). The translation of research into practice involves all health care disciplines. Gagnon, Labarthe, Legare, et al. (2011) found that one third of Canadians are affected by one of the six most common chronic conditions: heart disease, chronic obstructive pulmonary disease (COPD), diabetes, mood disorders, cancer, and arthritis. However, the implementation of research-based practice guidelines has been incomplete, highlighting the difficulty of translating research into practice. For example in the case of diabetes, even if several efficient strategies to prevent or delay diabetes complications exist, these strategies are suboptimally implemented in practice; that is, less than one half of the patients received the recommended lab tests and procedures. Only 50% of Canadians suffering from heart disease receive proven therapies on a regular basis. We might believe that once a research study is published in a journal, clinicians read it immediately and then nurses or policymakers use it to improve practice. Often, that is not the case. The CIHR (2013) supports research, capacity building, and knowledge translation, and it is through its Evidence Informed Healthcare Renewal initiative that multiple researchers and decision makers work together to advance the current state of knowledge, generate novel and creative solutions, and contribute to evidence-informed decision making about health care renewal in Canada.

Research provides the foundation for nursing practice improvement. Examples include preoperative teaching, pain management, child development assessment, falls prevention, pressure-ulcer risk detection, incontinence care, and family-centred care in critical care units. Rycroft-Malone, Seers, Titchen, et al. (2004) proposed that research informed by evidence comes from local data, professional knowledge, experiential knowledge, and patient experience. In addition, various researchers suggest that the best evidence combines theoretical, experiential, and tacit knowledge derived from professional experience and patient preferences (Benner, Hughes, & Sutphen, 2008). According to Brownson, Baker, Leet, et al. (2010), EBP involves integration of professional clinical expertise with best available clinical evidence from research. Nurses need to systematically evaluate nursing studies to decide what interventions should be implemented to improve the outcomes of care. Practices that were once thought to be the standard of care may quickly become outdated. Some practices may have been carried out for many years without ever being examined for their scientific basis or effectiveness. The latest research findings need to be incorporated into procedures and clinical practice guidelines (systematically developed statements of practice that assist practitioners and patients make appropriate clinical decisions) using an evidence-based model.

The integration of research into practice by knowledge users and practice into research by researchers bodes well for future implementation of EBP and, thus, improved health care (Gagnon et al., 2011). The Evidence section on page 431 illustrates how research can be incorporated into organizational practices.

EXERCISE 22-1

Identify a common activity that is part of your nursing practice, and determine whether any research supports that particular intervention or nursing care activity.

Nursing research designs can be categorized in several ways, such as basic versus applied, qualitative versus quantitative, cross-sectional versus longitudinal, experimental versus descriptive, and retrospective versus prospective. Regardless of the design, some research is ready for implementation and other research may not yet be ready to warrant a change in practice. Some decisions should not be based on the results of quantitative research alone but, instead, should be integrated with data from qualitative research when applied to a particular practice situation. The quality of care and the quality of patient outcomes can be dramatically improved with the implementation of EBP. Patients, those entrusted to our care, are deserving of practices that are based on the best available evidence. Examining the evidence for a particular practice generally needs to go beyond examining the results of a single study. A single, well-designed study might be adequate for recommending and implementing a practice change at times. However, developing an EBP requires the development of a clearly written clinical question and a more thorough search of the literature including a comprehensive review of single studies, meta-analyses, meta-syntheses, critically appraised topics, and systematic reviews.

Also, the evidence must be appraised and placed in the context of patient, family, and community values. Nurse managers or leaders may not necessarily be the ones actually conducting research, evaluating research evidence, or developing clinical practice guidelines, but they will be facilitating the application of research findings in practice. Key concepts for facilitating improved nursing outcomes include research utilization, EBP, diffusion of innovations, translating research into practice, evaluation of evidence, organizational strategies (for translating research into practice), and issues for nurse managers and leaders faced with implementing these processes.

RESEARCH UTILIZATION

Research utilization is the process of synthesizing, disseminating, and using research-generated knowledge to influence or change existing practices (Burns & Grove, 2009). Research utilization is different from, but complementary to, research. Although individual nurses may apply research findings to their own practice, nurses' broader responsibility to society includes activating the change process in translating research into practice. Research can be used for a variety of purposes: enlightenment, implementation of a research-based protocol, or the widespread adoption of standards based on research findings. Ultimately, multiple factors influence how a particular research finding is adopted, translated into practice, and sustained in practice.

Nurse researchers have a distinguished record of facilitating research utilization in clinical practice that has gone beyond dissemination through publication in research journals, but the gap of adapting research into practice still exists. Squires, Hutchinson, Bostrom, et al. (2011) recently conducted a systematic review to identify and analyze how nurses have used research findings in practice over the past 40 years. According to this review, nurses reported a moderate-high use of research, a level that remained relatively consistent over time until the early 2000s. The relatively unchanged self-reporting and the absence of studies to assess the effects of research use by nurses on patient outcomes is troubling with the increasing emphasis on EBP and easy access to electronic resources in research.

Many research utilization models in nursing were developed in the 1970s and 1980s. One of the first was the Stetler-Marram model developed in 1976, which now includes the facilitation of EBP (Stetler, 2001).

Originally, research utilization consisted of evaluating research and determining its applicability to practice; in the 1990s, this focus changed to finding research-based solutions to a problem. Stetler's (2001) research utilization model provides direction for an individual and for group members. It has implications for nurses in leadership roles responsible for patient care management. According to Stetler, the preparatory steps of research utilization sustain EBP. Stetler's model consists of five phases: preparation, validation, comparative evaluation or decision making, translation or application, and evaluation (Figure 22-1). The preparatory phase involves searching, sorting, and selecting sources of evidence, defining external factors influencing the application of a research finding, and defining internal factors diminishing objectivity. The second phase, validation, focuses on utilization with an appraisal of study findings rather than the critique of a study's design. This phase includes completing review tables to facilitate understanding each study and to facilitate decision making. The third phase,

comparative evaluation and decision making, involves making a decision about the applicability of the studies by synthesizing cumulative findings; evaluating the degree and nature of other criteria, such as risk, feasibility, and readiness of the finding; and actually making a recommendation about using the research. The fourth phase, translation and application, involves practical aspects of implementing the plan for translating the research into practice at the individual, group, department, or organizational level. Multiple strategies are recommended for the implementation of change. It is important to be sure that translating the research finding into practice does not exceed what the evidence warrants. The last phase includes an evaluation, which can be informal or formal and may include a cost–benefit analysis. Evaluation can include whether the research innovation was implemented as intended and goal achievement. Stetler's model focuses heavily on the change process to facilitate the successful translation of research into practice.

The knowledge-to-action model (Figure 22-2) developed by Straus, Tetroe, and Graham (2009) has been adopted by the CIHR as a model promoting the application of research and the process of knowledge translation in Canada.

The authors suggest this model is iterative, dynamic, and complex; it ranges from knowledge creation through multiple stages of action toward implementation. The action cycle consists of seven key steps, commencing with the identification of the problem (gap). This critical element of the action cycle acts as the foundation for the remaining stages in the knowledge-to-action cycle, as programs will be tailored to address the specifics of the gap. The next step in the cycle (once the gap has been identified) is adapting the research to the local context. Localizing knowledge requires an assessment of the barriers and key facilitators to knowledge implementation, as barriers and facilitators are analyzed and interwoven into the strategic initiative. Knowledge translation interventions need to be selected, tailored, and implemented based on the best research evidence or practices when dealing with a problem. Sustainability of knowledge through action ensures the continued implementation of innovative, evidence-based research in end-user programs and clinical practice guidelines. Adapting clinical practice guidelines for local use means that knowledge and the best evidence have been translated

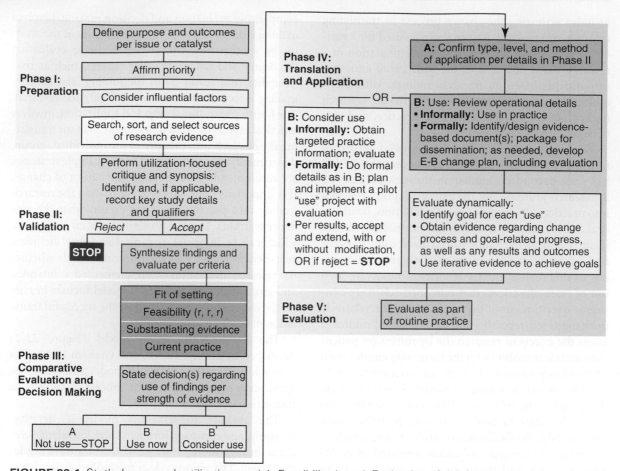

FIGURE 22-1 Stetler's research utilization model. *Feasibility (r, r, r),* Evaluation of *r*isk factors, need for *r*esources, and *r*eadiness of others involved.

into a set of specific recommendations for end users. This next section of the knowledge-to-action process deals with possible intervention directions one might face when determining the best possible approach in knowledge translation strategies. Therefore, it is imperative that research findings be communicated to those who can use the research effectively through program implementation in specific practice settings. Linkages and exchange activities such as face-to-face outreach visits and opinion leadership conferences are based on social interactions, relationships, and networks (Straus et al., 2009).

In 2006, a CIHR-funded study used participatory action research to understand a rural East Coast community's knowledge about their children's health. A conceptual knowledge translation framework and the

Ottawa Model of Research Use were applied to translate the knowledge gathered into action (Campbell, 2010). The graphical depiction of "applying knowledge to generate action" (Figure 22-3 on page 418.) incorporates the activities of community members and researchers working collaboratively to translate community knowledge and research into health promotion programs. The results indicated that the knowledge translated must be relevant, appropriate, applicable, timely, and reasonable to the needs of the users.

According to Straus, Tetroe, and Graham (2009), "Failures to use evidence from research to make informed decisions in healthcare are evident across all groups of decision-makers, including healthcare providers, patients, informal caregivers, managers and policymakers" (p. 165). One Canadian example of

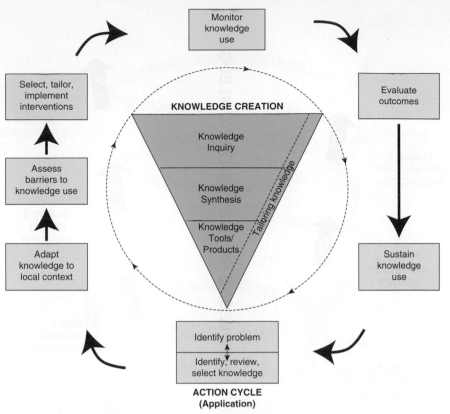

FIGURE 22-2 Straus, Tetroe, and Graham's knowledge-to-action model.

this gap in research to practice is the underprescribing of statins to reduce the risk of mortality and morbidity, which has been cited in several randomized trials (LaRosa, He, & Vupputuri, 1999; Majumdar, McAlister, & Furberg, 2004), while antibiotics continue to be overprescribed in children with upper respiratory tract symptoms (Arnold & Straus, 2005).

EVIDENCE-BASED PRACTICE

Evidence-based practice (EBP) is the integration of the best research evidence with clinical expertise and the patient's unique values and circumstances in making decisions about the care of individual patients (Straus, Richardson, Glasziou, et al., 2005). Ingersoll (2000) developed one of the first definitions for evidence-based nursing practice: "the conscientious, explicit, and judicious use of theory-derived, research-based information on making decisions about care delivery to individuals or groups of patients and in consideration of individual needs and preferences" (p. 151). EBP integrates current research on best practices, clinical expertise, and patient values to optimize patient outcomes as well as quality of life (Sackett, Straus, Richardson, et al., 2000). In EBP, clinical problems or gaps drive the search for solutions based on the best available evidence, which is then translated into practice. EBP is a broader, more encompassing view of research utilization. It is focused on searching for and evaluating the best evidence to address a particular clinical practice problem. A number of models exist for creating and implementing EBP, all based on the following five key essential elements (Moyer & Elliott, 2004): (1) ask a clinical question, (2) acquire the evidence, (3) appraise the evidence, (4) apply the evidence, and (5) assess the outcomes. Precisely articulating a clinical question is the first step in the process. Once the question is confirmed, an electronic literature search must be undertaken to acquire the existing evidence specific to the issue being researched. Critically analyzing the

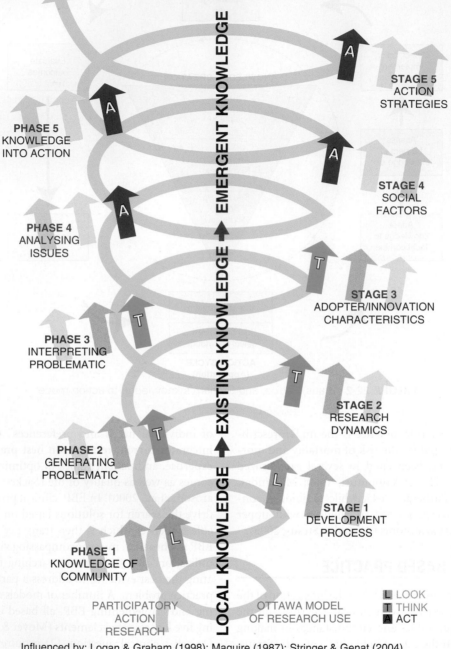

FIGURE 22-3 Conceptual Framework: Applying knowledge to generate action.

existing information on this topic is essential due to the volume of information available. At this time, a mechanism needs to be in place to disseminate the results of this research through communication and education to help identify necessary processes and outcome measures that should be assessed prior to any changes in a clinical practice site. Measuring process and outcome changes is a key step in the EBP model. Information systems play a key role in this process by measuring daily practice against evidence-based guidelines, standards, or protocols. The stage of evaluation is not a one-time activity with such changes so it needs to be ongoing, reflective, and iterative. The role of the organization in implementing EBP is illustrated by S. J. Brown (2008) in the Literature Perspective.

LITERATURE PERSPECTIVE

Resource: Brown, S. J. (2008). Time to move on: Definitions of evidence-based practice. *Journal of Nursing Care Quality, 23*, 201. http://dx.doi.org/10.1097/01.NCQ.0000324582.67180.4b

Using a definition of evidence-based practice (EBP) based on definitions of evidence-based medicine is limiting because those definitions do not accommodate EBP as it is practised in clinical settings in which nurses work. Evidence-based medicine focuses on individual clinicians using research evidence for individual patients, whereas nurses typically practise within an organizational context and are part of an interdisciplinary team. Many nurses providing direct care have not had the educational preparation for the use of EBP. Workplace pressures may also affect the use of EBP.

Implications for Practice
EBP models in nursing need to include a broader-based organizational approach that more accurately reflects the use of evidence-based standards of care for patient populations and the nurse's use of research evidence for patient-care decisions.

EBP, including evidence-based medicine, is derived from the work of Archie Cochrane. He described the lack of knowledge about health care treatment effects and advocated for the use of proven treatments. Subsequently, the Cochrane Collaboration was established at Oxford University in 1993. About that time, Gordon Guyatt and his colleagues at McMaster University authored a series of articles in the *Journal of the American Medical Association* known as the *Users' Guides to the Medical Literature*. These articles provided a foundation for teaching evidence-based medicine. Since then, the EBP movement has grown exponentially with the establishment of centres, resources on the Web, and grants given specifically to advance the translation of research into practice. A number of evidence-based nursing centres have been established around the world. The Joanna Briggs Institute, based in Australia, has a network of collaborating centres and evidence-based synthesis and utilization groups around the world. These centres have teams of researchers who critically appraise evidence and then disseminate protocols for the use of evidence in practice. PubMed Central Canada (http://pubmedcentralcanada.ca/pmcc/) provides free access to an online digital archive of full-text peer-reviewed research publications in health and life sciences. Resources for evidence-based health care are listed in Box 22-1. Many nursing education programs incorporate EBP into their curricula.

Our understanding of how evidence is used in practice is evolving and, in response, associated terminology is changing. Increasingly, nursing and other health-based literature is using the phrase

BOX 22-1 RESOURCES FOR EVIDENCE-BASED HEALTH CARE

Canadian Business and Current Affairs (CBCA) Database: http://www.lib.uwo.ca/business/cbca.html
Centre for Evidence-Based Medicine Toronto: http://ktclearinghouse.ca/cebm/
Centre for Reviews and Dissemination (CRD): http://www.york.ac.uk/inst/crd/
The Cochrane Collaboration: http://www.cochrane.org
Cochrane Database of Systematic Reviews (CDSR): http://www.cochrane.org/editorial-and-publishing-policy-resource/cochrane-database-systematic-reviews-cdsr
Database of Abstracts of Reviews of Effects (DARE): http://onlinelibrary.wiley.com/o/cochrane/cochrane_cldare_articles_fs.html
Government Information: MacOdrum Library, Carleton University: http://www.library.carleton.ca/find/government-information
Health Technology Assessment (HTA) Database: http://www.cochrane.org/editorial-and-publishing-policy-resource/health-technology-assessment-database-hta
National Guideline Clearinghouse: http://www.guideline.gov
National Institute for Health and Clinical Excellence: http://www.nice.org.uk
PubMed Central Canada: http://pubmedcentralcanada.ca/pmcc/
Scottish Intercollegiate Guidelines Network (SIGN): http://www.sign.ac.uk

"evidence-informed" rather than "evidence-based" to describe decision making about the care of patients based on health-related research. Evidence-informed practice recognizes that decisions are not always made solely based on research and that other factors influence decision making, such as local indigenous knowledge, cultural and religious norms, and clinical judgement. You will notice in this textbook that we primarily use "evidence-informed" to convey that broader understanding of decision making. As the terminology evolves, you will find that sometimes terms are used interchangeably. For example, the CNA's NurseONE Web site discusses "strategies to promote evidence-based practice/evidence-informed decision-making by nurses" (http://www.nurseone.ca/Default .aspx?portlet=StaticHtmlViewerPortlet&plang=1& ptnme=Strategies to promote evidence-based practice). The discussion of EBP in this chapter is important to enhance understanding of how the term entered nursing's language and how it is changing.

Various organizations have developed evidence-based standards of practice and clinical guidelines. The Oncology Nursing Society and the Registered Nurses' Association of Ontario have developed tool-kits for EBP, while the CNA has a comprehensive Web site (http://www.nurseone.ca/Default.aspx?portlet= StaticHtmlViewerPortlet&stmd=False&plang=1& ptdi=1798) offering clinical practice guidelines for over 20 nursing-specific primary care topics. Societal factors such as the rising cost of health care, quality improvement initiatives, and the pressures to avoid errors have resulted in an increased emphasis on research as a basis for practice decisions. Nurses and other health care providers are called upon to use evidence in practice in the midst of an exponentially expanding scientific knowledge base.

Nursing research exists on a continuum, and not all research is ready for, or of a quality that is appropriate for, implementation, or it may not be ready for implementation in a particular setting. However, the quality of care and the quality of the outcomes of care can be dramatically improved with the implementation of evidence-based nursing practices. Nurses are heeding the call to develop evidenced-based practices. Burns and Grove (2011) suggest current research could be a systematic analysis of a treatment, a service, or an intervention to produce the most effective outcome. The steps toward engaging in effective research to inform a health-practice context are similar to any decision-making process (including the nursing process):

1. Define the issue or the problem.
2. Search the appropriate research evidence efficiently.
3. Critically and efficiently appraise the available resources.
4. Interpret information and synthesize the evidence.
5. Adapt the evidence and the resources to the local context.
6. Implement the evidence into practice, program, policy development, or decision making.
7. Evaluate the effectiveness of implementation efforts (Ciliska, Thomas, & Buffett, 2008).

The Ontario Public Health Association (2009) in collaboration with McMaster University developed a tool known as Towards Evidence Informed Practice (TEIP) in response to requests from Canadian health promoters for practical tools to facilitate the systematic search and application of reliable and relevant evidence to support programming in health promotion.

Nurse managers and leaders have a critical responsibility in promoting the use of the best evidence that informs practice. Resources for evidence-informed nursing are listed in Box 22-2.

BOX 22-2 **RESOURCES FOR EVIDENCE-BASED/ EVIDENCE-INFORMED NURSING**

Canadian Nurses Association's Online Primary Care Toolkit: Evidence-Based Practice: http://www.nurseone.ca/Default. aspx?portlet=StaticHtmlViewerPortlet&plang=1&ptdi=514
The Joanna Briggs Institute: http://joannabriggs.org
The Sarah Cole Hirsch Institute for Best Nursing Practices Based on Evidence: http://fpb.case.edu/Centers/Hirsh/
Oncology Nursing Society Evidence-Based Practice Resource Area (EBPRA): https://www2.ons.org/Research/EBPRA
The Registered Nurses' Association of Ontario Nursing Best Practice Guidelines: http://rnao.ca/bpg

---

EXERCISE 22-2

Select a clinical guideline appropriate for implementation in your clinical setting (see the Canadian Nurses Association Online Primary Care Toolkit (http://www.nurseone.ca). Identify as many strategies as possible for disseminating the guideline's key points to staff nurses at your facility or a facility where you have your clinical experiences. Compare your list of strategies with that of a colleague.

DIFFUSION OF INNOVATIONS

The now classic theory of diffusion of innovations (Rogers, 2003) describes how innovations spread through society, occurring in stages: knowledge, persuasion, decision, implementation, and confirmation. This theory, highlighted in the Theory Box, provides a useful model in planning for the integration of evidence into practice over time.

An innovation might be continued because of the positive reinforcement received when outcomes are favourable. An innovation also might be discontinued—for example, when a better idea is adopted or when disenchantment occurs because of dissatisfaction with the process or outcome.

An intervention's characteristics can influence its adoption. These include the relative advantage (whether it is better than what it replaces), compatibility (consistency with values, experiences, needs), complexity (difficulty in understanding its use), trialability (the degree to which it can be easily tested), and observability (the ease of seeing the results) (Rogers, 2003).

Widespread media attention to a particular finding can be instrumental in the adoption of a practice change. Extensive publicity accompanied the publication of a study about family presence during emergency procedures and resuscitation (Meyers, Eichhorn, Guzzetta, et al., 2000). Publication of the study was accompanied by press releases and television news stories. Since then, the research was replicated and expanded to other settings (Smith, Hefley, & Anand, 2007), thus strengthening the scientific basis for the innovation and facilitating the practice of allowing families to be present during resuscitation. Hatfield, Gusic, Dyer, et al. (2008) found that the administration of oral sucrose to babies receiving their 2-month and 4-month immunizations reduced their pain scores. Their study received wide publicity in media outlets. Thus parents were alerted about the importance of asking that this simple pain management strategy be implemented for their infants when being immunized.

Nurse researchers write clinical articles in addition to research articles. Many journals that are directed toward clinicians provide nurses with easy-to-understand summaries of studies from the general health care and nursing research literature. Nursing schools develop press releases when researchers

THEORY BOX

Rogers' Diffusion of Innovations Theory

STAGE	KEY IDEA	ACTIVITIES
Knowledge	Exposure to an innovation and how it functions	The process includes seeking and analyzing information. Literature reviews are focused on addressing practice problems. Information can be disseminated through journals, conferences, educational programs, audiovisual or electronic media, journal clubs, or other outlets.
Persuasion	Development of attitudes about an innovation through psychological involvement and selective perception	Informal communication networks are used to facilitate change. Positive or negative attitudes can develop. An event or activity can be used to spark interest in moving from a favourable attitude to behaviour change.
Decision	Commitment to adoption	The innovation can be adopted, adopted and then discontinued, rejected outright, or not even considered by the organization at this stage.
Implementation	Putting the innovation into practice	Change agents provide support for the implementation process. Behaviour changes as the innovation is adopted. Key features of an innovation are identified to evaluate its effectiveness. Problems with implementing the innovation are addressed. Change and modification (reinvention) occur to use the innovation in a particular practice environment. Reinvention facilitates the sustainability of the innovation.
Confirmation	Evaluating the innovation	A decision is made about continuing or discontinuing the innovation. The innovation, if adopted, is integrated into the organization's practices.

Data from Rogers, E. M. (2003). *Diffusion of innovations* (5th ed.). New York, NY: Free Press, pp. 171–195.

publish studies, which are then used by the media for their news articles. For example, Rachel Jones (2008) conducted research on the use of urban soap opera videos delivered on a handheld device to convey messages about HIV risk reduction in young adult urban women. Publicity in various media outlets in the community, her receipt of a *New York Times* award, and the Web site Stop HIV—Women's Power Against HIV/AIDS (http://ncs.newark.rutgers.edu/media-gallery/detail/942/998) have increased the visibility of this important public health problem.

EXERCISE 22-3

Locate a research column in a clinical nursing journal. Identify one study that has implications for your practice. Retrieve the original article to learn more about the patient population, details of the study design, and results.

The translation of research into practice requires that nurse managers and leaders understand group dynamics, individual responses to innovation and change, and the culture of their health care organization. Rogers (2003) categorized people according to how quickly they are willing to adopt an innovation. Box 22-3 describes these categories. Understanding the characteristics of innovation adopters is critical when planning to introduce new practices based on research evidence.

Nursing as a profession has an obligation to the public to condense the 17-year typical time frame from

BOX 22-3	**CHARACTERISTICS OF INNOVATION ADOPTERS**

TYPE	CHARACTERISTICS
Innovators	They thrive on change, which may be disruptive to the unit stability.
Early adopters	They are respected by their peers and thus are sought out for advice and information about innovations and changes.
Early majority	They prefer doing what has been done in the past but eventually will accept new ideas.
Late majority	They are openly negative and agree to the change only after most others have accepted the change.
Laggards	They prefer keeping traditions and openly express their resistance to new ideas.

Data from Rogers, E. M. (1995). *Diffusion of innovations* (4th ed.). New York, NY: Free Press.

the discovery to the adoption of a research finding. Those committed to the EBP movement in nursing have attempted to speed up the adoption of innovations. Rogers' (2003) theory of diffusion of innovations is useful in helping us understand how research can be disseminated to the larger community. It also provides guidance on how to take advantage of organizational dynamics to accelerate the process.

The diffusion of an innovation does not necessarily follow a linear path. External factors may sometimes contribute to the adoption of an innovation. These may include the development of standards regarding the practice that are widely disseminated, cost-effectiveness studies, changes in the products or technology, the publication of clear and compelling evidence, and changes in staff members and leadership at an institution. A meta-analysis of the use of saline and the elimination of a low-dose heparin (Heparin) flush solution for capped angiocatheters is a well-known example of compelling evidence for innovation diffusion (Goode, Titler, Rakel, et al., 1991). A meta-analysis statistically combines the results of similar studies to determine whether the aggregated findings are significant. Although some institutions continued to use heparin flushes for a number of years, their use became less common and all but disappeared in the late 1990s. The decreased use of heparin flushes was considerably later than one would expect, given the compelling nature of the evidence. This example illustrates the particular challenges in implementing an EBP when more than one discipline is involved. The innovation needed to be communicated to nurses. Nurses also needed to convince physicians and the institutional hierarchy that using heparin was no longer appropriate. For some institutions, it was not until the costs were analyzed and concerns were raised about complications from small doses of heparin that the transition to saline flushes was finally accomplished. This research has been extended to central line catheters in adults and capped peripheral and central line catheters in children and neonates. A systematic review of heparin use in peripheral intravenous catheters in neonates indicated that because of variations in the neonates' clinical conditions and treatments, a recommendation to use heparin could not be made (Shah, Ng, & Sinha, 2005). The American Society of Health-System Pharmacists (2006) concurred about the lack of clarity in using heparin in intravenous catheters placed in children and neonates. Unfortunately, heparin's continued use has led to several widely publicized serious and deadly errors. Thus, careful analysis of research results, the timely implementation of important findings, and ongoing clinical research are critical to the nurse's role in promoting patient safety.

Another example of innovation diffusion is a review of the evidence for intramuscular injection technique conducted by Malkin (2008). The practice of administering intramuscular injections for pain management to adults in acute care settings has virtually disappeared with the use of the intravenous and epidural routes. Malkin rightfully emphasized that nurses learn the technique in their initial nursing program but may never subsequently question their practice in using this technique. Intramuscular injections are widely used in many settings throughout the world to deliver long-acting antibiotics; biologicals such as immune globulins, vaccines, and toxoids; and hormonal agents. The use of the dorso-gluteal site is no longer recommended, yet we do not know what proportion of nurses continue to use this technique. This review provides nurses with an evidence-based research-based standard that takes on even more significance because of wide variation among nurses in injection technique.

Madsen, Sebolt, Cullen, et al. (2005) questioned the practice of listening to the bowel sounds of abdominal surgery patients to assess the return of gastrointestinal motility. They concluded that the presence or absence of bowel sounds was not associated with any interventions. The authors recommended that problems experienced by patients after abdominal surgery that indicate absent bowel motility (e.g., nausea, abdominal distention) can be treated with interventions such as administering an antiemetic or inserting a nasogastric tube. A practice guideline was developed and evaluated by the research team outlining the steps in gastrointestinal assessment. Astute practitioners should observe for the subsequent adoption of these guidelines by nurses in other health care facilities and whether textbooks continue to mention the assessment of bowel sounds for patients after abdominal surgery.

Fetzer's (2002) meta-analysis of 20 studies demonstrated that the pain of venipuncture and intravenous line insertion could be reduced in 85% of the population (adults and children) with the use of an eutectic mixture of local anesthetics (EMLA) cream. This practice has not been widely adopted; this practice was illustrated by a study conducted in a large urban pediatric setting that indicated that minor procedures are commonly performed without pain management (MacLean, Obispo, & Young, 2007). A stumbling block described by practitioners is the length of time required for the EMLA to take effect. This issue is also indicative of the relative value placed on patient comfort and patient satisfaction and the challenge in using research to change pain management practices.

TRANSLATING RESEARCH INTO PRACTICE

Research takes a long time to be translated into practice. Consider the classic example of scurvy. James Lancaster demonstrated that lemon juice supplements eliminated scurvy in sailors in 1601, and James Lind replicated that finding in 1747. However, it was not until 1795 that the British navy added a citrus-juice supplement to the diet of its sailors (S. R. Brown, 2005). In nursing, medication tickets or small cards were first used in 1910 to facilitate the administration of medications. One hundred years later, some institutions are still using these tickets as reminders for some aspects of their medication-administration or treatment-administration systems despite evidence of the potential for error through their loss or duplication. This issue is indicative of a much broader problem related to the limited use of electronic health records. According to Geibert (2006), "Technology is the bridge to integrating EBP [evidence-based practice] into patient care" (p. 132).

Although interest in research utilization in nursing paralleled the development of nursing as a research-based discipline, the actual translation of research into practice has not been as rapid. The seminal work of Funk, Champagne, Wiese, et al. (1991) in categorizing barriers to research utilization according to the research itself, the nurse, the setting or organization, and presentation demonstrated that nurses perceived the most significant barrier to be organizational support, particularly time to use and conduct research. Nearly 10 years later, barriers to using research in Australia included access to research, anticipated outcomes of research use, organizational support, and support from others (Retsas, 2000). Some of these same barriers exist today.

The conceptual structure of research utilization includes direct, indirect, and persuasive aspects of research utilization (Estabrooks, 1999). An example of direct research utilization consists of actually using recommended interventions to prevent ventilator-associated pneumonia. An indirect research utilization example is when a nurse reads a research report and then has greater understanding of a person's response to diabetic teaching. An example of persuasive research utilization is when nurses work to implement an institutional change in practice such as using pH paper to test nasogastric tube placement. Different strategies should be used to achieve different research utilization goals.

When planning to translate a research finding into practice, nurses need to know what types of strategies have been most successful. It is also helpful to know how much time commitment was involved, how often the strategy was used, how long the treatment lasted, and whether the results were sustainable. Nurses are now testing the effectiveness of specific interventions within an organizational context and evaluating adherence to evidence-based guidelines. For example, although results may be good from a particular protocol used in a randomized controlled trial to decrease ventilator-associated pneumonia, those same results may not be as dramatic when the protocol is implemented at institutions with varying resources and degrees of commitment to implementing the protocol. Nurses need to pay careful attention to the development of a clinical protocol or an evidence-based guideline and also address the implementation process. For example, implementation of these guidelines with regard to pain management continues to be challenging. The implementation of an evidence-based pain management protocol for older adults with hip fractures not only improves the quality of pain management for these patients but also reduces hospital costs (Brooks, Titler, Ardery, et al., 2009; Titler, Herr, Brooks, et al., 2009). This evidence-based protocol used multi-faceted strategies including practitioners' review and "reinvention" of the evidence-based guideline, quick reference guides, and clinical reminders. In addition, the use of opinion leaders and change champions, a 3-day train-the-trainer educational program, and educational outreach for physicians and nurses was incorporated into the protocol. The intervention had a strong effect on nurse practice but had less effect on physician practices (Titler et al., 2009).

Dobbins, Ciliska, Estabrooks, et al. (2005) evaluated the strength of the research evidence for various strategies that promote behavioural change among health care providers. Consistently effective strategies included academic detailing or educational outreach visits (providing health care providers with accurate information in face-to-face visits), reminders, multi-faceted interventions, and interactive education meetings and workshops. Strategies having mixed effects included audit and feedback, local opinion leaders, local consensus processes, and patient-mediated interventions. Strategies having little or no effect included the distribution of educational materials and didactic educational programs. The key point here is that active involvement leads to greater success. In a systematic review of interventions to increase nurses' research use, only four studies met inclusion criteria (Thompson, Estabrooks, Scott-Findlay, et al., 2007). Educational meetings led by an opinion leader and formation of interdisciplinary committees were effective at increasing research use. Clearly, such limited evidence illustrates the need for additional research to examine best practices in increasing nurses' use of research.

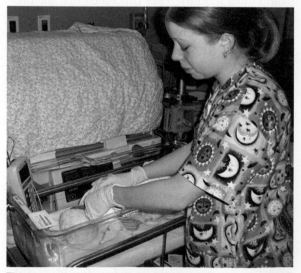

The purpose of gathering and analyzing evidence is to improve patient care.

The public and government agencies will increasingly expect that research findings be implemented, particularly when that implementation can lead to significant improvements in patient outcomes and cost savings.

Evidence-based nursing involves a fundamental shift in philosophy. Rather than relying on nurses (be they clinicians, managers, or administrators) to read the research and apply it to practice, nurses are now expected to analyze practice problems and identify the research that will help them answer questions about how they should go about delivering care.

EVALUATION OF EVIDENCE

Evidence is best evaluated with a systematic process. The EBP steps are illustrated in Box 22-4. The first steps in the implementation of EBP are creating a spirit of inquiry and identifying the problem so that the relevant information can be obtained. The clinical question can be put into the widely used PICOT format of *patient population, intervention or interest area, comparison intervention or issue of interest, outcome,* and *time* to facilitate searching for the appropriate evidence (Melnyk, Fineout-Overholt, Stillwell, et al., 2010; Thabane, Thomas, Ye, et al., 2009). These steps are illustrated in Box 22-5.

Identifying the question may be the most challenging part of the process. Different strategies can be used to identify practice problems. For example, one might conduct a survey of staff members or use a focus group methodology. Conducting a staff survey would necessitate that staff members have sufficient knowledge of research and EBP to understand what is desired. The data from surveys or focus groups, or even informal interviews with staff, can be examined along with patient outcome data for a particular setting to address relevant practice problems. Collaborating with nurses and extending that to collaboration with members of other disciplines to identify desired outcomes will enhance the ultimate success of an evidence-based project. This is because the staff members who will eventually be involved in implementing the practice are involved in its design and conception. Once the clinical question has been identified, writing it down will help in moving on to the next step of gathering evidence.

BOX 22-4   STEPS IN EVIDENCE-BASED PRACTICE

1. Cultivate a spirit of inquiry.
2. Ask the burning clinical question in PICOT (patient population, intervention or interest area, comparison intervention or issue of interest, outcome, and time) format.
3. Search for and collect the most relevant best evidence.
4. Critically appraise the evidence (i.e., rapid critical appraisal, evaluation, and synthesis).
5. Integrate the best evidence with one's clinical expertise and patient preferences and values in making a practice decision or change.
6. Evaluate outcomes of the practice design or change based on evidence.
7. Disseminate the outcomes of the EBP (evidence-based practice) decision or change.

From Melnyk, B. M., & Fineout-Overholt, E. (2011). Making the case for evidence-based practice and cultivating a spirit of inquiry. In B. M. Melnyk & E. Fineout-Overholt (Eds.), *Evidence-based practice in nursing and healthcare: A guide to best practice* (pp. 3–24). Philadelphia, PA: Lippincott, Williams & Wilkins.

BOX 22-5   ASKING THE RIGHT QUESTION: THE PICOT FORMAT

Patient population — What is the patient population or the setting? This could be adults, children, or neonates with a certain health problem; or home care versus an acute care setting.

Intervention/interest Area — What is the intervention? This can be an intervention or a specific area of interest (e.g., postoperative complications, the experience of postoperative pain).

Comparison — What is a comparison intervention? This is what the intervention might be compared with, such as a treatment, or the absence of a risk factor.

Outcome — What are the results? There might be multiple strategies to measure the results, such as complication rate, satisfaction, a nursing diagnosis, or a nursing quality indicator.

Time — What is the time frame for this intervention? Is time a relevant factor for this particular evaluation? For example, are you interested in short-term or long-term outcomes?

Adapted from Thabane, L., Thomas, T., Ye, C., et al. (2009). Posing the research question: Not so simple. *Canadian Journal of Anaesthesia, 56,* 71–79. http://dx.doi.org/10.1007/s12630 008-9007-4

EXERCISE 22-4

Here is an example of how to apply the PICOT format.

Example question: Can listening to sedative music for 45 minutes at bedtime over a 3-month period influence sleep duration and sleep quality among older adults in a long-term care facility?

Using the PICOT format this question can be broken up as follows:

P = Older adults in a long-term care facility

I = Listening to sedative music

C = Usual care (no music at bedtime)

O = Improved sleep duration and enhanced sleep quality

T = 45 minutes every day for 3 months

Now try to organize these research questions into the PICOT format.

1. Can the frequency and duration of visitation by family members influence recovery of older adult patients in critical care units?

2. Do compression stockings help prevent distension of veins in women over 65 years old who travel long distances?

3. Are pediatric patients who are rewarded for cooperating during nursing procedures more cooperative during subsequent nursing procedures than pediatric patients who are not rewarded?

Develop a clinical question using the PICOT format. Do a search in the Cumulative Index to Nursing and Allied Health Literature (CINAHL) (http://www.ebscohost.com/nursing/products/cinahl-databases) with the key PICOT terms.

The third step of the process is searching for and collecting evidence. A number of databases are available to search for evidence. Some databases contain preprocessed evidence, such as abstracts of studies and systematic reviews of evidence. Others contain citations for original single studies. Commonly used databases are listed in Box 22-6. Obtaining a librarian's assistance to navigate the databases is helpful because the databases are constantly being upgraded with new features. Several of the suggested readings that appear on the Evolve website (http://evolve.elsevier.com/Canada/Yoder-Wise/leading/) include more details on locating research evidence. Preprocessed evidence can also be located in the evidence-based/evidence-informed resources listed in Boxes 22-1 and 22-2 (see pp. 419 and 420).

The evidence for a particular practice problem can come from a single research study, an integrative review of the literature, a meta-analysis, a meta-synthesis, a clinically appraised topic, a clinical guideline, or a systematic review. Sometimes a single research study might be appropriate for application to a particular problem. For other clinical questions, there might be multiple guidelines from different organizations on essentially the same clinical problem with

BOX 22-6   COMMONLY USED DATABASES AND SEARCH PLATFORMS FOR NURSING

Evidence Based Practice Resources
http://hsl.mcmaster.ca/resources/topic/eb/nurse.html

An Introduction to Evidence Based Practice for Nursing Students (McMaster University)

CINAHL Cumulative Index to Nursing and Allied Health Literature
http://www.ebscohost.com/cinahl/

A comprehensive nursing and allied health abstract database that includes some full-text material such as state nursing journals, nurse practice acts, research instruments, government publications, and patient education material from 1982 to the present

Clinical Decision-Making (Evidence-Based Health Care)
http://www.mcgill.ca/library/find/subjects/health/evidence

Access to sources for background information, core and additional databases, and drug information (McGill Univ..sity, Life Sciences Library)

EBSCO
http://www.ebscohost.com

A search platform for a variety of databases including CINAHL and MEDLINE. By institutional subscription.

NurseONE
http://www.nurseone.ca

NurseONE.ca is a personalized interactive Web-based resource that provides nurses in Canada with access to current and reliable information to support their nursing practice, manage their careers, and connect with colleagues and health care experts.

OVID
http://www.ovid.com

A search platform for a variety of databases including CINAHL and MEDLINE. By institutional subscription and individual pay-per-view.

PsycINFO
http://www.apa.org/pubs/databases/psycinfo/index.aspx

Abstract database of the behavioural sciences and mental health literature from the 1800s to the present. By institutional subscription or individual article purchase.

PubMed
http://www.ncbi.nlm.nih.gov/pubmed

The abstract database of the National Library of Medicine, providing access to over 15 million citations from the 1950s to the present. Links to publishers' websites for many articles. Free.

slightly different recommendations. DiCenso, Ciliska, and Guyatt (2005) describe a hierarchy for rating the strength of evidence for treatment decisions as follows:

1. Unsystematic clinical observations
2. Physiological studies (e.g., blood pressure, bone density)
3. Single observational study addressing important patient outcomes
4. Systematic review of observational studies addressing important patient outcomes
5. Randomized trial
6. Systematic review of randomized trials

A hierarchy of preprocessed evidence (i.e., evidence from a single research study to systems that integrate and regularly update EBP) originally developed by Haynes (2001) and adapted by Collins, Voth, DiCenso, et al. (2005) is illustrated in Figure 22-4. Researchers examining evidence and developing guidelines use a variety of different rating systems that include a hierarchy and key quality domains. Rating evidence is a rapidly growing field. No single established method of rating evidence is best for all situations. Ultimately, whoever conducts the analysis will have to make some decisions about the strength of the evidence and whether it can be applied to a particular patient population. What is important is that once the evidence has been located, an appropriate and systematic method for rating or appraising the evidence is used. This rating system should include an analysis of whether the evidence can be applied to a particular clinical situation.

Appraisal tools exist for evaluating different types of evidence from a single qualitative study, qualitative meta-syntheses, descriptive studies, and randomized clinical trials to systematic reviews. The suggested readings provide examples. These appraisal tools generally include a series of steps for evaluating the quality of the research that is specific to the study design, type of review or guideline, or strategy for determining the applicability of the evidence to one's practice. AGREE Collaboration (2001), an international collaboration of researchers and policymakers, provides a tool for evaluating clinical guidelines. Key elements of such appraisal tools include an assessment of the reliability and validity of the evidence.

Much of the EBP literature has been devoted to evaluating randomized clinical trials. A randomized controlled trial (RCT) includes at least two groups where study participants are randomly assigned to either the control group or the intervention group in order to test a treatment's effectiveness. Generally, it is preferable that such studies are double-blinded, meaning that the participants and those who are evaluating the outcomes do not know who has received the

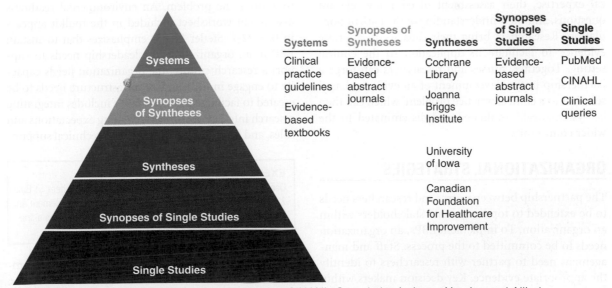

Systems	Synopses of Syntheses	Syntheses	Synopses of Single Studies	Single Studies
Clinical practice guidelines	Evidence-based abstract journals	Cochrane Library	Evidence-based abstract journals	PubMed
		Joanna Briggs Institute		CINAHL
Evidence-based textbooks				Clinical queries
		University of Iowa		
		Canadian Foundation for Healthcare Improvement		

FIGURE 22-4 Hierarchy of preprocessed evidence. *CINAHL,* Cumulative Index to Nursing and Allied Health Literature.

treatment. Although this design is generally considered the gold standard in terms of ranking individual studies, the number of RCTs conducted in nursing has been limited. Also, in certain clinical trials, blinding the recipients to a nursing intervention may be difficult to accomplish. An RCT is not always an appropriate design for answering a particular research question. Hence it is important that the appraisal method examine the rigour or the quality of the research in accordance with standards for that type of study.

Once the evidence has been appraised, this information needs to be integrated with clinical expertise and the preferences and values of patients, families, and communities in making the change. For example, in evaluating a research-based protocol for teaching oncology patients about preparing for a bone marrow transplant, the amount and type of information that would be desired by the patient need to be considered. In this instance, a qualitative research study might provide guidance for decision making. For certain types of interventions, the inclusion of patient preferences might not be appropriate, as in the example of implementing a protocol for the reduction of ventilator-associated pneumonia. Determining patient preferences depends on the nature of the intervention or change that is proposed.

The sheer quantity and complexity of information available indicate that nurses in direct practice need to collaborate with researchers. Nurses bring their clinical expertise, their assessment of clinically relevant questions, and their understanding of the patient population. Researchers bring their capacity to appraise evidence to facilitate its application to the clinical setting. Together, nurses and researchers can forge a partnership in the development of an evidence-based solution to a clinical practice problem, which can then be systematically evaluated and disseminated to the wider community.

ORGANIZATIONAL STRATEGIES

The partnership between nurses and researchers needs to be extended to top leaders and stakeholders within an organization. To implement EBPs, an organization needs to be committed to the process. Staff and management need to partner with researchers to identify the appropriate evidence. Key decision makers within the organization then need to receive the evidence in

a usable format. For example, in deciding whether it is best for nurses to administer preprocedure sedation or for parents to administer sedatives to children before their arrival in a department for a procedure, one needs to consider the evidence, the safety of the procedure, and the risks of unmonitored or parent-administered sedation, particularly if the child is being transported to the procedure in the back seat of a car. Providing key organizational decision makers with evidence regarding the safety of such a practice would be critical for decision making.

Nurse managers and leaders need to understand the organizational context for using research evidence. Lomas (2004) identifies the specific characteristics and competencies for creating the demand for research knowledge:

- Ability to understand the research and the decision-making environment
- Ability to find and assess relevant research
- Mediation and negotiation skills
- Communication skills
- Credibility

The Registered Nurses' Association of Ontario (RNAO, 2012) released a comprehensive toolkit to assist nurses in the implementation of evidence-based guidelines. The toolkit describes strategies for working with key stakeholders and stresses their early involvement because of their understanding of the extent of the problem, unmet needs, and motivation required to address the problem. An environmental readiness assessment worksheet included in the toolkit appears in Box 22-7. Stetler (2003) emphasizes that to sustain EBP in an organization, the leadership needs to support a research culture, the organization needs capacity to engage in EBP, and an infrastructure needs to be created to facilitate EBP. The latter includes integrating research into key documents, creating expectations and roles, and providing recognition and technical support.

EXERCISE 22-5

Use the environmental readiness assessment worksheet in Box 22-7 to assess the capacity of your organization to implement an evidence-based guideline. Identify one strategy to address a specific barrier to implementation.

The adoption of EBPs ultimately depends on a complex interaction of individual and organizational factors. Outside of nursing, factors associated with the adoption

BOX 22-7   ENVIRONMENTAL READINESS ASSESSMENT FOR THE IMPLEMENTATION OF A CLINICAL PRACTICE GUIDELINE (CPG)

ELEMENT	QUESTION	FACILITATORS	BARRIERS
Structure	To what extent does decision-making occur in a decentralized manner? Is there enough staff to support the change process?		
Workplace culture	To what extent is the CPG consistent with the values, attitudes and beliefs of the practice environment? To what degree does the culture support change and value evidence?		
Communication	Are there adequate (formal and informal) communication systems to support information exchange relative to the CPG and the CPG implementation processes?		
Leadership	To what extent do the leaders within the practice environment support (both visibly and behind the scenes) the implementation of the CPG?		
Knowledge, skills, and attitudes of target group	Does the staff have the necessary knowledge and skills? Which potential target group is open to change and new ideas? To what extent are they motivated to implement the CPG?		
Commitment to quality management	Do quality improvement processes and systems exist to measure results of implementation?		
Availability of resources	Are the necessary human, physical, and financial resources available to support implementation?		
Interdisciplinary relationships	Are there positive relationships and trust between and among the disciplines that will be involved or affected by the CPG?		

Registered Nurses' Association of Ontario. (2002). *Toolkit: Implementation of clinical practice guidelines.* Toronto, Canada: Registered Nurses Association of Ontario.

of innovation include larger organizational size, presence of a research champion, less traditionalism, and uncommitted organizational resources. Organizational determinants that positively influence research utilization by nurses include staff development, opportunity for nurse-to-nurse collaboration, staffing, and support services; less research utilization has been associated with increased emotional exhaustion and higher rates of patient and nurse adverse events (Cummings, Estabrooks, Midodzi, et al., 2007). Nurse managers and administrators are increasingly called upon to support individual nurses, implement strategies to enhance individuals' use of evidence, and create an organizational infrastructure that promotes EBP.

ISSUES FOR NURSE MANAGERS AND LEADERS

Some of the issues faced by nurse managers and leaders include a lack of resources, limited expertise of staff members with respect to EBP, lack of knowledge about nursing research, and limited time for researching and

planning. Not all organizations can hire a full-time nurse researcher. Some organizations may choose not to employ clinical nurse specialists, which is short-sighted in view of the potential benefits of improved patient outcomes and cost savings because of a reduction in adverse outcomes. However, this resource limitation is a reality faced in many organizations. Regardless, it is important to remember that using the best available evidence can be most successful in a partnership model. Therefore, working with nurse researchers at a local college or university could be valuable. Box 22-8 provides an abstract on a study by Ford, Rolfe, and Kirkpatrick (2011) on the process used to implement a Best Practice Guideline for patient-centred care through a partnership among clinical nurse specialists, primary health care nurse practitioners, and nurse educators in a Canadian teaching hospital. Faculty can partner with staff in a facility to provide consultation for a specific patient-care problem, and agencies can partner together to address a specific practice problem.

Collaboration is a critical organizational attribute ensuring that EBPs are incorporated into nursing care.

BOX 22-8	IMPLEMENTING A BEST PRACTICE GUIDELINE THROUGH A PARTNERSHIP AMONG HEALTH CARE PROVIDERS
Purpose	To implement the RNAO Best Practice Guideline (BPG) on Client-Centred Care (CCC) to make a positive impact on patient care through evidenced-based practice.
Background	In a Canadian teaching hospital, most practice guidelines are prescriptive, but this BPG was informed by elements of narrative theory, nursing models, and experiential learning from patients, families and nurses.
Outcomes	This process resulted in a 12-week course: "The Telling of Our Practice-Client-Centred Care." Evidence of sustainability and the BPG were disseminated through research, patient safety workshops, nursing staff orientation, and professional development activities focusing on quality of work and falls prevention.
Conclusion	Linkages made from a variety of nursing practice sites under the CCC brought organizational mandates, specific subject matter and current evidenced based guidelines into a culture of caring and change, which helped form new relationships across all sectors in this teaching facility. Patient care improved as did work life for all staff.

Ford, P. E. A., Rolfe, S., & Kirkpatrick, H. (2011). A journey to patient-centered care in Ontario, Canada: Implementation of a Best-Practice Guideline. *Clinical Nurse Specialist, 25*, 198–206. http://dx.doi.org/10.1097/NUR.0b013e318221f506

Collaboration within the organization should involve the interdisciplinary health care team. For example, the adoption of suctioning guidelines should include all members of the health care team involved in suctioning, including nurses, pulmonologists, hospitalists, and respiratory therapists. Ideally, documentation is integrated and focused on patient outcomes in order to improve practice.

Another organizational issue is that many nurses might not have had research and/or statistics courses in their basic nursing education. It is also possible that nurses may have had research courses many years ago and have not since used their research knowledge. Even if they did take a statistics course, nurses, nurse managers, and administrators might not be familiar with the critical appraisal of evidence. Nurses on a clinical unit might not be familiar with reading research or with using advanced search strategies for locating evidence for a particular practice problem. This might be especially true for nurses who have been out of school for a long time and have not had the opportunity to develop computer literacy skills. Information on evidence-based nursing as an approach has only recently been incorporated into nursing research textbooks. Therefore, a first step in developing the capacity to evaluate evidence for practice can be facilitated by starting a journal club that meets once a month. Journal clubs involve reading a relevant research article and discussing how it might be applied to the practice situation. Although a number of general and specialty nursing research journals exist, *Evidence-Based Nursing* and *Worldviews on Evidence-Based Nursing* are specifically devoted to evidence-based nursing practice. *Implementation Science* is a journal devoted specifically to the examination of strategies to promote the incorporation of research findings into routine health care. The resulting discussion at a journal club can be used as a springboard for the identification of clinical practice problems. Even small hospitals have libraries and perhaps a part-time librarian who can assist with gathering information and identifying useful articles for the journal club's agenda. Nurses returning to school for advanced education have access to a university library, as do nurses who are employed as adjunct faculty in nursing programs.

When translating research into practice, conduct an evaluation to document outcomes. It is preferable to collect outcomes data before implementing a protocol in order to have a basis for comparison. Collecting outcomes data is especially important when it is not possible to carry out an experimental design in which the intervention is implemented in one setting but not another. This may be the case because of sample size considerations or staff of different units casually talking with one another about the intervention. It is also important to consider whether the implementation of an EBP will turn into a research project. A research project is usually considered to be focused on the generation of new knowledge. Quality improvement activities and the adoption of EBPs might not meet the standards of a research project, and the results might not be generalizable to other settings (Newhouse, 2007). Regardless, nurses preparing to engage in an activity that might be considered a research project should consult with the organization's institutional review board early in the planning phase, regardless of whether data are collected directly from patients, medical records, or staff members.

Nurses, other health care providers, and the public might not be familiar with nursing research or evidence-based nursing. Therefore, it is important to publicize key nursing research findings. When nursing research is publicized in the media or through news alerts, be sure to communicate these findings to key organizational decision makers. Sending e-mails, posting articles, and providing resources helps people learn for themselves. Joining a professional association and a specialty association and signing up for alerts from key agencies provide nurses with access to the latest news, research, and standards. Research has a much better chance of being implemented if key stakeholders have the opportunity to understand its relevance.

It may be necessary to introduce concepts related to translating research into practice in small increments. For example, a first step might be incorporating research into the revision of procedures and employer guidelines as they come up for review. Subsequently, nurses and key stakeholders can be asked to identify clinical practice problems that create challenges in providing care in order to develop an evidence-based solution. Multiple strategies are needed to implement research findings. Multiple strategies are needed to change a culture to one that is driven by research and evidence-based standards for practice. Finally, if one should have the opportunity to implement an EBP, as much consideration needs to be given to planning for implementation as protocol development. Advance planning should include a thorough and frank discussion of the barriers and facilitators, as well as how to minimize the barriers and maximize the facilitators. Also, strategies to sustain the adoption of the practice over time need to be considered. Although the implementation of EBP is a very complex process, the increased emphasis on the use of scientifically based evidence creates an exciting opportunity for nurses to demonstrate the value of nursing in improving patient care and health care outcomes.

A SOLUTION

After an hour of trying to comfort the male patient, it became clear to Jade that he was simply (or not so simply) scared: scared of being in a strange place, scared of strangers hovering over him, and scared of his physical situation. The patient would aggressively jump straight up in bed with his eyes bulging and barely able to catch his breath. Every time this happened, Jade would have to forcefully restrain his body at the shoulders (to protect the open fracture). After reflecting on the situation, Jade knew that there had to be nonpharmacological interventions that could be helpful. After using multiple warm blankets, repositioning, and other nonpharmacological comfort measures, Jade pulled up a chair and sat at the patient's bedside. Jade gestured to him to "try to get some sleep" and made the action of putting her head on her hands as you would do for a child. He slowly reached over, grabbed Jade's hand, took a deep breath, and closed his eyes. His breathing slowed and he, for once, looked somewhat relaxed. Jade sat there holding his hand for 20 minutes until he appeared to finally be asleep. Jade used her other hand to remove the tight grip

he had on her and started to quietly tip-toe out of the room. Jade got to the door and was startled by an ear-piercing loud scream. It scared her, as well as her colleagues at the desk who came running over to help, thinking something was wrong. It was him telling her to "close the door." He *could* speak and knew exactly what he wanted. There was nothing "difficult" about him, he was just trying to tell them how he was feeling. Before Jade left the room and closed the door, he repeated Jade's gesture of "try to get some sleep" and smiled. Jade giggled as she turned off the light and, yes, closed the door.

While this situation is not unique, it made Jade reflect on how often we are too quick to judge and rely heavily on labels. Initially, the patient was labelled as "difficult," "schizophrenic," and "aggressive." It's not always easy to look beyond those labels, but if you do, it's well worth it.

Would this be a suitable approach for you? Why or why not?

THE EVIDENCE

Avery and Schnell-Hoehn (2010) described the clinical nurse specialist as essential to the "development, implementation, and evaluation of evidenced-informed clinical pathways used by care providers for a defined cardiac population" (p. 76). The cardiac sciences clinical nurse specialists studied worked collaboratively with nurse practitioners, cardiac staff, and Regional Health Authorities to conduct an audit of patient care, undertake a comprehensive literature review, make revisions to current clinical pathways, and make recommendations for nursing practice prior to implementing evidenced-informed research on current practice guidelines for cardiac patients. The clinical nurse specialists looked at the "big picture" in understanding population health needs, gaps in services, and how to improve health outcomes (p. 78).

NEED TO KNOW NOW

- Identify the most common practice problems in a clinical setting.
- Update practice by using the latest evidence.
- Work together with other nurses, key stakeholders, and colleagues across disciplines to adopt an EBP.

- Evaluate the results of a practice change.
- Communicate successes to colleagues, patients, families, and the public.

CHAPTER CHECKLIST

Society increasingly demands that health care be based on the best available evidence. Nurses have a societal obligation to use practices that are based on sound scientific evidence. The time from scientific discovery or publication of research to implementation in practice is lengthy and needs to be shortened. Nurses can speed up this process by using scientifically based strategies to facilitate the translation of research into practice. The nurse manager needs to understand the organizational context for the implementation of evidence-based protocols. Multiple strategies need to be developed to enhance the use of evidence as the foundation for nursing care delivery. Ongoing engagement is needed with nurses, nurse managers, and nurse leaders to see the relevance and importance of translating research into practice. We cannot continue to "only do what we know" when the issue of life and death truly is determined by nurses at the bedside. Every nurse needs to foster the mantra that research does belong in the forefront of everyday practice.

- Research is an integral part of professional nursing practice and part of every nurse's obligation under the Canadian Nurses Association's code of ethics (CNA, 2008).
- Research utilization is critical to an organization:
  - Synthesis, dissemination, and use of research are three distinct efforts.
  - Nurse researchers have a long history of developing demonstration or pilot projects to enhance research utilization.
  - Stetler's (2001) research utilization model incorporates elements of EBP and focuses heavily on the change process to facilitate translation of research into practice. The model's steps include preparation, validation, comparative evaluation or decision making, translation or application, and evaluation.
  - The knowledge-to-action framework is recognized by CIHR as the accepted model of knowledge translation.

- Evidence-based practice is the driving force in today's health care approaches:
  - Research-based information is used to make decisions.
  - Patient needs and preferences are considered.
  - EBP is broad in scope in that it involves appraising the evidence to address a specific clinical practice problem, whereas research utilization involves applying the findings from a particular study in practice.
- Rogers' (2003) diffusion of innovations theory is a useful framework for understanding how innovations are diffused throughout an organization. The stages of the innovation adoption process are knowledge, persuasion, decision, implementation, and confirmation.
- According to Rogers (1995), innovation adopters can be classified as follows: innovators, early adopters, early majority, late majority, and laggards.
- Using research evidence should be done in a systematic manner:
  1. Ask the relevant clinical question.
  2. Acquire the evidence.
  3. Appraise the evidence.
  4. Integrate the evidence with clinical expertise; patient, family and community preferences; and values.
  5. Assess the outcomes.
- Developing a relevant clinical question is enhanced by using the PICOT format.
- An organizational or environmental assessment of the capacity for evidence-based/evidence-informed practice will facilitate the translation of research into practice. An organizational assessment includes the following:
  - Access to resources for evidence
  - Capacity to appraise evidence
  - Adaptability in providing key leaders with summarized evidence

- Capacity to demonstrate applicability of the evidence to key leaders
- Evidence-based/evidence-informed practice is a strategy to answer clinical practice questions in real-world settings.
- The characteristics and competencies required for creating the demand for research knowledge are as follows:
  - Ability to understand the research and decision-making environment

- Ability to find and assess relevant research
- Mediation and negotiation skills
- Communication skills
- Credibility
- Collaboration
- Strategies to enhance individuals' abilities in using evidence, support for individual nurses' efforts to use research, as well the establishment of an organizational infrastructure will promote the use of EBPs.

TIPS FOR DEVELOPING SKILL IN APPLYING EVIDENCE TO PRACTICE

- Make a personal commitment to read research articles.
- Complete an online tutorial in EBP.
- Use your clinical experiences to develop relevant clinical questions.
- Obtain assistance from researchers, advanced practice registered nurses, and nurse leaders.

- Use the patient population, intervention or interest area, comparison intervention or issue of interest, outcome, and time (PICOT) format to search for evidence on a clinical practice problem.
- Create or join a journal club to encourage your colleagues to join you in learning about EBP and evaluating research evidence.

℮volve WEBSITE

Visit the Evolve website for Suggested Readings, Internet Resources, and additional resources related to the content in this chapter: http://evolve.elsevier.com/Canada/Yoder-Wise/leading/.

REFERENCES

AGREE Collaboration. (2001). Appraisal of guidelines for research & evaluation (AGREE) instrument. Retrieved from http://apps.who.int/rhl/agreeinstrumentfinal.pdf.

American Society of Health-System Pharmacists. (2006). ASHP therapeutic position statement on the institutional use of 0.9% sodium chloride injection to maintain patency of peripheral indwelling intermittent infusion devices. *American Journal of Health-System Pharmacy, 63*, 1273–1275. doi:10.2146/ajhp060094

Arnold, S., & Straus, S. E. (2005). Interventions to improve antibiotic prescribing practices in ambulatory care. *Cochrane Library, 4*. doi:10.1002/14651858.CD003539.pub2

Avery, L. J., & Schnell-Hoehn, K. N. (2010). Clinical nurse specialist practice in evidence-informed multidisciplinary cardiac care. *Clinical Nurse Specialist, 24*, 76–79. doi:10.1097/NUR.0b013e3 181cf5563

Benner, P., Hughes, R. G., & Sutphen, M. (2008). Clinical reasoning, decision making, and action: Thinking critically and clinically. In R. G. Hughes (Ed.), *Patient safety and quality: An evidence-based handbook for nurses.* Rockville, MD: Employer for Healthcare Research and Quality (US). Retrieved from http://www.ncbi.nlm.nih.gov/books/NBK2643/.

Brooks, J. M., Titler, M., Ardery, G., et al. (2009). Effect of evidence-based acute pain management practices on inpatient costs. *HSR: Health Services Research, 44*, 245–263. doi:10.1111/j.1475-6773.2008.00912.x

Brown, S. J. (2008). Time to move on: Definitions of evidence-based practice. *Journal of Nursing Care Quality, 23*, 201. doi:10. 1097/01.NCQ.0000324582.67180.4b

Brown, S. R. (2005). *Scurvy: How a surgeon, a mariner, and a gentleman solved the greatest medical mystery of the age of sail.* New York, NY: St. Martin's Press.

Brownson, R. C., Baker, E. A., Leet, T. L., et al. (2010). *Evidence-based public health* (eBook). n.p.: Oxford University Press.

Burns, N., & Grove, S. K. (2009). *The practice of nursing research: Conduct, critique, and utilization* (6th ed.). St. Louis, MO: Saunders.

Burns, N., & Grove, S. K. (2011). *Understanding nursing research: Building an evidence-based practice* (5th ed.). Maryland Heights, MO: Elsevier Saunders.

Campbell, B. (2010). Applying knowledge to generate action: A community based knowledge translation framework. *Journal of Continuing Education in the Health Professions 30*,(1), 65–71. doi:10.1002/chp.20058

Canadian Institutes of Health Research. (2009). About knowledge translation. Retrieved from http://www.cihr-irsc.gc.ca/e/29418.html.

Canadian Institutes of Health Research. (2013). Evidence-informed healthcare renewal. Retrieved from http://www.cihr-irsc.gc.ca/e/43628.html.

Canadian Nurses Association. (2007). *Framework for the practice of registered nurses in Canada*. Ottawa, ON: Author. Retrieved from http://www.cna-aiic.ca/CNA/practice/scope/default_e.aspx.

Canadian Nurses Association. (2008). *Code of ethics for registered nurses (2008 centennial edition)*. Toronto, ON: Author. http://www.cna-nurses.ca/CNA/practice/ethics/code/default_e.aspx.

Canadian Nurses Association. (2014). CNA's online primary care toolkit. Retrieved from http://www.nurseone.ca/Default.aspx?portlet=StaticHtmlViewerPortlet&stmd=False&plang=1&ptdi=1798.

Canadian Nurses Association & Registered Nurses Association of Ontario. (2010). *Nurse fatigue and patient safety*. Ottawa, ON: Author. Retrieved from http://www2.cna-aiic.ca/CNA/practice/safety/full_report_e/files/fatigue_safety_2010_report_e.pdf.

Ciliska, D., Thomas, H., & Buffett, C. (2008). *An introduction to evidence-based public health and a compendium of critical appraisal tools for public health practice*. Hamilton, ON: National Collaborating Centre for Methods and Tools.

College and Association of Registered Nurses of Alberta. (2005). *Scope of practice for registered nurses*. Edmonton, AB: Author. Retrieved from https://www.nurses.ab.ca/Carna-Admin/Uploads/Scope%20of%20Practice.pdf.

Collins, S., Voth, T., DiCenso, A., et al. (2005). Finding the evidence. In A. DiCenso, G. Guyatt, & D. Ciliska (Eds.), *Evidence-based nursing: A guide to clinical practice* (pp. 20–43). St. Louis, MO: Mosby.

Cummings, G. G., Estabrooks, C. A., Midodzi, W. K., et al. (2007). Influence of organizational characteristics and context on research utilization. *Nursing Research 56*, S24–S39. doi:10.1097/01.NNR.0000280629.63654.95

DiCenso, A., Ciliska, D., & Guyatt, G. (2005). Introduction to evidence-based nursing. In A. DiCenso, G. Guyatt, & D. Ciliska (Eds.), *Evidence-based nursing: A guide to clinical practice* (pp. 3–19). St. Louis, MO: Mosby.

Dobbins, M., Ciliska, D., Estabrooks, C., et al. (2005). Changing nursing practice in an organization. In A. DiCenso, G. Guyatt, & D. Ciliska (Eds.), *Evidence-based nursing: A guide to clinical practice* (pp. 172–200). St. Louis, MO: Mosby.

Estabrooks, C. A. (1999). The conceptual structure of research utilization. *Research in Nursing and Health, 22*, 203–216. doi:10.1002/(SICI)1098-240X(199906)22:3<203::AID-NUR3>3.0.CO;2–9

Fetzer, S. J. (2002). Reducing venipuncture and intravenous insertion pain with eutectic mixture of local anesthetic: A meta-analysis. *Nursing Research, 51*(2), 119–124.

Ford, P. E. A., Rolfe, S., & Kirkpatrick, H. (2011). A journey to patient-centered care in Ontario, Canada: Implementation of a Best-Practice Guideline. *Clinical Nurse Specialist, 25*, 198–206. doi:10.1097/NUR.0b013e318221f506

Funk, S. G., Champagne, M. T., Wiese, R. A., et al. (1991). Barriers: The barriers to research utilization scale. *Applied Nursing Research, 4*, 39–45. doi:10.1016/S0897-1897(05)80052-7

Gagnon, M.-P., Labarthe, J., Legare, F., et al. (2011). Measuring organizational readiness for knowledge translation in chronic care. *Implementation Science, 6*, 1–10. doi:10.1186/1748-5908-6-72

Geibert, R. C. (2006). The journey to evidence: Managing the information infrastructure. In K. Malloch & T. Porter-O'Grady (Eds.), *Introduction to evidence-based practice in nursing and health care* (pp. 125–148). Boston, MA: Jones & Bartlett.

Goode, C. J., Titler, M., Rakel, B., et al. (1991). A meta-analysis of effects of heparin flush and saline flush: Quality and cost implications. *Nursing Research, 40*(6), 324–330.

Hatfield, L. A., Gusic, M. E., Dyer, A. M., et al. (2008). Analgesic properties of oral sucrose during routine immunizations at 2 and 4 months of age. *Pediatrics, 121*, 327–334. doi:10.1542/peds.2006-3719

Haynes, R. B. (2001). Of studies, syntheses, synopses, and systems: The "4S" evolution of services for finding current best evidence. *ACP Journal Club, 134*, A11–A13. doi:10.1136/ebm.6.2.36

In conversation about nursing research. (2010). *Canadian Nurse,106* (2), 21–25. Retrieved from http://www.canadian-nurse.com/en/articles/issues/2010/february-2010/in-conversation-about-nursing-research?page=4.

Ingersoll, G. (2000). Evidence-based nursing: What it is and what it isn't. *Nursing Outlook, 48*, 151–152. doi:10.1067/mno.2000.107690

International Council of Nurses. (2007). Nursing research (position statement). Retrieved from http://www.icn.ch/images/stories/documents/publications/position_statements/B05_Nsg_Research.pdf.

Jones, R. (2008). Soap opera video on handheld computers to reduce young urban women's HIV sex risk. *AIDS and Behavior, 12*, 876–884. doi:10.1007/s10461-008-9416-y

LaRosa, J. C., He, J., & Vupputuri, S. (1999). Effect of statins on risk of coronary disease: A meta-analysis of randomized controlled trials. *JAMA, 282*, 2340–2346. doi:10.1001/jama.282.24.2340

Lomas, J. (2004). It takes two to tango: The importance of joint knowledge production for research use. *Canadian Health Services Research Foundation*. Presentation at the Ministerial Summit on Health Research and Global Forum, Mexico City, Mexico.

MacLean, S., Obispo, J., & Young, K. D. (2007). The gap between pediatric emergency department procedural pain management treatments available and actual practice. *Pediatric Emergency Care, 23*, 87–93. doi:10.1097/PEC.0b013e31803

Madsen, D., Sebolt, T., Cullen, L., et al. (2005). Listening to bowel sounds: An evidence-based practice project. *American Journal of Nursing, 105*(12), 40–49. Retrieved from http://www.jstor.org/stable/29745966.

Majumdar, S. R., McAlister, F. A., & Furberg, C. D. (2004). From knowledge to practice in chronic cardiovascular disease: A long and winding road. *Journal of American College of Cardiology, 43*, 1738–1742. doi:10.1016/j.jacc.2003.12.043

Malkin, B. (2008). Are techniques used for intramuscular injection based on research evidence? *Nursing Times, 104*(50–51), 48–51.

Melnyk, B. M., & Fineout-Overholt, E. (2011). Making the case for evidence-based practice and cultivating a spirit of inquiry. In B. M. Melnyk & E. Fineout-Overholt (Eds.), *Evidence-based practice in nursing and healthcare: A guide to best practice* (pp. 3–24). Philadelphia, PA: Lippincott, Williams & Wilkins.

Melnyk, B. M., Fineholt-Overholt, E., Stillwell, S. B., et al. (2010). Evidence-based practice: Step-by-step: The seven steps of evidence-based practice. *American Journal of Nursing, 110*, 51–53. doi:10.1097/01.NAJ.0000366056.06605.d2

Meyers, T. A., Eichhorn, D. J., Guzzetta, C. E., et al. (2000). Family presence during invasive procedures and resuscitation: The experience of family members, nurses, and physicians. *American Journal of Nursing, 100*(2), 32–43.

Moyer, V. A., & Elliott, E. J. (Eds.). (2004). *Evidence-based pediatrics and child health* (2nd ed.). London, UK: BMJ Publishing Group.

Newhouse, R. (2007). Diffusing confusion among evidence-based practice, quality improvement, and research. *Journal of Nursing Administration, 37*, 432–435. doi:10.1097/01.NNA.0000285156.58903.d3

Ontario Public Health Association. (2009). *Towards evidence-informed practice: TEIP program evidence tool—revised June 2010.* Toronto, ON: Author. Retrieved from http://www.google.ca/search?q=Ontario+Public+Health+Association.+%282009%29.+Towards+Evidence-Informed+Practice.

Pate, M. F. D. (2013). Nursing leadership from the bedside to the boardroom. *AACN Advanced Critical Care, 24*(2), 186–193.

Polit, D. F., & Beck, C. T. (2008). *Nursing research: Generating and assessing evidence for nursing practice.* Philadelphia, PA: Lippincott Williams & Wilkins.

Registered Nurses' Association of Ontario. *Toolkit: Implementation of clinical practice guidelines.* Toronto, Canada: Registered Nurses Association of Ontario.

Registered Nurses' Association of Ontario. (2012). *Toolkit: Implementation of Best Practice Guidelines* (2nd ed.). Toronto, ON: Author. Retrieved from http://rnao.ca/bpg/resources/toolkit-implementation-best-practice-guidelines-second-edition.

Retsas, A. (2000). Barriers to using research evidence in nursing practice. *Journal of Advanced Nursing, 31*, 599–606. doi:10.1046/j.1365-2648.2000.01315.x

Rogers, E. M. (1995). *Diffusion of innovations* (4th ed.). New York, NY: Free Press.

Rogers, E. M. (2003). *Diffusion of innovations* (5th ed.). New York, NY: Free Press. doi:10.1001/jama.288.3.321

Rycroft-Malone, J., Seers, K., Titchen, A., et al. (2004). What counts as evidence in evidence-based practice? *Journal of Advanced Nursing, 47*(1), 81–90.

Sackett, D. L., Straus, S. E., Richardson, W. S., et al. (2000). *Evidence-based medicine: How to practice and teach EBM* (2nd ed.). New York, NY: Churchill Livingstone.

Shah, P. S., Ng, E., & Sinha, A. K. (2005). Heparin for prolonging peripheral intravenous catheter use in neonates. *Cochrane Database of Systematic Reviews, 4.* doi:10.1002/14651858.CD002774.pub2

Smith, A. B., Hefley, G. C., & Anand, K. J. (2007). Parent bed spaces in the PICU: Effect on parental stress. *Pediatric Nursing, 33*(3), 215–221.

Squires, J., Hutchinson, A. M., Bostrom, A., et al. (2011). To what extent do nurses use research in clinical practice? A systematic review. *Implementation Science, 6*, 1–17. doi:10.1186/1748-5908-6-21

Stetler, C. B. (2001). Updating the Stetler model of research utilization to facilitate evidence-based practice. *Nursing Outlook, 49*, 272–279. doi:10.1067/mno.2001.120517

Stetler, C. B. (2003). Role of the organization in translating research into evidence-based practice. *Outcomes Management, 7*(3), 97–103.

Straus, S. E., Richardson, W. S., Glasziou, P., et al. (2005). *Evidence-based medicine: How to practice and teach EBM* (3rd ed.). Edinburgh, UK: Churchill Livingstone.

Straus, S. E., Tetroe, J., & Graham, I. (2009). Defining knowledge translation. *Canadian Medical Association Journal, 181*, 165–168. doi:10.1503/cmaj.081229

Thabane, L., Thomas, T., Ye, C., et al. (2009). Posing the research question: Not so simple. *Canadian Journal of Anaesthesia, 56*, 71–79. doi:10.1007/s12630-008-9007-4

Thompson, D. S., Estabrooks, C. A., Scott-Findlay, S., et al. (2007). Interventions aimed at increasing research use in nursing: A systematic review. *Implementation Science, 2*, 1–16. doi:10.1186/1748-5908-2-15

Titler, M. G., Herr, K., Brooks, J. M., et al. (2009). Translating research into practice intervention improves management of acute pain in older hip fracture patients. *Health Services Research, 44*, 265–287. doi:10.1111/j.1475-6773.2008.00913.x (2002).

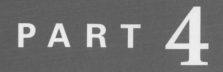

Interpersonal and Personal Skills

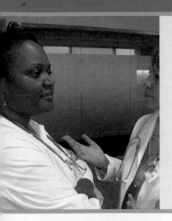

Understanding and Resolving Conflict

Victoria N. Folse
Adapted by Jayne Naylen McChesney and Heather D. Wilson

Appropriate conflict-handling strategies are essential in professional nursing practice because conflict cannot be eliminated from the workplace. To resolve conflicts, nurse leaders must be able to determine the nature of a particular issue, choose an appropriate approach for each situation, and implement a course of action. This chapter focuses on maximizing the nurse manager and leader's ability to deal with conflict by providing effective strategies for conflict resolution.

OBJECTIVES

- Use a model of the conflict process to determine the nature and sources of perceived and actual conflict.
- Assess preferred approaches to conflict, and commit to be more effective in resolving future conflict.
- Determine which of the five approaches to conflict is the most appropriate in different situations.
- Identify conflict management techniques that will prevent lateral violence from occurring.

TERMS TO KNOW

accommodating	compromising	lateral violence
avoiding	conflict	mediation
bullying	horizontal violence	negotiation
collaborating	interpersonal conflict	organizational conflict
competing	intrapersonal conflict	

After 3 years of working as a licensed practical nurse, Antonia decided to return to school to obtain her registered nurse (RN) degree. Throughout her studies, Antonia continued to work as a licensed practical nurse on the same rehabilitative unit. There were a total of 35 beds, the workload was heavy, and 4 beds were specifically designated for individuals with head injuries. The unit was busy but generally functioned well with a team of licensed practical nurses, special care aides, and an RN who was in charge each shift. Antonia always had good relationships with her co-workers, which she felt were based on mutual trust and respect.

After completing her degree, Antonia was hired as an RN on the same unit. Antonia thought this opportunity would help her solidify her nursing skills and help her transition into a new role on a unit in which she felt comfortable and confident. On Antonia's first shift as the RN in charge, she noticed that the licensed practical nurse colleagues she had worked with were now avoiding eye contact with her during report. Following report, there was a conversation about the upcoming staff party. Antonia was ignored when she asked for the address of the party. Again later in the shift, Antonia called the team together to inform them of an unexpected admission to their unit. Antonia delegated responsibility to a licensed practical nurse

to complete a head-to-toe assessment and measure vital signs on the newly admitted patient in order to be prepared for the physician rounds. When the physician arrived, Antonia checked the patient's chart for the assessment data, and no assessment data had been completed. When she addressed the issue with the licensed practical nurse, she verbally attacked Antonia and claimed that Antonia never delegated any task to her. She informed Antonia that she could complete her own assessments from now on. When the licensed practical nurse stormed off, Antonia immediately went to the washroom where she could be alone. Antonia was devastated and disappointed that her co-worker whom she thought was also a friend was not supportive. Antonia avoided the licensed practical nurse for the remainder of the shift and then booked a sick day the next day because she just could not face more conflict with her colleagues. Over the next few days, Antonia reflected on her choices of going back to school and her decision to take an RN job on the same unit she had worked previously.

What conflict resolution strategies could Antonia use to effectively manage this situation?

INTRODUCTION

Conflict is a disagreement in values or beliefs within oneself or between people that causes harm or has the potential to cause harm. Conflict is a catalyst for change and has the ability to stimulate either detrimental or beneficial effects. If properly understood and managed, conflict can lead to positive outcomes and practice environments, but if it is left unattended, it can have a negative impact on both the individual and the organization (Mitchell, Ahmed, & Szabo, 2014; Stanton, 2012). Positive outcomes of well-managed conflict include strengthened relationships among intraprofessional teams and with colleagues. Some of the first authors on organizational conflict (e.g., Blake & Mouton, 1964; Deutsch, 1973; Duffy, 1995) claimed that a complete resolution of conflict might, in fact, be undesirable because conflict can stimulate growth, creativity, and change.

Conflict is inherent in clinical environments in which nursing responsibilities are driven by patient needs that are complex and frequently changing (Latham, Ringl, & Hogan, 2013; Sherman & Pross, 2010). Health care providers are exposed to high stress levels from increased demands on an ever-limited

and aging or inexperienced workforce, a decrease in available resources, a more acutely ill patient population, and a profound period of change in the practice environment (Antoniazzi, 2011). Nurses employed in healthy practice environments report more positive job experiences and fewer concerns about quality care. Healthy practice environments and positive self-evaluations (self-esteem, self-efficacy, locus of control, and emotional stability) predicted nurses' constructive conflict management and, in turn, greater team effectiveness (Mazurek Melnyk, Hrabe, & Szalacha, 2013; Zerwekh & Zerwekh Garneau, 2011). Favourable self-evaluation was also a predictor of quality leader–staff relationships, empowerment, and job satisfaction for nurse managers (Canadian Nurses Association [CNA], 2009; Roche, Diers, Duffield, et al., 2010). Moreover, health care settings with positive nurse–physician relations are associated with better patient outcomes and increased satisfaction with nursing (Friese & Manojlovich, 2012).

In professional practice environments, unresolved conflict among nurses is a significant issue resulting in job dissatisfaction, absenteeism, and turnover. The complexity of the health care workplace compounds the impact that caregiver stress and unresolved conflict have on patient safety. Successful organizations are proactive in anticipating the need for conflict resolution and innovative in developing conflict resolution strategies that apply to all members (Berwick, 2011; Mitchell et al., 2014).

An important factor in the successful management of stress and conflict is a better understanding of its context within the practice environment. The diverse workforce in health care settings today reveals varying characteristics and work values, which influence the relationships among health care providers and can at times lead to conflict (Leiter, Price, & Spence Laschinger, 2010; Wolff, Ratner, Robinson, et al., 2010).

Nurse managers and leaders have a growing responsibility to effectively manage the nursing workforce by creating cultures that embrace diversity (Wolff et al., 2010). They must lead by example and strive to co-construct a climate of shared work goals and outcomes with the common purpose of delivering quality, safe nursing care (CNA, 2009; Wolff et al., 2010). The literature reflects that nurses continue to prefer not to confront conflict directly and will avoid, compromise, and even withdraw in hopes of spontaneous resolution (Blair, 2013; Jackson, Hutchinson, Peters, et al., 2013). Emotions of empathy, compassion, and caring should not be suppressed, but neither should assertive communication or behaviour. The stereotypical self-sacrificing behaviour seen in avoidance and accommodation is strongly supported by the altruistic nature of nursing (Blair, 2013). Avoidance may be a temporary leadership strategy during times of high stress, and it may seem relatively harmless; however, it can leave followers with the perception that their leader is abstaining from active leadership (Jackson et al., 2013) Avoidance leadership impacts the well-being of nurses and diminishes their commitment to the organization.

TYPES OF CONFLICT

The recognition that conflict is a part of everyday life suggests that mastering conflict management strategies is essential for overall well-being and personal and professional growth. Determining the type of conflict present in a specific situation is important because the more accurately conflict is defined, the more likely it will be resolved. The three types of conflict are as follows: intrapersonal, interpersonal, or organizational; a combination of types can also be present in any given conflict.

Intrapersonal conflict occurs within a person when confronted with the need to think or act in a way that seems at odds with one's sense of self. Questions often arise that create a conflict over priorities, ethical standards, and values. When a nurse manager decides what to do about the future (e.g., *Do I want to pursue an advanced degree or start a family now?*), conflict arises between personal and professional priorities. Some issues present a conflict over comfortably maintaining the status quo (e.g., *I know my operating room [OR] nurse leader prefers the OR over the surgical day care centre; Should I ask him to manage the centre anyway, since I need someone with his skills at the centre?*). Taking risks to confront people when needed (e.g., *Would recommending a change in practice that I learned about at a recent conference jeopardize unit governance?*) can produce intrapersonal conflict and, because it involves other people, may lead to interpersonal conflict.

Interpersonal conflict occurs between and among patients, family members, nurses, physicians, and members of other departments. Conflicts occur that focus on a difference of opinion, priority, or approach with others. A nurse manager may be called upon to assist two nurses in resolving a scheduling conflict or issues surrounding patient assignments. Members of health care teams often have disputes over the best way to treat particular cases or disagreements in determining how much information is necessary for patients and families to have about their illness. According to Johansen (2012), interpersonal conflicts were the most common and problematic type of conflict encountered by nurses in the workplace.

Organizational conflict arises when discord exists about policies and procedures, personnel codes of conduct, or accepted norms of behaviour and patterns of communication. Some organizational conflict is related to hierarchical structure and role differentiation among employees. Nurse managers and their staff often become embattled in institution-wide conflict concerning staffing patterns and how they affect the quality of care. Complex ethical and moral dilemmas may arise over the allocation of limited resources and funding for health care delivery (e.g., access to health care resources in remote areas versus densely populated urban centres). A major source of organizational conflict stems from strategies that promote more participation and autonomy of staff nurses. Increasingly, nurses are charged with balancing direct patient care with active involvement in organizational initiatives surrounding quality patient care. Nurses who perceive themselves as working in a healthy environment that promotes collaboration are more likely to report enhanced employee well-being and effective conflict management strategies (Bennett & Sawatzky, 2013; Longo, 2010). The following are other "forces" that contribute to effective conflict management in the practice environment:

- Organizational structure (nurses' involvement in shared decision making)
- Management style (nursing leaders create an environment supporting participation, encourage and value feedback, and demonstrate effective communication with staff)
- Personnel policies and programs (efforts to promote nurse work–life balance)
- Image of nursing (nurses effectively influencing system-wide processes)
- Autonomy (nurses' inclusion in governance leading to job satisfaction, personal fulfillment, and organizational success)

EXERCISE 23-1

Recall a situation in which conflict between or among two or more people was apparent. Describe verbal and nonverbal communication and how each person responded. What was the outcome? Was the conflict resolved? Were any issues left unresolved?

STAGES OF CONFLICT

Conflict proceeds through four distinct stages: frustration, conceptualization, action, and outcomes (K. W. Thomas, 1992). The ability to resolve conflicts productively depends on understanding these stages (Figure 23-1) and successfully addressing thoughts, feelings, and behaviours that form barriers to resolution. As one navigates through the stages of conflict, moving into a subsequent stage may lead to a return to and change in a previous stage. To illustrate, consider the example of nurses in a cardiac step-down unit who are asked to pilot a new hand-off protocol for the

Frustration ↔ Conceptualization ↔ Action ↔ Outcomes

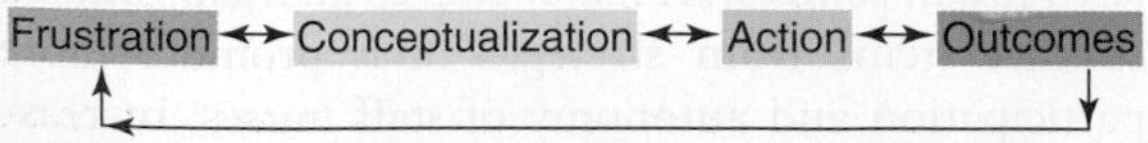

FIGURE 23-1 Stages of conflict.

next 6 weeks. The pilot stimulates intense emotions because the unit is already inadequately staffed (frustration). A hand-off protocol is the transfer of patient care from one care provider, unit, or team to another, and it is critical to ensuring continuity of care and patient safety (Matney, Maddox, & Staggers, 2014). Two nurses on the cardiac unit interpret this conflict as a battle for control with the nurse educator, and a third nurse thinks it is all about professional standards (conceptualization). A nurse manager facilitates a discussion with the three nurses (action); she listens to the concerns and presents evidence about the potential effectiveness of the new hand-off protocol. All agree that the real conflict comes from a difference in goals or priorities (new conceptualization), which leads to less negative emotion and ends with a much clearer understanding of all the issues (diminished frustration). The nurses agree to pilot the hand-off protocol after their ideas have been incorporated into the plan (outcome).

Frustration

When people or groups perceive that their goals may be blocked, frustration results. This frustration may escalate into stronger emotions, such as anger and deep resignation. For example, a nurse may perceive that a postoperative patient is noncompliant or uncooperative, when in reality the patient is afraid or has a different set of priorities at the start from those of the nurse. At the same time, the patient may view the nurse as controlling and uncaring, because the nurse repeatedly asks if the patient has used his incentive spirometer as instructed. When such frustrations occur, it is a cue to stop and clarify the nature and cause of the differences.

Conceptualization

Conflict arises when there are different interpretations of a situation, including a different emphasis on what is important and what is not, and different thoughts about what should occur next. Everyone involved develops an idea of what the conflict is about, and individual views may or may not be accurate. Viewpoints may result from an instant conclusion, or may be developed over time. Everyone involved has an individual interpretation of what the conflict is and why it is occurring. Most often, these interpretations are dissimilar and involve the person's own perspective, which is based on personal values, beliefs, and attitudes.

- Regardless of the accuracy of variously held viewpoints, conceptualization forms the basis for everyone's frustration. The way in which individuals perceive and define the conflict has a great deal of influence on the approach to resolution and outcomes. For example, within the same conflict situation, some individuals may see a conflict between a nurse manager and a staff nurse as insubordination and become angry at the threat to the leader's role. Others may view it as trivial complaining, voice criticism (e.g., "We've been over this new protocol already; why can't you just adopt the change?"), and withdraw from the situation. Such differences in conceptualizing the issue block its resolution. Thus it is important for each person to clarify "the conflict as I see it" and "how it makes me respond" before those involved can define the conflict, develop a shared conceptualization, and resolve their differences. The following questions can help advance to shared conceptualization and a resolution:

- What is the nature of our differences?
- What are the reasons for those differences?
- Does our leader endorse ideas or behaviours that add to or diminish the conflict?
- Do I need to be mentored by someone, even if that individual is outside my own department or work area, to successfully resolve this conflict?

Action

A behavioural response to a conflict follows the conceptualization. This may include seeking clarification about how another person views the conflict, collecting additional information that informs the issue, or engaging in dialogue about the issue. As actions are taken to resolve the conflict, the way that some or all involved conceptualize the conflict may change. Successful resolution frequently stems from identifying a common goal that unites individuals (e.g., quality patient care, good working relations). It is important to understand that people are always taking some action regarding the conflict, even if that action is avoidance, deliberately delaying action, or choosing to do nothing. The longer that ineffective actions continue, the more likely people will experience frustration, resistance, or even hostility. The more appropriately actions match

the nature of the conflict, the more likely that the conflict will be resolved in a timely manner with desirable results.

Outcomes

Tangible and intangible consequences result from actions taken and have significant implications for the work setting. Outcomes include (1) the conflict being resolved with a revised approach, (2) stagnation of any current movement, or (3) no future movement. Appropriately selected and effectively deployed conflict management strategies minimize destructive effects and maximize constructive outcomes (Saltman, O'Dea, & Kidd, 2006).

Constructive conflict results in successful resolution that leads to the following:
- Professional and organizational growth
- Problem resolution
- Unification of groups and improved team functioning
- Productivity increases
- Increases in employee commitment

Unsatisfactory resolution is typically destructive and results in the following:
- Negativity, resistance, and increased frustration that inhibit movement
- Decrease in or absence of resolutions
- Group divisions and weakened relationships
- Decreased productivity
- Decreased employee satisfaction levels

Assessing the degree of conflict resolution is useful for improving individual and group skills in resolutions. Two general outcomes are considered when assessing the degree to which a conflict has been resolved: (1) the degree to which important goals were achieved and (2) the nature of the subsequent relationships among those involved (Box 23-1; J. Hurst & Kinney, 1989).

CATEGORIES OF CONFLICT

Categorizing and determining the root cause of a conflict can help define an appropriate course of action toward its resolution. Conflicts arise from discrepancies in four areas: facts, goals, approaches, and values. Sources of fact-based conflicts are external written sources and include job descriptions, hospital policies, and provincial and territorial standards of practice.

BOX 23-1	ASSESSING THE DEGREE OF CONFLICT RESOLUTION

1. Quality of decisions?
   a. How creative are resulting plans?
   b. How practical and realistic are they?
   c. How well were intended goals achieved?
   d. What surprising results were achieved?
2. Quality of relationships?
   a. How much understanding has been created?
   b. How willing are people to work together?
   c. How much mutual respect, empathy, concern, and cooperation has been generated?

Adapted from Hurst, J., & Kinney, M. (1989). *Empowering self and others.* Toledo, OH: University of Toledo.

Objective data can be provided to resolve a disagreement generated by discrepancies in information. Goal conflicts often arise from competing priorities (e.g., desire to empower employees versus control through micromanagement); often, focusing on a common goal (e.g., quality patient care) can aid conflict resolution. Even when agreement exists on a common goal, different ideas about the best approach to achieve that goal may ignite conflict. For example, if the unit goal is to reduce costs by 10%, one leader may target overtime hours and another may eliminate the budget for continuing education. Values, opinions, and beliefs are much more personal, thus generating disagreements that can be threatening and adversarial. Because values are subjective, value-based conflicts sometimes remain unresolved. In these circumstances, professionals should find ways for competing values to coexist, such as agreeing to disagree.

A pessimist sees the difficulty in every opportunity; an optimist sees the opportunity in every difficulty.
—*Winston Churchill*

APPROACHES TO CONFLICT RESOLUTION

Understanding the ways in which health care providers respond to conflict and the current states of incivility and moral distress in various health care domains is an essential first step in identifying effective strategies to help nurses constructively handle conflicts in the practice environment (Clark, 2013; Edmonson, 2010; Longo, 2010). Five distinct approaches can be used in conflict resolution: avoiding, accommodating, competing, compromising, and collaborating (K. W. Thomas & Kilmann, 1974, 2002). These approaches can be viewed within the dimensions of assertiveness (satisfying one's own concerns) and cooperativeness (satisfying the concerns of others). Most people tend to employ a combined set of actions that are appropriately assertive and cooperative, depending on the nature of the conflict situation (K. W. Thomas, 1992). See the conflict self-assessment in Box 23-2.

EXERCISE 23-2

Self-assessment of preferred conflict-handling approaches is important. As you read and answer the 30-item conflict survey in Box 23-2, think of how you respond to conflict in professional situations. After completing the survey, tally, total, and reflect on your scores for each of the five approaches. Consider the following questions:

- Which approach do you prefer? Which do you use least?
- What determines if you respond in a particular manner?
- Considering the reoccurring types of conflicts you have, what are the strengths and weaknesses of your preferred conflict-handling styles?
- Have others offered you feedback about your approach to conflict?

Avoiding

Avoiding, or withdrawing, is very unassertive and uncooperative because people who avoid neither pursue their own needs, goals, or concerns immediately nor assist others to pursue theirs. Avoidance as a conflict management style only ensures that conflict is postponed or prolonged, and conflict ignored may escalate in intensity. That is not to say that all conflict must be addressed immediately as some issues require considerable reflection before strategies can be selected and action taken. The positive side of withdrawing may be postponing an issue until a better time or simply walking away from a "no-win" situation (Box 23-3). The self-assessment in Box 23-4 will help you recognize your own avoidance behaviours and use them more effectively.

Accommodating

When accommodating, people neglect their own needs, goals, and concerns (unassertive) while trying to satisfy those of others (cooperative). This approach has an element of being self-sacrificing and simply

BOX 23-2 CONFLICT SELF-ASSESSMENT

Directions: Read each of the following statements. Assess yourself in terms of how often you tend to act similarly during conflict at work, at clinical placements and at school. Place the number of the most appropriate response in the blank in front of each statement. Put *1* if the behaviour is never typical of how you act during a conflict, *2* if it is seldom typical, *3* if it is occasionally typical, *4* if it is frequently typical, or *5* if it is very typical of how you act during conflict.

_____ 1. Create new possibilities to address all important concerns.
_____ 2. Persuade others to see it and/or do it my way.
_____ 3. Work out some sort of give-and-take agreement.
_____ 4. Let other people have their way.
_____ 5. Wait and let the conflict take care of itself.
_____ 6. Find ways that everyone can win.
_____ 7. Use whatever power I have to get what I want.
_____ 8. Find an agreeable compromise among people involved.
_____ 9. Give in so others get what they think is important.
_____ 10. Withdraw from the situation.
_____ 11. Cooperate assertively until everyone's needs are met.
_____ 12. Compete until I either win or lose.
_____ 13. Engage in "give a little and get a little" bargaining.
_____ 14. Let others' needs be met more than my own needs.
_____ 15. Avoid taking any action for as long as I can.
_____ 16. Partner with others to find the most inclusive solution.

_____ 17. Put my foot down assertively for a quick solution.
_____ 18. Negotiate for what all parties value and can live without.
_____ 19. Agree to what others want to create harmony.
_____ 20. Keep as far away from others involved as possible.
_____ 21. Stick with it to get everyone's highest priorities.
_____ 23. Argue and debate over the best way.
_____ 23. Create some middle position everyone agrees to.
_____ 24. Put my priorities below those of other people.
_____ 25. Hope the issue does not come up.
_____ 26. Collaborate with others to achieve our goals together.
_____ 27. Compete with others for scarce resources.
_____ 28. Emphasize compromise and trade-offs.
_____ 29. Cool things down by letting others do it their way.
_____ 30. Change the subject to avoid the fighting.

Conflict Self-Assessment Scoring

Look at the numbers you placed in the blanks on the conflict assessment. Write the number you placed in each blank on the appropriate line below. Add up your total for each column, and enter that total on the appropriate line. The greater your total is for each approach, the more often you tend to use that approach when conflict occurs at work. The lower the score is, the less often you tend to use that approach when conflict occurs at work.

COLLABORATING	COMPETING	COMPROMISING	ACCOMMODATING	AVOIDING
1._____	2._____	3._____	4._____	5._____
6._____	7._____	8._____	9._____	10._____
11._____	12._____	13._____	14._____	15._____
16._____	17._____	18._____	19._____	20._____
21._____	22._____	23._____	24._____	25._____
26._____	27._____	28._____	29._____	30._____
Total _____	Total _____	Total _____	Total _____	Total _____

Throughout the rest of this section, there are descriptions of each approach and related self-assessment and commitment-to-action activities. Use the scores you received above to think about how you do and could handle conflict at work. Most important, consider if your pattern of frequency tends to be consistent or inconsistent with the types of conflicts you face. That is, does your way of dealing with conflict tend to match the situations in which that approach is most useful?

Hurst, J. B. (1993). *Conflict self-assessment.* Toledo, OH: Human Resource Development Center, University of Toledo.

obeying orders or serving other people. For example, a co-worker requests that you cover her weekends during her children's holiday break. You had hoped to visit friends from college, but you know how important it is for her to have more time with her family, so you agree. Box 23-5 lists some appropriate uses of accommodation.

Individuals who frequently use accommodation may feel disappointment and resentment because they "get nothing in return." This is a built-in by-product of the overuse of this approach. The self-assessment in Box 23-6 asks you to examine your current use of accommodation and challenges you to think of new ways to use it more effectively.

BOX 23-3 APPROPRIATE USES OF AVOIDANCE

1. When facing trivial and/or temporary issues, or when other far more important issues are pressing.
2. When there is no chance to obtain what one wants or needs, or when others could resolve the conflict more efficiently and effectively
3. When the potential negative results of initiating and acting on a conflict are much greater than the benefits of its resolution
4. When people need to "cool down," distance themselves, or gather more information

BOX 23-4 AVOIDANCE: SELF-ASSESSMENT AND COMMITMENT TO ACTION

If You Tend to Use Avoidance Often, Ask Yourself the Following Questions:
1. Do people have difficulty getting my input into and understanding my view?
2. Do I block cooperative efforts to resolve issues?
3. Am I distancing myself from significant others?
4. Are important issues being left unidentified and unresolved?

If You Seldom Use Avoidance, Ask Yourself the Following Questions:
1. Do I find myself overwhelmed by a large number of conflicts and a need to say "no"?
2. Do I assert myself even when things do not matter that much? Do others view me as an aggressor?
3. Do I lack a clear view of what my priorities are?
4. Do I stir up conflicts and fights?

Commitment to Action
What two new behaviours would increase your effective use of avoidance?
1.
2.

BOX 23-5 APPROPRIATE USES OF ACCOMMODATION

1. When other people's ideas and solutions appear to be better, or when you have made a mistake
2. When the issue is far more important to the other(s) person than it is to you
3. When you see that accommodating now "builds up some important credits" for later issues
4. When you are outmatched and/or losing anyway; when continued competition would only damage the relationships and productivity of the group and jeopardize accomplishing major purpose(s)
5. When preserving harmonious relationships and avoiding defensiveness and hostility are very important
6. When letting others learn from their mistakes and/or increased responsibility is possible without severe damage

BOX 23-6 ACCOMMODATION: SELF-ASSESSMENT AND COMMITMENT TO ACTION

If You Use Accommodation Often, Ask Yourself the Following Questions:
1. Do I feel that my needs, goals, concerns, and ideas are not being attended to by others?
2. Am I depriving myself of influence, recognition, and respect?
3. When I am in charge, is "discipline" lax?
4. Do I think people are using me?

If You Seldom Use Accommodation, Ask Yourself the Following Questions:
1. Am I building goodwill with others during conflict?
2. Do I admit when I have made a mistake?
3. Do I know when to give in, or do I assert myself at all costs?
4. Am I viewed as unreasonable or insensitive?

Commitment to Action
What two new behaviours would increase your effective use of accommodation?
1.
2.

Competing

When **competing**, people pursue their own needs and goals at the expense of others. Sometimes people use whatever power, creativeness, or strategies that are available to "win." Competing may also take the form of standing up for your rights or defending important principles, as when opposition to mandatory overtime is voiced (Box 23-7).

People whose primary approach to addressing conflict is through competition often react by feeling threatened, acting defensively or aggressively, or even resorting to cruelty in the form of cutting remarks, deliberate gossip, or hurtful innuendo. Competition within work groups can generate ill will, favour a win–lose stance, and compel people to a stalemate. Such behaviours force people into a corner from which there is no easy or graceful exit. Use Box 23-8 to help you learn to use competing more effectively.

1. When quick, decisive action is necessary
2. When important, unpopular action needs to be taken, or when trade-offs may result in long-range, continued conflict
3. When an individual or group is right about issues that are vital to group welfare
4. When others have taken advantage of an individual's or group's non-competitive behaviour and now are mobilized to compete about an important topic

| BOX 23-8 | COMPETING: SELF-ASSESSMENT AND COMMITMENT TO ACTION |

If You Use Competing Often, Ask Yourself the Following Questions:
1. Am I surrounded by people who agree with me all the time and who avoid confronting me?
2. Are others afraid to share themselves and their needs for growth with me?
3. Am I out to win at all costs? If so, what are the costs and benefits of competing?
4. What are people saying about me when I am not around?

If You Seldom Compete, Ask Yourself the Following Questions:
1. How often do I avoid taking a strong stand and then feel a sense of powerlessness?
2. Do I avoid taking a stand so that I can escape risk?
3. Am I fearful and unassertive to the point that important decisions are delayed and people suffer?

Commitment to Action
What two new behaviours would increase your effective use of competing?
1.
2.

Compromising

Compromising involves both assertiveness and cooperation on the part of everyone and requires maturity and confidence. Negotiation is a learned skill that is developed over time. A give-and-take relationship results in conflict resolution, with the result that each person can meet his or her most important priorities as much of the time as possible. Compromise is very often the exchange of concessions as it creates middle ground. This is the preferred means of conflict resolution during union negotiations, in which each side is appeased to some degree. With this approach, nobody gets everything he or she thinks he or she needs, but a sense of energy exists that is necessary to build important relationships and teams.

Negotiation and compromise are valued approaches. They are chosen when less accommodating or avoiding is appropriate (Box 23-9). Compromising is a blend of both assertive and cooperative behaviours although it calls for less finely honed skills for each behaviour than does collaborating. Negotiation, which involves conferring with others to bring about a settlement of differences, is somewhat like trading (e.g., "You can have this if I can have that" as in "I will chair the regional committee on improving morale if you send me to the hospital's leadership training classes next week so I can have the skills I need to be effective"). Compromise is one of the most effective behaviours used by nurse managers and leaders because it supports a balance of power between themselves and others in the work setting. The self-assessment in Box 23-10 will help you become more aware of your own use of negotiation and compromise and improve it.

| BOX 23-9 | APPROPRIATE USES OF COMPROMISE |

1. When two powerful sides are committed strongly to perceived mutually exclusive goals
2. When temporary solutions to complex issues need to be implemented
3. When conflicting goals are "moderately important" and not worth a major confrontation
4. When time pressures people to expedite a workable solution
5. When collaborating and competing fail

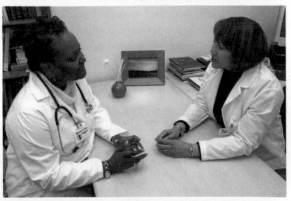

Compromise supports a balance of power between self and others in the workplace.

BOX 23-10 NEGOTIATION/ COMPROMISE SELF-ASSESSMENT AND COMMITMENT TO ACTION

If You Tend to Use Negotiation Often, Ask Yourself the Following Questions:

1. Do I ignore large, important issues while trying to work out creative, practical compromises?
2. Is there a "gamesmanship" in my negotiations?
3. Am I sincerely committed to compromise or negotiated solutions?

If You Seldom Use Negotiation, Ask Yourself the Following Questions:

1. Do I find it difficult to make concessions?
2. Am I often engaged in strong disagreements, or do I withdraw when I see no way to get out?
3. Do I feel embarrassed, sensitive, self-conscious, or pressured to negotiate, compromise, and bargain?

Commitment to Action

What two new behaviours would increase your compromising effectiveness?

1.
2.

Collaborating

Collaborating refers to a group of people working together to achieve a common goal. Although the most time-consuming approach to conflict resolution, it is the most creative. It is both assertive and cooperative because people work creatively and openly to find a solution that most fully satisfies all important concerns and goals to be achieved. Collaboration involves analyzing situations and defining the conflict at a higher level where shared goals are identified and commitment to working together is generated (Box 23-11). When nurses use cooperative conflict management approaches, decision making becomes a collective process in which action plans are mutually understood and implemented. For example, when nurses and physicians work together, they can collaborate by asking, "What is the best thing we can do for the patient and family right now?" and "How does each of us fit into the plan of care to meet their needs?" This requires discussion about the plan, how it will be accomplished, and who will make what contributions toward its achievement and proposed outcomes. Use the self-assessment in Box 23-12 to determine your own use of collaboration.

BOX 23-11 APPROPRIATE USES OF COLLABORATION

1. When seeking creative, integrative solutions in which both sides' goals and needs are important, thus developing group commitment and a consensual decision
2. When learning and growing through cooperative problem solving, resulting in greater understanding and empathy
3. When identifying, sharing, and merging vastly different viewpoints
4. When being honest about and working through difficult emotional issues that interfere with morale, productivity, and growth

BOX 23-12 COLLABORATION: SELF-ASSESSMENT AND COMMITMENT TO ACTION

If You Tend to Collaborate Often, Ask Yourself the Following Questions:

1. Do I spend valuable group time and energy on issues that do not warrant or deserve it?
2. Do I postpone needed action to get consensus and avoid making key decisions?
3. When I initiate collaboration, do others respond in a genuine way, or are there hidden agendas, unspoken hostility, and/or manipulation in the group?

If You Seldom Collaborate, Ask Yourself the Following Questions:

1. Do I ignore opportunities to cooperate, take risks, and creatively confront conflict?
2. Do I tend to be pessimistic, distrusting, withdrawing, and/or competitive?
3. Am I involving others in important decisions, eliciting commitment, and empowering them?

Commitment to Action

What two new behaviours would increase your collaboration effectiveness?

1.
2.

At the onset of conflict, involved collaborating individuals can carefully analyze situations to identify the nature and reasons for conflict and choose an appropriate approach. For example, a conflict arises when a staff nurse and a charge nurse on a psychiatric unit disagree about how to handle a patient's complaints regarding the staff nurse's delay in responding to the patient's requests. At the point that they reach agreement that it is the staff nurse's responsibility and decision to make, collaboration has occurred. The nurse leader might say, "I didn't realize your plan of care was to respond to the patient at predetermined intervals or that you told the patient that you would check on her every 30 minutes. I can now inform the patient that I know about and support your approach." Or the staff nurse and nurse leader might talk and subsequently agree that the staff nurse is too emotionally involved with the patient's problems and that it may be time for her to withdraw from providing care and enlist the support of another nurse, even temporarily. Discussion can result in collaboration aimed at allowing the staff nurse to withdraw appropriately. Another, less-desirable choice could be to compete and let the winner's position stand (e.g., "I'm in charge; I'm going to assign another nurse to this patient to preserve our patient satisfaction scores" or "I know what is best for this patient; I took care of her during her past two admissions").

DIFFERENCES OF CONFLICT-HANDLING STYLES AMONG NURSES

The way in which nurses respond to conflict has changed very little in the past 20 years. Previous studies suggest that avoidance and accommodation remain the predominant choices for staff nurses and that the prevalent style for nurse managers is compromise, despite the emphasis placed on collaboration as an effective strategy for conflict management (Iglesias & Vallejo, 2012; Mahon & Nicotera, 2011). See the Research Perspective for a discussion about the correlation between emotional intelligence and the preferred conflict-handling styles among nurses. Professional nurses often avoid conflict when they fear a consequence (Johansen, 2012). Nurses sometimes choose to avoid conflict because they fear that engaging in conflict or even attempting to resolve conflict may jeopardize their career advancement (Johansen, 2012; Mahon & Nicotera, 2011). It is interesting to note that newly graduated nurses are especially vulnerable to workplace conflict and report being unprepared to handle it (Latham et al., 2013). Students most frequently use avoidance and compromise as strategies to manage conflict (Pines, Rauschhuber, Norgan, et al., 2012). See also Chapter 27 for how these student approaches coincide with role transition.

RESEARCH PERSPECTIVE

Resource: Morrison, J. (2008). The relationship between emotional intelligence competencies and preferred conflict-handling styles. *Journal of Nursing Management, 16*(8), 974–983. doi:10.1111/j.1365-2834.2008.00876.x

The purpose of this study was to determine if a relationship exists between emotional intelligence and the preferred conflict-handling styles of registered nurses in a health care setting. Emotional intelligence (EI) is the capacity to understand one's own feelings as well as the feelings of others and includes self-control, persistence, and motivation. It has been previously demonstrated that individuals who exhibit more emotional self-control can handle conflicting circumstances more effectively. A total of 92 nurses, over half of whom had graduated within the past 4 years, participated in the study. Nurses indicated that they chose the accommodating style most frequently and used collaborating infrequently. Results showed that higher levels of EI positively correlated with collaborating and negatively with accommodating.

Implications for Practice

With the dynamic changes in health care today and the expanding role of the professional nurse, recognizing the issues affecting conflict in the practice environment is essential. Understanding how emotional intelligence levels and conflict skills correlate can be used to reduce conflict and improve interpersonal relationships in the practice environment. When conflict is approached with high levels of EI, interpersonal skills are enhanced. Thus, effective nurses and nursing leaders can enhance their EI competencies as a way of addressing conflict issues affecting the profession. EI development training can target the problems of conflict and stress in the practice environment.

Researchers have generally found that nurses and physicians do not routinely collaborate with each other during conflict situations (Brooks, Polis, & Phillips, 2014). Conflicts between nurses and physicians may be intensified because of communication breakdowns that prevent clarification of roles and issues where practice domains overlap (Brooks et al., 2014). Furthermore, when asked to describe working relationships with physicians, nurses frequently reported power imbalance as a dominant theme that supported major impediments to improving nurse–physician collaborative behaviours (Longo, 2010; Nair, Fitzpatrick, McNulty, et al., 2012). Compromising strategies were found to be the most common conflict-handling approach to nurse–physician interactions. A positive correlation existed between how long nurses had functioned in a leadership position and how often they chose collaborating as a strategy for dealing with disruptive behaviours and resolving conflict with physicians (Hendel, Fish, & Berger, 2007). These findings further emphasized that conflict is disruptive and influences clinical practice environments and patient safety (Brooks et al., 2014). Health care organizations need to strengthen healthy professional relationships and foster an organizational culture that embraces collaborative practice to safeguard positive patient outcomes.

THE ROLE OF THE LEADER

Encouraging positive working relations among health care providers requires effective conflict management as an integral part of the practice environment (Lachman, Murray, Iseminger, et al., 2012). The role of the nurse leader is to foster a practice environment that encourages open communication, collaborative practices for achieving mutual goals, and constructive approaches to conflict management (Ceravolo, Schwartz, Foltz-Ramos, et al., 2012).

Nurse leaders promote positive clinical practice environments by promoting conflict prevention and supporting conflict resolution (Ceravolo et al., 2012). Nurse leaders model professionalism and empower their followers by coaching newer nurses to think strategically about conflict resolution strategies and to respond to conflict in a timely manner and with carefully selected approaches. Disrespectful communications or miscommunications are common elements of conflict that can often be resolved with collaboration, active listening, and respectful assertive communication (Ceravolo et al., 2012). Nurse leaders encourage collaboration by modelling open and honest communication and demonstrating commitment to address conflict in a timely fashion (Blair, 2013; Spence Laschinger, Cummings, Wong, et al., 2014).

The Canadian Nurses Association (2009) supports the need for nurse leaders to be present in all nursing practice settings at all levels, including the front line. Many front-line nurses report feeling unprepared to take on leadership roles and have identified the need for organizations to provide ongoing education and competency development to enhance leadership abilities in front-line nurses (Sherman, Schwarzkopf, & Kiger, 2011). Nurses at the front

line are often change agents. They coordinate, integrate, and facilitate interprofessional and intraprofessional teamwork to ensure that quality patient care is provided (Porter-O'Grady, 2011). Front-line nurse leaders must have strong communication and organizational skills and must be approachable and nonjudgemental.

The health care workforce today is made up of individuals from four generations, and generational differences in values, traits, expectations, communication style, and behaviour influence professional relationships (Leiter, Price, & Spence Laschinger, 2010). These intergenerational tensions can sometimes lead to conflict. Leaders can help establish workplace cultures that acknowledge generational

LITERATURE PERSPECTIVE

Resource: Almost, J. (2006). Conflict within nursing environments: Concept analysis. *Journal of Advanced Nursing, 53*(4), 444–453. doi:10.1111/j.1365-2648.2006.03738.x

A concept analysis of conflict in nursing work environments was conducted using the evolutionary approach. Results following an exhaustive review of the literature published from 1980 to 2004 included a conceptual diagram of antecedents and consequences of conflict (Figure 23-2). Sources of conflict originate from individual characteristics, interpersonal factors, and organizational dynamics. Individual differences, typically generated by differing opinions and values, create potential conflict. Demographic dissimilarity (e.g., gender, educational levels, age, race, ethnicity) can stimulate conflict as well. Interpersonal factors such as distrust, perceptions of injustice or disrespect, and inadequate or poor communication style can lead to conflict. Organizational factors including the interdependence among team members and the changes that result from restructuring can set the stage for conflict within the practice environment.

Similarly, the effects of unresolved conflict are visible in individual characteristics, interpersonal factors, and organizational dynamics. Individual effects include job stress and dissatisfaction, absenteeism, and intent to leave, whereas interpersonal factors such as hostility and avoidance are dominant. The organizational impact of negative conflict management includes reduced productivity and ineffective teamwork.

Implications for Practice
Sources of conflict within the practice environment must be anticipated and addressed to enhance organizational effectiveness. Health care leaders must engage in conflict management strategies to prevent or resolve conflict within nursing environments to ensure quality and safety.

differences by highlighting and building on the strengths this diversity brings while concurrently emphasizing common goals (Keepnews, Brewer, Kovner, et al., 2010). One way to promote a positive work setting is to promote conflict prevention and ensure conflict resolution (Almost, 2006) (see the Literature Perspective).

Nurses in managerial and leadership positions spend inadequate time on conflict resolution. Many do not feel qualified or sufficiently experienced to deal with conflict (Becher & Visovsky, 2012). Moreover, some staff can be difficult to work with, so managers must remain focused on the problem and not the personalities of the team members. Nurse managers must quickly address and intervene in

conflict and lateral violence. Nurse managers must also remain cognizant of other pitfalls of effective conflict resolution. For example, nurse managers commonly avoid conflict in the workplace by delaying responding to colleagues' concerns voiced in staff meetings, not replying to voice mails or e-mail messages, or cancelling or postponing important meetings. However, if this behaviour is known and continues, conflict remains and the avoiding behaviour becomes acceptable and leads to poor outcomes for the individuals involved, patients, and the organization (Stanton, 2012). Avoidance leads to poor communication, which negatively influences patient outcomes (Johansen, 2012). To reduce conflict and the incidence of workplace violence, the leader must

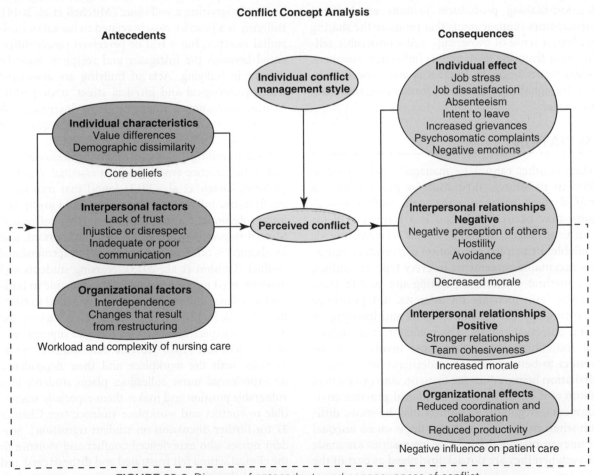

FIGURE 23-2 Diagram of antecedents and consequences of conflict.

empower followers to create a respectful practice climate while at the same time set acceptable standards of behaviour (Spence Laschinger et al., 2014). Longo (2010) has suggested that promoting healthy work environments requires organizations and nurse leaders to implement sound policies such as zero-tolerance policies that support cultures that do not tolerate disruptive behaviours leading to conflict. Healthy work environments require a committed leader and organizational support.

Working in teams is an important part of health care delivery. Negative relationships among colleagues can disrupt team performance, ultimately compromising patient safety (Becher & Visovsky, 2012). For teams to be successful, they need to work independently of managers, receiving direction and interventions when needed. Functional teams working together will initiate meetings and implement decision-making procedures (actions emphasizing participatory management) that promote the sharing of ideas, a sense of ownership, and a noticeable self-direction from the team and its individual members. When teams begin to lose focus and cohesiveness, they are signalling the need for further direction from a manager.

MEDIATION

When conflict cannot be managed easily by those close to its source, mediation—a process using a trained third party to assist with conflict resolution—may occur. Mediation is a learned skill for which advanced training and/or certification is available. Principled negotiation can produce mutually acceptable agreements in every type of conflict. The method involves separating the people from the problem; focusing on interests, not positions; inventing options for mutual gain; and insisting on using objective criteria. The mediator is an impartial individual who assists those involved in the conflict to better hear and understand one another. Mediation helps reduce the focus on who can control whom and on a "winner." In clinical practice environments, negotiating conflicts may be more difficult when at least one of the parties is on an unequal or uneven playing field. These inequalities are made worse when they are not acknowledged as part of the problem.

MANAGING LATERAL VIOLENCE AND BULLYING

A significant source of interpersonal conflict in the workplace stems from lateral violence—"psychological harassment evidenced by verbal abuse, intimidation, exclusion, unfair assignments, denial of access to opportunities, and withholding of information" (Morse, 2008). *Lateral violence* is often used interchangeably with horizontal violence, which is "an act of aggression that's perpetuated by one colleague toward another colleague" (Longo & Sherman, 2007). Nurses direct dissatisfaction toward one another through various behaviours. The literature identifies several common forms of lateral violence such as criticizing a colleague, belittling or making hurtful comments to or about a colleague in front of others, complaining about a colleague, rolling eyes, or simply ignoring a colleague (Mitchell et al. 2014). Bullying is a practice closely related to lateral or horizontal violence, but a real or perceived power differential between the instigator and recipient must be present in bullying. Acts of bullying are associated with psychological and physical stress, underperformance, professional disengagement, increased job turnover, and the potential for diminished quality of care (Vessey, DeMarco, Gaffney, et al., 2009).

Understanding the sources of intraprofessional conflict in the practice environment is essential. Gordon, Melrose, Janzen, et al. (2013) found that transitioning from one nursing role to another could precipitate intraprofessional conflict between nursing colleagues. Mutual respect between colleagues is important, and its absence is often at the centre of intraprofessional conflict (Gordon et al., 2013). Nursing students and inexperienced nurses are especially vulnerable to horizontal violence and are generally not prepared to effectively handle it (Latham et al., 2013). Newly graduated nurses can experience a lack of collegial support and, in fact, Johnson (2010) reveals that students' unfamiliarity with the workplace and their dependence on experienced nurse colleagues places students in a vulnerable position and makes them especially susceptible to conflict and workplace violence (see Chapter 27 for further discussion on student transition). Student nurses who experienced conflict and violence in the clinical setting felt frustrated and disheartened and reported that the experience was destructive to their self-image (King-Jones, 2011). Lateral violence affects newly licensed nurses' job satisfaction and stress, as well as their intent to remain in their current position or the nursing profession (C. Thomas, 2010; Woelfle & MaCaffrey, 2007).

Lateral violence may be a symptom of extremely demanding clinical practice environments (Spence Laschinger et al., 2014). The CNA and the Canadian Federation of Nurses Unions (CFNU) (2007) jointly affirmed that workplace violence includes actual and attempted incidents of verbal and psychological abuse (including bullying), and that such violence negatively affects all health care providers, patients, and organizations. The CNA and CFNU recommend that leaders in health care organizations address unacceptable behaviours, advocate for collaborative and all-inclusive practice environments, and seek to eliminate violence.

Collaborative conflict resolution must be encouraged and supported, but a mechanism for confidential reporting is also necessary (Schaffner, Stanley, &

Hough, 2006). Increased awareness and education sessions on conflict resolution are other key elements for establishing positive professional practice environments. Leadership training is essential and builds competencies in how to recognize and defend against lateral violence (Johansen, 2012).

EXERCISE 23-3

Consider a conflict you would describe as "ongoing" in a clinical setting. Reflect on the issue in terms of the concepts presented in this chapter. Consult with some people involved in the conflict to get their historical perspective on this issue. Once you have gathered the details, consider the following questions:

- What are their positions and years of experience?
- How are resources, time, and personnel wasted on mismanaging this issue?
- What blocks the effective management of this issue?
- What currently aids in its management?
- What new things and actions would add to its management in the future?

💡 A SOLUTION

Conflict is uncomfortable and unnerving, but learning about conflict and developing conflict resolution strategies can help you effectively handle these situations. Antonia analyzed the way she was dealing with the negativity in the workplace and, after completing a conflict self-assessment, she realized that she was avoiding the conflict. Her ability to care for patients was being impacted by the bullying, and Antonia knew she needed to get help. Antonia approached her nurse manager, and without naming individuals, described the conflict she was having. The nurse manager told Antonia that she had a right to a workplace free of psychological violence and that the hospital was committed to preventing such a workplace. The nurse manager referred Antonia to free counselling through the human resources department and assured her that her complaint would be followed up on. Antonia felt that she had been heard and that her feelings and thoughts were important to the nurse manager. Antonia is seeing a counsellor and is attending assertiveness training classes, which is helping her develop the skills to manage the conflict better.

Was this approach effective in this situation? Does this approach to handling conflict align with your preferred conflict management style? Why or why not?

■ THE EVIDENCE

Conflict is inherent in the professional practice environment and has both positive and negative outcomes for nurses and other health care providers, organizations, and even patients. Lateral violence is toxic to the profession. Lateral violence causes physical and psychological effects on nurses, as well as negative outcomes for patients. Nurses must speak out and advocate for respectful and nonviolent treatment of all health care staff, patients, residents, and their friends and families

(CNA & CFNU, 2007) The need for a culture change to abolish lateral violence has been endorsed by a number of professional organizations, including the Canadian Nurses Association, the Canadian Federation of Nurses Unions, and the International Council of Nurses. Nurses must enhance their knowledge and skills to eliminate hostile work environments, workplace intimidation, reality shock for new graduates, and accepted notions of "nurses eating their young."

NEED TO KNOW NOW

- Know how to assess conflict and its circumstances to determine which approach to conflict resolution is potentially most effective.
- Identify and offer appropriate behaviours to prevent or resolve conflict in your practice environment.

- Evaluate your practice environment for situations reflecting lateral violence. Be proactive and know how to respond to a colleague who demonstrates lateral violence.

CHAPTER CHECKLIST

A more thorough understanding of conflict within the professional practice environment will enable the nurse to prevent or successfully manage nonproductive conflict. Navigating desirable conflict within the work environment will promote change resulting in organizational growth and personal and professional enrichment of nurses.

- The three types of conflict are as follows:
  - Intrapersonal
  - Interpersonal
  - Organizational
- The conflict process progresses through four stages:
  - Frustration:
    - Blocked goals lead to frustration.
    - Frustration is a cue to stop and clarify differences.
  - Conceptualization:
    - The way a person perceives a conflict determines how he or she reacts to the frustration.
    - Differences in conceptualizing an issue can block resolution.
  - Action:
    - Intentions, strategies, plans, and behaviour are formulated.

- Outcomes:
  - They include both tangible and intangible consequences.
- When assessing how well a conflict has been resolved, one must consider the following:
  - The quality of decisions, including the degree to which important goals were achieved by assessing the outcomes
  - The quality of relationships, including how willing people involved in the conflict are to work together
- The five modes of conflict resolution are as follows:
  - Avoiding
  - Accommodating
  - Competing
  - Compromising
  - Collaborating
- Each mode of conflict resolution can be viewed along two dimensions:
  - From uncooperative to highly cooperative
  - From unassertive to highly assertive
- The role of the nurse leader is to foster a practice environment that encourages open communication, collaborative practices for achieving mutual goals, and constructive approaches to conflict management.

TIPS FOR ADDRESSING CONFLICT

- Communicate to yourself and others that conflict is a naturally occurring and beneficial process for individuals and organizations, typically marked by frustration, different conceptualizations, a variety of approaches to resolving it, and ongoing outcomes.
- Assess the work environment to see what behaviours are endorsed and fostered by the leaders. Determine if these behaviours are worthy of imitation.

- Determine any similarities and differences in facts, goals, methods, and values in sorting out the different conceptualizations of a conflict situation.
- Assess the degree of conflict resolution by reflecting on the quality of the decisions (e.g., creativity, practicality, achievement of goals, breakthrough results) and the quality of the relationships (e.g., understanding, willingness to work together, mutual respect, cooperation).

- Reflect on your preferred strategies for resolving conflict (e.g., which of the five approaches do you not use often enough and which do you overuse?) and assess each situation to match the best approach for that type of conflict regardless of which is your favourite approach.
- Assist others around you in assessing conflict situations and determining how they can best approach them.
- Commit to addressing and confronting disruptive behaviours.

- View conflict as an opportunity to grow as a person and a professional.
- Model collaborative conflict resolution practices.
- Do your part in fostering a healthy work environment that embraces diversity and inclusion.
- Speak out about violence to help increase awareness and knowledge.
- Advocate for "zero tolerance" policies.

℮volve WEBSITE

Visit the Evolve website for Suggested Readings, Internet Resources, and additional resources related to the content in this chapter: http://evolve.elsevier.com/Canada/Yoder-Wise/leading/.

REFERENCES

Almost, J. (2006). Conflict within nursing environments: Concept analysis. *Journal of Advanced Nursing, 53*(4), 444–453. doi:10.1111/j.1365-2648.2006.03738.x

Antoniazzi, C. D. (2011). Respect as experienced by registered nurses. *Western Journal of Nursing Research, 33*(6), 745–766. doi:10.1177/0193945910376516

Becher, J., & Visovsky, C. (2012). Horizontal violence in nursing. *MEDSURG Nursing, 21*(4), 210–232.

Bennett, K., & Sawatzky, J. A. (2013). Building emotional intelligence: A strategy for emerging nurse leaders to reduce workplace bullying. *Nursing Administration Quarterly, 37*(2), 144–151. doi:10.1097/NAQ.0b013e318286de5f

Berwick, D. (2011). Preparing nurses for participation in and leadership of continual improvement. *Journal of Nursing Education, 50*(6), 322–327. doi:10.3928/01484834-20110519-05

Blair, P. (2013). Lateral violence in nursing. *Journal of Emergency Nursing, 39*(5), e75–e78. doi:10.1016/j.jen.2011.12.006

Blake, R. R., & Mouton, J. S. (1964). *Solving costly organization conflict.* San Francisco, CA: Jossey-Bass.

Brooks, A. M. T., Polis, N., & Phillips, E. (2014). The new healthcare landscape: Disruptive behaviors influence work environment, safety and clinical outcomes. *Nurse Leader, 12*(1), 39–44.

Canadian Nurses Association. (2009, October). Position statement: Nursing leadership. Retrieved from http://www.nanb.nb.ca/PDF/CNA_Nursing_Leadership_2009_E.pdf.

Canadian Nurses Association & Canadian Federation of Nurses Unions. (2007). Joint position statement: Workplace violence. Retrieved from https://nursesunions.ca/sites/default/files/workplace_violence_position_statement_cna-cfnu_0.pdf.

Ceravolo, D. J., Schwartz, D. G., Foltz-Ramos, K. M., et al. (2012). Strengthening communication to overcome lateral violence. *Journal of Nursing Management, 20*(5), 599–606.

Clark, C. (2013). *Creating and sustaining civility in nursing education.* Indianapolis, IN: Sigma Theta International.

Deutsch, M. (1973). *The resolution of conflict: Constructive and destructive processes.* New Haven, CT: Yale University Press.

Duffy, E. (1995). Horizontal violence: A conundrum for nursing. *Journal of the Royal College of Nursing, 2*(2), 5–17.

Edmonson, C. (2010). Moral courage and the nurse leader. *Online Journal of Issues in Nursing, 15*(3). doi:10.3912/OJIN.Vol15No03Man05

Friese, C. R., & Manojlovich, M. (2012). Nurse–physician relationship in ambulatory oncology settings. *Journal of Nursing Scholarship, 44*(3), 258–265. doi:10.1111/j.1547-5069.2012.01458.x

Gordon, K., Melrose, S., Janzen, K. J., et al. (2013). Licensed practical nurses becoming registered nurses: Conflicts and responses that can help. *Clinical Nursing Studies, 1*(4), 1–8. doi:10.5430/cns.v1n4p1

Hendel, T., Fish, M., & Berger, O. (2007). Nurse/physician conflict management mode choices: Implications for improved collaborative practice. *Nursing Administration Quarterly, 31*(3), 244–253. doi:10.1097/01.NAQ.0000278938.57115.75

Hurst, J., & Kinney, M. (1989). *Empowering self and others.* Toledo, OH: University of Toledo.

Hurst, J. B. (1993). *Conflict self-assessment.* Toledo, OH: Human Resource Development Center, University of Toledo.

Iglesias, M. E. L., & Vallejo, R. B. B. (2012). Conflict resolution styles in the nursing profession. *Contemporary Nurse, 43*(1), 73–80.

Jackson, D., Hutchinson, M., Peters, K., et al. (2013). Understanding avoidant leadership in healthcare: Findings form a secondary analysis of two qualitative studies. *Journal of Nursing Management, 21*(3), 572–580. doi:10.1111/j.1365-2834.2012.01395.x

Johansen, M. L. (2012). Keeping the peace. Conflict management strategies for nurse managers. *Nursing Management, 43*(2), 50–54. doi:10.1097/01.NUMA.0000410920.90831.96

Johnson, M. (2010). The bullying aspect of workplace violence in nursing. *JONA's Healthcare Law, Ethics and Regulation, 12*(2), 36–42. doi:10.1097/NHL.0b013e3181e6bd19

Keepnews, D. M., Brewer, C. S., Kovner, C. T., et al. (2010). Generational differences among newly licensed registered nurses. *Nursing Outlook, 58*(3), 155–163. doi:10.1016/j.outlook.2009.11.001

King-Jones, M. (2011). Horizontal violence and the socialization of new nurses. *Creative Nursing, 17*(2), 80–86. doi:10.1891/1078-4535.17.2.80

Lachman, V., Murray, J. S., Iseminger, K., et al. (2012). Doing the right thing: Pathways to moral courage. *American Nurse Today, 7*(5), 24–29.

Latham, C. L., Ringl, K., & Hogan, M. (2013). Combating workplace violence with peer mentoring. *Nursing Management, 44*(9), 30–38. doi:10.1097/01.NUMA.0000429005.47269.f9

Leiter, M. P., Price, S. L., & Spence Laschinger, H. K. (2010). Generational differences in distress, attitudes and civility among nurses. *Journal of Nursing Management, 18*(8), 970–980. doi:10.1111/j.1365-2834.2010.01168.x

Longo, J. (2010). Combating disruptive behaviors: Strategies to promote a healthy work environment. *Online Journal of Issues in Nursing, 15*(1). doi:10.3912/OJIN.Vol15No01Man05

Longo, J., & Sherman, R. O. (2007, March). Levelling horizontal violence. *Nursing Management*, 34–36, 50+.

Mahon, N. M., & Nicotera, A. M. (2011). Nursing and conflict communication: Avoidance as preferred strategy. *Nursing Administration Quarterly, 35*(2), 152–163. doi:10.1097/NAQ.0b013e31820f47d5

Matney, S. A., Maddox, L. J., & Staggers, N. (2014). Nurses as knowledge workers: Is there evidence of knowledge in patient handoffs? *Western Journal of Nursing Research, 36*(2), 171–190. doi:10.1177/0193945913497111

Mazurek Melnyk, B., Hrabe, D. P., & Szalacha, L. A. (2013). Relationships among work stress, job satisfaction, mental health and healthy lifestyle behaviors in new graduate nurses attending the nurse athlete program. *Nursing Administration Quarterly, 37*(4), 278–285. doi:10.1097/NAQ.0b013e3182a2f963

Mitchell, A., Ahmed, A., & Szabo, C. (2014). Workplace violence among nurses, why are we still discussing this? Literature review. *Journal of Nursing Education and Practice, 4*(4), 147–150. doi:10.5430/jnep.v4n4p147

Morrison, J. (2008). The relationship between emotional intelligence competencies and preferred conflict-handling styles. *Journal of Nursing Management, 16*(8), 974–983. doi:10.1111/j.1365-2834.2008.00876.x

Morse, K. J. (2008). Lateral violence in nursing [Editorial]. *Nursing2014 Critical Care, 3*(2), 4.

Nair, D. M., Fitzpatrick, J. K., McNulty, R., et al. (2012). Frequency of nurse–physician collaborative behaviors in acute care hospital. *Journal of Interprofessional Care, 26*(2), 115–120. doi:10.3109/13561820.2011.637647

Pines, E. W., Rauschhuber, G. H., Norgan, J. D., et al. (2012). Stress resiliency, psychological empowerment and conflict management styles among baccalaureate nursing students. *Journal of Advanced Nursing, 68*(7), 1482–1493. doi:10.1111/j.1365-2648.2011.05875.x

Porter-O'Grady, T. (2011). Leadership at all levels. *Nursing Management, 42*(5), 32–37. doi:10.1097/01.NUMA.0000396347.49552.86

Roche, M., Diers, D., Duffield, C., et al. (2010). Violence toward nurses, the work environment, and patient outcomes. *Journal of Nursing Scholarship, 42*(1), 13–22. doi:10.1111/j.1547-5069.2009.01321.x

Saltman, D. C., O'Dea, N. A., & Kidd, M. R. (2006). Conflict management: A primer for doctors in training. *Postgraduate Medical Journal, 82*, 9–12. doi:10.1136/pgmj.2005.034306

Schaffner, M., Stanley, K., & Hough, C. (2006). No matter which way you look at it, it's violence. *Gastroenterology Nursing, 28*(6), 75–76. doi:10.1097/00001610-200601000-00019

Sherman, R., & Pross, E. (2010). Growing future nurse leaders to build and sustain healthy work environments at the unit level. *Online Journal of Issues in Nursing, 15*(1). doi:10.3912/OJIN.Vol15No01Man01

Sherman, R., Schwarzkopf, R., & Kiger, A. J. (2011). Charge nurse perspectives on frontline leadership in acute care environments. *International Scholarly Research Network Nursing, 2011*. doi:10.5402/2011/164052

Spence Laschinger, H. K., Cummings, G. C., Wong, C. A., et al. (2014). Resonant leadership and workplace empowerment: The value of positive organizational cultures in reducing workplace incivility. *Nursing Economics, 32*(1), 5–16.

Stanton, K. (2012). Resolving workplace conflict. Retrieved from http://nursing.advanceweb.com/Editorial/Content/PrintFriendly.aspx?CC=260175.

Thomas, C. (2010). Teaching nursing students and newly registered nurses strategies to deal with violent behaviors in the professional practice environment. *The Journal of Continuing Education in Nursing, 41*(7), 299–308.

Thomas, K. W. (1992). Conflict and conflict management: Reflections and update. *Journal of Organizational Behavior, 13*(3), 265–274. doi:10.1002/job.4030130306

Thomas, K. W., & Kilmann, R. H. (1974). *Thomas-Kilmann Conflict Mode Instrument*. Tuxedo, NY: Xicom.

Thomas, K. W., & Kilmann, R. H. (2002). *Thomas-Kilmann Conflict Mode Instrument* (revised edition). Mountain View, CA: CPP.

Vessey, J. A., DeMarco, R. F., Gaffney, D. A., et al. (2009). Bullying of staff registered nurses in the workplace: A preliminary study for developing strategies for the transformation of hostile to healthy workplace environments. *Journal of Professional Nursing, 25*(5), 299–306. doi:10.1016/j.profnurs.2009.01.022

Woelfle, C. Y., & McCaffrey, R. (2007). Nurse on nurse. *Nursing Forum, 42*(3), 123–131. doi:10.1111/j.1744-6198.2007.00076.x

Wolff, A. C., Ratner, P. A., Robinson, S. L., et al. (2010). Beyond generational differences: A literature review of the impact of relational diversity on nurses' attitudes on work. *Journal of Nursing Management, 18*(8), 948–969. doi:10.1111/j.1365-2834.2010.01136.x

Zerwekh, J., & Zerwekh Garneau, A. (2011). *Nursing today: transition and trends* (7th ed.). St. Louis, MO: Elsevier Saunders.

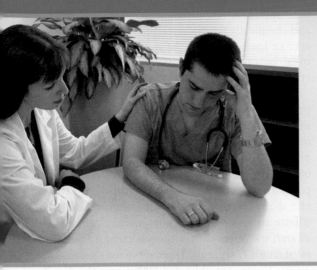

Managing Personal/ Personnel Problems

Karren Kowalski
Adapted by Jayne Naylen McChesney and
Heather D. Wilson

This chapter discusses various personal and personnel problems that nurse managers and leaders must face in all nursing settings. It offers specific tips and tools on ways to intervene, coach, correct, and document problem behaviours. Emphasis is placed on effective communication, both written and verbal.

OBJECTIVES

- Describe common personal/personnel problems.
- Describe how clarifying role expectations can help resolve personnel problems.
- Understand strategies that are useful in approaching specific personnel problems.
- Describe how to document performance problems.
- Understand the steps involved in progressive discipline.
- Describe the guidelines that should be followed when terminating an employee.
- Value the leadership aspects of the role of the novice nurse.

TERMS TO KNOW

absenteeism	nonpunitive discipline	role strain
chemical dependency	progressive discipline	role stress
grievance		

Brooklyn started her new job as a resource float pool nurse with a shift on the mother baby unit. While taking care of Tessa and her newborn, Brooklyn noticed that the newborn was jittery and having difficulties with breastfeeding, even after several attempts. Brooklyn was engaged in caring for Tessa and had spent considerable time reassuring her and offering suggestions on positioning the newborn at the breast. Later in the shift, Miranda, the nurse manager, was checking in on Brooklyn and her patients and noticed that Tessa's newborn was jittery. After discussing the progress of the newborn's breastfeeding and determining the birth weight with Brooklyn, Miranda inquired about the newborn's blood sugar level. Brooklyn had not checked the newborn's blood sugar level, as she was unaware of the protocol. Brooklyn felt terrible and questioned her competency to continue working on the mother baby unit.

Consider the above scenario from the viewpoint of nurse manager Miranda. What are your thoughts about this situation, and how might you manage it?

INTRODUCTION

Novice nurses require orientation, ongoing guidance, mentoring, and sometimes additional education resources; however, they also have a responsibility to apply their knowledge and critical thinking in clinical practice (Chandler, 2012). Novice nurses might also require coaching regarding when to ask for guidance and when to directly involve leaders to ensure patients are safe. The nurse manager should engage with followers and be aware of how the care team is functioning in order to provide guidance and any necessary support. Ultimately, the nurse manager needs to actively support quality care, general safety, and optimal patient outcomes (Hughes, 2008).

Many health care settings in Canada deliver care using a team approach, and so nurse managers often lead a team consisting of various health care providers, such as licensed practical nurses and special care aides. Nurse managers also assume responsibility for other staff members, such as housekeeping staff, dietary service workers, and other allied health professionals. The role of the nurse manager or leader can be rewarding and satisfying, yet it also involves challenges that require specific knowledge, skills, and attitudes. Some of these challenges include absenteeism,

uncooperative or unproductive employees, clinical incompetence, employees with emotional problems, and chemically dependent employees. If a nurse manager or leader wants to be successful, these problems must be carefully managed while minimizing their effects on patient care and staff morale.

Documentation is an integral part of professional practice and is a critical aspect of patient care. Equally important is accurate and thorough documentation of performance problems or any conflict within the professional practice environment (College of Nurses of Ontario, 2013; Longo, 2010). The nurse manager's goals are to empower followers (employees) to maintain the highest standards of patient care and to contribute to a supportive, safe environment in which all staff members deliver quality care and attain work satisfaction (Espinoza, Lopez-Soldana, & Stonestreet, 2009). Nurses are obligated to preserve the dignity of all and promote justice even when addressing difficult issues and taking action that potentially creates moral distress (Canadian Nurses Association [CNA], 2008; Edmonson, 2010). In this chapter, it is from this perspective that we examine specific employee problems, the nurse manager or leader's role in addressing such problems, and the responsibilities of the novice nurse.

PERSONAL/PERSONNEL PROBLEMS

Absenteeism

One of the most frustrating personnel problems for nurse managers is absenteeism, which is the rate at which an individual misses work on an unplanned basis. Inadequate staffing adversely affects patient care both directly and indirectly. When an absent caregiver is replaced by another who is unfamiliar with the routines, the employee's morale is impacted and patient care may not meet established standards. Working with inadequate staffing or working overtime to cover for absent workers creates physical and mental stress for the care provider team and the leader. Replacement or float personnel often need more supervision, which not only is costly but also may decrease productivity and the quality of patient care. Indirectly, co-workers may become resentful about being forced to assume heavier workloads and/or may be pressured to work extra hours. Chronic absenteeism may lead to increased staff conflicts, decreased morale, and eventually increased absenteeism among the entire staff.

Research indicates that nurse leaders prefer to avoid conflict and negative behaviour by acknowledging concerns but abstaining from action, providing an ambivalent response, and failing to address concerns (Jackson, Hutchinson, Peters, et al., 2013). However, nurse leaders must model and confront persistent absenteeism and discuss the situation directly with the employee (refer to Chapter 23) by verbalizing their concerns:

- "I feel concerned when I see that you have been absent 3 days this month."
- "Can you see how excessive absences affect the smooth functioning of the unit, the workload of other team members, and the safety of patients?"
- "This rate of absences cannot continue. What is your plan for addressing this situation?"

Absenteeism costs the organization money; replacement of absent personnel by temporary personnel or overtime paid to other employees has significant repercussions. When labour costs are excessive, those costs compromise support for other creative efforts of the unit, such as staff education or the ability to purchase new equipment. Also, as care delivery systems become more complex and technically oriented, nurse managers realize that technology is not a substitute for human caregivers. Caregivers cannot be replaced with machines.

Absenteeism is not always related to organizational issues, and it cannot be totally eliminated. There are always unplanned illnesses, accidents, bad weather, sick family members, a death in the family, and even jury duty, all of which are legitimate reasons for missing work and beyond the control of management. Difficult situations can lead to chronic stress for the employee, which makes it difficult for him or her to concentrate and perform job duties (Edmonson, 2010). Absenteeism may also indicate an employee's dissatisfaction with work; dissatisfied staff may in fact be completely disengaged, which can lead to increased absences. Work dissatisfaction is of particular concern because a disengaged nurse potentially puts patients at risk. If the nurse manager or leader believes that an issue is related to work dissatisfaction, team meetings and one-on-one discussion may lead to insight about the sources of the issue. Such discussions provide an excellent opportunity for novice nurses to actively listen, learn, speak up, and advocate for certain issues. If retention of employees is the organizational goal,

any underlying workplace issues should be identified. Doing so may help the organization implement strategies to prevent the loss of dissatisfied employees. Some employees who convey that they are consistently dissatisfied with their jobs may continually disrupt the overall unit and are difficult to manage. The Evidence section on page 470 looks at predictors of short-term absenteeism.

Investigating and determining the specific reasons and root causes of an employee's absence from work can address absenteeism. Wallace (2009) identified typical examples that lead to absenteeism, including personal circumstances such as sick and dependent family members, poor health, job stress, or high work demands such as long hours, excessive workload, lack of control over work, and poor support from managers. These stressors directly impact the care provider team and contribute to an unhealthy work environment. Some of the consequences are low morale, disengaged nurses and care providers, decreased productivity, and decreased quality of care (Ritter, 2011). When nurses stop being accountable for professional quality practice, it compromises their responsibility to uphold professional nursing practice standards. This is detrimental to patients, organizations, and ultimately the nursing profession.

With role theory as a framework, absenteeism has been linked to role stress and role strain. Absence from work is a way of withdrawing from an undesirable situation short of actually leaving, and many employees increase their absenteeism just before submitting their resignation. If a health care provider is experiencing some form of role stress—a condition in which role demands are conflicting, irritating, or impossible to fulfill—it might be manifested through absenteeism (Tucker, Weymiller, Cutshall, et al., 2012). Role stress has negative consequences for both the nurse and the organization (Garrosa, Moreno-Jimenez, Rodriguez-Munoz, et al., 2011). Role strain, the subjective feeling of discomfort experienced as a result of role stress, may be reflected by (1) withdrawal from interaction, (2) reduced involvement with colleagues and the organization, (3) decreased commitment to the mission and the team, and (4) job dissatisfaction. All of these could be manifested through absenteeism. With this framework, management of absenteeism is based on the belief that competent role performance requires interpersonal competence. "Role competence is the ability of a person in an interdependent position, which is ongoing in time, to carry out lines of action that are task and interpersonally effective" (Hardy & Conway, 1988, p. 195). Role behaviour occurs in a social context rather than in isolation. Therefore, the nurse manager needs to understand the culture, the current situation, the context surrounding the situation, and the change needed to better support change. When employees are satisfied with their work, they are more committed to their co-workers and their employer.

One approach to address absenteeism is nonpunitive discipline, which is a disciplinary measure, usually verbal, describing existing standards and goals to which the parties agreed; pay is not withheld, and the employee agrees either to adhere to the standards in the future or to be terminated. A model for behavioural change using nonpunitive discipline appears in Figure 24-1. This model demonstrates how undesirable behaviours, such as absenteeism, can be successfully altered. Box 24-1 identifies specific steps that are involved in nonpunitive discipline.

This model of nonpunitive discipline allows employees to rid themselves of role stress by clarification of role expectations and assumptions. Employees can attain satisfaction and gain a sense of control by understanding that a problem may not be related to their inadequate performance but, rather, a lack of clarification of role expectations within the organization. Most organizations provide orientation to novice nurses so that they can learn organizational policies, procedures, and performance expectations. Competency skills checklists like the example in Table 24-1 on page 462, are useful tools that document nurse's skills. All nurses including novice nurses have a responsibility to ask questions when they do not understand or when they need support and guidance (CNA, 2008).

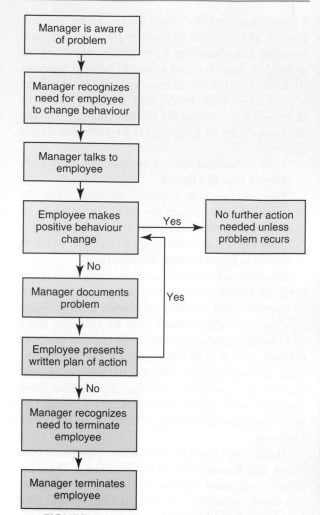

FIGURE 24-1 Model for behavioural change.

EXERCISE 24-1

Interview a nurse manager or leader in your local health region and inquire about their experience with absenteeism. Find out what strategies and processes the nurse manager or leader uses when dealing with chronic absenteeism. What are the possible consequences for employees who are chronically absent from work?

Uncooperative or Unproductive Employees

The problem of uncooperative or unproductive employees can be another challenge for nurse managers. Hersey, Blanchard, and Johnson (2008) identified two major dimensions of job performance that relate to this problem: motivation and ability. Employee motivation is a significant element in organizational performance (Lambrou, Kontodimopoulos, & Niakas, 2010). The type and intensity of employee motivation vary according to personal needs and professional goals. Nurse managers can support professional nurses and employees with motivation problems by being fully present and visible on the unit. They have a significant influence on the work environment to

BOX 24-1   STEPS TO CLARIFY ROLE EXPECTATIONS

Step 1: Remind the employee of the performance expectations and the employment policies of the employer. Sometimes an employee does not know or has forgotten the existing standards, and a reminder or verbal warning with no threats or discipline is all that is needed. It is important that the employee understands his or her responsibility and accountability to the organization's policies and procedures. Regulated nurses also have an obligation to professional practice standards. Consult relevant collective agreements in advance of this conversation and be sure to follow all required stipulations. There should be written and signed documentation of all conversations, and copies should be given to the employee and also placed on his or her human resources file.

Step 2: When the verbal warning does not result in behaviour change, state the issues clearly in a written letter of warning to the employee. These verbal and written warnings must be clear, straightforward communication that includes details and statements of the exact problem, as well as the goals to which both the nurse manager and the employee agree. The employee may agree that the behaviour in question is not acceptable and may volunteer to change and meet the performance expectations. Even if agreement exists between the employee and the employer, the warning must be made to the employee. An employee has a right to support and guidance while striving to meet the performance expectations and you and the organization must collaboratively determine the exact supportive measures required.

Step 3: If the verbal or written warning does not influence the employee to make the necessary behavioural changes, consult with human resources and refer to the relevant collective agreement for your province or health region as to the next steps in handling the situation. Ensure that thorough documentation exists on each and every meeting with the employee, and file it accordingly. It is important to recognize that collective agreements vary from province to province and health region to health region, and that there are different collective agreements within each profession. For example, the collective agreement for registered nurses in Saskatchewan is different from the collective agreement for registered nurses in Alberta.

Step 4: If the employee decides not to meet the performance expectations and adhere to standards and no physical or mental diagnosed limitations exist, termination usually results. All contracts and written agreements must be maintained and copies provided to the employee, employer, and the organization's human resources department.

Organizational policies on termination as well as collective agreements are usually transparent processes that the employee is made aware of early on in the discipline process. Nurse managers need to know and understand the general processes, although human resources departments oversee the termination process.

Occasionally, grievances are filed against organizations. A **grievance** is "an allegation, usually by an individual (employee), but sometimes by the union or management, of misinterpretation or misapplication of a collective bargaining agreement or of traditional work practices" (Doherty, 1989). Collective agreements provide employees with the right to grieve most decisions against them, and the local union supports the employee throughout the grievance process (see Chapter 5 for more information on collective agreements). Typically, in these types of situations, human resources consults with legal services, whose recommendations are taken into account throughout the termination process. Disciplinary and termination processes are complex, and nurse managers should not attempt to handle them on their own but rather consult with human resources and/or legal services.

---

promote a work ethic, mutual respect, and collegial interpersonal relationships by engaging with their team. They can also model and demonstrate commitment and support to followers by providing necessary resources to support safe, quality care.

If an employee is uncooperative or unproductive because of a lack of knowledge or ability, education is an appropriate intervention. Through observations and conversations with employees, the nurse manager can observe and determine the employee's strengths and areas requiring growth. Frequent errors in judgement or techniques are often an indication of lack of knowledge, skill, or critical thinking. Nurse managers must document all variances or untoward events after discussing them with the employee. Citing problem behaviours allows nurse managers to identify possible trends with specific employees. All nurses and employees have a right to clear expectations, appropriate supervision, and ongoing feedback with the opportunity to demonstrate improvement (CNA, 2009). Nurse managers can provide coaching and mentoring to enhance skills, abilities, and attitudes in their followers (Batson & Yoder, 2012). Corrective action is easier to pursue, and resolution is more effective with this strategy. When the problem is determined to result from a need for more education or training, the nurse manager can work with various educational resources such as the clinical nurse educator to help the employee improve his or her skills. Most employees are receptive and extremely cooperative in such situations because they want to improve and meet job expectations. However, some employees may deny that they need help or may be too embarrassed to ask for help because they believe doing so shows weakness

TABLE 24-1   EXAMPLE OF A SKILLS CHECKLIST

Purpose

1. The clinical skills inventory is a three-phase tool to enable the newly hired registered nurse (RN) and the nurse manager to determine individual learning needs, verify competency, and plan performance goals.
2. The RN will complete the self-assessment of clinical skills during the first week of employment. The RN will use the appropriate scale to document current knowledge of clinical skills.
3. The nurse manager will document observed competency of the orientee or delegate this to a peer. All columns must be completed on the inventory level.
4. At the end of orientation, the new RN and the manager will use the inventory to identify performance goals on the plan sheet. The skills inventory will be in a specified place on the nursing unit so that it is available to the manager and other RNs. It should be updated at appropriate intervals as specified by the manager.

Scale for Self-Assessment

1 = Unfamiliar/never done
2 = Able to perform with assistance
3 = Can perform with minimal supervision
4 = Independent performance/proficient

Score for Validation of Competency

1 = Unable to perform at present
2 = Able to perform with assistance
3 = Progressing/repeat performance necessary
4 = Able to perform independently

CLINICAL SKILLS (EXAMPLES)	SELF-ASSESSMENT			VALIDATION			
	SCALE	DATE	COMMENT	SCORE	DATE	INITIALS	COMMENT
Epidural catheter care							

Nasogastric tube
  Insertion
  Management							

Preoperative care/teaching							
Postoperative care/teaching							

Plan Sheet for Skills Inventory

Name _____
Date _____

Goals	Date to Be Completed
_____	_____
_____	_____
_____	_____
_____	_____
_____	_____
_____	_____
_____	_____

Orientee's signature _____
Manager's signature _____
Date _____

or reflects negatively on their relationships with their peers and their leaders.

Immature Employees

Sometimes an unproductive employee simply lacks maturity. This lack of maturity may be described as *emotional intelligence underdevelopment* that results in difficulty forming collegial relationships, difficulty controlling emotions, and an unwillingness to collaborate with colleagues (Harris & Roussel, 2010; Strickland, 2000). Immature employees can be regulated care providers, such as registered nurses, or unregulated care providers, such as special care aides. They demonstrate a lack of insight into their behaviour and how their behaviours impact others.

Sometimes immaturity in an employee may not be readily apparent. However, it may manifest in the following actions: defiance, testing of workplace guidelines, passivity or hostility, or little appreciation for management decisions. The challenge for the nurse manager is not to react in frustration but to demonstrate a high level of professionalism and continue to engage with the employee in a professional manner. If the nurse manager focuses on identifying the root cause of the undesirable behaviour, he or she will be better able to find the right solution and be better prepared to address the issue as a whole. For example, if an employee states, "Administration is always making decisions to make our jobs harder," rather than making a hostile or defensive comment in reply, the nurse manager could take the employee aside and say, "I notice that you seem to be angry about this new policy. Let's talk about it some more." Immature employees either act immaturely all of the time or regress to an immature level when stressed. It is important to keep in mind that this employee may be displaying dynamics rooted in unresolved personal matters and that the behaviour is not a personal attack on the nurse manager. An effective strategy to manage this situation is to confront the employee with a nonthreatening, collaborative approach to discuss the specific problem and define acceptable behaviour expectations and also outline consequences for nonadherence to policies and procedures. Generally, employees comply with specific performance expectations but will push boundaries and test management in other areas. As this testing occurs, the nurse manager must continue to communicate performance expectations clearly and

frequently and offer suggestions for improvement. Immature employees usually have challenges in the workplace because of a desire to control everything, a lack of self-worth, and an inability to control their emotions and behaviours. Facilitating goal accomplishment, building relationships, and offering praise when appropriate are effective strategies to empower followers/employees. Chapter 3 addresses generational differences and Chapter 10 addresses workforce diversity, if they are factors to consider.

EXERCISE 24-2

You are a nurse manager of a 70-bed Alzheimer and dementia unit. It is a locked unit and the staffing includes registered nurses, licensed practical nurses, and resident assistants. One of the registered nurses, Adriana, reports to you that another nurse, Kelly, is inappropriately using restraints on one of the residents because the resident was continually following the nurse around on the unit and asking too many questions.

As the nurse manager, how would you manage this situation? Is this a professional practice issue?

Clinical Incompetence

Clinical incompetence is possibly one of the most serious and complex problems that the nurse manager encounters. Due to the complexity of these types of situations, the nurse manager usually requires the support and consultation services of human resources personnel and the local professional regulatory body. Clinical incompetence may be obvious immediately after hire, or over a period of time it may become evident that the nurse is unable to the meet the expected practice competencies according to the CNA (2007).

Some nurses are reluctant and unwilling to report instances when they witness clinical incompetence because they fear repercussions. Peternelj-Taylor and Yonge (2003) suggested that nurses may feel ambivalence about their loyalties in these types of situations. They may feel forced to choose between their collegial relationships, their loyalty to their chosen profession, and their moral integrity, as well as adhering to their responsibilities to patients and the organization (Peternelj-Taylor & Yonge, 2003).

When a nurse manager becomes aware that one nurse covers for the mistakes of another, the nurse manager must offer support, guidance, and resources such as additional education, but ultimately must hold the followers accountable to do what is morally right.

Bowen & Weil (2011) reported that less than 10% of nurse leaders use the CNA code of ethics (2008) to counsel followers and colleagues. The nurse manager has a responsibility to create an environment where ethical issues are openly discussed and addressed (Bowen & Weil, 2011). The nurse manager must guide and support followers to find courage and be accountable in morally distressing situations (Edmonson, 2010). All RNs have a professional responsibility to address and report inappropriate and unprofessional behaviour (College of Registered Nurses of British Columbia [CRNBC], 2012a, 2012b). The CNA code of ethics (2008) outlines ethical issues and a nursing regulatory body practice advisor can be an excellent resource to support nurses through difficult situations. Ignoring and avoiding practice violations contributes to unsafe nursing practice, which jeopardizes patient care and ultimately patient safety. Canadian nursing regulatory bodies take practice violations very seriously; a practice violation can lead a nurse to be reprimanded or, in some cases, have his or her nursing licence revoked.

Most health care organizations use skills checklists or a competency evaluation program to ascertain that their employees have and maintain essential skills and abilities necessary for their position. A skills checklist is one way to determine basic clinical competency (Table 24-1). This checklist typically includes a list of basic skills and essential skills for safe nursing practice. Any type of skills review should be directly linked to quality-improvement indicators. Moreover, the purpose and process of the skills review should be explained to the staff nurse, which may increase the staff nurse's motivation and commitment. When the nurse manager explains the purpose and process of the skills review, he or she demonstrates respect for the staff nurse; a nurse manager who engages the staff nurse in the process may help motivate the employee. The skills review may require the employee to undertake a self-assessment of specific skills or competencies and then perform a return demonstration for the nurse educator or manager to validate adequate competency of the skills. If the nurse manager determines that an employee is have difficulty meeting performance expectations and cannot perform a skill adequately, he or she may choose to work alongside the nurse while delivering direct patient care, giving the nurse manager a chance to observe the nurse's strengths and support areas requiring growth. It can be helpful for the staff nurse to develop a learning portfolio to document the strengths and areas requiring growth, not just skills (CNA, 2013). For example, some nurses struggling with time management or medication administration may benefit from coaching, formal mentoring, or other more formal education. The nurse manager must document and keep detailed records of all meetings with the staff nurse to have a paper trail and clear documentation for future reference should further counsel and/or reprimand or termination be necessary. When managing ancillary personnel, the nurse manager supports the team by being present in the clinical environment, being available, and being approachable.

Emotional Problems

Emotional problems among nursing personnel may affect not only the individual involved but also co-workers and, indirectly, patients. The nurse manager must be aware that certain behaviours, such as poor judgement, increased errors, increased absenteeism, decreased productivity, and a negative attitude, may be manifestations of emotional problems in employees. Research indicates that nursing can take a toll on the psychosocial and physical health of the nurse (Sabo, 2011). Emotional problems include a broad range of problems that have serious effects on a person, including emotional exhaustion and burnout, compassion fatigue, and posttraumatic stress disorder (PTSD) (even though it is recognized as a mental health disorder) (CNA, 2010, 2012; Czaja, Moss, & Mealer, 2012; Sabo, 2011).

A nurse manager began hearing complaints from patients about a nurse named Noemi. Patients were saying that Noemi was abrupt and uncaring with them. The nurse manager had not received any complaints about Noemi before this time, so she questioned Noemi about why this was occurring. Noemi reported that her mother was very ill and she was so worried about her and so upset that she could not sleep and was extremely tired lately. She went on to say that she was having trouble being sympathetic with complaining patients when they did not seem to be as sick as her mother.

When an employee's behaviour changes significantly, personal problems with which the person cannot cope may be the cause. The nurse manager is not and should not be a counsellor to the staff but must intercede, not only to support the staff member with personal problems but also to maintain the adequate functioning of the unit. In dealing with the employee who exhibits behaviours that indicate emotional problems, the nurse manager assists the individual obtain professional help to cope with the problem. The individual's work setting and schedule may need to be adjusted, which may necessitate support from other nurses and staff to minimize negative effects on the care team and on patient care. The nurse manager acknowledges that an employee is experiencing emotional difficulties and yet the standards of practice for quality patient care cannot be compromised. It is reassuring for staff to witness the care and concern shown to a co-worker who is in a difficult situation. Staff can interpret that similar support would be given to them if they were in a difficult situation.

It is important for the nurse manager or leader to be supportive, caring, empathic, and encouraging with an emotionally troubled employee. Many organizations have employee assistance programs (EAPs)

to which the nurse manager or leader should refer employees.

The Literature Perspective describes a counselling service and the positive effects that supportive resources play in the retention of nurses. Throughout the process, nurse managers or leaders must consult with human resources about any potential legal implications. Nurse managers should always remember that various resources are available to assist employees that experience personal problems. They should never feel required to know all of the legal implications regarding employment policies. Rather, they must know that help is available and how to access it.

EXERCISE 24-3

As a nurse manager in a community health centre, you have just attended a meeting that was requested by several of your staff nurses. They expressed concern regarding another nurse colleague, Christine, who has come to work tearful several times during the past week. They report that Christine spends a lot of time in the bathroom when she is at work, and her eyes are red and swollen as if she has been crying when she comes out of the bathroom. Her co-workers have offered to support her, but she has refused to discuss her distress with her colleagues. Christine's colleagues express concern and ask you to help her.

Take a moment to reflect on the role of the nurse manager in this situation. What is your response to the group of concerned colleagues? How would you manage this situation?

LITERATURE PERSPECTIVE

Resource: Luquette, J. S. (2005). The role of on-site counseling in nurse retention. *Oncology Nursing Forum, 32*(2), 234–236. doi:10.1188/05.ONF.234-236

This article describes various aspects of an on-site counselling service and how it demonstrates value to nurses. The key cornerstone beliefs of the service are confidentiality, minimal financial cost, professionalism of the provider, and convenient appointment times and office locations. Services can be both group and individually based. To be effective, the services must be available when nurses work and also be available by phone. Confidentiality is critical, and it is helpful when the support services are offered in a confidential location. In addition, the employee assistance program should include a broad range of services including crisis intervention and conflict resolution.

Implications for Practice
The availability of on-site counselling during any work schedule allows charge nurses and nurse managers to refer individuals for support in a timely fashion. An on-site employee assistance program (EAP) understands the nature of the work of the employees it serves, which enhances its services. Although an on-site EAP is convenient, some employees fear a breach of confidentiality and prefer to seek external assistance for their problems. Most organizations can accommodate the employee's request for external assistance.

Chemical Dependency

Chemical dependency among nurses and other health care providers is a serious global problem that puts patients and co-workers at risk (Berg, Dillon, Sikkink, et al., 2012). Chemical dependency is a psychophysiological state in which an individual requires a substance, such as medications or alcohol, to prevent the onset of symptoms of abstinence. An employee practising while impaired with a chemical substance adversely affects staff morale by increasing stress on other staff members when they have to assume heavier workloads to cover for the chemically dependent employee who is not performing at full capacity or who is often absent. Patient safety is jeopardized for many reasons, including that nursing colleagues and staff are often focusing more on the problems of a co-worker than on those of the patients (LaSala & Bjarnason, 2010; New, 2014). Novice nurses must be aware of their professional and ethical responsibility to report incidents in which peers or team members exhibit signs of chemical dependency. According to professional nursing standards throughout Canada, nurses have a responsibility to identify, report, and address actual or potential unsafe practices, such as when nurses are under the influence of a chemical substance (CNA, 2007; Saskatchewan Registered Nurses Association, 2013). This responsibility includes taking action in all situations where patient safety and the well-being of any other group of people are potentially compromised (CNA, 2008; Edmonson, 2010). The nurse manager must professionally intervene and handle the situation while abiding by organization policies and professional practice standards that are aligned with ethical and morally responsible care and ensure that situations are handled consistently (Edmonson, 2010; New, 2014).

The *Health Professions Acts* and professional nursing standards and competencies vary across Canada. The underlying expectation is that members of any health care profession recognized in Canada will always act to protect the public's interest (CNA, 2009). Some of Canada's provinces and territories have a mandatory "duty to report" clause, which imposes reporting requirements on registrants of the health professional regulatory body (see also Chapter 5). As is true of all nurses, nurse managers must uphold the nursing practice standards of the province or territory in which they practise. Also, they should be familiar with the legal and safety risks associated with employing a nurse who has a chemical dependency (CNA, 2009). Nurse managers handle situations involving the chemical dependency of unregulated care providers according to organizational policies. Consultation with human resources personnel is critical to ensure adherence with organizational expectations.

In Canadian health care organizations and most unionized environments, there is a concerted effort to support affected individuals by offering support in seeking treatment versus immediately terminating the employee (CNA, 2009). Identifying an employee with a chemical dependency is usually difficult, as one of the primary symptoms is denial. Employees may also display obvious behavioural changes that are different from the behaviours the employee normally exhibited (New, 2014). Those different behaviours include lying, stealing, sudden and unusual neglect of personal appearance, an unusual interest in patients' pain control, frequent changes in jobs and shifts, and an increase in absenteeism and tardiness (College of Registered Nurses of Nova Scotia, 2008; New, 2014).

Nurse managers have a responsibility to use due diligence and address concerns and suspicions of chemical dependence or abuse in all employees (CNA, 2009). Open and supportive leadership is critical, but the nurse manager must consider the legal, ethical, and potential regulatory aspects of these situations (LaSala & Bjarnason, 2010). Referring an employee who is struggling with chemical dependency for treatment demonstrates supportive action. In addition, the nurse manager must consider if a report should be made to the provincial or territorial nursing regulatory body about the matter. For example, if a nurse is terminated for ongoing substance abuse and the nursing regulatory body of that province or territory is not notified, the nurse may be able to continue to practise nursing and put patients and colleagues at risk. Nursing regulatory bodies have a responsibility to protect the public, but they also have an obligation to support nurses in meeting standards of practice (CNA, 2009; Nurses Association of New Brunswick, 2011).

Canada has rehabilitation programs available for nurses who suffer from an addiction so that they may return to nursing once rehabilitated. Nurse managers are sometimes involved with monitoring the return-to-work process once the rehabilitative therapy is complete. Action plans, monitoring guidelines, and follow-up expectations are collaboratively established with the employee, the health care organization, and the nurse manager (Angres, Bettinardi-Angres, & Cross, 2010). Sometimes, provincial or territorial nursing regulatory bodies impose sanctions on the nurse who suffers from an addiction. For example, a nurse who has been through rehabilitation for narcotics substance abuse may be allowed to work in a setting in which narcotics are never used, or the nurse may have a restricted nursing licence and not be permitted to administer any controlled substances or narcotics. This type of situation can be difficult for health care teams, colleagues, and nurse managers; however, if handled positively, professionally, and openly, it can further enhance the team's cohesiveness and have minimal impact on patient care. If the nurse manager models professional ethics while offering empathy, he or she can de-escalate the associated distress and disorganization (National Business Group on Health, 2009; Tanga, 2011). It is always prudent for the nurse manager to seek guidance from other senior leaders and human resources consultants when faced with such challenges. The nurse manager is responsible for establishing and fostering an environment that supports professional practice (Cornett, 2009).

DOCUMENTATION

Documentation of all conversations and meetings with employees regarding their personnel problems should be accurately documented in detail and kept in employees' human resources file. From a regulatory and legal perspective, it is imperative that nurse managers maintain detailed documentation logs. Mooney (2013) suggested that writing reports and documentation is the most important step in the process of dealing with an employee who has emotional problems or substance abuse issues.

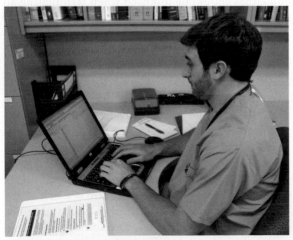

Documentation of all meetings and communication with employees is an important aspect of the nurse manager's role.

Documentation cannot be left to memory! At the time that an employee is involved in a difficult situation or when an employee receives a compliment or exceeds expectations, a notation should be made and kept in the employee file. This entry must include the date, time, and a brief description of the incident. Along with this information, the nurse manager should keep a log or summary sheet of all reported errors, unusual incidents, and wrongdoings/mistakes. This documentation can reveal patterns of individual's problem areas, areas of excellence in individual performance, and overall organizational problematic areas. The nurse manager who engages with followers and carefully keeps records about organizational functioning has greater control and influence in the management of employee problems. Box 24-2 describes the

BOX 24-2   DOCUMENTATION OF PERFORMANCE PROBLEMS

- Description of incident—an objective statement of the facts related to the incident
- Actions—statements describing the plan to correct and/or prevent future problems
- Follow-up—dates and times that the plan is to be carried out, including required meeting with the employee

Example

Several patients reported that Rebecca, one of the registered nurses, was "curt" and "gruff" and seemed uncaring with them. I called Rebecca into my office and reiterated the complaints that I had received, including the specifics of times and incidents. I reminded Rebecca about what my expectations were relating to patient care, emphasizing the importance of a caring attitude with all patients. We discussed what the possible cause of Rebecca's behaviour might be, such as problems at home or lack of sleep. Rebecca denied being curt or gruff but agreed that some of her mannerisms might be misinterpreted. I suggested to Rebecca that perhaps she needed to be particularly aware of her body language and to soften her tone of voice. After discussing this incident and reminding Rebecca of the importance of caring in nursing, I cited the policy regarding behaviour and told Rebecca that this behaviour would not be tolerated. I told Rebecca we needed to meet once a week to discuss how the week had gone and to determine how she was interacting with the patients assigned to her. I also told Rebecca I would be checking with patients to see what they had thought of Rebecca, pointing out that I do this routinely.

These weekly meetings are to be conducted for 6 weeks, followed by monthly meetings for a 3-month period. If problems do not recur, the meetings will be discontinued after this time.

Jean-Paul Martin, RN, MSN
Hospital Nurse Manager

content and format for such documentation and provides an example.

PROGRESSIVE DISCIPLINE

When an employee's performance falls below the acceptable standard despite corrective measures that have been implemented, nurse managers have a responsibility to follow through with some form of discipline. Usually collective agreements and human resources policies outline the process for progressive discipline to correct unprofessional conduct. The nurse manager must document all interactions with the employee to ensure that strategic processes and procedures are followed according to the corresponding collective agreement. If the employee in question is unionized, he or she has the right to be accompanied by a union representative at disciplinary meetings.

Progressive discipline consists of evaluating performance and providing feedback within a specified structure of increasing sanctions. Progressive discipline must be handled according to organizational policies. Inappropriate discipline is not only detrimental to the relationship between the leader and the followers but can directly contravene collective agreements. The sanctions, which progress from least severe to most severe, are described in Box 24-3. Harassment, sexual abuse of a patient, and chemical substance abuse by an employee are examples of unacceptable workplace behaviour and professional misconduct that usually involve progressive discipline and termination.

TERMINATION

In some situations, despite the best efforts of the nurse manager, the employee issue or disruptive behaviour may continue. In such cases, sometimes no choice exists but to terminate the employee. Front-line nurse managers play a critical role in human resources management of employees and staff nurses (Pegram, Grainger, Sigsworth, et al., 2013). Nurse managers are responsible for assisting employees in achieving their maximum potential. Terminating an employee is one of the most difficult functions of the manager role (Lachman, Murray, Iseminger, et al., 2012). The following

---

BOX 24-3   STEPS IN PROGRESSIVE DISCIPLINE

1. Discuss the problem in detail with the employee.
2. Reprimand the employee. A verbal reprimand usually precedes a written one, but some organizations issue both a verbal and a written reprimand simultaneously, depending on the issue. Documentation must include evidence that the wrongdoing or misconduct was brought to the attention of the employee, and best practices would indicate that both the nurse manager and employee sign the documentation (Crigger & Godfrey, 2014). By signing the documentation, the employee is not stating that he or she agrees with the reprimand but, rather, that he or she is aware of the reprimand. It is important that the process is transparent and that all documentation is kept in the employee's human resources file.
3. Suspend the employee if the problem persists (depending on the corresponding collective agreement). The consequences vary according to the collective agreement but might include time away from work, mandatory education courses, and possibly the need to report to the provincial or territorial nursing regulatory body (for registered nurses and licensed practical nurses) (Brous, 2012). Explain the rationale for the disciplinary action so that there is no surprise for the employee. At this point, the employee often realizes the magnitude and seriousness of the problem based on the resulting discipline.
4. Allow the employee to return to work with written conditions regarding problem behaviour and strict follow-up.
5. Terminate the employee (subject to the guidelines of the corresponding collective agreement) if the problem recurs following rehabilitation. Human resources must be consulted regarding this process.

---

guidelines should be followed when terminating an employee:

1. The provisions of human resources policies and procedures and relevant collective agreements must be followed.
2. All communication between the employee and employer and incidents must be accurately documented in detail and show evidence of due process. Documentation provides a paper trail of the specifics of the incident and details of conversations between the employer and employee and should be considered a legal document. When nurse managers do not maintain relevant documents, there is a lack of evidence to support management decisions regarding discipline or termination. Documentation should include evidence that the employee was aware of the position expectations, was offered guidance on how to meet expectations, and was given opportunities

to improve. It should also include specific examples of how the employee was not meeting performance expectations. Documentation is time consuming, but it is a necessary aspect of management.

3. Throughout the disciplinary process and in the event of termination, human resources personnel must be consulted, and legally binding collective agreements must be followed.

Terminating an employee follows extensive investigation and due process. Other suggestions on terminating an employee the right way are outlined in Box 24-4. Situations that may warrant immediate dismissal include theft, violence in the workplace, and willful abuse of a patient. The following example illustrates an incident that led to the immediate termination of an employee.

Alyssa, an RN with 4 years' experience, worked at a community mental health clinic. She recently completed the professional development session on using Social Media: Risks & Professional Obligations offered by her employer and the local registered nurse regulatory body.

Two months following the session, Alyssa posted several pictures on her Facebook page of a patient she cared for at the community mental health clinic. The pictures were accompanied by derogatory, demeaning comments. Alyssa's postings

had a nasty tone and contained inappropriate vulgar terms. Management became aware of the Facebook postings and deemed them as an unethical use of social media. The nurse manager consulted with the regional human resources department, and the nurse was immediately terminated.

In this example, the nurse did not abide by the CNA code of ethics (2008) and contravened one of the primary values, to preserve the dignity of all. Alyssa's inappropriate use of social media also violated a very basic organizational policy by breaching the confidentiality of the patient. Alyssa did not act as a moral agent nor did she act in the best interest of the patient.

EXERCISE 24-5

Explore your provincial or territorial nursing regulatory body Web site. Locate and examine the professional nursing practice standards and identify what potential incidents might call for immediate termination from a nursing position. Is substance abuse one of those causes?

CONCLUSION

All employees, including nurse managers, need to support and foster a positive and healthy work environment. Organizations must implement a zero-tolerance policy for unethical or disruptive behaviour among co-workers. All employees should be empowered to have a voice and speak out against unethical or disruptive behaviour.

BOX 24-4   TERMINATING THE RIGHT WAY

The termination of employees should be planned with forethought to avoid any potential problems. Steps should be taken to avoid the possibility of violence during employee separation. A key step is protecting the employee's dignity and avoiding humiliation. The reasons for termination should be clear and leave no room for debate. All details of the process of termination should be prearranged, including timing, the room used, and who is present. The room should provide privacy but not contain any objects that could be used as a weapon. The person being terminated should not be blocked from accessing the exit door. Termination notices and severance cheques along with any other documentation should be on hand. Arrangements should be made to clean out the person's desk or locker. There should be no reason for the person to return to the worksite. This saves everyone from embarrassment and any potential scenes. It is important to try to determine how the person will react to make appropriate arrangements. If there is a perceived need, a security officer or off-duty police officer can be called to stand by.

Adapted from Winfeld, L. (2001). *Training tough topics.* New York, NY: American Management Association.

💡 A SOLUTION

Nurse manager Miranda determined that the root cause of Brooklyn's mistake was a lack of knowledge regarding the specific needs and protocols on the specialized hospital unit. Miranda collaborated with Brooklyn and the unit's nurse educator to compile a specific skills checklist and develop a training module for new hires and nurses from the resource float pool who occasionally work on the mother baby unit. Miranda followed up by having float nurses, newly hired nurses, and regular staff nurses complete a questionnaire to determine their knowledge about unit policies and procedures as well as maternal child nursing.

Would this be a suitable approach for you? Why or why not? Reflecting on this scenario, consider other strategies to support casual float nurses who provide nursing care on units that they are not familiar with.

THE EVIDENCE

Davey, Cummings, Newburn-Cook, et al. (2009) sought to identify predictors of short-term absenteeism in staff nurses. Such absenteeism contributes to lack of continuity in patient care and decreases staff morale, which is costly to a health care organization. A systematic review of studies conducted from 1986 to 2006 led to the inclusion of 16 peer-reviewed research studies. The authors found that individual nurses' "history of prior absences," "work attitudes" (e.g., job satisfaction, organizational commitment, and work involvement), and "retention factors" (e.g., shared governance) reduced absenteeism. By contrast, poor leadership, "burnout," and "job stress" increased absenteeism. It became clear that the reasons underlying absenteeism are still poorly understood and that a robust theory for nurse absenteeism is lacking. Further theory development and research are needed.

NEED TO KNOW NOW

- The human resources department is an essential resource for nurse managers. The collaborative problem solving and decision making between nurse managers and human resources personnel are critical to consistent and effective management and leadership.
- Successful nurses
  - Have a positive attitude about patients and families.
- Demonstrate respect for all co-workers, from housekeeping staff to the CEO.
- Participate in open discussion and decision making that is fair and reflects the organizational mission.
- Recognize and celebrate the contributions of co-workers.
- Practise according to organizational policies and their professional code of ethics.

CHAPTER CHECKLIST

To obtain satisfaction from working with people, a nurse manager or leader must be knowledgeable about employee and personnel issues that are common in the work setting. The nurse manager or leader must be able to detect, prevent, and correct problems that affect nursing care and staff morale. Accurate and factual documentation and follow-up actions are key elements in the successful management of all personnel issues.

- Absenteeism's detrimental effects are as follows:
  - Patient care may be below standard.
  - Replacement personnel require additional supervision.
  - Absenteeism may increase among the entire staff.
  - Financial management of the unit suffers adverse effects.
- Effective strategies to reduce absenteeism include the following:
  - Enhance nurses' job satisfaction.
  - Undertake nonpunitive discipline.
- The problem of uncooperative or unproductive employees are related to motivation and ability.
- Praise and affirmation are often the most effective strategies for an employee who lacks maturity.
- Clinical incompetence is a highly correctable problem for nurse managers:
  - Clinical incompetence may be masked by co-workers' enabling behaviour.
  - A skills checklist helps determine basic clinical competency and pinpoint the need for additional training and education.
  - A comprehensive competency program may include not only a skills checklist but also a means for evaluating the critical-thinking ability of the employee.
- When emotional problems are evident, the nurse manager must assist the employee in getting professional help.
- The nurse manager is responsible for early recognition of chemical dependency and referral for treatment when appropriate.
  - The nurse manager must do the following:
    - Uphold the professional standards for nursing practice.

- Be familiar with the laws of the province or territory regarding chemical dependent employees.
- Know the health care organization's personnel policy on chemical dependency.
- Possible warning signs of chemical dependency are as follows:
  - Behavioural changes such as mood swings
  - Lying and theft
  - Sudden and unusual neglect of personal appearance
  - Unusual interest in patients' pain control
  - Increased absenteeism and tardiness
- Documentation of problems must include the following:
  - A description of the incident
  - A description of the manager's actions
  - A plan to correct/prevent future occurrences
  - Dates and times of follow-up measures
- Progressive discipline may be used when other corrective measures have failed. Steps in progressive discipline (subject to collective agreements) are as follows:
  - Discuss the problem in detail with the employee.
  - Reprimand the employee (first verbally, then in writing).
  - Suspend the employee if the problem persists.
  - Allow the employee to return to work, with written stipulations regarding problem behaviour.
  - Terminate the employee (subject to the guidelines of the corresponding collective agreement) if the problem continues or recurs following rehabilitation.

TIPS FOR DOCUMENTING PROBLEMS

- Identify the incident and related facts.
- Describe the actions taken by the nurse manager when the problem was identified.
- Develop an action plan for everyone involved.
- Schedule a follow-up meeting to evaluate the progress of the action plan.
- Provide detailed, objective, and accurate information in documentation.

evolve WEBSITE

Visit the Evolve website for Suggested Readings, Internet Resources, and additional resources related to the content in this chapter: http://evolve.elsevier.com/Canada/Yoder-Wise/leading/.

REFERENCES

Angres, D. H., Bettinardi-Angres, K., & Cross, W. (2010). Nurses with chemical dependency: Promoting successful treatment and reentry. *Journal of Nursing Regulation*, *1*(1), 16–20. Retrieved from https://jnr.metapress.com.

Batson, V. D., & Yoder, L. H. (2012). Managerial coaching: A concept analysis. *Journal of Advanced Nursing*, *68*(7), 1658–1669. doi:10.1111/j.1365-2648.2011.05840.x

Berg, K. H., Dillon, K. R., Sikkink, K. M., et al. (2012). Diversion of drugs within health care facilities, a multiple-victim crime: Patterns of diversion, scope, consequences, detection and prevention. *Mayo Clinic Proceedings*, *87*(7), 674–682. doi:10.1016/j.mayocp.2012.03.013

Bowen, D. J., & Weil, P. A. (2011). ACHE's code of ethics highlights challenges faced by healthcare leaders. *Healthcare Executive*, *26*(4), 39–42. Retrieved from http://issuu.com/healthcareexecutive.

Brous, E. (2012). Common misconceptions about professional licensure. *American Journal of Nursing*, *112*(10), 55–59. doi:10.1097/01.NAJ.0000421027.92789.95

Canadian Nurses Association. (2007). *Framework for the practice of registered nurses in Canada*. Ottawa, ON: Author. Retrieved from https://www.cna-aiic.ca/~/media/cna/page%20content/pdf%20en/2013/07/25/13/53/rn_framework_practice_2007_e.pdf.

Canadian Nurses Association. (2008). *Code of ethics for registered nurses (2008 centennial edition)*. Toronto, ON: Author. Retrieved from http://www.cna-aiic.ca/~/media/cna/files/en/codeofethics.pdf.

Canadian Nurses Association. (2009). Position statement: Nursing leadership. Retrieved from http://www.cna-aiic.ca/~/media/cna/page%20content/pdf%20en/2013/07/26/10/52/ps110_leadership_2009_e.pdf.

Canadian Nurses Association. (2010). Position statement: Taking action on nurse fatigue. Retrieved from http://www.nanb.nb.ca/PDF/CNATaking_Action_on_Nurse_Fatigue_E.pdf.

Canadian Nurses Association. (2012). Fact sheet: Nurse fatigue. Retrieved from https://www.cna-aiic.ca/~/media/cna/page%20content/pdf%20en/2013/07/26/10/39/fact_sheet_nurse_fatigue_2012_e.pdf.

Canadian Nurses Association. (2013). Building my online portfolio. Retrieved from http://www.nurseone-inf-fusion.ca/Default.aspx?portlet=StaticHtmlViewerPortlet&&ptdi=1304.

Chandler, G. E. (2012). Succeeding in the first year of practice. *Journal for Nurses in Staff Development*, *28*(3), 103–107. doi:10.1097/NND.0b013e31825514ee

College of Nurses of Ontario. (2013). *Professional conduct, professional misconduct,* Toronto, ON: Author. Retrieved from http://www.cno.org/Global/docs/ih/42007_misconduct.pdf.

College of Registered Nurses of British Columbia. (2012a). *Assisting nurses with significant practice problems.* Vancouver, BC: Author. Retrieved from https://www.crnbc.ca/Standards/Lists/StandardResources/354AssistingNursesPracticeProblems.pdf.

College of Registered Nurses of British Columbia. (2012b). *Professional practice standards for registered nurses and nurse practitioners.* Vancouver, BC: Author. Retrieved from https://crnbc.ca/Standards/Lists/StandardResources/128Professional Standards.pdf.

College of Registered Nurses of Nova Scotia. (2008). *Problematic substance use in the workplace: A resource guide for registered nurses.* Halifax, NS: Author. Retrieved from https://www.crnns.ca/documents/Problematic%20Substance%20Use%20Resource%20Guide.pdf.

Cornett, P. (2009). Managing the difficult employee: A reframed perspective. *Critical Care Nursing Quarterly, 32*(4), 314–326. doi:10.1097/CNQ.0b013e3181bad3a0

Crigger, N., & Godfrey, N. S. (2014). Professional wrongdoing: Reconciliation and recovery. *Journal of Nursing Regulation, 4*(4), 40–45. Retrieved from http://jnr.metapress.com.

Czaja, A. S., Moss, M., & Mealer, M. (2012). Symptoms of posttraumatic stress disorder among pediatric acute care nurses. *Journal of Pediatric Nursing, 27*(4), 357–365. doi:10.1016/j.pedn.2011.04.024

Davey, M. M., Cummings, G., Newburn-Cook, C. V., et al. (2009). Predictors of nurse absenteeism in hospitals: A systematic review. *Journal of Nursing Management, 17*(3), 312–330. doi:10.1111/j.1365-2834.2008.00958.x

Doherty, R. E. (1989). *Industrial and labour relations terms: A glossary* (6th ed.). Ithaca, NY: ILR Press.

Edmonson, C. (2010). Moral courage and the nurse leader. *Online Journal of Issues in Nursing, 15*(3). doi:10.3912/OJIN.Vol15No03Man05

Espinoza, D., Lopez-Saldana, A., & Stonestreet, J. (2009). The pivotal role of the nurse manager in healthy workplaces: Implications for training and development. *Critical Care Nurse Quarterly, 32*(4), 327–334. doi:10.1097/CNQ.0b013e3181bad528

Garrosa, E., Moreno-Jimenez, B., Rodriquez-Munoz, A., et al. (2011). Role stress and personal resources in nursing: A cross-sectional study of burnout and engagement. *International Journal of Nursing Studies, 48*(4), 479–489. doi:10.1016/j.ijnurstu.2010.08.004

Hardy, M. E., & Conway, M. E. (1988). *Role theory: Perspectives for health professionals* (2nd ed.). Norwalk, CT: Appleton & Lange.

Harris, J. L., & Roussel, L. (2010). *Initiating and sustaining the clinical nurse leader role: A practical guide.* Sudbury, MA: Jones & Bartlett Learning.

Hersey, P., Blanchard, K., & Johnson, D. E. (2008). *Management of organizational behavior: Utilizing human resources* (9th ed.). Englewood Cliffs, NJ: Prentice Hall.

Hughes, R. G. (2008). *Patient safety and quality: An evidence-based handbook for nurses.* Rockville, MD: U.S. Department of Health and Human Services.

Jackson, D., Hutchinson, M., Peters, K., et al. (2013). Understanding avoidant leadership in health care: Findings from a secondary analysis of two qualitative studies. *Journal of Nursing Management, 21*(3), 572–580. doi:10.1111/j.1365-2834.2012.01395.x

Lachman, V. D., Murray, J. S., Iseminger, K., et al. (2012). Doing the right thing: Pathways to moral courage. *American Nurse Today, 7*(5), 24–29. Retrieved from http://www.americannursetoday.com.

Lambrou, P., Kontodimopoulos, N., & Niakas, D. (2010). Motivation and job satisfaction among medical and nursing staff in a Cyprus public general hospital. *Human Resources for Health, 8*(26). Retrieved from http://www.human-resources-health.com/content/8/1/26.

LaSala, C. A., & Bjarnason, D. (2010). Creating workplace environments that support moral courage. *Online Journal of Issues in Nursing, 15*(3). doi:10.3912/OJIN.Vol15No03Man04

Longo, J. (2010). Combating disruptive behaviors: Strategies to promote a healthy work environment. *Online Journal of Issues in Nursing, 15*(1). doi:10.3912/OJIN.Vol15No01Man05

Luquette, J. S. (2005). The role of on-site counseling in nurse retention. *Oncology Nursing Forum, 32*(2), 234–236. doi:10.1188/05.ONF.234-236

Mooney, D. H. (2013). Investing and making a case for drug diversion. *Journal of Nursing Regulation, 4*(1), 9–13. Retrieved from http://jnr.metapress.com.

National Business Group on Health. (2009, August). An employer's guide to workplace substance abuse: Strategies and treatment recommendations. Retrieved from https://www.businessgrouphealth.org/pub/f3151957-2354-d714-5191-c11a80a07294.

New, K. (2014). Preventing, detecting, and investigating drug diversion in health care facilities. *Journal of Nursing Regulation, 5*(1), 18–25. Retrieved from http://jnr.metapress.com.

Nurses Association of New Brunswick. (2011). *Recognition and management of problematic substance use in the nursing profession.* Fredericton, NB: Author. Retrieved from http://www.nanb.nb.ca/downloads/Recognition%20and%20Management%20of%20Problematic%20Substance%20Use%20in%20the%20Nursing%20Profession_E_New%20Cover.pdf.

Pegram, A. M., Grainger, M., Sigsworth, J., et al. (2013). Strengthening the role of the ward manager: A review of the literature. *Journal of Nursing Management, 22*(2). doi:10.1111/jonm.12047

Peternelj-Taylor, C. A., & Yonge, O. (2003). Exploring boundaries in the nurse-client relationship: Professional roles and responsibilities. *Perspectives in Psychiatric Care, 39*(2), 55–66. doi:10.1111/j.1744-6163.2003.tb00677.x

Ritter, D. (2011). The relationship between healthy work environment and retention of nurses in a hospital setting. *Journal of Nursing Management, 19*(1), 27–32. doi:10.1111/j.1365-2834.2010.01183.x

Sabo, B. (2011). Reflecting on the concept of compassion fatigue. *Online Journal of Issues in Nursing, 16*(1). doi:10.3912/OJIN.Vol16No01Man01

Saskatchewan Registered Nurses Association. (2013). *Standards and foundation competencies for the practice of registered nurses.* Regina, SK: Author. Retrieved from http://www.srna.org/images/stories/Nursing_Practice/Resources/Standards_and_Foundation_2013_06_10_Web.pdf.

Strickland, D. (2000). Emotional intelligence: The most potent factor in the success equation. *Journal of Nursing Administration, 30*(3), 112–117. Retrieved from http://jnr.metapress.com.

Tanga, H. Y. (2011). Nurse drug diversion and nursing leaders responsibilities: Legal, regulatory, ethical, humanistic and practical considerations. *JONA's Healthcare Law, Ethics & Regulation, 13*(1), 13–16. doi:10.1097/NHL.0b013e31820bd9e6

Tucker, S. J., Weymiller, A. J., Cutshall, S., et al. (2012). Stress ratings and health promotion practices among RNs: A case for action. *Journal of Nursing Administration, 42*(5), 282–292. doi:10.1097/NNA.0b013e318253585f

Wallace, M. (2009). Occupational health nurses: The solution to absence management. *American Association of Occupational Health Nurses Journal, 57*(3), 122–127. Retrieved from http://aaohn.org/practice/journal.html.

Winfeld, L. (2001). *Training tough topics.* New York, NY: American Management Association.

Workplace Violence and Incivility

Yolanda Babenko-Mould

Nurses working in hospitals and other health care facilities are at a disproportionally high risk for physical violence because of the very nature of their job. Health care workers screen patients and their visitors to the best of their ability, but one never knows who will walk through the door and in what mental state. To maintain personal safety and an environment free from the potential of physical violence, nurses must be alert to signs of trouble. Not all health care workplace violence is of a physical nature or from patients or their families; like any other workplace, health care settings are subject to horizontal violence and incivility. Horizontal violence includes intimidating or derisive behaviour between and among staff, managers, or physicians; it interferes with optimal job performance and negatively affects the delivery of high-quality patient care. Research suggests that workplace violence and incivility can be prevented if people are aware of warning signs and understand how to effectively deal with potentially problematic situations. No organization can completely prevent or eliminate workplace violence and incivility, but with proper planning and effective programs, the opportunities for such occurrences can be dramatically reduced.

OBJECTIVES

- Categorize the types of violence and incivility that can occur in the workplace.
- Understand the risk factors for potential violence or disruption.
- Understand how to conduct an organizational workplace violence assessment.
- Describe interventions that can help prevent horizontal violence and incivility.

TERMS TO KNOW

bullying	incivility	lateral violence
horizontal violence	interpersonal conflict	toxic workplace

Sophie, a nurse, had been recording a report for the change of shift in the "reporting room" on a medical–surgical unit at approximately 6:00 when she heard loud yelling and what sounded like smashing metal. She immediately ran out into the dimly lit hallway to see her colleague, Louisa, at the end of the hall, standing just inside the brightly lit entrance of the clean utility room, wearing a uniform that was now covered in blood. Next to Louisa was a man who had been admitted to the unit from the emergency department while Sophie was recording the report. The male patient turned away from Louisa and glared at Sophie. Then, he began to run at Sophie. He was not wearing his hospital gown. Louisa yelled at Sophie to back up against the wall. Sophie did just that, but in doing so was helpless as the patient came closer. He approached Sophie, looked into her eyes, but it seemed that he was not really seeing her. He kept running down the hall. Louisa ran after him.

What do you think you would do if you were Sophie?

INTRODUCTION

Workplace violence and incivility in health care have emerged as important safety issues over the past decade. Workplace violence is seen on a continuum from threats or intimidation to its most extreme form, homicide. Violence, whether by persons outside or within an organization, has been shown to have negative effects including increased job stress, reduced productive work time, decreased morale, increased staff turnover, and loss of trust in the organization and its management. The purpose of this chapter is to increase awareness of the risk factors for violence and incivility in health care facilities and to enhance consideration of strategies for decreasing or preventing those events in the workplace.

DEFINING WORKPLACE VIOLENCE AND INCIVILITY

The Canadian Centre for Occupational Health and Safety (CCOHS, 2014a) conducts research, carries out projects, and publishes information on workplace health and safety to carry out a vision of "creating a work world without pain, loss, or tragedy." The CCOHS works with industry and labour organizations to understand and improve worker safety and health in Canada. Although one might assume that workplace violence is related specifically to acts that cause physical injury, the CCOHS (2014c) defines *workplace violence* as "any act in which a person is abused, threatened, intimidated or assaulted in his or her employment." Box 25-1 provides examples of workplace violence.

Workplace violence does not only occur in the work setting. It can take place at any off-site location (i.e., home, business conference) that is associated with work. For instance, receiving a harassing e-mail or telephone call at home from a former patient or co-worker would be considered as a form of workplace-related violence.

In recent years, additional descriptions of workplace violence have been added. Horizontal violence is "an act of aggression that's perpetuated by one colleague toward another colleague" (Longo & Sherman, 2007). Lateral violence, which is often used interchangeably with *horizontal violence*, refers to "psychological harassment evidenced by verbal abuse, intimidation, exclusion, unfair assignments, denial of access to opportunities, and withholding of information" (Morse, 2008). Other terms associated with this type of violence include bullying, which is a practice closely related to lateral or horizontal violence, but a real or perceived power differential between the instigator and recipient must be present in bullying. Interpersonal conflict occurs between and among patients, family members, nurses, physicians, and members of other departments. These behaviours exist in what has

---

BOX 25-1   TYPES OF VIOLENCE

Workplace violence includes these broad categories:
- **Threatening behaviour:** For example, shaking fists, destroying property or throwing objects; verbal or written threats and any expression of an intent to inflict harm
- **Harassment:** Any behaviour that demeans, embarrasses, humiliates, annoys, or alarms a person and is known or would be expected to be unwelcome. It includes verbal abuse (swearing, insults, or condescending language), disrespectful gestures, intimidation, bullying, or other inappropriate activities
- **Physical attacks:** The act of hitting, shoving, pushing, or kicking someone

Rumours, pranks, arguments, property damage, vandalism, sabotage, theft, psychological trauma, anger-related incidents, rape, arson, and murder are also examples of workplace violence.

Based on Canadian Centre for Occupational Health and Safety. (2014b). Violence in the workplace: Awareness, p. 9. Retrieved from http://author.vubiz.com/fModules/5595EN/LMSStart.html?vModId=5595EN.

been termed toxic workplaces, which are organizations in which people feel devalued or dehumanized and in which disruptive behaviour often flourishes. Incivility includes a wide range of behaviours from ignoring, to rolling one's eyes, to yelling, and eventually to personal attacks, both physical and psychological. The term *bullying* is often subsumed under the term *incivility*. Workplace violence and incivility can also occur from patients, or from members of the public who don't have a direct connection to the organization, but have criminal intent.

Scope of the Problem

The true scope of workplace violence in health care is difficult to determine. The International Council of Nurses (2009) has indicated that nurses are the health care workers most at risk for workplace violence; female nurses are most vulnerable to experiencing violence in the workplace. A Statistics Canada report on workplace violence (Shields & Wilkins, 2009) noted that in 2005, 34% of nurses in Canada who were employed in acute or long-term health care organizations reported being physically abused by a patient, while 47% reported that they had experienced emotional abuse at work. Nurses who reported abuse were often male; had less experience; usually worked non-day shifts; and perceived staffing or resources as inadequate, nurse–physician relations as poor, and co-worker and supervisor support as low. Another Statistics Canada report (de Léséleuc, 2004) noted that of the 356 000 incidents of workplace violence that took place in the provinces, 33% were reported by health care or social assistance workers. A shortage of national data on workplace violence exists, which means that accurate data for health care alone and nursing in particular are hard to determine. Workplace violence in health care facilities is unsettling, nonetheless.

A key concern is that the true rate of workplace violence is much higher because many incidents might not be reported, especially when violence does not result in physical injury or is verbal in nature (e.g., intimidation or bullying). Underreporting is thought to be related to nursing perceptions that assaults with or without injuries are "part of the job." One survey found that 80% of the 1377 nurse respondents from the United States and 17 other countries reported having experienced some form of violence within the work setting (Hader, 2008). Verbal rather than physical forms of violence were reported most often. According to the survey, the perpetrator was a patient 53.2% of the time, with nurse colleagues a close second at 51.9% of the time. The ranking of those who experienced violence was as follows: physicians (49%), visitors (47%), and other health care workers (37.7%). Nearly 8 out of 10 (79.7%) nurses observed their colleagues being the primary target of this violence, and well over half (56.1%) had personally been the target. Many earlier studies with similar findings demonstrate the need to examine the causes of workplace violence and develop programs and strategies to improve personal safety in the workplace. In particular, attention needs to be paid to the causes and remedies for lateral violence issues.

Ensuring a Safe Workplace

Although legislation or regulations to address the prevention of workplace violence exist in each province and territory, their content is not consistent across Canada. Most recently, Bill 168 gained royal assent by the Legislative Assembly of Ontario as an amendment to the *Occupational Health and Safety Act* in relation to violence and harassment in the workplace. The CCOHS has published voluntary guidelines for workers in health care and several other high-risk professions. Although not all employers across Canada are legally obligated to follow the CCOHS guidelines, the *Canada Occupational Health and Safety Regulations* and any derivative of the acts that exist in the provinces or territories generally mandate employers to comply with workplace hazard-specific standards. Employers have a general duty to provide their employees with a workplace free from recognized hazards likely to cause death or serious physical harm. Consequences can occur if such measures are not adhered to. For instance, an organization can be cited if its leaders fail to address such hazards. The CCOHS (2013) developed a *Violence in the Workplace Prevention Guide* to help organizations develop violence prevention plans. Several provinces are also enacting or developing laws, standards, or recommendations that address health care workplace security and safety.

The Canadian Nurses Association (CNA, 2009) position statement on leadership in nursing calls for nurse leaders to create and sustain practice environments that are free of violence for patients, families, and health care providers. The position statement cites studies that suggest intimidating and disruptive behaviours contribute to poor patient satisfaction and preventable adverse outcomes. The CNA's *Code of Ethics for Registered Nurses* (2008) includes the following core responsibilities central to ethical nursing practice: promoting health and well-being; preserving dignity; promoting justice; being accountable; and providing safe, compassionate, competent, and ethical care. Provincial and territorial nursing associations and regulatory bodies have developed practice standards that are drawn from the CNA code of ethics. These standards articulate the role of nurses in promoting safe and healthy practice environments for those that are in their care and for their nursing colleagues. For instance, the College of Nurses of Ontario (2009) practice standards include accountability, ethics, knowledge application, leadership, and relationships. Thus, when nurses engage in any form of workplace violence toward patients or other health care providers, they are in effect breaching the ethics and standards of their profession. Further, if nurses are the victims of or witnesses to workplace violence, they have a duty and right to report the situation and to seek support to address the incident, as required. Given the profession's standards and code of ethics, it is evident that nurses' and patients' well-being are to be considered a priority in all health care settings.

The Cost of Workplace Violence

Our knowledge of the scale of workplace violence remains incomplete because no consistent system of data collection exists in Canada (de Léséleuc, 2004). Data regarding less severe forms of workplace violence are particularly sparse. Even less clear is the financial toll workplace aggression exacts on businesses. In the United States, a Workplace Violence Research Institute study estimated that the aggregate cost of workplace violence to US employers was more than US$36 billion as a result of expenses associated with lost business and productivity, litigation, medical care, psychiatric care, higher insurance rates, increased security measures, negative publicity, and loss of employees (Kaufer & Mattman, 1996). The annual direct and indirect costs in the United States of workplace incivility and violence are US$23.8 billion (Sheehan, McCarthy, Barker, et al., 2001, as cited in Laschinger, Wong, Regan, et al., 2013). Although Canadian figures for the overall costs of workplace violence in health care are not currently available, if one applies the US per capita costs to the Canadian population, then the costs of workplace violence to Canadian businesses are similarly exorbitant. The costs from lost work time and wages, reduced productivity, medical costs, workers' compensation payments, legal and security expenses, and the costs to patients may be difficult to estimate but are clearly excessive when compared with the cost of prevention.

Gates, Gillespie, and Succop (2011) found that workplace violence led to costs associated with nurses' health and well-being. Gates et al. (2011) noted that of the 230 emergency department nurses who participated in their study, 94% experienced at least one episode of post-traumatic stress disorder in relation to an incident of violence in the practice setting. Gates et al. (2011) also stated that nurses' levels of stress in the workplace were associated with decreased productivity.

Other costs of workplace violence include increased staff turnover rates. A meta-analysis of 66 studies on bullying in nursing found that workplace violence was associated with "both job-related and health- and well-being-related outcomes, such as mental and physical health problems, symptoms of post-traumatic stress disorder, burnout, increased intentions to leave, and reduced job satisfaction and organizational commitment" (Nielsen & Einarsen, 2012, p. 309). Loss of the organizational investment required to train qualified staff as well as the departure of experienced existing staff can increase operating expenses and reduce the quality of care. Pearson and Porath (2009) suggest that cost estimates should consider how many times people report they are sick when they are really avoiding bad behaviour as well as decreases in productivity because employees no longer feel comfortable in the environment. The costs of absenteeism alone mount rapidly. When nurses begin to stay away from the practice setting because of workplace violence issues, it is plausible that they are considering leaving the setting altogether. Research has demonstrated that stress, burnout, and incidences of incivility in the workplace are linked with intentions to leave the practice setting (Oyeleye, Hanson, O'Connor, et al., 2013). Studies have yet to capture the full cost of workplace violence in its many forms. More measurement is also needed to assess the cost and effectiveness of known intervention strategies.

Making a Difference

So what is the nurse in a leader, manager, or follower role to do given the serious and complex issue of violence in the workplace? Making a difference includes promotion of an organizational culture of safety, developing and implementing a safety strategy, providing training programs, predicting problems, and using technology (e.g., to monitor isolated places) to reduce the incidence of violence. A culture of safety includes health care providers, patients, and their families. When workplace violence occurs in the practice setting, both nurses' and patients' health and well-being are at risk. If nurse leaders' and nurses' time and energy are being directed away from patient care because of workplace violence issues, then the implications for patients could range from decreased attention to patient pain control needs, lack of or receipt of incorrect treatments, and potentially even death (Emergency Care Research Institute, 2009). When considering the issue of workplace violence from a nurses' perspective, given the gravity of the issue and the myriad of negative personal and professional outcomes it can have, strategies to prevent being victimized by violence in any practice setting are critical.

PREVENTION STRATEGIES

The old adage "an ounce of prevention is worth a pound of cure" is particularly relevant when dealing with workplace violence. Preventing even one act of violence can save money and time and diminish the possible negative psychological impact of such an event (Ostrofsky, 2012). By taking a proactive approach that includes preventing violence, organizations can also avoid being victimized. To address the issue of violence, it is necessary to recall that violence can be perpetuated by co-workers, managers, patients, former employees, or members of the public not aligned with the organization (CCOHS, 2014b). Thus, the types of violence that may be encountered and the signs that portend a potentially violent situation might differ depending on who is the perpetrator. In short, prevention is the right thing to do for people and for the organization.

Identifying Risk Factors

Although anyone working in health care is at risk of becoming a victim of violence, those with direct patient contact are at a higher risk. Violence is also a frequent occurrence in psychiatric and geriatric settings. Hospital-based violence can take place either horizontally, among nurses, or can be directed at nurses by patients or their families as a result of feeling frustration or anger. Such acts are usually related to feelings of vulnerability, stress, and loss of control that accompany illness. Many factors have been identified that can increase the risk of violence erupting in health care facilities. The US-based Occupational Safety and Health Administration (OSHA, 2004) identified risk factors for workplace violence in health care facilities. These factors are listed in Box 25-2.

Other risk factors for violence include the location of the facility, its size, and the type of care provided. Assaults may occur when service is denied, when a patient is involuntarily admitted, or when a health care

---

BOX 25-2   RISK FACTORS FOR VIOLENCE IN HEALTH CARE FACILITIES

- Low staff levels, especially during visiting hours and meal times
- Transportation of patients between areas within a facility
- Long wait times for patient care
- Overcrowded, uncomfortable waiting areas
- Solo work in an area isolated from other staff
- Solo work in an area with no backup or way to get assistance, such as communication devices or alarm systems
- Poor environmental design
- Inadequate security
- Lack of staff training in handling potentially violent situations
- Lack of policies for preventing and managing crises with potentially violent individuals
- Unrestricted movement of patients or visitors
- Poorly lit corridors, rooms, parking lots, or other areas
- Prevalence of handguns or other weapons among patients, their families, or friends
- Increasing presence of gang members, drug or alcohol abusers, trauma patients, or distraught family members
- Use of hospitals or health care facilities for holding criminals, violent individuals, and the acutely mentally disturbed
- An increase in the number of chronically mentally ill patients being released without adequate resources for follow-up care
- Availability of money or medications within the facility

Adapted from Occupational Safety and Health Administration. (2004). *Guidelines for preventing workplace violence for health care and social service workers* (OSHA Publication No. 3148-01R). Washington, DC: U.S. Department of Labor. Retrieved from https://www.osha.gov/Publications/OSHA3148/osha 3148.html.

worker attempts to set limits on eating, drinking, or use of tobacco or alcohol.

Similar to the nursing process, prevention of workplace violence begins with a systematic assessment. Assessing risk and planning for prevention of workplace violence call for input and expertise from a variety of staff. A risk assessment based on a multidisciplinary team approach to workplace violence prevention is often the most effective. A team with representation from administration, staff, security, facilities engineering, human resources, legal counsel, and risk management is needed to address risks from all perspectives. The *Violence in the Workplace Prevention Guide* developed by the CCOHS (2013) provides readers with a step-by-step, common-sense approach to assessing and reducing existing and potential areas of workplace violence. The Ontario Ministry of Labour has also developed an online resource to assist individuals and groups to create programs and policies to support a healthy work environment free of workplace violence called *Developing Workplace Violence and Harassment Policies and Programs: A Toolbox* (2013). In addition, in the United States, OSHA's *Guidelines for Preventing Workplace Violence for Health Care and Social Service Workers* (2004) provides a comprehensive assessment with checklists adapted from the American Nurses Association's (ANA) (2002). *Promoting Safe Work Environments for Nurses* document to assist with the process. The checklists are in-depth, are very applicable to the Canadian context, and are helpful to nurse managers and leaders to conduct a broad assessment of the practice context (Box 25-3).

When looking at possible threats or hazards, those from within an organization also must be considered. Determining if current employees pose a danger in the workplace is a critical factor that is often overlooked. In addition to personal and psychological factors, behaviours can be observed in employees that may be related to violence or aggression in the workplace (Paludi, Nydegger, & Paludi, 2006). The most obvious of these is a previous history of aggression and substance abuse. Screening potential employees through background inquiries and references can help reduce these risks. Paludi et al. (2006) also advise of warning signs that can alert employers of problems with current employees that warrant intervention to prevent a violent incident.

No profile or litmus test exists to identify whether a current employee might become violent. It is

---

BOX 25-3   WORKPLACE VIOLENCE PROGRAM CHECKLISTS

OSHA with the ANA have provided comprehensive checklist documents that can help nurse managers and leaders conduct an organizational workplace violence assessment. The checklist titles are provided here. The checklists provide detailed step-by-step instructions to conduct an in-depth assessment and establish a monitoring program. To see the complete document, go to https://www.osha.gov/Publications/OSHA3148/osha3148.html.

Checklist 1: Answer organizational assessment questions regarding management commitment and employee involvement

Checklist 2: Analyze workplace violence records.

Checklist 3: Identify environmental risk factors for violence.

Checklist 4: Assess the influence of day-to-day work practices on occurrences of violence.

Checklist 5: Ensure post-incident response.

Checklist 6: Assess employee and supervisor training.

Checklist 7: Undertake recordkeeping and evaluation.

Adapted from American Nurses Association. (2002). *Promoting safe work environments for nurses.* As cited in Occupational Safety and Health Administration. (2004). *Guidelines for preventing workplace violence for health care and social service workers* (OSHA Publication No. 3148-01R). Washington, DC: U.S. Department of Labor. https://www.osha.gov/Publications/OSHA3148/osha3148.html.

---

important for employers and employees alike to remain alert to problematic behaviour that, in combination, could point to possible violence. Because no one behaviour in and of itself suggests a greater potential for violence, behaviours must be looked at in totality. Problem situations and circumstances that may heighten the risk of violence can involve a particular event or employee or the workplace as a whole.

EXERCISE 25-1

Assess several practice settings for workplace violence risks. Can you identify any of the risks listed in Box 25-2? What security measures are currently in place? Can any of the identified risks be improved? How? How safe would you feel in the different geographical areas?

Once the risk assessment is completed, the next step is to analyze the data and prioritize the problems that need to be addressed. Priorities can be established by asking a few basic questions: What are the risks? Who might be harmed and how? What is the level of risk? What measures need to be taken to reduce or eliminate risk? Do changes need to be implemented now or later? Once the priorities are set, the business of designing or improving prevention programs can begin.

EXERCISE 25-2
What elements do you think represent a healthy workplace or practice environment? Consider a practice setting where you were employed or where you were a student that you feel represents such "healthy" elements. What was it like to work and learn in such a setting? What were the relationships like among health professionals, among nurses, and among nurses and the nursing leadership? In what ways do you think that such a healthy practice environment ultimately influenced the quality of patient care and patient outcomes? What is your role as a current or soon-to-be nurse in contributing to the development and sustainability of a healthy practice environment?

HORIZONTAL VIOLENCE: THE THREAT FROM WITHIN

Horizontal violence includes a wide variety of behaviours, from verbal abuse to physical aggression between co-workers. This term, although commonly used, may be limiting because it suggests that the violence is perpetrated between those at the same level of authority. It may be better termed *relational aggression*, which involves bullying using psychological and social behaviours between people at the same or different levels (Dellasega, 2009).

Horizontal violence and its effects have been reported in nursing literature for more than 20 years. A review of five research studies published between 2003 and 2004 on horizontal violence found that horizontal violence is experienced by all nurses, regardless of their degree of work experience (Woelfle & McCaffrey, 2007). Many of the research studies found infighting and a general lack of support among nurses to be common occurrences. The studies also indicated that new graduates were likely to experience horizontal violence, which resulted in high absentee rates and thoughts of leaving nursing after the first year. *Nursing2011* conducted a survey to identify how often nurses experience or witness horizontal violence. In all, 82% or 778 of survey respondents reported having witnessed or experienced horizontal violence either daily or weekly (Dumont, Meisinger, Whitacre, et al., 2012). Nurse peers were most often cited as the perpetrators of horizontal violence, and supervisors were cited as next to highest (Dumont et al., 2012). Findings from this survey caused the researchers to ask this question: How can nurses treat patients kindly and give them the respect they need when they treat each other so poorly? In light of the looming nursing shortage, these consistent findings among nurses were cause for concern.

Many theories exist as to why horizontal violence takes place in nursing. Historically, horizontal violence in nursing was considered to be a result of nursing's traditional hierarchical structure, the oppression of nursing as a profession, or feminism (Farrell, 2001). However, since workplace aggression is common in other professions as well, it is most likely the result of a complex myriad of individual, social, and organizational characteristics (Farrell, 2001; Hutchinson, Vickers, Jackson, et al., 2006). More recently, bullying in the workplace has been linked to worker burnout and decreased access to empowering structures in the work environment, including access to information, resources, supports, and opportunities (Laschinger, Grau, Finegan, et al., 2010). When nurses are more structurally empowered, they report fewer incidents of bullying (Laschinger et al., 2010), which supports the proposition that empowering work environments have the potential to decrease incidents of workplace violence of the horizontal type (see the Research Perspective for more on building empowering work environments). Regardless of the reasons why it happens, the concerns are that impaired intrapersonal relationships between nurses at work can cause errors, accidents, and poor work performance (Gates et al., 2011) and that those relationships may play a significant role in attrition (Johnson, 2009). In a classic survey on workplace intimidation published by the Institute for Safe Medication Practices (2003), almost half of the 2095 respondents recalled being verbally abused when questioning or clarifying medication prescriptions. This intimidation led some health care providers to refrain from questioning a medication order to avoid confrontation with the prescriber. The results of the survey had professional health care and nursing organizations issue calls to action to address all types of workplace violence in the interest of promoting a safe and respectful work environment that promotes the delivery of high-quality care instead of threatening it. Shortly after the release of the Institute's report, the International Council of Nurses (ICN, 2006) published a position statement on health care workplace violence, which included the following assertion:

> Violence in the workplace threatens the delivery of effective patient services and, therefore, patient safety. If quality care is to be provided, nursing personnel must be ensured a safe work environment and respectful treatment. Excessive workloads, unsafe working conditions, and inadequate support can be considered forms of violence and incompatible with good practice.

🔍 RESEARCH PERSPECTIVE

Resource: Laschinger, H. K. S., Leiter, M. P., Day, A., et al. (2012). Building empowering work environments that foster civility and organizational trust. Testing an intervention. *Nursing Research*, *61*(5), 316–235. doi:10.1097/NNR.0b013e318265a58d

The authors studied the impact of a workplace intervention (a Civility, Respect, and Engagement in the Workplace [CREW] program) on nurses' empowerment, experiences of incivility, and trust in nursing management. The 6-month-long CREW program was instituted in eight acute care hospital units across two provinces. A total of 33 units were control groups. The CREW program involved weekly unit meetings that were facilitated by a CREW "expert." At the meetings, management and nursing staff would develop goals to achieve positive interpersonal relationships, and strategies were selected from the CREW toolkit to support the achievement of the goals. The process for enacting strategies was also outlined in the weekly planning meetings. Participants in the control and intervention groups completed measures to assess perceptions of structural workplace empowerment, rates of supervisor and co-worker incivility, and trust in management. Initially, it appeared that the intervention and control group measurement scores were similar. However, in-depth statistical analysis demonstrated that over time, in comparison to the control group, the intervention group scores were significantly improved for overall empowerment and trust in management, and reported rates had significantly decreased over time for supervisor and co-worker incivility.

Implications for Practice
The authors noted that the CREW program showed promising results in supporting management and staff to foster and sustain positive professional relationships. The authors underscored that empowering work environments are associated with decreased levels of incivility. Empowering environments have been associated with enhanced psychological empowerment, which in turn influences nurses' use of empowering behaviours, job satisfaction, and nurse-assessed quality of care (Purdy, Laschinger, Finegan, et al., 2010). Therefore, managers who make a concerted effort to enhance access to support, resources, opportunities for growth and learning, and information related to the broader organization give nurses a greater opportunity to find more meaning and self-efficacy in their role. Further, managers who engage in empowering behaviours, such as involving nurses in decision making and problem solving on the unit, and provide timely feedback about performance foster greater job satisfaction for nurses. Finally, when nurses partner with management to create and sustain strategies to enhance relationships, such as those in the CREW program, the number of incidents of workplace incivility will decrease, which can ultimately lead to better patient outcomes.

In 2008, the Center for American Nurses published a position paper stating that no place exists in a professional practice environment for horizontal violence and bullying among nurses or health care providers overall. These disruptive behaviours are toxic to the nursing profession and have a negative impact on retention of quality staff. Horizontal violence and bullying should never be considered as a normal part of socialization in nursing or be accepted in professional relationships. The Literature Perspective below discusses nursing student experiences with incivility. The Center for American Nurses asserts that all health care organizations should implement a zero tolerance policy on disruptive behaviour as well as a professional code of conduct and educational and behavioural interventions to assist nurses in addressing disruptive behaviour. The Canadian Nurses Association partnered with the Canadian Federation of Nurses Unions (2008) to publish a joint position statement about workplace violence, noting that "it is the right of all nurses to work in an environment that is free from violence" (p. 1). With professional groups in both Canada and the United States calling for change from within nursing, we must examine how to implement that change.

📖 LITERATURE PERSPECTIVE

Resource: Anthony, M., & Yastik, J. (2011). Nursing students' experiences with incivility in clinical education. *Journal of Nursing Education, 50*(3), 140–144.

A qualitative study was conducted with 21 nursing students in focus group settings to explore students' experiences of incivility in the clinical setting and to understand their views about how nursing programs should attend to the topic and issue of incivility. Students' comments reflected themes of exclusion and being dismissed by nursing staff, along with being subjected to rude and hostile behaviour from staff. Students also shared positive experiences, such as when staff took the initiative to include students in learning opportunities involving patient care. Students felt that they would benefit from more preparation about the challenges they might face in the practice setting related to incivility. They also felt that nursing programs could better liaise with nurse leaders and nursing staff in the practice setting so that staff are aware of students' course goals and level of knowledge and skill at the outset of the clinical experience. Students also felt that when clinical instructors were respected by nursing staff, by extension, they were treated well by staff.

Implications for Practice
The findings of the study suggest that healthy work environments exist when nursing staff, nurse leaders, educators, and nursing students recognize that their individual and collective efforts are contributing factors to such environments. Finally, when organizational structures support a healthy work environment, then opportunities can exist for staff nurses to practise in a more inclusive and civil manner.

CONCLUSION

Workplace violence and incivility affect us all. The burden is borne not only by victims but also by their co-workers, their families, their employers, and every worker at risk of such acts. Workplace violence and incivility also have real consequences for patients and patient safety. Although we know that, each year, workplace violence in Canada results in deaths, injuries, and financial costs, our understanding of workplace violence in health care is still in its infancy. Much remains to be done in the area of research, particularly in data collection and interventions for horizontal violence. Without basic information on who is most affected and which prevention measures are effective in what settings, we can expect only limited success in addressing these problems. The first steps have been taken, but a number of key issues have been identified that require future research. All nurses and health care leaders need a broader understanding of the scope and impact of workplace violence and incivility to reduce the human and financial burden of these significant public health problems.

💡 A SOLUTION

Sophie ran to the nurses' station and called for security and for the emergency department physician to come to the unit. Then, she ran back down another hall where she could hear the man yelling at Louisa in a patient room. When Sophie entered the room, the man was in what had been an empty bed and Louisa and another nurse, Beth, were standing close to him. The patient was holding the bed linens up to his chest and was yelling incoherently at the two nurses. Louisa, who had blood all over the front of her uniform, had not been seriously physically injured. Beth's hair was dishevelled and she was not wearing her glasses. The nurses were speaking calmly to the patient, trying to reassure him that he was safe and that nobody was going to harm him. Within what felt like mere seconds, security personnel had entered the room with the emergency department physician. The physician had a copy of the patient's blood work that had been drawn just before he was admitted to the unit. The patient's blood glucose was dangerously low. The physician verbally ordered medication to increase the patient's blood glucose level. While we waited in the room with the patient, the physician and one of the nurses kept responding to the patient in a calm manner. Louisa, Beth, and Sophie stepped away from the patient's bed to give him a feeling of space. The ordered medication arrived very quickly and was administered by the physician via injection. Within less than 1 minute, the patient's behaviour was completely altered. He was confused about where he was and what was going on. He apologized profusely, as he came to realize that he was not wearing clothing, saw that security personnel were in the room, and saw the blood on Louisa's uniform. Beth explained to the patient that his blood glucose had been very low, which caused him to act out of character, but that she and the other nurses would continue to provide the care necessary for him to feel safe. The patient was not moved to another room, as that was felt to be too disruptive for him at the time.

After the incident, Sophie learned how the situation unfolded. When the patient was admitted to the unit, Beth was starting an IV on him when he accused her of taking his glasses. He believed that Beth's glasses were his own. Thus, he grabbed Beth's hair and physically took off her glasses. Beth was in pain from having her hair severely torn at, so she called for help. That is when Louisa entered the patient's room and tried to move the patient's hand from the hold he had on Beth's hair. Next, the patient began to tear the IV catheter out, which caused what looked like the loss of a lot of blood on Louisa's uniform. The patient then leapt out of bed, tore off his hospital gown, and began chasing Louisa down the hallway. That was the point when Sophie observed the patient and Louisa down the hall.

At the time of this situation, Sophie was a student nurse. What she learned from this experience is that the situation was addressed effectively by a team of health care providers in collaboration. The patient's dignity was respected throughout the incident, and he was never physically restrained. Communication techniques and body language skills were used to try and de-escalate the situation, while a medically therapeutic intervention was enacted. When the patient's behaviour returned to normal, the nursing staff did not demean or cast blame on the patient. Instead, they took even more time with the patient to ensure he felt safe and respected. Recognizing the patient's humanity in this situation helped make a tangible difference in the outcome.

How might you have dealt with this situation in the practice setting?

THE EVIDENCE

Workplace violence is recognized as a significant problem within health care. Reviews of nursing literature indicate that violence in the workplace is a significant reason why many nurses leave their jobs and, in some cases, the profession of nursing. With growing concern about a nursing shortage, nurse leaders need to implement effective intervention programs that can foster a healthier workplace. Education has been the main intervention used in the past, but little research has been done to evaluate its effectiveness.

A study by Oostrom and van Mierlo (2008) sought to evaluate the effectiveness of an aggression management training program. A three-part training program was offered to voluntary participants. The program consisted of a variety of teaching methods. The participants were asked to complete a questionnaire developed to evaluate the training. Based on a principal component analysis, two separate scales were constructed: insight into assertiveness and aggression and ability to cope with adverse working situations. The results of the study showed considerable and significant improvement on both scales. The improvements persisted after the training and indicated an enduring change in knowledge and behaviour. The participants' scores on ability to cope showed further increase after the training. From this finding, the researchers concluded that aggression management training may be an effective instrument in the fight against workplace violence.

NEED TO KNOW NOW

- Know how to access the workplace safety plan in your area of practice.
- Be aware of your surroundings at all times, keeping in mind that you are at increased risk for violence.
- Use an assessment tool to help you identify behaviours that predict violence.
- Practise what to say to stop workplace bullying.

CHAPTER CHECKLIST

Nursing research indicates that violence in any form can drain nurses of their enthusiasm for their work and undermine efforts to create a satisfied workforce. At a time when we are facing a nursing shortage, it is imperative to prevent or eliminate workplace violence and incivility in health care.

- All nurses—leaders, managers, and followers—must be aware of the potential for all forms of violence and incivility. They must also strive to not participate in horizontal violence, which weakens nursing as a profession. The key to preventing violence is understanding the potential for it and implementing interventions to minimize that potential.
- Workplace violence and incivility in health care are important safety issues.
- Workplace violence includes threatening behaviour, harassment, and physical attacks. It can be perpetuated by co-workers, managers, patients, former employees, or members of the public not aligned with the organization.
- Key organizations are calling for action to reduce workplace violence, including the following:
  - Canadian Centre for Occupational Health and Safety
  - Canadian Nurses Association
  - International Council of Nurses
  - Institute for Safe Medication Practices
- The risk factors for violence in health care facilities must be assessed when planning for prevention.
- Horizontal violence is experienced by all nurses, regardless of their degree of work experience.
  - Regardless of why it happens, the concerns are that impaired intrapersonal relationships can cause errors, accidents, and poor work performance.
- When nurses are more structurally empowered, they report fewer incidents of bullying.

TIPS FOR PREVENTING WORKPLACE VIOLENCE

- Take advantage of education offered on workplace violence. If education is not offered, ask your employer to consider providing it.
- Make a personal commitment not to participate in any behaviours that perpetuate horizontal violence.
- Practise precautionary strategies and analyze workplaces for safety risk factors.

evolve WEBSITE

Visit the Evolve website for Suggested Readings, Internet Resources, and additional resources related to the content in this chapter: http://evolve.elsevier.com/Canada/Yoder-Wise/leading/.

REFERENCES

Statutes

Canada Occupational Health and Safety Regulations, SOR/86-304.

Occupational Health and Safety Act, RSO 1990, c. O.1.

Texts

American Nurses Association. (2002). *Promoting safe work environments for nurses.* n.p.: Author.

Anthony, M., & Yastik, J. (2011). Nursing students' experiences with incivility in clinical education. *Journal of Nursing Education, 50*(3), 140–144.

Canadian Centre for Occupational Health and Safety. (2013). Violence in the workplace prevention guide. Retrieved from http://www.ccohs.ca/products/publications/violence.html.

Canadian Centre for Occupational Health and Safety. (2014a). About CCOHS. Retrieved from http://www.ccohs.ca/ccohs.html.

Canadian Centre for Occupational Health and Safety. (2014b). Violence in the workplace: Awareness. Retrieved from http://author.vubiz.com/fModules/5595EN/LMSStart.html?vModId=5595EN.

Canadian Centre for Occupational Health and Safety. (2014c). Violence in the workplace: Warning signs. Retrieved from http://www.ccohs.ca/oshanswers/psychosocial/violence_warning_signs.html.

Canadian Nurses Association. (2008). *Code of ethics for registered nurses (2008 centennial edition).* Toronto, ON: Author. Retrieved from https://www.cna-aiic.ca/~/media/cna/files/en/codeofethics.pdf.

Canadian Nurses Association. (2009). Position statement: Nursing leadership. Retrieved from http://cna-aiic.ca/~/media/cna/page-content/pdf-en/ps110_leadership_2009_e.pdf.

Canadian Nurses Association & Canadian Federation of Nurses Unions. (2008). Joint position statement: Workplace violence. Retrieved from https://nursesunions.ca/sites/default/files/workplace_violence_position_statement_cna-cfnu_0.pdf.

Center for American Nurses. (2008). Policy statement on lateral violence and bullying in the workplace. Retrieved from http://www.mc.vanderbilt.edu/root/pdfs/nursing/center_lateral_violence_and_bullying_position_statement_from_center_for_american_nurses.pdf.

College of Nurses of Ontario. (2009). Professional standards. Retrieved from http://www.cno.org/Global/docs/prac/41006_ProfStds.pdf?epslanguage=en.

de Léséleuc, S. (2004). *Criminal victimization in the workplace* (Canadian Centre for Justice Statistics Profile Series). Ottawa, ON: Statistics Canada. Retrieved from http://www.statcan.gc.ca/pub/85f0033m/85f0033m2007013-eng.pdf.

Dellasega, C. (2009). Bullying among nurses. *American Journal of Nursing, 109*(1), 52–58.

Dumont, C., Meisinger, S., Whitacre, M. J., et al. (2012, January). Horizontal violence survey report. *Nursing2012,* 44–49. doi:10.1097/01.NURSE.0000408487.95400.92

Emergency Care Research Institute. (2009, March). Disruptive practitioner behavior. *Healthcare Risk Control.* Retrieved from https://www.ecri.org/Documents/PSA/May_2009/Disruptive_practitioner_behavior.pdf.

Farrell, G. (2001). From tall poppies to squashed weeds: Why don't nurses pull together more? *Journal of Advanced Nursing, 35*(1), 26–33.

Gates, D., Gillespie, G., & Succop, P. (2011). Violence against nurses and its impact on stress and productivity. *Nursing Economics, 29*(2), 59–66.

Hader, R. (2008). Workplace violence survey 2008. *Nursing Management, 39*(7), 13–19.

Hutchinson, M., Vickers, M., Jackson D., et al. (2006). Workplace bullying in nursing: Towards a more critical organizational perspective. *Nursing Inquiry, 15,* 118–126.

Institute for Safe Medication Practices. (2003). Survey on workplace intimidation. Retrieved from http://www.ismp.org/Survey/surveyresults/Survey0311.asp.

International Council of Nurses. (2006). Position statement: Abuse and violence against nursing personnel. Retrieved from http://www.icn.ch/images/stories/documents/publications/position_statements/C01_Abuse_Violence_Nsg_Personnel.pdf.

International Council of Nurses. (2009). *Violence: A worldwide epidemic* [Fact sheet]. Geneva, Switzerland: Author. Retrieved from http://www.icn.ch/images/stories/documents/publications/fact_sheets/19k_FS-Violence.pdf.

Johnson, S. (2009). Workplace bullying: Concerns for nurse leaders. *Journal of Nursing Administration, 39*(2), 84–90.

Kaufer, S., & Mattman, J. (1996). *The cost of workplace violence to American businesses.* Palm Springs, CA: Workplace Violence Research Institute.

Laschinger, H. K. S., Grau, A., Finegan, J., et al. (2010). New graduate nurses' experiences of bullying and burnout in hospital settings. *Journal of Advanced Nursing, 66*(12), 2732–2742. doi:10.1111/j.1365-2648.2010.05420.x

Laschinger, H. K. S., Leiter, M. P., Day, A., et al. (2012). Building empowering work environments that foster civility and organizational trust. Testing an intervention. *Nursing Research, 61*(5), 316–325. doi:10.1097/NNR.0b013e318265a58d

Laschinger, H. K. S., Wong, C., Regan, S., et al. (2013). Workplace incivility and new graduate nurses' mental health: The protective role of resiliency. *The Journal of Nursing Administration, 43*(7/8), 415–421. doi:10.1097/NNA.0b013e31829d61c6

Longo, J., & Sherman, R. O. (2007, March). Levelling horizontal violence. *Nursing Management,* 34–36, 50+.

Morse, K. J. (2008). Lateral violence in nursing [Editorial]. *Nursing2014 Critical Care, 3*(2), 4.

Nielsen, M. B., & Einarsen, S. (2012). Outcomes of exposure to workplace bullying: A meta-analytic review. *Work and Stress, 26*(4), 309–332. doi:10.1080/02678373.2012.734709

Occupational Safety and Health Administration. (2004). *Guidelines for preventing workplace violence for health care and social service workers* (OSHA Publication No. 3148–01R). Washington, DC: U.S. Department of Labor. Retrieved from https://www.osha.gov/Publications/OSHA3148/osha3148.html.

Ontario Ministry of Labour. (2013). *Developing workplace violence and harassment policies and programs: A toolbox.* Author. Retrieved from https://www.labour.gov.on.ca/english/hs/pubs/wvps_toolbox/index.php.

Oostrom, J., & van Mierlo, H. (2008). An evaluation of an aggression management training program to cope with workplace violence in the healthcare sector. *Research in Nursing & Health, 31*, 320–328.

Ostrofsky, D. (2012). Incivility and the nurse leader. *Nursing Management*, 18–22. doi:10.1097/01.NUMA.0000422892.06958.51

Oyeleye, O., Hanson, P., O'Connor, N., et al. (2013). Relationship of workplace incivility, stress, and burnout on nurses' turnover intentions and psychological empowerment. *Journal of Nursing Administration, 43*(10), 536–542. doi:10.1097/NNA.0b013e31 82a3e8c9

Paludi, M., Nydegger, R., & Paludi, C. (2006). *Understanding workplace violence: A guide for managers and employees*. Westport, CT: Praeger.

Pearson, C., & Porath, C. (2009). *The cost of bad behavior: How incivility is damaging your business and what to do about it.* London, UK: Portfolio.

Purdy, N., Laschinger, H. K. S., Finegan, J., et al. (2010). Effects of work environments on nurse and patient outcomes. *Journal of Nursing Management, 18*, 901–913. doi:10.1111/j.1365-2834.2010.01172.x

Shields, M., & Wilkins, K. (2009). Factors related to on-the-job abuse of nurses by patients. *Health Reports, 20*(2), 1–13. Retrieved from http://www.statcan.gc.ca/pub/82-003-x/2009002/article/10835-eng.pdf.

Woelfle, C., & McCaffrey, R. (2007). Nurse on nurse. *Nursing Forum, 42*(3), 123–131.

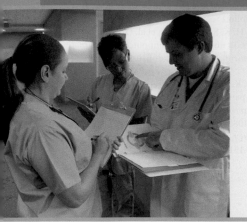

Practising and Leading in Interdisciplinary Settings

Erin Wilson

Nurses are integral members of an interprofessional team. While effective collaboration is a complex process, the outcomes can positively impact patients, health care providers, organizations, and the health care system overall. This chapter considers the nursing role in interdisciplinary settings and reviews how legislation and regulation of nurses can influence interdisciplinary and interprofessional teams. It identifies a framework for interprofessional collaboration as well as barriers and facilitators of collaboration. It also examines how nursing leadership can provide the backbone for effective teams.

OBJECTIVES

- Define interdisciplinary team and interprofessional team.
- Understand the role and boundaries of nurses' scope of practice in your province or territory as well as how the scope of practice overlaps with that of other health care providers.
- Understand the complexity of effective interdisciplinary collaboration and nurses' role on an interprofessional team in providing patient-centred care.
- Identify the purpose of the National Interprofessional Competency Framework.
- Describe strategies to enhance collaboration.
- Understand how team leaders can facilitate successful collaboration.
- Understand how structures and processes influence the functioning of interdisciplinary and interprofessional teams.

TERMS TO KNOW

accountability	interdisciplinary team	scope of practice
collaboration	interprofessional team	unregulated care providers
collaborative practice	patient-centred care	(UCPs)
delegation	role clarity	

❓ A CHALLENGE

Thomas is a registered nurse (RN) on a general surgery ward. He is speaking with the physiotherapist about Mrs. Haley's progress with walking and reviewing medications that might interfere with her balance. Suddenly a breathless porter approaches Thomas asking why Mrs. Haley isn't in X-ray for her fluoroscopy-guided procedure. Thomas was completely unaware this procedure had been booked. Just then, Mrs. Haley begins retching and her daughter is asking when her mother had last received Gravol (dimenhydrinate). Thomas is pretty sure his colleague Layla, an RN, gave Mrs. Haley a p.r.n. dose while Thomas was on his break, but when he checks the medication administration record, nothing is recorded. The physiotherapist would like to know when Mrs. Haley might attend a physiotherapy appointment, the porter has his hands on Mrs. Haley's chair

ready to wheel her to radiology, and her daughter is holding Mrs. Haley's head over a kidney basin while she vomits. Thomas feels overwhelmed: Should he search for Layla to see if Mrs. Haley had any dimenhydrinate, or try to find out what procedure Mrs. Haley has booked in radiology, or assist Mrs. Haley while she is sick, or direct the physiotherapist as to when Mrs. Haley might attend physiotherapy?

Identify the interpersonal, organizational, and systemic components of this scenario that could be improved by better interdisciplinary care. What do you think you would do if you were Thomas?

INTRODUCTION

In 1978, the Declaration of Alma-Ata identified that primary health care and improvement in health of the world's populations would rely in part on the ability of health care providers to work in teams (World Health Organization, 1978). In the intervening decades, policymakers in Canada have identified effective interdisciplinary collaboration as a national priority (Curran, 2007; Laschinger, 2007), and currently every jurisdiction in Canada is implementing interdisciplinary teams in a variety of settings (Advisory Committee on Health Delivery and Human Resources [ACHDHR], 2009). The rationale for this shift toward interdisciplinary care is directly related to changes in the Canadian health care landscape: the aging population has increasingly complex and comorbid illnesses (Curran, 2007); health human resources are facing shortages (Baranek, 2005); and it is clear that no single health care provider can adequately address patient needs in the twenty-first century (Reeves, Macmillan, & van Soeren, 2010). The benefits of interdisciplinary care are reduced duplication of services, decreased fragmentation of care, and improved quality of care for patients (Litaker, Mion, Planavsky, et al., 2003). The implementation and integration of interprofessional teams within Canada's health care system can allow health care providers to work to their full scope of practice and create innovative, sustainable ways of providing high-quality health care for all Canadians.

Despite the laudable benefits of interprofessional collaboration, in practice they have remained elusive

(Hills, Mullett, & Carroll, 2007). Barriers to collaboration include policies (including policy overload), funding, power inequalities, and overlapping scopes of practice (Baranek, 2005; Martin-Misener & Valaitis, 2009; Reeves et al., 2010). This chapter examines the nurse's role as an interdisciplinary or interprofessional team member and considers how some of the barriers to effective collaboration might be reduced or eliminated.

CONCEPTS AND DEFINITIONS

Interdisciplinary Team to Interprofessional Team

An interdisciplinary team comprises members from different clinical disciplines who have specialized knowledge, skills, and abilities. Members often work alongside one another and may or may not collaborate closely on patient care. This has been the traditional way health care providers work "together" in hospitals.

An interprofessional team comprises "different healthcare disciplines working together towards common goals to meet the needs of a patient population. Team members divide the work based on their scope of practice; they share information to support one another's work and coordinate processes and interventions to provide a number of services and programs" (Virani, 2012, p. 3).

Interprofessional care provides an increased ability to be innovative, to better understand the local context, to promote sustainable solutions, and to see the "big picture" (Lasker & Weiss, 2003). Effective interprofessional teams demonstrate clear and frequent communication, respect, the ability to resolve conflict, a shared understanding of "health," shared protocols or best practices, and an understanding of all members' roles within the team (Canadian Interprofessional Health Collaborative [CIHC], 2010; Laschinger, 2007; Sargeant, Loney, & Murphy, 2008).

While interdisciplinary teams are more recognizable in health care service provision in Canada today, nurses must be leaders in advancing interprofessional teams for their synergistic effects and potential to reorient health care services, versus maintaining the status quo of the coordinated care of interdisciplinary teams. As Sargeant et al. (2008) note, working "alongside" is not enough to effect change.

Collaborative Practice and Collaboration

Collaborative practice is "an inter-professional process for communication and decision making that enables the separate and shared knowledge and skills of the care providers to synergistically influence the client/patient care provided" (Way, Jones, & Busing, 2000, p. 3). Collaboration has been described as a complex, voluntary, and dynamic process with underlying concepts of power, interdependency, sharing, partnership, and process (D'Amour, Ferrada-Videla, San Martin Rodriguez, et al., 2005). Through collaboration, interdisciplinary teams should be able to accomplish more than individuals working alone or in tandem. Care for patients could occur more seamlessly between institutions and communities, health promotion and illness prevention could be included for all patient encounters, health care providers could be able to stay informed of new evidence, and health outcomes could be improved (CIHC, 2010; Jones & Way, 2007).

THE RISE OF DISTINCT DISCIPLINES

Historically, professions developed through craft guilds first formed in the 1500s "to protect and promote their members' interests through the ownership of knowledge" (Reeves et al., 2010, p. 259). Noticeably, this approach is contrary to interdisciplinary collaboration. From these guilds arose the health care professions. Nursing did not professionalize until almost a century after medicine; thus, the division of work was not intentionally determined but was instead moulded over time through the influence of political and economic factors (Reeves et al., 2010). Today, health care

providers continue to be educated in "silos" (Jones & Way, 2007), with little understanding of the role or scope of other health professions. Within individual disciplines, students learn discipline-specific frameworks and theories, ways of defining health, methods for solving problems, technical terminology, and documentation techniques. These factors reinforce the cohesion among professionals in their own discipline and are, in fact, central to professional development (D'Amour et al., 2005; Hall, 2005; Hills et al., 2007).

SCOPE OF PRACTICE

The Canadian Nurses Association (CNA, 1993) defines scope of practice as "activities nurses are educated and authorized to perform, as established through legislated definitions of nursing practice complemented by standards, guidelines and policy positions issued by professional nursing bodies" (p. 15). In Canada, nursing scopes of practice have remained purposefully broad, avoiding a splintering into various specialties. The discipline recognizes that nurses should not and cannot be defined by tasks or lists of skills, and that nursing scopes of practice have changed throughout the decades to reflect the emergence of other health professions (Baranek, 2005).

Although the broad scope of nursing practice has many benefits, it has led to difficulty with interpretation. Consider, for example, the role of a registered nurse in a remote area of Canada. In addition to requiring knowledge commonly understood to be in the realm of nursing practice, this nurse also provides expertise and skills such as suturing, diagnosing some illnesses, and prescribing some medications—a scope of practice that is considerably different from urban nurses. The expansion of the role of nurse into areas that overlap with medicine raises the question why some registered nurses are considered capable of performing tasks in one setting but not another (CNA, 1993). In most provinces and territories, a nurse's authority to perform these activities (considered outside the legislative scope of nursing practice) is "covered" by extensive use of delegation or "transfer of function" from physicians (CNA, 1993; Wearing & Nickerson, 2010). Consistently, the physicians who sign delegation orders never meet the nurses carrying out the orders or the patients who receive the nurses' care. It may be that the physician perhaps presumes that it is the employer's responsibility to ensure the nurse is competent to provide the required care, while the employer places a large portion of the onus on the nurse and, thus, the nursing regulatory body. The development of mechanisms that expand the activities of registered nurses without clarifying responsibility and accountability (the obligation to account for one's actions) has been a cause for concern. For example, in response, the BC provincial government moved to a new restricted activities framework that required a review of the scopes of practice of all health professions in the 1990s (Wearing & Nickerson, 2010).

> **EXERCISE 26-1**
> Visit your provincial or territorial nursing regulatory body or professional association website. Read the professional and practice standards and scope of practice statements, then ask two or more colleagues how they stay current with the requirements of the regulatory body, and what is required for continuing competence once in practice.

Widespread concern also exists over the clarity of scopes of practice in a number of health professions (Baranek, 2005). Such concerns promise to be increasingly complex because nursing practice is experiencing rapid growth in scope of practice. Certified practice in British Columbia is one example, and in Ontario the premier recently promised an expanded scope of practice for registered nurses and registered practical nurses to improve access for patients (Government of Ontario, 2013).

In the 1990s, a period of consultation on health professional regulation began in several provinces, and legislation for the scope of practice of regulated health care providers was revised. Ontario, Alberta, and British Columbia have adopted a common framework known as a "restricted activities" or "controlled acts" model that provides a consistent approach to registration, continuing competence, discipline, and restricted activities for the health care professions (College and Association of Registered Nurses of Alberta [CARNA], 2005; College of Nurses of Ontario [CNO], 2014; College of Registered Nurses of British Columbia [CRNBC], 2010). What makes this model distinct from the model of licensure still used in other provinces and territories is that nurses are not bound by exclusive scopes of practice (Baranek, 2005). That is, the model licenses specific acts rather than a particular role. More than one profession can perform the same act, or parts of the act (e.g., prescribing medication). If an act is not controlled, it can be performed by anyone (Baranek, 2005).

The controlled acts model has several benefits over the licensure model: it allows professionals to perform to the range of their competency and abilities; it recognizes that scope of practice is not static and does not have firm boundaries; it places greater emphasis on standards and competence; and it increases flexibility in allowing patients more choice in providers and employers more innovation in optimal skill mix, while protecting the public from harm (Baranek, 2005; CARNA, 2005; CNO, 2014; CRNBC, 2010). While each of these benefits is important and arguably necessary, the legislative reform to recognize overlapping competencies has caused role confusion, further competition over "turf" for various health care providers, and difficulty in optimizing skill mix (Baranek, 2005). Additionally, legal reporting requirements must be exceptionally clear to members of an interdisciplinary team. Numerous legislative acts (e.g., those that relate to the reporting of child abuse, gunshot wounds, and adverse events) (see also Chapter 5) identify several health professions as having a legal obligation to report occurrences of these events. Health care providers (including nurses), employers, and patients can be uncomfortable with the shades of grey that accompany competency-based practice. It can lead to diminished professional identity (Baranek, 2005) that in turn can undermine role clarity, which is essential in understanding inclusion on an interdisciplinary team.

A FRAMEWORK FOR INTERPROFESSIONAL COLLABORATION

If nurses and other team members are going to be successful collaborators, they need to not only understand their own and others' roles but also use common terminology as a platform for communication. However those who have examined the evidence regarding effective interprofessional collaboration found most literature to be descriptive, and many of the studies did not identify a theoretical framework to guide effective collaboration (Martin-Misener & Valaitis, 2009; Zwarenstein & Reeves, 2006).

In an effort to advance interprofessional collaboration, the Canadian Interprofessional Health Collaborative (CIHC) has produced a National Interprofessional Competency Framework (Figure 26-1). The framework consists of six competency domains that "highlight the knowledge, skills, attitudes and values that together shape the judgments that are essential for interprofessional collaborative" (CIHC, 2010, p. i). The six

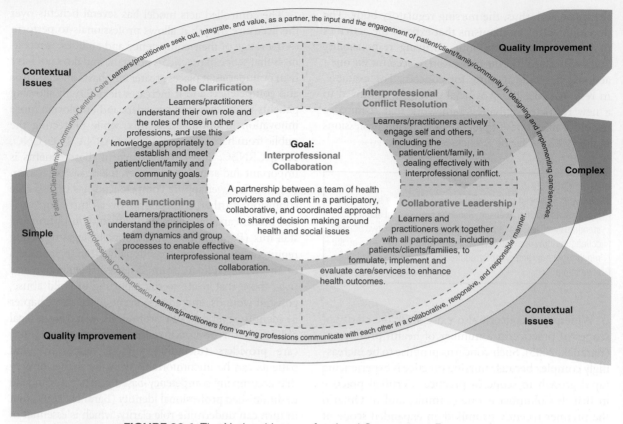

FIGURE 26-1 The National Interprofessional Competency Framework.

competency domains are as follows: interprofessional communication; patient/family/community-centred care; role clarification; team functioning; collaborative leadership and interprofessional conflict resolution (CIHC, 2010). In every situation, the domains of patient/family/community-centred care and interprofessional communication are relevant and consistently influence and support the other four domains (CIHC, 2010). This framework was designed so that any professional can learn and apply the competencies, regardless of skill or practice setting. The CIHC views interprofessional learning as an additive and continuous process that begins prelicensure (CIHC, 2010).

When considering the competencies required to achieve interprofessional collaboration, it is also important to identify the factors which influence collaboration. Martin-Misener and Valaitis (2012) described the factors influencing collaboration between primary care and public health, which can be organized in three separate layers: interactional, organizational, and systemic (Figure 26-2). Leaders, managers, and followers have important roles in facilitating interprofessional collaboration at the organizational and interpersonal levels of their health care settings.

Nurses are integral members of any team, regardless of the setting. Whether they are part of a palliative care team, an operating theatre team, or a public health team, nurses have an important role. By incorporating the framework reviewed here, nurses and other members of the interdisciplinary team can identify common ground, name the barriers and facilitators facing their particular team, and progress toward effective collaboration that can be beneficial

---

EXERCISE 26-2

Ask three staff nurses to identify the top three team members they communicate with most frequently (i.e., unit clerks, social workers, physicians), and then ask which team member is easiest to talk with, and why they think that is so.

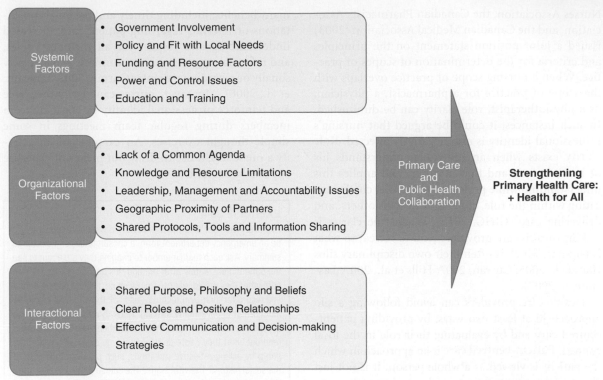

FIGURE 26-2 Factors influencing collaboration between primary care and public health.

to patient outcomes, health care providers, and their organization.

MOVING FORWARD IN COLLABORATIVE PRACTICE

When collaboration is ineffective or unsuccessful, disciplinary silos are reinforced and turf protection escalates. Such environments contribute to workplace stress and affect patient care (Laschinger, 2007). Consider the example of the pediatric cardiac surgery inquest of 12 deaths in 1994 at a Winnipeg hospital. Nurses raised serious and legitimate concerns about problems they had noticed, but were not taken seriously (Grinspun, 2007):

> Even when a series of deaths occurred in rapid succession, there was not a timely and appropriate response within the surgical team, the Child Health program, the medical and administrative structures of the [hospital], the death review processes of the [Office of the Chief Medical Examiner], and the complaints/investigation processes of the [College of Physicians & Surgeons of Manitoba]. (p. 87)

In the report of the inquest, Justice Sinclair clarified that the nurses were not treated as full, equal members of the surgical team in the pediatric surgery program (Sinclair, 2000).

EXERCISE 26-3
Find out whether your current place of practicum or work has a whistle-blower policy. If it does, describe the policy's purpose and who it protects. If it does not, provide reasons why the organization should have a whistle-blower policy.

Although most instances of ineffective collaboration do not lead to as serious and tragic an outcome as described above, we are reminded that although complex health problems have created greater interdependencies among health care providers, working collaboratively can be challenging (D'Amour, et al., 2005). As previously mentioned, one strategy to enhance collaboration is to clarify roles. Role clarification is commonly addressed by defining scopes of practice and is one of the reasons that the Canadian

Nurses Association, the Canadian Pharmacists Association, and the Canadian Medical Association (2003) issued a joint position statement on the principles and criteria for the determination of scopes of practice. When a nursing scope of practice overlaps with the scope of practice for a pharmacist, a physician, or a physiotherapist, role clarity can be diminished. In such instances, it could be argued that nursing's professional identity is also negatively affected. Role clarity exists when an individual understands his or her own role and that of others and applies this understanding while performing the role, communicating within the role, collaborating with others, and delivering care (CIHC, 2010). When role clarity is lacking, health care providers tend to retreat to what is familiar, which is often their own disciplinary silos (Baranek, 2005; Curran, 2007; Hills et al., 2007; Laschinger, 2007).

Health care providers can avoid following a silo approach in at least two ways: by providing patient-centred care and by evaluating their role in the local context. Patient-centred care is an approach in which the patient is viewed as a whole person; it is not just about delivering services and involves advocacy, empowerment, and respecting the patient's autonomy, voice, self-determination, and participation in decision making. Innovative and practical solutions to patient care can be found if nurses and other members of the interdisciplinary team consistently ask themselves, *What is best for the patient?* This approach requires operationalization of the concept of "working with" versus "taking care of" patients (Lasker & Weiss, 2003). Thus, it requires acceptance of the patient's choice of provider and the patient's values and beliefs regarding treatment choices, as well as the incorporation of the patient's health care agenda with the professional's agenda of providing high-quality evidence-informed care.

Nurses on interdisciplinary or interprofessional teams should evaluate their role and professional identity within a local context (i.e., within their own team). All team members should be clear about what they bring to the health care and team process (Baranek, 2005; Laschinger, 2007). This clarity can be facilitated by co-location and engagement. Although simply grouping a variety of health care providers together in the same building will not create a team (Hills et al., 2007), co-location can have many benefits, including timely and personal consultations or referrals regarding patient care, increased understanding and respect for all members' roles, and informal opportunities to connect, whether personally or regarding patients (Curran, 2007; Sargeant, et al., 2008). Moreover, nurses can clarify their role and reinforce professional identity by engaging team members during regular team meetings in some simple thought exercises. An example of an activity a nurse might use to draw out niches of expertise appears in Exercise 26-4.

EXERCISE 26-4

Ask every member of a team to review a patient report. It might be an emergency department form, a consult letter, or a discharge summary. Ask each team member to imagine they are about to see the patient immediately after reading this document. Ask them to note what they would want to follow up on, ask the patient about, and record for their own records. Also ask them to note any information that is particularly striking. Allow 5 minutes for everyone to read the report and make their notes, then have team members read out what they wrote down. Encourage discussion within the group by asking reflective questions, such as, Who took note of the social history? The vital signs? The course of the hospital stay? Who wrote down that they would update the patient chart when they noticed a new medication was added for the patient's blood pressure? Who wrote down that they would follow up with the patient regarding the strong family history of breast cancer? In this fashion, and through similar recurring scenarios, members of the interdisciplinary team can not only draw out some of the subtle differences their roles bring to patient care but also recognize their synergy as they see the different contributions each professional makes to patient care.

Undoubtedly, the tension between maintaining one's professional identity and participating in collaborative care in an interdisciplinary setting will remain for some time. However, in practice, nurses and other team members must strive to reduce this tension. Maintaining teams that are co-located in flexible, innovative environments is not only beneficial in and of itself, but "the proposed solutions for improving teamwork mirror those for ensuring [a] healthy work environment" (Laschinger, 2007, p. 45). All team members must strive to engage in mutually respectful communication, which includes transparency and disclosure with all team members, as well as patients (CIHC, 2010). Finally, nurses must incorporate a framework such as the National

Interprofessional Competency Framework (CIHC, 2010) to help all team members understand the domains they might work on together to achieve the synergy of effective collaboration that can improve patient care and outcomes.

LEADING INTERDISCIPLINARY OR INTERPROFESSIONAL TEAMS

Providing leadership to an interdisciplinary or interprofessional team is complex (Reeves et al., 2010), and doing so may call for qualities not found in a more traditional type of leader (Lasker & Weiss, 2003). The Research Perspective provides an example of the complexities involved in leading teams.

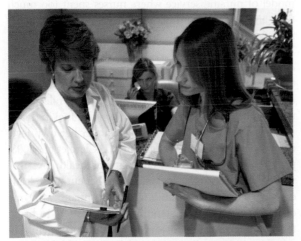

Nurse leaders face complex decisions when leading interdisciplinary or interprofessional teams.

To facilitate successful collaboration, team leaders must be able to inspire, engage, and motivate; they must be able to establish and articulate a vision and purpose to the team and greater community, and

be open and inclusive in their language and actions (French, 2004; Lasker & Weiss, 2003).

In interprofessional practice, leadership might be more effective when it is shared. For example, one team member might lead others to carry the work forward, while another team member might ensure that patients and families are staying connected to the team and that the work of the team has meaning and impact for the key team player—the patient (CIHC, 2010). Teams might also choose to rotate leadership or choose leaders in different situations based on the contextual or experiential knowledge of the proposed leader. Either of these leadership models may help redistribute the hierarchal power that is common in health care settings. Regardless, leaders must be able to apply principles that will support and enhance successful collaborative efforts, as well as anticipate conflicts such as power hierarchies, role ambiguity, and competing priorities (CIHC, 2010). Team leaders may or may not be part of management. Leadership and management, although not the same, are interdependent (French, 2004).

Followers have a symbiotic relationship with leaders (Whitlock, 2013). Followers are not subordinates but individuals who use their judgement to decide which leader they feel motivated to help be successful (Thomas, 2012). An exemplary follower has strong critical-thinking skills, is participative and competent, and feels motivated when engaged in interesting and challenging work (Thomas, 2012). The effectiveness of leaders depends on relationships between leaders and followers that develop through motivating and inspiring others, as opposed to managing and controlling them (Batcheller, 2012).

🔍 RESEARCH PERSPECTIVE

Resource: Lingard, L., McDougall, A., Levstik, M., et al. (2012). Representing complexity well: A story about teamwork, with implications for how we teach collaboration. *Medical Education, 46,* 869–877. doi:10.1111/j.1365-2923.2012.04339.x

Researchers in this ethnographic study aimed to produce a rich description of how teamwork happens in a distributed team. The setting was a solid-organ transplant unit of a tertiary care hospital in Canada. Thirty-nine team members consented to participate, and data collection involved 162 hours of observation, 30 field interviews, and 17 formal interviews. The study employed activity theory and the concept of "knotworking" to explore how

Continued

the team worked through challenges or barriers. It also employed the concept of "boundary" to examine how interactions within the team are shaped by organizational and professional boundaries. The results identified the different challenges faced by different parts of the team: the "core" transplant team, the "interservice" team (where challenges were identified between the core transplant team and other clinicians or services within the hospital), and "outside" challenges between the core team and clinical or administrative or social supports outside the hospital. The results of this study are presented in a nontraditional manner in that a patient story is related to the reader with supporting observational and interview data to highlight the complexities and challenges of the team involved in a transplant patient's care.

Implications for Practice

This study revealed the difficulty faced by interdisciplinary teams and the type of emerging challenges that need to be addressed and resolved daily in health care settings in order to provide timely, safe patient care. The division of labour can be fluid, as can the authority and roles of team members, who may be distributed across time and space in a single setting. Most important, this study highlighted how roles are sometimes fluid or blurred within teams. The intricacies of working within an interdisciplinary team as described in this article can help nurses in novice and leadership roles alike better understand the different priorities and motives of team members, which can help resolve everyday tensions and conflict in any patient care setting.

Leadership development, particularly in relation to teams, should begin in nursing prelicensure programs (French, 2004; Oandasan, 2007). Ideally, based on the National Interprofessional Competency Framework (CIHC, 2010), collaborative leadership could be included as a competency that might be taught to multiple health disciplines synchronously, preparing future graduates with the skills to collaborate and lead in interdisciplinary practice.

It is imperative for leaders of interdisciplinary or interprofessional teams to ensure that structures and processes to allow teams to function optimally are in place (Curran, 2007; LeClerc, Doyon, Gravelle, et al., 2008; Xyrichis & Lowton, 2008). Structures would include administrative support, adequate meeting space, dedicated times for team members to meet, and a culturally safe practice environment (Curran, 2007; LeClerc, et al., 2008). Processes would include mutually dependent team goals, needs assessments, team activities to engage the community, and quality improvement efforts (CIHC, 2010; Martin-Misener &

Valaitis, 2009; Xyrichis & Lowton, 2008). An important process that is often absent in interdisciplinary practice settings is evaluation. Interdisciplinary or interprofessional teams should incorporate processes and indicators that evaluate how their efforts affect patient, health care provider, and system outcomes (ACHDHR, 2009; Jones & Way, 2007; Martin-Misener & Valaitis, 2009).

In some environments, leaders are responsible for human resources planning or implementing care delivery models. In such environments, the leader of a team might heed two lessons that relate to nursing. The first is to have adequate full-time nursing staff on the team. Understandably, teams are able to be more cohesive if the core group is employed full time and has daily opportunities to interact. From the perspective of patient-centred care, nurses who can care for the same patients every day will know them better than casual or agency-employed nurses who are frequently reassigned between shifts (Grinspun, 2007). The second lesson is interwoven with the first, which involves planning for an optimal skill mix, or the combination of team members who have the capacity and competence to produce the best level of health care services. LeClerc et al. (2008) described the implementation of a care delivery model based on an optimal skill mix at a continuing care facility. The facility went from delivering care according to a traditional model of nursing service where nurses spent too much time and effort "coordinating, delegating and supervising" (p. 67) to an autonomous–collaborative model, in which the time spent by nurses in a 24-hour period on non-nursing duties was reduced from 9.75 hours to 2.85 hours. The autonomous–collaborative model allowed team members to work together while maintaining accountability for care provision, making each nurse "responsible for determining his or her own level of knowledge, skill and judgment" (LeClerc et al., 2008, p. 69). As this example indicates, patients, health care providers, and the health care system can benefit when leaders have a clear understanding of team members' scope of practice. That understanding allows leaders to bring together health care providers with an appropriate skill mix that can be applied to a care delivery model that is safe and effective and acknowledges abilities and judgement.

An interdisciplinary or interprofessional team may include unregulated personnel who are also involved in providing direct care to patients. Unregulated care providers (UCPs) are unregulated caregivers who perform a variety of tasks (see also Chapters 5 and 8).

Settings where unregulated care providers (such as care aides, home support workers, or community health representatives) are commonly employed include long-term care, home care, and nursing stations. In such settings, registered nurses are often responsible to delegate tasks regarding patient care to these team members. Delegation refers to "achieving performance of care outcomes for which you are accountable and responsible by sharing activities with other individuals who have the appropriate authority to accomplish the work" (Yoder-Wise, 2011, p. 523). To delegate safely, a registered nurse must be aware of the scope of practice and ability of the delegatee, communicate effectively, and seek a degree of trust in the delagator-delegatee relationship (Yoder-Wise, 2011). The regulatory bodies of several provinces (e.g., Nunavut and Northwest Territories, Nova Scotia, New Brunswick, Ontario, Manitoba, Alberta, British Columbia) provide registrants with frameworks or practice guidelines for delegation to unregulated care providers.

EXERCISE 26-6
Scenario A
Three months ago, you accepted your first job as a registered nurse in a community-based long-term care facility in Moncton, New Brunswick. Yesterday, you delegated the administration of a heparin injection and a dressing change for a leg ulcer to a patient care aide. Today, you delegate the same tasks to a different patient care aide who was also hired about 3 months ago. She tells you she has only ever given one injection before and has never cared for someone with a leg ulcer. What do you do?

Scenario B
You are a registered nurse in northern Saskatchewan. Your job requires you to spend 1 week in one community and the following week in a different community that is a 45-minute drive away. You are available by phone for the community health representative when you are not in the community. Today, the community health representative calls you to say a mother has brought her child to the clinic with a rash and she is pretty sure it is chicken pox. The community health representative asks you if she may dispense calamine lotion and acetaminophen (Tylenol©) to the mother. What do you do?

WORKING "WITH" VERSUS "ALONGSIDE" OTHERS

An important issue that has not yet been addressed is how to achieve the ideal of collaboration, interdisciplinary practice, shared decision making, and visionary leadership to practice. Many health care team members have congenial and collegial relationships, and some have real partnerships that have been achieved due to many factors, not the least of which is sustained effort. However, in order for these working partnerships to become the status quo versus an ideal that we aspire to, all nurses must endorse and enact power redistribution (Grinspun, 2007). In order to move from working "alongside" to working "with" other professionals and patients, nurses must notice and recommend changes to existing power differentials. Some authors have described Canada's current top-down approach to health care as being physician-driven and have demonstrated how, in an interdisciplinary team, nonphysician team members "frequently judged their contributions to client care in relation to the physician's practice" (Hills et al., 2007, p. 131). For example, nonphysician team members who spent time reviewing medications and providing health education to a patient did not consider their contribution to comprehensive, high-quality patient care; instead, "these activities were valued for saving the physician's time" (Hills et al., 2007, p. 131).

In Canada, nurses represent the largest group of health care providers (Canadian Institute of Health Information, 2010), and they are included in almost every interdisciplinary and interprofessional team. All nurses, and particularly those in formal or informal leadership positions, must advocate for moving beyond recurring debates of professional competition to focus on the opportunities afforded by linking interprofessional care to improved patient-centred care (Reeves et al., 2010). Bringing the focus back to what is best for the patient can be an excellent catalyst for change to structures and values, and propel nurses to act beyond the walls of their organizations to research, educate, and lead reforms at a policy and systems level.

CONCLUSION

Practising and leading in an interdisciplinary setting is complex and yet necessary to meet the health care needs of Canadians in the twenty-first century. Nurses are integral to championing the implementation and integration of innovative, sustainable collaborative teams that have a shared goal of providing high-quality patient-centred care.

A SOLUTION

Interpersonal components: Keeping Mrs. Haley's well-being at the centre of Thomas's decisions, he helps the daughter tend to her, tells the physiotherapist he will phone her in 30 minutes, and asks the porter to quietly get Layla so that he can ask about the last dose of dimenhydrinate. Thomas communicates to Mrs. Haley and her daughter that he will be getting medication for her nausea and emesis as soon as he establishes a safe dose for an antiemetic based on the last dose she received. Thomas apologizes for the wait and provides reassurance that it will be sorted quickly. This addresses themes of shared purpose, maintaining good relationships, and effective communication and decision making (Martin-Misener & Valaitis, 2009).

Organizational components: A clear structure exists for reporting when one leaves and returns from breaks, with attention to prompt documentation in addition to a verbal report. While uncertainty regarding Layla's medication administration to Mrs. Haley may be an oversight, consistent use of a reporting structure can decrease this and other oversights. Additionally, if dimenhydrinate is not controlling Mrs. Haley's symptoms, there should be a clear and easy way to obtain an order for a different, more suitable medication. This addresses themes of accountability, common agendas, and shared protocols (Martin-Misener & Valaitis, 2009).

Systemic components: With regards to the X-ray that has been booked in radiology, interorganizational electronic booking systems should be accessible to direct-care providers so that they can check these databases along with other appointments to ensure patients are ready for their appointments in a timely manner. Such systems should be programmed so that cross-referencing is allowed; that is, to ensure the patient does not have an appointment booked with another department at the same time, such as physiotherapy. This addresses themes of information infrastructure, education and training, funding, and government involvement; in fact, most of these themes are interconnected (Martin-Misener & Valaitis, 2009).

What other components would you address and how?

THE EVIDENCE

A pilot project assigned seven students from different health care educational programs to the same site for clinical rotations and included organized case-based discussions between the students of different professions. Cragg, Hirsh, Jelley, et al. (2010) described the opportunity given to students to share different perspectives and appreciate the contributions of other professions at a clinical site that was already known to have supportive administration and good communication channels. The participating students represented four professional groups that included nursing, physiotherapy, medicine, and spiritual care, and the program ran for 12 weeks, with weekly sessions attended between five and twelve times. Pre- and post-qualitative and quantitative data were collected through semi-structured interviews and a scale to measure interprofessional attitudes was also applied.

At the end of the pilot project, the students reported that they would practise differently as a result of the project. They also noted important learning outcomes, including the recognition of different approaches, values, and terminology of different professions.

This pilot project, although small, highlighted how prelicensure exposure to other health care providers can increase understanding of roles on an interdisciplinary team, and can be a cost-effective way to promote interprofessional education. As a result of this project, weekly interprofessional rounds were started on an inpatient unit and continued after the students completed their rotation.

NEED TO KNOW NOW

- Understand the elements of successful collaboration.
- Be familiar with provincial or territorial legislation that impacts nursing practice and how your regulatory body or professional association regulates this legislation for nurses. Know whether the legislation is designed to affect several health professions or just nursing.

- Consider what you bring to the health care process. What aspects of care do others on your team contribute? What is missing? Who should provide the "missing pieces"?
- Reflect on how you will add your voice to those of other nurses across Canada. Be aware of the role of the Canadian Nurses Association and how its mission, vision, and mandate might be different from that of your regulatory body.

CHAPTER CHECKLIST

Practising and leading in interdisciplinary settings is a dynamic process throughout which nurses play a critical role. In some settings, nurses may be the health care providers who not only see patients the most but also interact with the greatest variety of professionals who are also involved in patient care. For this reason, nurses must step forward and take a leadership role in interdisciplinary care. They must also demonstrate the competencies of interprofessional practice and educate others in how to apply them. At the interpersonal, team, organizational, and systemic levels, nurses must seek to bring clarity to their roles, acknowledge what other health care providers and staff bring to patient care, families, and communities, and be comfortable with the shades of grey in overlapping scopes of practice.

- Practice in interdisciplinary settings requires flexibility and knowledge.

- Nurses must be prepared to enact power redistribution, as effective collaboration cannot occur within an imbalanced hierarchy.
- Interprofessional teams must work toward a shared goal or purpose in order to be effective. This goal should include patient-centred care.
- Regular meetings, open communication, and orientation of all team members are essential to effective collaboration.
- Building a trusting relationship takes time and has tremendous value in working effectively.
- Legislation and regulation provide the legal structure for nurses; the Canadian Nurses Association's *Code of Ethics for Registered Nurses* provides the ethical structure.

TIPS FOR PRACTISING AND LEADING IN INTERDISCIPLINARY SETTINGS

- Be knowledgeable of all team members' roles and competencies.
- Use the National Interprofessional Competency Framework to identify and apply competencies for interdisciplinary practice.
- Be sure to engage in evaluation to assess the team's accomplishments.

- Maintain open and respectful communication practices.
- Pay attention to employee retention and what keeps professionals happy and healthy in their work environment.
- Keep the patient at the centre of your decisions in an effort to provide high-quality patient care and decrease professional competition.

evolve WEBSITE

Visit the Evolve website for Suggested Readings, Internet Resources, and additional resources related to the content in this chapter: http://evolve.elsevier.com/Canada/Yoder-Wise/leading/.

REFERENCES

Advisory Committee on Health Delivery and Human Resources. (2009). *How many are enough? Redefining self-sufficiency for the health workforce. A discussion paper.* Ottawa, ON: Health Canada.

Baranek, P. M. (2005). *A review of scopes of practice of health professions in Canada: A balancing act.* Toronto, ON: Health Council of Canada.

Batcheller, J. (2012). Learning how to dance: Courageous followership: A CNO case study. *Nurse Leader, 10*(2), 22–24.

Canadian Institute of Health Information. (2010, December 9). Canada's nursing workforce grows 9% in five years [Press release]. Retrieved from http://www.cihi.ca/cihi-ext-portal/internet/en/document/spending+and+health+workforce/workforce/nurses/release_09dec2010.

Canadian Interprofessional Health Collaborative. (2010). A national interprofessional competency framework. Retrieved from http://www.cihc.ca/files/CIHC_IPCompetencies_Feb1210.pdf.

Canadian Nurses Association. (1993). *The scope of nursing practice: A review of issues and trends.* Ottawa, ON: Author. Retrieved from http://ners.unair.ac.id/materikuliah/scope_nursing_practice_e.pdf.

Canadian Nurses Association, Canadian Pharmacists Association, & Canadian Medical Association. (2003). Joint position statement: Scopes of practice. Retrieved from http://www.cna-aiic.ca/~/media/cna/page-content/pdf-en/10%20-%20ps66_scopes_of_practice_june_2003_e.pdf.

College and Association of Registered Nurses of Alberta. (2005). *Health Professions Act: Standards for registered nurses in the performance of restricted activities.* Edmonton, AB: Author. Retrieved from http://www.nurses.ab.ca/Carna-Admin/Uploads/HPA_Restricted_Activities.pdf.

College of Nurses of Ontario. (2014). *RHPA: Scope of practice, controlled acts model.* Toronto, ON. Retrieved from http://www.cno.org/Global/docs/policy/41052_RHPAscope.pdf.

College of Registered Nurses of British Columbia. (2010). *Overview of Health Professions Act, Nurses (Registered) and Nurse Practitioners Regulation, CRNBC bylaws.* Vancouver, BC: Author. Retrieved from https://www.crnbc.ca/crnbc/documents/324.pdf.

Cragg, B., Hirsh, M., Jelley, W., et al. (2010). An interprofessional rural clinical placement project. *Journal of Interprofessional Care, 24*(2), 207–209.

Curran, V. (2007). Collaborative care. *Synthesis series on sharing insights.* Ottawa, ON: Health Canada.

D'Amour, D., Ferrada-Videla, M., San Martin Rodriguez, L., et al. (2005). The conceptual basis for interprofessional collaboration: Core concepts and theoretical frameworks [Review]. *Journal of Interprofessional Care, 19*(Suppl. 1), 116–131. doi:10.1080/13561820500082529

French, S. (2004). Challenges to developing and providing nursing leadership. *Canadian Journal of Nursing Leadership, 17*(4), 37–40.

Government of Ontario. (2013). Enhancing the role of Ontario nurses [Press release]. Retrieved from http://news.ontario.ca/opo/en/2013/04/enhancing-the-role-of-ontario-nurses.html.

Grinspun, D. (2007). Healthy workplaces: The case for shared clinical decision making and increased full-time employment. *Healthcare Papers, 7*(special issue), 85–91.

Hall, P. (2005). Interprofessional teamwork: Professional cultures as barriers. *Journal of Interprofessional Care, 1*(Suppl.), 188–196.

Hills, M., Mullett, J., & Carroll, S. (2007). Community-based participatory action research: Transforming multidisciplinary practice in primary health care. *Pan American Journal of Public Health, 21*(2/3), 125–135.

Jones, L., & Way, D. (2007). Healthy workplaces and effective teamwork: Viewed through the lens of primary healthcare renewal. *Healthcare Papers, 7*(special issue), 92–97.

Laschinger, H. K. (2007). Building healthy workplaces: Time to act on the evidence. *Healthcare Papers, 7*(special issue), 42–45.

Lasker, R. D., & Weiss, E. S. (2003). Creating partnership synergy: The critical role of community stakeholders. *Journal of Health and Health Services Administration*, 2003(Summer), 119–139.

LeClerc, C. M., Doyon, J., Gravelle, D., et al. (2008). The autonomous–collaborative care model: Meeting the future head on. *Canadian Journal of Nursing Leadership, 21*(2), 63–75.

Lingard, L., McDougall, A., Levstik, M., et al. (2012). Representing complexity well: A story about teamwork, with implications for how we teach collaboration. *Medical Education, 46*, 869–877. doi:10.1111/j.1365-2923.2012.04339.x

Litaker, D., Mion, L., Planavsky, L., et al. (2003). Physician–nurse practitioner teams in chronic disease management: The impact on costs, clinical effectiveness, and patients' perception of care [Clinical trial randomized controlled trial research support, non-U.S. Gov't]. *Journal of Interprofessional Care, 17*(3), 223–237. doi:10.1080/1356182031000122852

Martin-Misener, R., & Valaitis, R. (2009). *A scoping literature review of collaboration between primary care and public health: A report to the Canadian Health Services Research Foundation.* n.p. Retrieved from http://fhs.mcmaster.ca/nursing/documents/MartinMisener-Valaitis-Review.pdf.

Oandasan, I. (2007). Teamwork and healthy workplaces: Strengthening the links for deliberation and action through research and policy. *Healthcare Papers, 7*(special issue), 98–103.

Reeves, S., Macmillan, K., & van Soeren, M. (2010). Leadership of interprofessional health and social care teams: A socio-historical analysis. *Journal of Nursing Management, 18*(3), 258–264. doi:10.1111/j.1365-2834.2010.01077.x

Sargeant, J., Loney, E., & Murphy, G. (2008). Effective interprofessional teams: "Contact is not enough" to build a team. *Journal of Continuing Education in the Health Professions, 28*(4), 228–234. doi:10.1002/chp.189

Sinclair, C. M. (2000). *Report of the Manitoba pediatric cardiac surgery inquest: An inquiry into twelve deaths at the Winnipeg Health Sciences Centre in 1994.* Winnipeg, MB: Provincial Court of Manitoba.

Thomas, S. (2012). Followership: Leadership's partner. *Canadian Journal of Medical Laboratory Sciences, 74*(4), 8–10.

Virani, T. (2012). *Interprofessional collaborative teams.* Ottawa, ON: Canadian Health Services Research Foundation. Retrieved from http://www.cfhi-fcass.ca/Libraries/Commissioned_Research_Reports/Virani-Interprofessional-EN.sflb.ashx.

Way, D., Jones, L., & Busing, N. (2000). *Implementation strategies: "Collaboration in primary care—family doctors & nurse practitioners delivering shared care."* Ottawa, ON: Ontario College of Family Physicians. Retrieved from http://www.eicp.ca/en/toolkit/hhr/ocfp-paper-handout.pdf.

Wearing, J., & Nickerson, V. (2010). Establishing a regulatory framework for certified practices in British Columbia. *Journal of Nursing Regulation, 1*(3), 38–43.

Whitlock, J. (2013). The value of active followership. *Nursing Management, 20*(2), 20–23.

World Health Organization. (1978). Declaration of Alma-Ata. International Conference on Primary Health Care, Alma-Ata, USSR, 6–12. Retrieved from http://www.who.int/publications/almaata_declaration_en.pdf.

Xyrichis, A., & Lowton, K. (2008). What fosters or prevents interprofessional teamworking in primary and community care? A literature review. *International Journal of Nursing Studies, 45*(1), 140–153. doi:10.1016/j.ijnurstu.2007.01.015

Yoder-Wise, P. (2011). *Leading and managing in nursing* (5th ed.). St. Louis, MO: Elsevier.

Zwarenstein, M., & Reeves, S. (2006). Knowledge translation and interprofessional collaboration: Where the rubber of evidence-based care hits the road of teamwork. *The Journal of Continuing Education in the Health Professions, 26*(1), 46–54. doi:10.1002/chp.50

Role Transition

Diane M. Twedell
Adapted by Judy Boychuk Duchscher
and Kandis Harris

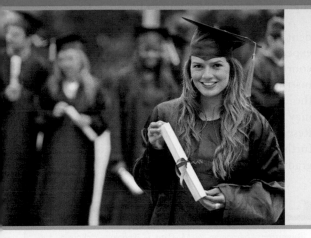

Role transition in nursing is the process of moving from one role, embedded within a framework of knowledge, to another. Managing the work done by others requires a fundamental understanding of the challenges inherent in making a role transition. The exercises in this chapter offer opportunities to recognize and build on your abilities to facilitate the evolution of the professionals under your direction.

OBJECTIVES

- Describe the stages of role transition for the new nursing graduate in the first year of practice.
- Describe what "ROLES" stands for and how each of its elements applies to role transition.
- Understand the phases of the professional role transition model: role preparation, role orientation, role integration, and role stabilization.
- Identify the challenges posed by role transition.
- Define strategies that can help promote role transition.

TERMS TO KNOW

mentorship	role integration	role stabilization
preceptorship	role negotiation	role strain
role discrepancy	role orientation	role stress
role expectations	role preparation	role transition

A CHALLENGE

On her first day, Claire walked into the nurses' report room, and all eyes zeroed in on her. She was absolutely certain that she had "NEWBIE" written across her forehead. One nurse turned to another and asked, "Who is she?" There were no more chairs in the room, so Claire stood throughout the entire report. She knew the routine from her student days, but this was different. Everyone spoke quickly and used many abbreviations that she did not understand. She could not keep up and got lost. Claire said to herself, *Whatever you do, don't look stupid.* Following report, Claire mustered up enough confidence to ask, "Who am I with today?" In response, Claire heard individual nurses say, "I took the last one, I need a break," "I have a really heavy patient load today, it wouldn't be a good shift with me," "I don't want her." And then, finally, like a breath of fresh air, Alexis said, "She can come with me today." Alexis smiled at Claire and asked, "Are you ready to roll?"

Alexis was wonderful about explaining tasks to Claire. However, Claire found it odd that Alexis never asked her a single question about where she had come from, what experience she had, or what competencies she wanted to work on. Nonetheless, Claire learned a lot as she shadowed Alexis during her shift. Alexis offered all kinds of advice, some of which Claire retained and some of which she did not understand. During the shift, some nurses asked who Claire was and some did not. Alexis introduced Claire to some patients and not to others. Claire hoped that Alexis would not ask her something that she did not know. Claire desperately wanted to look like she knew what she was doing.

Claire had been a strong student in school and looked forward to the challenge of her new role, even though she was a bit nervous about it. Although she was merely observing on her first day, she was beyond exhausted when her shift ended. She never met her unit's nurse manager or nurse educator. Alexis must have been occupied, since she did not say goodbye. Claire never got the opportunity to say to patients, "Good morning, my name is Claire and I will be the registered nurse working with you today." She was really looking forward to saying that. Maybe tomorrow.

What more could the nurse manager and Alexis have done to support Claire's transition into her new role?

INTRODUCTION

Role transition occurs when one moves from a role that is familiar (e.g., nursing student) to one that is unfamiliar (e.g., novice professional nurse). Necessarily, changes to the way a person interacts with and is perceived by others in a new role challenges his or her established professional identity. During the initial days and weeks of a formal role transition, that which was consistent, predictable, familiar, and stable is disrupted, inviting uncertainty and, with it, anxiety.

A new graduate makes a transition from the student role to the professional nurse role. While the expectations of students are clearly specified in course and clinical objectives and feedback from instructors and preceptors is consistent and explicit, the expectations for a new nurse as an employee may not be so clear. The Literature Perspective and Research Perspectives found in this chapter provide further information on role transitions for newly graduated nurses.

LITERATURE PERSPECTIVE

Resource: Chernomas, W. M., Care, D., Lapointe McKenzie, J. A., et al. (2010). "Hit the ground running": Perspectives on new nurses and nurse managers on role transition and integration of new graduates. *Nursing Leadership, 22*(4), 57–73. http://dx.doi.org/10.12927/cjnl.2010.21598

The Workplace Integration of New Nurses (WINN) project was instituted in 2006 through a partnership between the Winnipeg Regional Health Authority and the University of Manitoba. The mandate of this project was to assess the job satisfaction, work stress, and evolving development of new nurses who had access to a Transition Facilitator for the initial 13 months of their transition to professional practice. Facilitators were senior practising nurses who served as teachers, counsellors, and primary support persons for novices entering medical–surgical nursing directly out of their undergraduate BScN educational programs. Findings revealed three themes: (1) "know who I am" is the need for organizational recognition of what it is like to be a new nurse related to knowledge expectations, opportunities to practise, being welcomed and embraced as a new professional, and being accepted as being "in a transition"; (2) "know what I need" is the need for support and guidance from experienced nurses through knowledge sharing, skill coaching, assistance with problem solving, the provision of respectful feedback, and a willingness to teach; and (3) "I feel prepared but . . ." is a sense of being ready to enter practice but not feeling ready to take on the full weight of professional responsibility immediately upon entry in the workplace.

Implications for Practice
The idea of "hitting the ground running" is an adage often used in the nursing profession. This study, among others, provides strong evidence that this ideology does not "fit" with the developmental needs and evolving professional identity of the new nurse. Nurse managers, educators, and senior nurses must be sensitive to the challenges and time involved in professional role transition for new graduates and assist in intentionally integrating new practitioners into the workplace in a way that fosters their commitment and passion for nursing as a lifetime career.

RESEARCH PERSPECTIVE

Resource: Laschinger, H. K., Finegan, J., & Wilk, P. (2009). New graduate burnout: The impact of professional practice environment, workplace civility, and empowerment. *Nursing Economics, 27*(6), 377–383.

Creating supportive professional practice environments has become an increasing focus of workplaces across North America. The Magnet™ hospital concept identifies staffing, leadership, decision making, care models, and effective collaboration as characteristics that predict nurse-assessed adverse events, job satisfaction, burnout, and workplace empowerment. In this study, it was hypothesized that "new graduates who feel their work environments are supportive of professional nursing practice will also rate the level of civility among coworkers and their feelings of empowerment highly, which in turn will result in lower levels of burnout" (Laschinger et al., 2009, p. 379). Newly graduated participants in this study perceived their work environments to have moderate levels of overall Magnet™ characteristics and reported somewhat positive ratings of workplace civility in their work setting and low levels of conflict among nurses on their units. Conversely, they considered their workplaces only somewhat empowering and revealed alarming levels of emotional exhaustion (62% reported severe burnout). Laschinger and colleagues suggested that the evidence strongly supports the importance of working environments that "enable new graduates to practice according to professional standards learned in their educational programs" (p. 381). Subanalysis revealed that strong nursing leadership, adequate levels of staffing, and primary use of a nursing model of care (versus a medical model) significantly reduced the levels of emotional exhaustion in new graduates and further enhanced relations among unit nurses.

Implications for Practice

Strong linkages exist between supportive practice environments grounded in nursing models of care and workplace civility, empowerment, and reduced levels of burnout in newly graduated nurses.

RESEARCH PERSPECTIVE

Resource: Romyn, D. M., Linton, N., Giblin, C., et al. (2009). Successful transition of the new graduate nurse. *International Journal of Nursing Scholarship, 6*(1), Article 34, 1–15. http://dx.doi.org/10.2202/1548-923X.1802

The authors undertook discussion groups across Alberta with 14 new graduates and 133 staff nurses to better understand what constitutes "readiness for practice" in newly graduated nurses. Five additional new graduates and 34 staff nurses, employers, and educators provided input by fax or e-mail. The findings suggested that it takes a newly graduated nurse approximately 12 months to acquire the sense of self-assurance and confidence needed to care for complex caseloads. The new graduates quickly become aware of the disparity between the nurse they "thought" they could be and the reality of enacting their high practice standards in the context of a dynamic and highly charged professional environment.

Implications for Practice

Employers, nurse managers, nurse educators, and senior colleagues of newly graduated nurses must remind one another that the workplace has changed. High levels of acuity, advancements in technology, and challenges to staffing strain the educational program's ability to adequately prepare graduates for today's workplace. While it is reasonable to expect graduates of nursing programs to be prepared for general practice at a novice level, it is not realistic to think that they will be ready to absorb the tensions of a system that even the most experienced nurses find taxing. Providing formal and extended mentorship programs, individualized and flexible orientations, fostering workplace cultures that embrace learning and recognize growth, and enhancing partnerships between "theory" and "practice" stakeholders will go a long way toward creating a context that empowers all nurses to practise quality care.

Not only new graduates face role transition. So too do other nurses who change roles. For example, the direct care nurse who decides to advance his or her education or scope of practice or perhaps branch out into the role of clinical educator or nurse manager is making a role transition. The same is true for the staff nurse who becomes a nurse manager or the staff nurse who moves from an acute care setting to a home health care agency. Regardless of the kind of transition, organizations play a key role in assisting employees through role transitions. Changes in roles can be either painful or exciting and depend largely on the work culture and support provided. According to Meleis (2010),

"human beings always face many changes throughout the lifespan that trigger internal processes . . . [and] are characterized by different dynamic stages, milestones, and turning points" (p. 11). Knowing what to expect during a transition can reduce stress and facilitate a healthy acceptance of the change over time.

TYPES OF ROLE TRANSITIONS

From Nursing Student to Practising Nurse

The transition from nursing student to practising nurse incorporates a journey of *becoming*, where new graduates progress through stages of *doing, being,* and *knowing.*

The stages of role transition that occur for new graduates during the initial 12 months of professional practice appear in Table 27-1. Stage 1, which takes place in the first 3 to 4 months of the new graduate's journey, is often an exercise in adjusting and adapting to the realities of the new workplace, professional life, and personal life. New professionals have little energy or time to lift their gaze from the very immediate issues or tasks set before them, and their "shock" (Figure 27-1) state demands a concerted focus on simply "surviving" the experience, without revealing their feelings of overwhelming anxiety or exposing their self-perceived incompetence.

Stage 2 of professional role transition for new graduates takes place over the next 4 to 5 months of the post-orientation period and is characterized by a consistent and rapid advancement in their thinking, knowledge level, and skill competency. As this period progresses and the new graduates gain a comfort level with their professional role and responsibilities, they are often confronted by inconsistencies and inadequacies within the health care system that serve to challenge their somewhat idealistic pregraduate notions of the profession. An increased awareness of the divergence between their professional "self" and the enactment of that self in their new role motivates a relative withdrawal of new graduates from their surroundings. The primary task for new graduates at this stage is to make sense of their role as a nurse relative to other health care providers and to find a balance between their personal and professional lives.

Stage 3, the final stage of transition for new graduates during the initial 12 months of their careers, is focused on achieving a separateness that both distinguishes them from the established practitioners around them and permits them to reunite with their larger community as professionals in their own right. With an increase in both familiarity and comfort in their nursing role, professional responsibilities, and relationships with co-workers, new graduates have the time and energy to begin a deeper exploration and critique of their professional landscape, making visible the more troubling aspects of their sociocultural and political work environments. If

TABLE 27-1	STAGES OF ROLE TRANSITION FOR THE NEW NURSING GRADUATE	
STAGE	**PROCESSES**	**THE EXPERIENCE**
Stage 1: Doing (3–4 months)	Learning Performing Concealing Adjusting Accommodating	• Is most comfortable in a *learning* role and least comfortable applying theory to practice • Often defaults to theory as that is what the new graduate knows • Feels that everything is new—even the familiar looks different • Is most concerned with the ability to *perform* tasks required; the objective is not to "stand out" but to focus on "what" and "how" • Is motivated by a desire for acceptance, so the new graduate *conceals* insecurities or feelings of inadequacy from colleagues • *Adjusts* to new roles, responsibilities, and relationships • Takes practice cues from surrounding nurses—more vulnerable to poor modelling and may choose to *accommodate* rather than challenge existing practices • Has an overwhelming sense of responsibility; finds decision making daunting
Stage 2: Being (4–5 months)	Searching Examining Doubting Questioning Revealing	• Begins a *search* for meaning in the role—asking "why" rather than "what" or "how" • Has increasing comfort with the role, relationships, responsibilities, and knowledge, which allows time to *examine* the workplace • Demonstrates a growing identity—asks *Who am I as a nurse?* that may feed *self-doubt* • Shows advanced thinking that motivates *questioning*; incongruence within the system is *revealed* and may be disturbing—engages in "bigger picture" thinking
Stage 3: Knowing (3–5 months)	Separating Recovering Exploring Critiquing Accepting	• Is exhausted from prior two stages, which can feed discouragement or disillusionment; *separates* from work in an attempt to *recover* energy and gain some perspective • Begins to think about the future; *explores* career possibilities • *Critiques* his or her work, colleagues, and profession, which is part of identity development • *Accepts* what he or she can while seeking to change what is considered untenable; seeks stability

Based on Boychuk Duchscher, J. (2008). A process of becoming: The stages of new nursing graduate professional role transition. *Journal of Continuing Education in Nursing, 39*(10), 441–450. http://dx.doi.org/10.3928/00220124-20081001-03

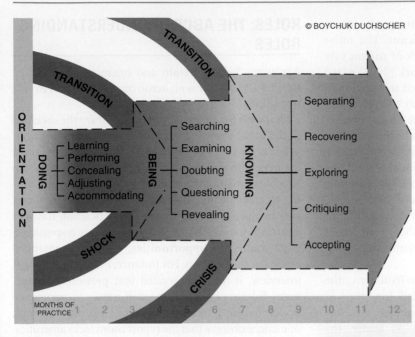

© BOYCHUK DUCHSCHER

FIGURE 27-1 Stages of transition model.

the transition experience to this point has been less than satisfactory for the new graduate, he or she may express dissatisfaction with work; this feeling is often fed by a residual exhaustion from prior stages. For some, this is simply a case of adjusting to the work world for the purpose of achieving a sense of job satisfaction. For others, the thought of sacrificing particular professional expectations and aspirations due to perceived inadequacies in the system within which they planned to spend their career can be terminally demotivating. Some new graduates may choose to search for alternative avenues of fulfillment (e.g., finding a new job, leaving the country, returning to school, or creating a distinct separation between work and home life).

From Practising Nurse to Nurse Leader or Manager

Accepting a nurse manager or other leadership position (e.g., an educator role) requires acceptance of three roles that involve complex processes. The roles of leader, manager, and follower are complex because they involve working with unique individuals in a rapidly changing environment. Examples of the people with whom they interact and the processes involved in each role are shown in Table 27-2. In nursing, each of these roles relates to patients.

TABLE 27-2	LEADER, MANAGER, AND FOLLOWER ROLES: THE PEOPLE AND PROCESSES INVOLVED	
ROLE	**PEOPLE WITH WHOM INTERACTIONS OCCUR**	**PROCESSES INVOLVED IN THE ROLE**
Leader	Persons being led Peers	Listening Encouraging Motivating Organizing Problem solving Developing Supporting
Manager	Persons under leaders' direction Nursing administrators Supervisors Regulatory bodies Faculty	Organizing Planning Budgeting Hiring Evaluating Reporting Disseminating Researching/writing
Follower	Supervisor Peers	Conforming Implementing Contributing Completing assignments Alerting

The transition from being a direct care nurse to being a nurse manager is significant. The nurse moves from leading the clinical work of patient care to leading a group of employees. Clark (2008) noted that "leadership is not simply granted to individuals and is not about responding passively to events. It is about creating possibilities that were absent before" (p. 30). McConnell (2008) says that a health care provider who takes on a managerial position is accepting a second occupation: "The professional who enters [leadership] must wear two hats" (p. 278). One role is as the professional on technical and clinical matters, and the other is as a generalist responsible for directing a diverse demographic that itself varies greatly in roles, responsibilities, relationships, and knowledge.

In the evolving health care environment, the nurse who provides direct care also functions as a leader, assuming the roles of manager and follower in relation to patient care. As *leader*, the direct care nurse recognizes the uniqueness of each patient, planning, implementing, and evaluating clinical progress over time. As *manager*, the direct care nurse links the patient and family to resources that optimize clinical outcomes. Health information is translated into a format that the patient can use to make informed decisions about treatment and self-care. Through collaboration with multiple disciplines, the nurse consults and makes referrals as needed, and facilitates continuity of care within the larger system. In the role of *follower*, the direct care nurse is accountable to a team and his or her supervisor for completing the work that is assigned. The nurse as a follower must practise within the policies and procedures of the organization and the standards of the profession. Finally, direct care nurses respect the authority of others and contribute to common organizational goals. In doing so, they recognize their accountability to persons above them on the organizational chart, recognize that leadership is provided by others within their environment, and support a collaborative approach to decision making.

Learning the leader, manager, and follower aspects of any new role can be overwhelming. Another approach to the complexity of role transition is the acronym *ROLES*, in which each letter represents a component common to all roles.

ROLES: THE ABCS OF UNDERSTANDING ROLES

Acronyms help us retain and organize information. **ROLES** (Box 27-1) is an acronym that is useful in role transition.

R **stands for responsibilities.** What are the specified duties in the position description for the new position? What tasks are to be completed? What decisions must the person in this position make? For example, the job of a nurse manager may involve 24-hour accountability, whereas the job of a staff nurse may involve direct care in a primary care setting. Every position has specific tasks for which the position holder is responsible.

O **stands for opportunities,** which are untapped aspects of the position. For instance, in the employment interview, it may be revealed that previous management did not encourage the staff nurses to participate in continuing education. Or, while touring the unit, one might observe that the report room lacks amenities. Or, in the course of following the care path of patients on the unit, it may become clear that a new method of delivering patient care may be appropriate for the unit. These possibilities represent opportunities for the new nurse to influence organizational and unit goals.

L **represents lines of communication,** which are at the heart of every nursing role. No matter what position an individual is in, it involves relationships with multiple individuals including supervisors and peers. Roles incorporate patterns of structured interaction among people in these groups and require that individuals be competent at receiving and sending messages. Being a skillful listener can be more important than being skillful in sending messages. Skill is required to communicate both the content and the intent of the message effectively. Only through reflective practice can one develop techniques of effective communication (see Chapter 19).

E **stands for expectations.** Expectations vary depending on one's goals and professional aspirations. Colleagues may expect a new nurse practitioner to be

BOX 27-1	"ROLES" ACRONYM

Responsibilities
Opportunities
Lines of communication
Expectations
Support

on call every weekend or a new graduate to work all major statutory holidays for the first year. New staff nurses may have specific expectations of their nurse managers related to feedback or promotion, or may respond differently to varying styles of management and leadership. The nursing executive or administrator in transition will likely have expectations about how the nurse managers under their supervision spend their time on the job—even about how much time they spend at work.

Finding out in advance what the explicit and implicit expectations are of the people with whom you are working can facilitate a smoother role transition by decreasing role ambiguity (Hardy, 1978). Hardy's work with role theory suggests a strong, positive, relationship between role ambiguity (one type of role stress—a condition in which role demands are conflicting, irritating, or impossible to fulfill) and role strain (the subjective feeling of discomfort experienced as a result of role stress). The major concepts of role theory are presented in the Theory Box below.

THEORY BOX

Hardy's Role Theory

THEORY/ CONTRIBUTOR	KEY IDEAS	APPLICATION TO PRACTICE
Hardy (1978) is credited with applying role theory to health care providers. A *role* is the expected and actual behaviours associated with a position. Role expectations are the attitudes and behaviours others anticipate that a person in the role will possess or demonstrate.	Role stress is a precursor to role strain. Role stress is associated with low productivity and performance. Role stress and role strain can lead a person to withdraw psychologically from the role. Clear, realistic role expectations can decrease the role stress for someone in a new role (e.g., a new nurse manager).	Clear, realistic role expectations can increase productivity.

Data from Hardy, M. E. (1978). Role stress and role strain. In M. E. Hardy & M. E. Conway (Eds.), *Role theory: Perspectives for health professionals* (pp. 73–109). New York, NY: Appleton-Century-Crofts.

There are also personal expectations related to performance in a new role. You have a mental image of an individual in this position; that image may well have motivated you to move your career in this direction. The process of role transition unfolds as the new employee identifies expectations, recognizes the similarities and differences with preconceptions, and evolves in the roles of leader, manager, and follower within their position.

S stands for support, which is closely tied to expectations about performance. All roles are shaped to some degree by the support and services others provide. The new acute care nurse in an urban setting often has colleagues readily available when a second opinion is needed, while the same nurse may feel lost when confronted with clinical issues during a home care visit or when working nights in a rural hospital. The nurse manager who must develop a unit's budget in a health care facility may have no accounting department to provide a detailed analysis of the facility's prior expenditures. Each role has some support available. When a new position is being considered, it is important to evaluate whether support is available in areas in which the new employee may lack fundamental knowledge or skills. When implementing a change in one's nursing role, seek out someone in the organization that can help you identify or even provide the support services that will facilitate your role transition.

ROLE TRANSITION PROCESS

One way to think about the way in which someone transitions to a new role is illustrated in Box 27-2.

STRATEGIES TO PROMOTE ROLE TRANSITION

Becoming a manager or assuming a new role often results in a change in professional identity. Such a transformation invokes stress as the person unlearns old roles and learns the management role. Several strategies can help an individual ease the strain and speed the process of role transition (Box 27-3).

Strengthen Internal Resources

A key strategy in promoting role transition is to recognize and draw on one's values and beliefs. Behaviour is influenced by values and beliefs. Clark (2008)

BOX 27-2   PROFESSIONAL ROLE TRANSITION MODEL FOR THE NEW NURSING GRADUATE

Unlearning old roles while learning new ones requires an identity adjustment over time. The persons involved must invest themselves in the process, which involves moving through the phases of role preparation, role orientation, role integration, and role stabilization (Boychuk Duchscher, 2012; see Figure 27-2 on page 507).

Role Preparation

During this phase of role transition, the individual gets ready to make a major change (assuming that this change is planned and its transition is anticipated). Time is spent exploring and seeking to understand what the new role will entail, the supports available to facilitate the role change, and to whom the incumbent will report and how. Role preparation entails education and socialization to the professional role within postsecondary and/or health care systems. In the case of the newly graduated nurse, time spent in senior clinical placements may serve as the preparatory period. In the case of a new nurse manager or educator, attempts may be made to "preview" the role by spending time working alongside someone who currently assumes that role. Developing accurate role expectations is the primary objective of the preparation phase of role transition, so it is important that the preparatory phase be as realistic and representative as possible. Role discrepancy speaks to the gap between role expectations and role performance, and can cause role frustration, leading to role stress and strain over time. Role discrepancy can ultimately be resolved by changing expectations of role performance or through adaptation to the differences over time, but it is obviously more desirable not to be in this position. If the role is valued and the differences are seen as tenable or amenable, a decision will most likely be made to stay in the role and sort out the discrepancies. This decision requires negotiation and a certain degree of conciliation by all parties.

Role Orientation

Role orientation constitutes a formal employment process whereby the expectations of the role are clearly identified and the new employee is introduced to the organizational structure within which he or she will be working. Orientation often includes some element of preceptorship (skill, role, or responsibility orientation) as well as mentorship (organizational, cultural, or professional process orientation). The length of time required to orientate to a new role will depend on the individual's existing familiarity with the role, confidence in performing the role in this new context, and degree of role discrepancy revealed during orientation. A new employee who gradually and progressively assumes the multiple elements of a new role (with planned debriefings and a concerted analysis of the factors contributing to both successes and challenges during the transition) is more likely to become successfully engaged in the new role.

Role Integration

During this phase of role transition, the individual undergoes significant adjustments to his or her perceptions about the role and reconciles discrepancies between the previous understanding of the role and what it is. Feedback and dialogue about the role discrepancies that take place during role integration (the process of adjusting perceptions of one's role and reconciling discrepancies between the previous understanding of the role and what it is) are essential for the individual to realign values that may have become displaced. Failure to undergo this phase may result in role frustration and disillusionment and, ultimately, role disengagement.

Significant to role integration is the consolidation of the individual's sense of accountability and responsibility for the role within the larger work context (unit, centre, or institution). Not uncommonly, skill competence improves during this phase, as does the capacity for independent decision making, judgement, and critical thinking. Tenure in the role has most likely exposed the individual to conflict and crisis, which has equipped him or her with the skills to solve fundamental problems and resolve basic conflicts that arise in the course of the role.

Role Stabilization

Role stabilization occurs as an individual matures in his or her performance of all facets of the role, to the point where he or she internalizes the role, performing it fluidly and with confidence. At this juncture, the individual has learned the behaviours that meet the role expectations, and these behaviours have become second nature. The energy previously expended learning the new role can be redirected toward optimizing the skills required in the role, understanding the gestalt of the role, and critically thinking about the judgements and decisions that are encompassed within the role. The focus shifts from distinction to discernment of role expectations, and energy is now spent accomplishing unit, institutional, or professional goals collaboratively with colleagues. Individuals who have internalized their roles have developed their own unique personal approaches to role performance and role satisfaction and feel valued for their contribution.

Unexpected Role Transition

Not every transition can be anticipated or predicted. Some changes are unexpected, and the individual must process the end of one way of being or doing prior to successfully integrating into another. In cases where an employee is terminated, a position is eliminated, or a job description changes dramatically, the response can be shock, disbelief, or possibly grief. In what amounts to a forced role transition, the individual may experience disorientation and confusion to the point of being unable to function. As the shock wears off, the individual may become angered by the change and may direct anger toward those who are perceived as instigating the role change. Conversely, the anger may be directed internally, leading to depression. If the individual is unable to acknowledge and talk about the loss he or she experienced as a result of the change, the period of grief may be extended or emotional baggage may be created that is carried into the next role. Grieving can eventually resolve into acceptance. Lessons learned from the experience are identified and internalized. A new role is sought, and the cycle begins again.

Health care is in a tumultuous state of affairs. Reorganizations, realignments, restructuring, and downsizing of the workforce are now commonplace. To be successful, work role restructuring must be undertaken with the same sensitivity afforded any significant life change. Role transition takes time, tremendous patience, and understanding.

notes that values and beliefs "shape how individuals think, and see the world, and the meanings they attribute to their experiences, actions and relationships with others" (p. 30). It is important while making any role transition to not lose sight of your own values and beliefs. A particular role or place of work is not suited for everyone. One must consider whether personal goals and professional fulfillment can best be achieved through that role, within that institution, or under the direction of that supervisor. One's commitment to the challenges of making a professional role transition can provide the desire to persevere during the process.

Clark (2008) notes that "nurses typically work according to two sets of values; professional values, which are determined by their code of professional conduct, and personal values" (p. 31). If an individual in transition understands his or her own personal values, these will help the person respond to situations and relationships. A person's worth does not depend on the quality or quickness of his or her adjustment to a new role. An exercise such as writing down short

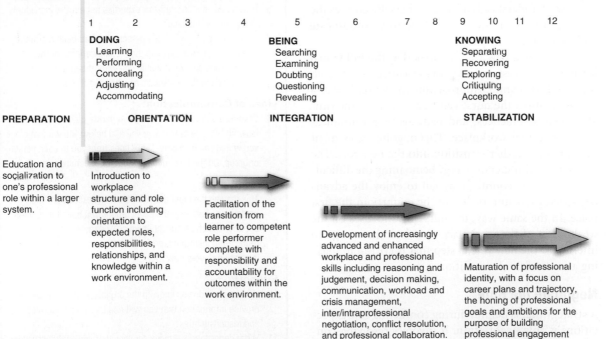

© BOYCHUK DUCHSCHER

FIGURE 27-2 Professional role transition for the new nursing graduate.

statements of self-belief or self-affirmations and post-ing them on a wall or fridge at home may be helpful as a visual reminder.

The rapid and constant changes occurring in health care dictate the need for flexibility. Successful transition into a new role within the health care system requires the willingness and ability to learn and master new skills, translate information, and adapt behaviour to new situations. The individual making the transition must also temper expectations of himself or herself, particularly in the early stages of change. Understanding transition as a process will help with flexibility.

Assess the Workplace

Taking on a new role is much like being an immigrant in a new country. An immigrant learns how to access the available resources to acclimate to the new environment. Cultural practices of the new country may seem strange or odd. Cultural differences are analyzed and decisions are made about which aspects to adopt. Subtle differences in communication patterns or group dynamics are also identified. Understanding the nuances of social interactions is often the most difficult aspect of acclimatising to a new country. The transition is smoother for the immigrant who understands himself or herself, assesses the new environment, and learns how to communicate within groups.

Navigating a new role requires that the individual learn how to access resources in the work context (unit, organization, clinic). Approaching the workplace as a foreign culture, the nurse can keenly observe the rituals, accepted practices, and patterns of communication within that workplace. This ongoing assessment promotes a speedier transition into the new role. The immigrant who spends energy bemoaning the difficulties of the new country may fail to enjoy the advantages that drew him or her to the country in the first place. In the same way, the nurse who focuses on the weaknesses of the workplace may lack the energy to internalize the new role, a step that is critical to making a successful role transition.

Negotiate the Role

A strategy that is helpful during conflicting role expectations is **role negotiation**. It involves resolving conflicting expectations about personal performance through communication. The ROLES assessment (see

Exercise 27-1) may identify areas of significant conflict. Writing down the expectations is the first step in resolving areas of conflict. It is important to review the expectations listed to determine whether they are realistic. Unrealistic expectations strongly held by others may require diplomatic re-education so that their expectations can become more realistic.

EXERCISE 27-1

ROLES Assessment

Assume that you are transitioning to a nurse manager role. Answer these questions about your new role.

Responsibilities:

1. From the position description, what are the responsibilities?
2. Is there support for the ongoing learning required during your transition?
3. For what decisions are you responsible, and will you be provided with the time and resources to grow into the role?
4. Consider information about the position that you learned during the interview. Also consider the responsibilities of individuals in similar roles that you have observed. Are there other responsibilities to add to your list?

Opportunities:

5. What opportunities for growth and professional development are supported in this workplace?
6. How could your strengths or expertise benefit the individuals in this new workplace?
7. Dream a little (or a lot). If a person who had been a patient on the unit were describing the nursing care to another potential patient, what would you want the first patient to say? Describe the workplace as you want it to be.

Lines of Communication:

8. Draw yourself in the middle of a separate piece of paper. Now fill in the people above you and below you with whom you would communicate. Draw lines from you to each person or group. On the line, identify the form of communication.

Expectations:

9. This may be the most difficult part to assess. List in short sentences or phrases the expectations you have for yourself and those each person (colleagues or direct supervisors) or group (unit, institution, professional group) may have for you in relation to your new role.

Support:

10. What people do you know in the organization who could provide information that you will need to fulfill your roles and responsibilities?
11. What departments provide services that you could access for assistance?

Next Steps:

Now compare the lists.

Place a star next to those expectations that are held by more than one person or group. For example, as a *new manager*, you might be expected to handle the budget of a unit in accordance with a vision that is determined by administrators outside your sphere of influence. As a *new nurse*, you might be expected to take a significantly larger workload than was expected of you as a student, while working collaboratively with other scopes of nursing practice, unregulated care providers, and allied health practitioners. As a *new educator*, you may be required to complete multiple unit-based orientations for practice areas outside of your experience or expertise.

Circle those items that could cause conflicts.

Refer to the Strategies to Promote Role Transition section in this chapter on how to resolve these conflicts.

Save your responses to these questions to review in 3 months. You may be surprised how your own perception of your ROLES may change over time.

Grow Through Preceptorship and Mentorship

While often used interchangeably, the terms *preceptorship* and *mentorship* are distinct. Preceptorship is "a period of practical experience and training for a trainee supervised by an expert or specialist in a particular field" (The Ottawa Hospital, n.d.). It is seen as an efficient and effective way to introduce an individual to a new role and its responsibilities (Myrick & Yonge, 2005). Most often used in the context of a student completing a clinical practicum or a newly graduated nurse making the initial role transition to professional practice, preceptorship focuses on the learning of tasks, skills, and routines necessary to perform one's role efficiently and effectively. Preceptorship is often distinguished from mentorship by its shorter tenure, narrower objectives, and differing supporter characteristics. The attributes of a good preceptor are grounded in a strong practice history relative to the specific role (direct care nurse, nurse manager, or nurse educator). Meanwhile, the attributes of a good mentor are grounded in advanced relational capacity and expertise in the role area balanced with a strong vision for how the person transitioning can develop and contribute professionally while growing personally through the enactment of the role. While one individual may serve as both a preceptor and mentor in any given transition support situation, preceptorship tends to be short lived, terminating once the knowledge and skills required to perform the role have been successfully transferred from preceptor to preceptee.

Mentorship "is a formal supportive relationship between two, or more, health professionals that has the potential to result in professional growth and development for both mentors and mentees" (Ontario Ministry of Health and Long-Term Care, 2014, p. 14). A mentor is there to "pick up the pieces" after the initial transition is complete and when the individual in transition becomes more aware of (and able to think about) the purpose, significance, and relative importance of their work. Mentors are an important component of a nurturing environment that promotes staff retention. They can be a tremendous source of guidance and support for new nurses, nurse managers, and nurse educators in transition, serving both career and psychosocial functions. Career functions are possible because the mentor has sufficient professional experience and organizational authority to facilitate the career of the mentee. Box 27-4 highlights some key functions of mentors during the role transition of new nursing graduates. The Robert Wood Johnson Nurse Executive Fellows program has identified five core competencies of leaders and mentors: interpersonal and communication effectiveness, risk taking and creativity, self-knowledge and self-renewal, inspiring and leading change, and strategic vision (Center for the Health Professions, 2009).

A mentor often creates opportunities for the mentee to achieve and advance and can provide encouragement and a needed sense of perspective for the mentee that originates out of the mentor's long-standing tenure in the role to which the mentee is transitioning. Mentors offer career guidance and emotional support. Through coaching activities, mentors provide information about how to improve role performance by offering feedback and "in the moment" guidance.

The mentor, as coach, facilitates critical thought, decision making, and judgement that is grounded in extended experience of the role being assumed by the mentee. The interpersonal connection between the mentor and the mentee is critical, as trust and mutual positive regard are required for the relationship to evolve. For this reason, it may be beneficial for mentees to choose their mentors. Mentors may offer counsel to mentees by providing opportunities for mentees to explore personal concerns as filtered through the knowing ear of the mentor. The relational aspects of effective mentorship partnerships or pairings include confidentiality, trust, and respect.

BOX 27-4   MENTORING NEW NURSING GRADUATES THROUGH TRANSITION

Role Preparation Phase (Pregraduate)

The relationship is primarily preceptorial in this phase.

Mentor functions:

- Introduce and establish terms of relationship
- Indicate that the responsibility for connection is mutual
- Encourage final practicum in unit to which the student will transition
- Educate the student on role transition stages/transition shock
- Facilitate socialization exercises (i.e., how to engage with other nurses)
- Foster partnerships between the educational institution and workplace
- Develop workplace engagement activities/strategies
- Explore work experiences with the student
- Redirect evaluation to self-appraisal strategies

Role Orientation Phase (1–3 months post-hire)

The focus is on skill assessment, skill practice for familiarity and performance confidence, and understanding work role expectations.

Mentor functions:

- Facilitate personal (nonworkplace) connection over 1–2 weeks with a focus on encouragement, support, and collegiality
- Assess career intentions (the desired professional trajectory)
- Undertake transition–knowledge framed orientation approaches
- Establish confidential new nurse peer support network
- Seek ongoing (every shift) feedback/performance appraisal by the nurse manager and educator, and the clinical support team

Role Transition Phase (3–6 months post-hire)

The focus is on progressive (complexity and volume) skill acquisition, time management, and conflict resolution/coping.

Mentor functions:

- Facilitate discussion on professional culture, work relationships
- Ensure that the clinical support team is well versed on transition shock and the stages of transition

- Initiate an interdisciplinary role knowledge sharing program
- Consider supernumerary employment
- Create flexible staffing/scheduling options
- Provide feedback/performance appraisal to move the mentee more toward self-reflection

Role Integration Phase (6–9 months post-hire)

The focus is on advanced clinical judgement/reasoning/decision making through experiential case study learning and care debriefing.

Mentor functions:

- Facilitate discussion on coping strategies, professional self-care, and big picture thinking about the health care system and its relationship to the workplace
- Ask mentee to consider interinstitutional employment flexibility as career growth option
- Encourage intellectual recovery strategies with a focus on life balance
- Optimize utilization of nursing clinicians and charge nurses

Role Stabilization Phase (10–12 months post-hire)

The focus is on guiding decisions and experiences through clinical consultation rather than directive approaches.

Mentor functions:

- Utilize multiple clinical coaches (e.g., other nurse experts)
- Facilitate professional development, practise introspection, and encourage a professional perspective
- Ask the mentee to consider charge nurse orientation toward the 12-month mark
- Facilitate advanced practice rotations (i.e., emergency department/critical care unit rotations)
- Review the career trajectory of the mentee and encourage professional planning
- Encourage the mentee to engage in professional association/workplace committee work

Modified with permission from Boychuk Duchscher, J. (2012). From surviving to thriving: Navigating the first year of professional nursing practice. Calgary, AB: Nursing the Future. Retrieved from http://www.nursingthefuture.ca/from_surviving_to_thriving.

EXERCISE 27-2

Role Transition Self-Assessment

Respond to each item using the following scale. Add up your score.

1 = Strongly disagree
2 = Disagree
3 = Unsure
4 = Agree
5 = Strongly agree

1. I am aware of the stages and phases of professional role transition.
2. I am responsible for my own professional development.
3. I feel confident about my ability to learn the skills I need to be effective in my new role.
4. I have the support I need to learn the responsibilities expected of me in this new role.
5. I feel confident in my ability to balance the multiple priorities and activities required of me in this role.
6. I have the resources to develop a personal network of support.

No magical score indicates your readiness for role transition. If you are unsure in every category, your score will be 6. A score of 25 or above indicates that you are confident that you can master the transition to your new role. If you currently have a mentor, ask that person to respond to each item to analyze your abilities. Compare those responses with your own. Do you have a realistic view of yourself?

Relationships between mentors and mentees vary because of individual characteristics and the career phase of each. During the early phases of a role transition, a mentee is concerned about competence and a mentor can provide valuable coaching. As the individual advances along the transition continuum, support from a mentor can prepare the individual for career advancement. A mentor nearing the end of his or her work career can find fulfillment in sharing knowledge with others while equally benefiting from the counsel of a recently retired colleague; and the mentorship cycle continues.

CONCLUSION

Professional role transitions—whether they be from nursing student to practising nurse or practising nurse to charge nurse, nurse manager, or nurse educator—pose new challenges. Nurses who make these transitions with minimal discomfort are reflective of role theory in action. Although nurses today are better prepared to take on a variety of roles throughout their careers, the breadth and scope of those roles are more challenging. Charge nurses and nurse managers are often responsible for mentoring and coaching new staff as they transition to their new roles. Facilitating a healthy transition takes time, should be framed on the evidence available about role transition, and requires strategic effort to achieve the best results possible.

Making a successful professional role transition is certainly worth the effort. Learning how to lead a life that is fulfilling, purposeful, and balanced is the intended outcome of role transition. Finding

synergy between your work and the level of commitment and integrity you strive for as a professional brings out the best in you and everyone you work with. A sense of role fulfillment and subsequent job satisfaction contributes significantly to the quality of any workplace and directly influences the quality of patient care.

A SOLUTION

The nurse manager could have set up a one-on-one meeting with Claire the day before her first shift, which would have allowed her to gain some familiarization of the unit. The nurse manager could have given Claire a tour around the unit, introduced her to some of the staff (e.g., other nurses, the ward clerk, cleaning personnel). The nurse manager could have shown Claire where to hang her coat, put her lunch, find her mailbox, etc. Doing so would have helped Claire feel less out of place on the first day of work. Additionally, the nurse manager could have introduced Claire to the unit educator. On that first shift, Alexis might have met Claire at the entrance to the hospital and walked with her to the unit. This would have allowed them to have a quick chat so they could get to know each other, making Claire feel a part of the team more quickly. Alexis might have benefited from having an understanding of role transition theories to maximize opportunities for mentoring and guiding. Lastly, as Claire settles in, it would be beneficial for the nurse manager (and the unit educator) to plan to periodically check in with Claire to ensure her successful integration into the unit.

Would this be a suitable approach for you? Why or why not?

THE EVIDENCE

Etheridge's (2007) descriptive, longitudinal, phenomenological study examined the perceptions of recent nursing graduates about learning to make clinical judgements. Semi-structured interviews were conducted to determine the meaning of making clinical nursing judgements. These interviews were conducted on three different dates: within a month after the end of a preceptor experience,

2 to 3 months later, and 8 to 9 months after the first interview.

Major components of learning to think like a nurse included building confidence, accepting responsibility, adapting to changing relationships with others, and thinking more clinically. Discussions with peers were a powerful experience for the individual nurses transitioning to their new role.

NEED TO KNOW NOW

- Be prepared to feel a certain amount of discomfort, anxiety, and loss during role transition. It can be disruptive.
- Keep in mind that professional role transition is a process that takes place in stages; new graduates, and those who support them, should understand these stages and target support resources accordingly (see http://www.nursingthefuture.ca/from_surviving_to_thriving for an important resource in supporting new nurses).
- Obtain a complete and detailed position description for the new role.
- Identify critical resources available in the organization to assist with role transition: nurse managers, nurse educators, clinical nurse specialists, preceptors, charge nurses, peers, employee assistance programs.
- Be open to feedback, and arrange for it on a regular basis.
- Identify a mentor in the first 1 to 3 months of a new role.
- Attend educational programs that expand your knowledge of the role.
- Recognize that role transition is as personal as it is professional; make sure those on whom you depend for support are aware of the influences this transition is having on your life.
- Be aware of the stages of role transition so that you can anticipate stress points during the process and seek help accordingly.

CHAPTER CHECKLIST

- Experiencing a role transition yourself or assisting a staff member to successfully integrate into a new role takes time and energy—two scarce resources for nurse managers. Knowing what to expect can speed up the process, maximize the outcome, and minimize the energy expenditure characteristic of professional role transition.
- Role transition is often a process of unlearning old roles while learning new ones.
- The stages of professional role transition for newly graduated nurses are doing, being, and knowing.
- Responsibilities, opportunities, lines of communication, expectations, and support (ROLES) are aspects common to all roles. When considering how to effectively navigate (or support others through) a role transition, gather information about each of these aspects.
- Managers are also leaders and followers.

- Unexpected role transitions are particularly challenging and often involve a grieving process.
- Role stress has its roots in discrepancies between role expectations and the reality of role enactment in the "real world."
- Role strain develops when the stressors contributing to a mismatch between expectation and reality go unacknowledged or are insufficiently addressed.
- Role negotiation involves resolving conflicting expectations about personal performance through communication.
- Commitment, character, self-respect, and flexibility are internal resources that can facilitate the process of role transition.
- Preceptors can assist in the understanding and performance of the tasks of a new role, and mentors are there to provide career guidance and emotional support.

TIPS FOR ROLE TRANSITIONING

- Anticipate and prepare for role changes. Role transition is a normal and healthy process.
- Identify the responsibilities, opportunities, lines of communication, expectations, and support for the new role.
- Understand that a transition involves changing roles, responsibilities, relationships, and knowledge and is at once physical, emotional, intellectual, sociocultural, and developmental.
- Use both external and internal resources to negotiate a role transition that supports and reinforces your life values and commitments.

evolve WEBSITE

Visit the Evolve website for Suggested Readings, Internet Resources, and additional resources related to the content in this chapter: http://evolve.elsevier.com/Canada/Yoder-Wise/leading/.

REFERENCES

Boychuk Duchscher, J. (2008). A process of becoming: The stages of new nursing graduate professional role transition. *Journal of Continuing Education in Nursing, 39*(10), 441–450. doi:10.3928/00220124-20081001-03

Boychuk Duchscher, J. (2012). *From surviving to thriving: Navigating the first year of professional nursing practice* (2nd ed.). Calgary, AB: Nursing the Future. Retrieved from http://www.nursingthefuture.ca/from_surviving_to_thriving.

Center for the Health Professions. (2009). *RWJ program eligibility.* Retrieved from http://www.futurehealth.ucsf.edu.

Chernomas, W. M., Care, D., Lapointe McKenzie, J. A., et al. (2010). "Hit the ground running": Perspectives of new nurses and nurse managers on role transition and integration of new graduates. *Nursing Leadership, 22*(4), 70–86. doi:10.12927/cjnl.2010.21598

Clark, L. (2008). Clinical leadership: Values, beliefs and vision. *Nursing Management, 15*(7), 30–35.

Etheridge, S. A. (2007). Learning to think like a nurse: Stories from new nurse graduates. *Journal of Continuing Education in Nursing, 38*(1), 24–30.

Hardy, M. E. (1978). Role stress and role strain. In M. E. Hardy & M. E. Conway (Eds.), *Role theory: Perspectives for health professionals* (pp. 73–109). New York, NY: Appleton-Century-Crofts.

Laschinger, H. K., Finegan, J., & Wilk, P. (2009). New graduate burnout: The impact of professional practice environment, workplace civility, and empowerment. *Nursing Economics, 27*(6), 377–383.

McConnell, C. R. (2008). The health care professional as a manager: Balancing two important roles. *The Health Care Manager, 27*(3), 277–284. doi:10.1097/01.HCM.0000318759.21654.d2

Meleis, A. I. (Ed). (2010). *Transitions theory: Middle-range and situation-specific theories in nursing research and practice.* New York, NY: Springer.

Myrick, F., & Yonge, O. (2005). *Nursing preceptorship: Connecting practice and education.* Philadelphia, PA: Lippincott Williams and Wilkins.

Ontario Ministry of Health and Long-Term Care. (2014, May). Guidelines for participation in the nursing graduate guarantee initiative. Retrieved from http://www.healthforceontario.ca/UserFiles/file/Nurse/Inside/ngg-participation-guidelines-jan-2011-en.pdf.

The Ottawa Hospital. (n.d.). Pain connect—The Ottawa Hospital Pain Clinic (TOHPC) preceptorship. Retrieved from https://www.ottawahospital.on.ca/wps/portal/Base/TheHospital/ClinicalServices/DeptPgrmCS/Departments/Anesthesiology/ChronicPainUnitTOHPainClinic/PainPreceptorship.

Romyn, D. M., Linton, N., Giblin, C., et al. (2009). Successful transition of the new graduate nurse. *International Journal of Nursing Education Scholarship, 6*(1), Article 34, 1–15. doi:10.2202/1548-923X.1802

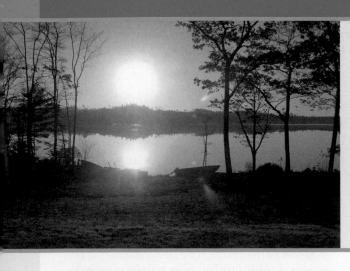

CHAPTER

28

Self-Management: Stress and Time

Catherine A. Hill
Adapted by Shelley L. Cobbett

This chapter examines the concept of self-management—the ability of individuals to actively gain control of their lives. Through self-management, the professional nurse can effectively order his or her day, engage in powerful persistence, and enjoy daily renewal. Three components of self-management are explored: stress management, time management, and meeting management. Methods for managing stress and organizing time are introduced. Practical exercises and suggestions for stress management and time management are presented that can be used for personal and professional situations to reduce stress and enhance efficiency.

OBJECTIVES

- Define self-management.
- Identify personal and professional stressors.
- Describe physical, mental, and emotional/spiritual strategies to manage stress.
- Understand the nurse manager's role in helping staff manage stress.
- Describe common time wasters.
- Identify time-management techniques that can help manage time more effectively.
- Describe tips for managing meetings effectively.

TERMS TO KNOW

agenda	general adaptation syndrome (GAS)	role stress
burnout	information overload	self-management
coping	overwork	time management
delegation	perfectionism	
employee assistance program (EAP)	procrastination	

Denise feels as if she does not get a break from the stress in her life. Just when she thinks things are becoming easier, she is side-swiped by another stressful event. Denise seems to have few stress-free days or periods in her life lately. She knows that stress is not good for her. She is employed full time at a level-one emergency department and finds that she faces ongoing pressure to work overtime to fulfill the unit's staffing requirements. Denise is also a part-time master in nursing student and has not been able to focus on her studies as much as she would like, which is causing her added stress. Denise has a partner and two children that she seems to rarely have any time for, which she knows is not fair to her family. She feels like she always has something to do, is unable to get to the things that she wants to do, and has little time for herself. It seems like a never-ending battle.

What do you think you would do if you were Denise?

INTRODUCTION

What should you do when you have tried your best, but things are not going well? What needs changing? Where do you begin? **Self-management** is the ability of individuals to actively gain control of their lives. It involves self-directed change to achieve important goals (Stuart & Laraia, 2008). As a nurse leader, your goals will require balancing personal and professional objectives and organizing your time and activities to reach them. A priority concern in nursing management is quality of patient care because of its positive correlation with job satisfaction (Teng, Hsiao, & Chou, 2010), staff recruitment, and retention (Bailey, 2009). Compared with other professions, nursing can be highly stressful. How the nurse perceives the stress is the result of personal characteristics and the work environment, including demographic characteristics, working situations, occupational roles, and personal resources (Wu, Chi, Chen, et al., 2010).

Nash (2009) investigated the relationships among nurse manager stress, hardiness, and leadership, and found that nurse managers with higher hardiness had a greater inclination for transformational leadership practices. The presence of hardiness behaviours is positively correlated with good health and performance, and negatively correlated with strain, denial, and avoidance behaviours (Maddi, 2013). To develop stress hardiness, we must actively improve our skills related to stress management, adaptive coping, healthy communication, and problem solving. Research has demonstrated that hardiness can be learned (Maddi, 2013).

The three key strategies for achieving self-management introduced in this chapter—stress, time, and meeting management—are important ways to do more with fewer resources. Time and stress are somewhat of a "chicken and egg" phenomenon—not enough time contributes to stress, and stress can erode efficiency and thus decrease time on task. The key lies in our ability to manage both time and stress, not only personally but also professionally. The outcome of effective self-management is hardiness and the ability to accomplish professional and personal goals.

UNDERSTANDING STRESS

Nurses have learned about the effect of stress on patients and how to teach them to manage its consequences. However, only one third of nurse managers have any sort of formal leadership or managerial training (Bailey, 2009) that would prepare them for dealing with multiple sources of stress at the same time. Nurses need to recognize the unique stressors in their professional and personal lives. Everyone experiences stress—the exhilaration of a joyous event, as well as the negative feelings and unpleasant physical symptoms that may be associated with a difficult life situation or even the anticipation of difficulty. Stress is the uncomfortable gap between how we would like our life to be and how it actually is. Nurses are not immune to the effects of stress. Learning what stress is, its dynamics, and some strategies to manage distress is a part of the personal and professional maturation of nurses.

Definition of Stress

In this chapter, *stress* is a consequence of or response to an event or stimulus and can be negative (distress) or positive (eustress). Each individual's interpretation determines whether the event is viewed as positive or threatening. In addition, stress management does not necessarily mean stress reduction. Preventive stress management is an important tool for promoting individual health, organizational health, and ultimately organizational performance (Hargrove, Quick, Nelson, et al., 2011). Preventive stress management activities exist at every level of the organization. However, effective preventive stress management is dependent on committed leadership. Stress management is a Canadian Nurses Association (CNA) (CNA, n.d.) competency for a registered nurse (it appears under Health and Wellness Competency HW-10). Stress management has important implications for the workplace because of its link to low absenteeism rates, improved quality of care, and increased productivity (Limm, Gundel, Heinmuller, et al., 2011). Nurses would benefit from learning to transform stress into a tool for achieving their full potential (Guimond-Plourde, 2011).

SOURCES OF JOB STRESS

Job stress can be defined as the physical and emotional responses that arise when job requirements do not match the abilities, resources, or needs of the worker. Work-related stress can lead to poor physical and emotional health and injury. Job stress can motivate us to learn new skills and master our jobs, or it can cause distress, which can lead to exhaustion, feelings of inadequacy, and failure. For example, the stress associated with an interview for a new position can be useful; it provides you with determination and gives you an "edge" that will help you think quickly and clearly and express your thoughts in ways that will benefit your interview process. However, having your car break down on the way to the interview creates distress when you realize that you will be late for your interview. As more is learned about the relationship of stress to physiological changes, stressors will become even easier to identify. When one looks at job-related stressors, the stressors fall into one of two categories: external sources (working conditions) and internal sources (worker characteristics).

External Sources

Occupational stress in nursing has been well-defined and documented. Work-related stressors, such as workload, rotating shifts, high patient acuity, inadequate staffing, ethical conflicts, dealing with death and acute illness, role ambiguity, the intensity of complexity compression, and job insecurity have all been associated with increased stress and burnout. Nursing burnout merits special attention from staff nurses, physicians, managers, and nursing leaders (Bogaert, Clarke, Roelant, et al., 2010). The nurse practice environment and its connection to stress and burnout is an extremely important leadership and organizational issue (Wolf, Triolo, & Ponte, 2008).

Change. Although the increased stress that results from change takes many forms, two underlying patterns appear to be constant. Often, nurses feel trapped by conflicting expectations. They expect to furnish care, to meet patients' needs, and to be nurturing. However, organizations require nurses to be managers of patient care and of systems, and value their contribution to efficiency and cost-effectiveness while simultaneously preserving quality of care. Because nurses cannot comply with both expectations, they experience considerable role conflict, frustration, and distress.

Social. Interpersonal relations can buffer stressors or can in themselves become stressors. Outside the work setting, home can be a refuge for harried nurses; however, stresses at home, when severe, can impair work performance and relationships among staff or even result in violence that may invade the workplace.

Changes in health care delivery systems, as well as the current nursing shortage, have reduced the number of professional nurses, often creating situations of minimally safe staffing levels. Consequently, some nurses lose supportive, collegial relationships that may have been established over many years. Many institutions now depend on supplemental staffing that can create a very transient nursing staff. In other situations, nurses are reassigned or they "float" to various patient-care units, which require that they work with unfamiliar staff. Thus, they may feel isolated or become unwillingly involved in dysfunctional politics on the unit. Such situations may also necessitate that nurses work with patients whose requirements for care may be unfamiliar, resulting in further stress related to patient safety concerns.

Persons in management-level positions may also become stressors. Communication may come from the top down, with little opportunity for nurses to participate in decisions that affect them directly or that they may need to implement without proper training or support. Nurses may experience distress from feelings of frustration and helplessness with this lack of opportunity for input to decisions.

In addition, disruptive behaviour poses considerable work stress. Although healthy workplaces include freedom from such behaviour, too many instances occur in health care settings. In addition to being stressful for nurses, such behaviour can disrupt patient safety efforts.

The Position. Upon entering nursing school, most students expect that caring for patients who are chronically or critically ill and for families who have experienced tragedy will be stressful. The current environment in many health care organizations, however, is more complex and is often characterized by overwork, a situation in which employees are expected to become more productive without additional resources. It is also characterized by the stresses inherent in nursing practice. In some settings, direct care nurses have been expected to stay beyond the designated assignment period, often with little or no notice. Some nurse managers experience stress in those situations and resort to threatening behaviours and statements, such as the potential for dismissal. These situations often escalate when direct care nurses do not believe they can deliver safe care and nurse managers exhaust creative ways to provide adequate coverage.

Role stress is a condition in which role demands are conflicting, irritating, or impossible to fulfill. It is an additional stressor for nurses and is associated with negative consequences for the individual and the organization (Garrosa, Moreno-Jimenez, Rodriguez-Munoz, et al., 2011). Role stress is particularly acute for new graduates, whose lack of clinical experience and organizational skills, combined with new situations and procedures, may increase feelings of overwhelming stress. Considering the relationship between burnout and turnover in the general nursing population (see the Research Perspective), high burnout of new graduates is particularly alarming in light of the severe nursing shortage (Laschinger, Finegan, & Wilk, 2009). Nursing the Future Bridge Clubs are available in almost every province and territory to assist new graduate nurses in fostering new and healthy ways to transition to the role of the professional nurse (http://nursingthefuture.ca/bridge_clubs/bridge_club _info). Role transition is also discussed in Chapter 27.

🔍 RESEARCH PERSPECTIVE

Resource: Poghosyan, L., Clarke, S. P., Finlayson, M., et al. (2010). Nurse burnout and quality of care: Cross-national investigation in six countries. *Research in Nursing and Health, 33,* 288–298. http://dx.doi.org/10.1002/nur.20383

This study explored the relationship of quality care and nurse burnout with a sample of 53 846 nurses from Canada, the United States, the United Kingdom, Germany, New Zealand, and Japan. Data were collected over a 6-year period using the Maslach Burnout Inventory and a single item reflecting nurse-rated quality of care. Higher levels of nurse burnout were associated with lower quality of care. However, the cross-sectional design and absence of data on processes of care preclude causal interpretations.

Implications for Practice
Reducing nurse burnout is an effective intervention for improving quality of care in hospitals and must be addressed.

Gender Roles. Approximately 94% of the nation's over 280 000 nurses are women (CNA, 2011), and many go home to traditionally gender-related responsibilities that may include household management, children, and aging parents. These additional responsibilities often contribute to the level of stress felt by the nurse. Thanks to Generation Y's entry into the workforce, greater emphasis on work–life balance has become increasingly important. This generation's needs include recognition, flexible work schedules, stability, adequate supervision, and opportunities for professional development (Lavoie-Tremblay, Leclerc, Marchionni, et al., 2010).

Rochlen, Good, and Carver (2009) found that, overall, men in the nursing profession were well adjusted and satisfied in their work roles and lives. They also found that greater gender-related work barriers were associated with higher levels of gender role conflict, less social support, lower job skills, and less work and life satisfaction. In addition, research indicates that males and females differ in their stress and coping processes when subjected to stress in a work context (Watson, Goh, & Sawang, 2011). For example, males and females identify, assess, and apply coping strategies differently. Thus, it is important for nurses to acknowledge gender differences in relation to stress and coping behaviours.

Internal Sources

Personal stress "triggers" are events or situations that have an effect on specific individuals. A personal trigger might be a specific event such as the death of a loved one, an automobile accident, losing a job, or getting married. These events are in addition to daily personal stressors such as working in a noisy environment, job dissatisfaction, or a difficult commute to work. Negative self-talk, pessimistic thinking, self-criticism, and overanalyzing can be significant ongoing stressors. These internal sources of stress usually stem from unrealistic self-beliefs (unrealistic expectations, taking things personally, all-or-nothing thinking, exaggerating, or rigid thinking), perfectionism, or the type-A personality.

As mentioned earlier in the chapter, an individual's ability to cope with stress has been shown to be influenced by his or her hardiness. Hardiness relates to both attitudes and strategies that facilitate turning stressful situations from potential disasters into opportunities for growth (Maddi, 2013). Whether you are a nurse manager or a staff nurse in the community, long-term care, or acute care setting, strategies and attitudes demonstrating hardiness are invaluable for managing stress in the health care environment. According to Maddi (2013), the three attitudes of hardiness are commitment, control, and challenge. *Commitment* keeps you involved and leads you to make your best effort; when you exert *control*, you see yourself in charge rather than passive; and if you consider change to be a regular part of life, you see it simply as a *challenge* (Bold, 2010).

Lifestyle choices, such as the use of caffeine, lack of exercise, poor diet, inadequate sleep and leisure time, and cigarette smoking, have a direct effect on the amount of one's stress. Recognizing that most of the stress an individual has is self-generated is the first step to dealing with it.

Dynamics of Stress

Stress may result from unrealistic or conflicting expectations, the pace and magnitude of change, human behaviour, individual personality characteristics, the characteristics of the position itself, or the culture of the organization. Other stressors may be unique to certain environments, situations, and persons or groups. Initially, increased stress produces increased performance. However, when stress continues to increase or remains intense, performance decreases. Selye's (1956, 1965) investigations of the nature of and reactions to stress have been very influential in the study of stress.

He described the concept of stress and developed the general adaptation syndrome (GAS), which is a theory detailing a predictable multi-stage response to stress (see Figure 28-1).

More recent investigations of the relationship among the brain, the immune system, and health (psychoneuroimmunology) have generated models that challenge Selye's general adaptation syndrome. Although Selye stated that all people respond with a similar set of hormonal and immune responses to any stress, studies using a response-based orientation indicate that stress is stimulus- and situation-specific, and depends on the individual (Rice, 2013). For example, Roy's (2008) adaptation model is a nursing model that uses stress and stressors as its theoretical underpinning. Roy defines a person as an open, adaptive system constantly interacting with his or her environment and using coping skills to deal with stressors. Unlike Selye's GAS, Roy's model suggests that each person's ability to deal with stress varies and depends on individual adaptive capacity (Roy, 2008).

Critical of stress research using predominantly (83%) male subjects, both human and animal, Taylor, Klein, Lewis et al. (2000) proposed a model of the female stress response, the "tend and befriend," as opposed to the male's "fight or flight" model. The "tend and befriend" response is an estrogen and oxytocin–mediated stress response that is characterized by caring for offspring and befriending those around in times of stress to increase chances of survival (Post, 2010). Women often reach out to others during times of stress, whereas men tend to isolate themselves (Post, 2010). With the vast majority of nurses being female, this model may be helpful to understanding stress responses nurses make in the health care environment.

Most nurses can easily recognize the origins of stress and its symptoms. For example, a health care employer may make demands on nurses, such as excessive work, that the nurses regard as beyond their capacity to perform. When they are unable to resolve the problem through overwork, with more staff, or by looking at the situation in another way, the nurses may feel threatened or depressed. They may also experience headache, fatigue, or other physical symptoms. If the stress persists, such symptoms may increase; nurses may attempt to cope by becoming apathetic or by

TABLE 28-1   SIGNS OF OVERSTRESS IN INDIVIDUALS

PHYSICAL	MENTAL	SPIRITUAL/EMOTIONAL

• Physical signs of ill health:
  • Increase in flu, colds, accidents
  • Change in sleeping habits
  • Fatigue
• Chronic signs of decreased ability to manage stress:
  • Headaches
  • Hypertension
  • Backaches
  • Gastrointestinal problems
• Unhealthy coping activities:
  • Increased use of drugs and alcohol
  • Increased weight
  • Smoking
  • Crying, yelling, blaming
	• Dread going to work every day
	• Rigid thinking and a desire to go by all the rules in all cases; inability to tolerate any changes
	• Forgetfulness and anxiety about work to be done; more frequent errors and incidents
	• Returning home exhausted and unable to participate in enjoyable activities
	• Confusion about duties and roles
	• Generalized anxiety
	• Decrease in concentration
	• Depression
	• Anger, irritability, impatience
		• Sense of being a failure; disappointed in work performance
		• Anger and resentment toward patients, colleagues, and managers; overall irritable attitude
		• Lack of positive feelings toward others
		• Cynicism toward patients, blaming them for their problems
		• Excessive worry, insecurity, lowered self-esteem
		• Increased family and friend conflict

resigning their positions. Table 28-1 outlines physical, mental, and spiritual/emotional signs of overstress in individuals.

Physical illnesses linked to stress include visceral adiposity, type II diabetes, cardiovascular disease (hypertension, heart attack, stroke), musculoskeletal disorders, psychological disorders (anxiety, depression), workplace injury, neuromuscular disorders (multiple sclerosis), suicide, cancer, ulcers, asthma, and rheumatoid arthritis. Stress can even cause life-threatening sympathetic stimulation.

STRESS MANAGEMENT

Individuals respond to stress by eliciting coping strategies that are a means of dealing with stress to maintain or achieve well-being. These strategies may be ineffective because of their reliance on methods such as withdrawal or substance abuse, or they may be effective in helping restore a greater sense of well-being and effectiveness. Some of these effective strategies are discussed here.

Stress Prevention

One effective way to deal with stress is to determine and manage its source. Discovering the origin of stress in patient care may be difficult because some environments have changed so rapidly that the nursing staff is overwhelmed trying to balance bureaucratic rules and limited resources with the demands of vulnerable human beings. When in distress, nurses may need to step back and look at the "big picture." By identifying daily stressors, the nurse can then develop a plan of action for management of the associated stress. This plan may include elimination of the stressor, modification of the stressor, or changing the perception of the stressor using a reframing technique (e.g., viewing mistakes as opportunities for new learning).

The theory of preventive stress management, discussed in Box 28-1, can be used to assess stressors in your nursing practice.

Considering the critical nature of nursing work and the potential for serious injury to others, many of the day-to-day activities of nursing can create workplace stress. Given the stressful nature of nursing, it is wise for the nurse to be alert to his or her own signs of stress and to develop lifestyle habits that help reduce stress. Adequate sleep, a balanced diet, regular exercise, and frequent interactions with friends are excellent stress-buffering habits to develop.

Shirey, McDaniel, Ebright, et al. (2010) studied nurse manager stress and coping experiences using a qualitative methodology with a sample of 21 nurse managers. Their findings suggested that addressing stress, coping, and the complexity of the nurse manager role requires individual and health system strategies. Individual factors (nurse experience), organizational context (organizational

BOX 28-1 THEORY OF PREVENTIVE STRESS MANAGEMENT

The theory of preventive stress management (TPSM) is a macro-level theory that is not discipline specific and helps explain or conceptualize potential relationships between stressors, stress responses, and outcomes of stress (Hargrove et al., 2011). In an organization, the stress cycle begins with stressors, moves to the stress response, and then to the outcomes. Stressors can be environmental or self-imposed. The stress response is activated when an individual is exposed to stressors. In terms of outcomes, positive stress responses can lead to eustress, whereas negative stress responses can lead to distress. The stages of an individual's response to stress are illustrated in Figure 28-1. Stress can originate from role factors, job stressors, and interpersonal demands (Hargrove et al., 2011). The TPSM includes three stages (primary, secondary, and tertiary) to help reduce stressors, moderate the stress response, and reduce the negative impact of distress (Hargrove et al., 2011). Nurse leaders have a responsibility to create and maintain healthy organizations in which nurses can thrive. Good leaders know how to minimize the negative impact of distress and maximize the positive impact of eustress.

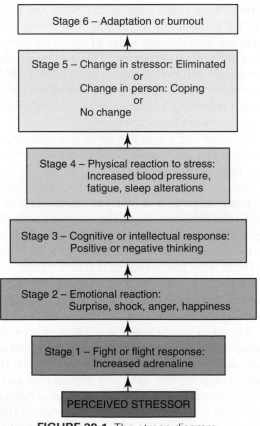

FIGURE 28-1 The stress diagram.

culture), and structural elements and systems (span of control, co-manager model, director of nursing empowerment) all influence nurse managers' perceptions of stress and their coping experiences. Minimizing stress for nurse managers can enhance their coping experiences, facilitate good decision making, and improve engagement and retention of nurse managers and staff nurses (Shirey et al., 2010).

LaMontagne, Keegel, Louie, et al. (2007) reviewed 90 reports on job-stress interventions between 1990 and 2005 and found that they could be divided into three levels of preventive stress management. Primary interventions included techniques for directly managing or changing the stressor; secondary interventions included actions designed to improve individual stress responses (e.g., those that improve individual coping); and tertiary interventions included actions aimed at treating the symptoms of distress (e.g., employee assistance programs). It is important to be aware of the stress that you experience and how you typically manage it. Analyze your stress experiences by completing Exercise 28-1.

EXERCISE 28-1

Identify the stress you experience and how you usually manage it. Create and complete a log at the end of each shift that includes the date, situation, your response, how you dealt with your response, and the evaluation of the situation. Ask yourself if the stress was good stress (eustress) or bad stress (distress). Review the log and note what stressors (e.g., people, technology, values conflict) were the most common. Do you encounter some on a regular basis? If so, try to formulate a plan to conquer the problems. You may need to role-play or get continuing education to improve a specific skill. You may need to simply break a task down into smaller pieces or to eliminate interruptions.

Identify how you most often react to stress: physically, mentally, and emotionally/spiritually. Then think about what more positive strategies could be used to deal with a similar situation.

Symptom Management

Unpredictable and uncontrollable change, coupled with immense responsibility and little control over the work environment, produces stress for nurses and other health care providers. Consequently, nurses may develop emotional symptoms such as anxiety, depression, or anger; physical alterations such as fatigue, headache, and insomnia; mental changes such as a decrease in concentration and memory; and behavioural changes such as smoking, drinking, crying, and swearing. The important factor is not the stressor but, rather, how the individual perceives the stressor and what coping mechanisms are available to mediate the hormonal response to the stressor.

Change is inevitable and permeates all areas of health care, sometimes on a daily basis. Knowing how you react to change and how you cope during periods of change can help you build a repertoire of strategies that you can easily apply to reduce your stress during times of change. Exercise 28-2 offers a personal analysis of change.

EXERCISE 28-2

This personal analysis of change exercise can be used when you are considering pursuing a personal or professional change. It helps you analyze your reaction to the planned change.

1. Write down the objective of the change that you want to make.
2. Objectively document the change that you want to pursue, including where the change will happen, when it will happen, and what you have to do to make it happen. Be specific; you have to be able to evaluate the change, so its factors need to be measurable.
3. Write a statement on how confident you are that you will achieve the planned change (on a scale of 1 to 10, with 1 being no confidence and 10 being complete confidence).

   As you begin the change, keep a log of your stress levels in relation to the change. Also record the stress-reducing behaviours you engage in to reduce your stress level, including how much your stress level changed afterward. After you complete the change, analyze your log of stress-reducing behaviours and note those that most effectively reduced your stress level.

Multiple "stress-buffering" behaviours can be elicited to reduce the detrimental effects of stress. The stressor-induced changes in the hormonal and immune systems can be modulated by an individual's behavioural **coping** response (the immediate response of a person to a threatening situation). Coping responses include leisure activities and taking time for self, decreasing or discontinuing the use of caffeine, positive social support, a strong belief system, a sense of humour, developing realistic expectations, reframing events, regular aerobic exercise, meditation, and use of the relaxation response.

Everyone needs to balance work and leisure in his or her life. Leisure time and stress are inversely proportional. If the time for work is more than 60% of

the time awake or if self-time is less than 10% of the time awake, stress levels will increase. Changes should be made to relieve stress, such as decreasing the number of work hours or finding more time for leisure activities. Caffeine is a strong stimulant and, in itself, a stressor. Slowly weaning off caffeine should result in better sleep and more energy. Positive social support can offer validation, encouragement, or advice. By discussing situations with others, one can reduce stress. A great deal of stress comes from our belief systems, which cause stress in two ways. First, behaviours result from them, such as placing work before pleasure. Second, beliefs may also conflict with those of other people, as may happen with patients from different cultures. Articulating beliefs and finding common ground will help reduce anger and stress. Humour is a great stress reducer and laughter a great tension reducer. A common source of stress is unrealistic expectations. Realistic expectations can make life feel more predictable and more manageable. *Reframing* is changing the way you look at things to make you feel better about them or to obtain a different perspective. Recognizing that there are many ways to interpret the same situation, taking the positive view is less stressful. Regular aerobic exercise is a logical method of dissipating the excess energy generated by the stress response.

Meditation to elicit the relaxation response can be beneficial. The benefits of practising relaxation techniques for 20 minutes daily include a feeling of well-being, the ability to learn how tension makes the body feel, and the sense that tension can be controlled. In cases of some stress-related disorders (e.g., hypertension), biofeedback may be used to monitor physiological relaxation processes. Exercise 28-3 outlines one systematic relaxation technique.

EXERCISE 28-3

This exercise can be used in the middle of a working day, the last thing at night, or at any time you feel tense or anxious. Review the information and strategies of "Meditation: A simple, fast way to reduce stress" at the Mayo Clinic website: http://www.mayoclinic.org/meditation/ART-20045858. Make a short list of steps to take, and put it in your smart phone, personal digital assistant (PDA), or notepad.

Applebaum, Fowler, Fiedler, et al. (2010) found a direct relationship between perceived stress and turnover intention. The results of their study indicated that it may not be the stress itself but the physical consequences of stress (missing lunch breaks, physical symptoms, excessive overtime) that cause nurses to leave their job. Similarly, Ritter (2011) found a link between healthy work environments and the retention of nurses in a hospital setting.

Social support in the form of positive work relationships may be an important way to buffer distress and provide a life-enhancing social network ("Understanding the stress," 2011). Although colleagues may form friendships, the workload and the shifting of staff from one unit to another often make it difficult to establish and maintain close relationships with peers. However, managers and co-workers who are supportive may improve morale in the workplace (Zangaro & Soeken, 2007) (see the Research Perspective below). Nurses in a new position or in an unfamiliar geographical area must anticipate that they will benefit from the security of being part of a group that can furnish emotional support. Without easily accessible family and friends, nurses need to be intentional about seeking new, supportive personal relationships. Positive coping strategies may also make nurses less likely to adopt potentially negative coping strategies such as withdrawing, lowering their standards of care, and abusing alcohol or other substances.

RESEARCH PERSPECTIVE

Resource: Zangaro, G. A., & Soeken, K. L. (2007). A meta-analysis of studies of nurses' job satisfaction. *Research in Nursing & Health, 30*, 445–458. http://dx.doi.org/10.1002/nur.20202

This study looked at the strength of the relationship between job satisfaction, autonomy, stress, and collaboration in 31 studies that included 14 567 subjects. Although the findings varied, job satisfaction correlated most strongly with job stress, followed by collaboration and autonomy. These findings have important implications for improving nurses' work environment.

Implications for Practice
Given the current nursing shortage, nurse job satisfaction and employee retention are very important to current health care industry demands for safe, effective, patient-centred, timely, efficient, and equitable care. Nurses and nurse managers in all settings are faced with resource constraints. Identifying and validating nurse perceptions about stress, collaboration, and autonomy facilitate accurate assessment and effective management of staff, turnover rates, and performance.

Burnout

Sometimes individuals cannot manage stress successfully through their own efforts and require assistance. Examples of behaviour related to stress that feels overwhelming appear in Table 28-1. Coping strategies, such as those described previously, may furnish temporary relief or none at all. With this level of distress, one can feel overwhelmed or helpless and may be at a greater risk for mental or physical illness. This constellation of emotions is commonly called *burnout.*

A classic definition of burnout is a "prolonged response to chronic emotional and interpersonal stressors on the job" (Maslach, Schaufeli, & Leiter, 2000, p. 398). The sources of the stressors may exist in the environment, in the individual, or in the interaction between the individual and the environment. Some stressors, such as employment termination, appear to be universal, whereas other stressors, such as meeting deadlines, are more personal. For example, some nurses thrive on goals and timetables, whereas others feel constrained and frustrated and thereby experience distress. Burnout is not an objective phenomenon as if it were the accumulation of a certain number and type of stressors. How the stressors are perceived and how they are mediated by an individual's ability to adapt are important variables in determining levels of distress.

People's psychological relationships to their jobs can be considered as a continuum between burnout (negative experience) and job engagement (positive experience). The three interrelated dimensions of this continuum are exhaustion–energy, cynicism–involvement, and inefficacy–efficacy (Maslach & Leiter, 2008). The exhaustion–energy dimension represents the basic individual strain of burnout, including feelings of being overextended and worn out. The cynicism–involvement dimension represents the interpersonal context of burnout, including negative, callous, or excessively detached responses to various aspects of the job. The inefficacy–efficacy dimension represents the self-evaluation component of burnout, including feelings of incompetence and a lack of achievement and productivity in work. The significance of this model is that it clearly places an individual's experience of strain within the social context of the workplace. Research on burnout uses the Maslach Burnout Inventory (Maslach & Jackson, 1981) to assess these three dimensions. Recent research has also turned to an examination of

TABLE 28-2	STRESS-MANAGEMENT STRATEGIES	
PHYSICAL	**MENTAL**	**EMOTIONAL/SPIRITUAL**
• Accept physical limitations • Modify nutrition: moderate carbohydrate and protein, high fruits and vegetables, low caffeine and sugar • Exercise: an enjoyable activity five times a week for 30 minutes • Make your physical health a priority • Nurture yourself: take time for breaks and lunch • Sleep: get enough in quantity and quality • Relax: use meditation, massage, yoga, or biofeedback	• Learn to say "no"! • Use cognitive restructuring and self-talk • Use imagery • Develop hobbies or activities • Plan vacations • Learn about the system and how problems are handled • Learn communication, conflict resolution, and time-management skills • Take continuing education courses • Learn to delegate	• Use meditation • Seek solace in prayer • Seek professional counselling • Participate in support groups • Participate in networking • Communicate feelings • Identify and acquire a mentor • Ask for feedback and clarification

the positive opposite of the three dimensions, or job engagement (Maslach & Leiter, 2008).

New Graduate Nurse Stress

New graduates entering the health care system face many challenges transitioning from the student role to the professional nurse role. Role transition is discussed in Chapter 27. Unruh and Zhang (2013) studied the influence of the hospital work environment on newly licensed registered nurses' commitment to nursing and intent to leave nursing. They reported that negative perceptions of the work environment were strong predictors of intent to leave nursing and that retention of newly licensed registered nurses can be improved through changes in the work environment that seek to reduce stress (Unruh & Zhang, 2013). Beecroft, Dorey, and Wenten (2008) found that 30% of new graduates had high turnover intentions, mainly as a result of the work environment. When the work environment is positive and offers empowerment, registered nurses are less likely to experience burnout and, therefore, more likely to remain in nursing (Wang, Kunaviktikul, & Wichaikhum, 2013). Given the current nursing shortage in Canada, nurse leaders need to ensure that nursing professional practice environments foster high-quality collegial working relationships to enhance the retention of new graduates.

RESOLUTION OF STRESS

Resolution of stress in its early stages can be accomplished through a variety of techniques. Nurses must

be able to reach a balance of caring for others and caring for self. Table 28-2 summarizes physical, mental, and emotional/spiritual strategies.

Social Support

Peers and followers can be supportive and help reduce stress by assisting with problem solving and by developing new perspectives. Family and friends can provide a safe haven and a vacation from stress. Social isolation increases stress. Social support allows one to be playful, have fun, laugh, and vent emotions.

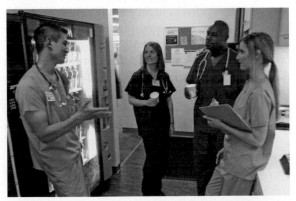

Peers and followers can be supportive and help reduce stress.

Counselling

Persistent, unpleasant feelings, problem behaviour, and helplessness during prolonged stress may suggest the need for assistance from a mental health professional. Examples of problem behaviours include tearfulness or angry outbursts over seemingly minor incidents, major changes in eating or sleeping patterns, frequent unwillingness to go to work, and substance abuse. In such cases, the aforementioned coping strategies afford only temporary relief; nurses with this level of distress feel overwhelmed and believe that their well-being cannot be maintained. In these stressful situations, nurses may feel helpless and require professional assistance from an advanced practice psychiatric nurse, clinical psychologist, psychiatrist, or other mental health worker.

In some organizations, **employee assistance programs (EAPs)** provide free, voluntary, confidential, short-term professional counselling and other services for employees either via in-house staff or by contract with a mental health counsellor. This type of counselling can be effective because the counsellors may already be aware of organizational stressors. Some nurses may have confidentiality concerns when using employer-recommended or employer-provided counselling services. Mental health professionals are bound by their professional standards of confidentiality. Nonetheless, there may be times when it is in the nurse's best interest to sign a release of information, such as when seeking employer accommodation for a certain physical or emotional problem.

Those who seek counselling outside of the workplace may be guided in their selection of mental health professionals by a personal physician, a knowledgeable colleague, their provincial nursing association or college, or by contacting the Canadian Mental Health Association. When the problem underlying the distress is ethical or moral, a trained pastoral counsellor may be helpful in addition to consulting the Canadian Nurses Association code of ethics (CNA, 2008). When private counselling is being arranged, the extended health coverage should be checked to determine mental health benefits and the payment limitations and types of providers eligible for reimbursement.

Leadership and Management

Although social support and counselling can alter how stressors are perceived, time management and effective leadership can modify or remove stressors. Nurse managers have limited formal authority as individuals in most organizations, although managerial groups may be able to influence policy and resource allocation.

Nurse managers can, however, control some environmental stressors on their units. First, nurse managers can examine their own behaviour as a source of subordinates' stress.

In some cases, a controlling or autocratic style of management is appropriate, such as in emergency situations and when working with a large percentage of new and inexperienced employees. For the most part, however, professional nurses need and want the latitude to direct their activities within their sphere of competence. "Letting go," or delegating, means that the nurse leader trusts the personal integrity and professional competence of the team. It does not mean abdicating accountability for achieving accepted standards of patient care and agreed-upon outcomes.

Assistance with problem solving is another way to reduce environmental stressors. Nurse leaders may provide technical advice, refer staff to appropriate resources, or mediate conflicts. Often, nurse leaders enable staff to meet the demands of their work more independently by providing time for continuing education and professional meetings to enhance competence.

Another way in which nurse leaders can reduce stress is to be supportive of staff. Support is not equated with being a friend but, rather, with helping one's peers accomplish good care, develop professionally, and feel valued personally. Leaders can ensure that the expected workload is in line with the nurses' capabilities and resources. They can work to ensure meaningfulness, stimulation, and opportunities for nurses to use their skills. Nurses' roles and responsibilities need to be clearly and publicly defined. Work schedules should be posted as far in advance as possible and should be compatible with what is known about patient safety. Encouraging innovation and experimentation, for example, can motivate staff and give them a sense of greater control over their environment. Affirming a good idea or finding resources to study or implement a promising new procedure or proposal by a staff nurse is supportive. In contrast, when staff members struggle with overwork and other stressors, support is recognizing the condition and helping the nurses avoid such passive coping strategies as feeling helpless or lowering standards of care in favour of active problem solving. Nurse leaders must be sensitive to the distress of the nursing staff and recognize it verbally without becoming counsellors, which is in conflict with their role.

Support may involve making nursing staff aware of resources that furnish counselling while being careful to avoid diagnostic labels and to maintain strict confidentiality. When distress relates to the personal life of subordinates, managers should focus on the effect of such situations on workplace performance—not on the events that have produced the stress.

In addition, leaders can enhance the workplace by dealing effectively with their own stressors. Maintaining a sense of perspective as well as a sense of humour is important. Some stressors, in fact, can be ignored or minimized by posing three questions:

1. "Is this event or situation important?" Stressors are not all equally significant. Do not waste energy on little stressors.
2. "Does this stressor affect me or my unit?" Although some situations that produce distress are institution-wide and need group action, others target specific units or activities. Do not borrow stressors.
3. "Can I change this situation?" If not, then find a way to cope with it or, if the situation is intolerable, make plans to change positions or employers. This decision may require gaining added credentials that may produce long-term career benefits.

Keeping stressful situations in perspective can enable nurses to conserve their energies to cope with stressful situations that are important, that are within their domain, or that can be changed or modified. Stress management interventions have been studied in relation to nurse leaders. Findings from a randomized control trial on the effects of a nurse leader mindfulness meditation course for managing stress demonstrated preliminary effectiveness in reducing self-reported stress symptoms among nurse leaders (Pipe, Bortz, Dueck, et al., 2009).

TIME MANAGEMENT

A very close relationship exists between stress management and time management. Time management is one method of stress prevention or reduction. Stress can decrease productivity and lead to poor use of time. Time management can be considered a preventive action to help reduce the elements of stress in a nurse's life.

Everyone has two choices when managing time: organize or "go with the flow." There are only 24 hours in every day, and it is clear that some people make better use of time than others do. *How* people use time makes some people more successful than others. The effective use of time-management skills thus becomes an even more important tool to achieve personal and professional goals. **Time management** is the appropriate use of tools, techniques, and principles to control time spent on low-priority needs and to ensure that time is invested in activities leading toward achieving desired, high-priority goals. More simply, time management is the ability to spend your time on the things that matter to you and your organization. That goal may also involve delegation. It is important to keep in mind that planning daily time-management strategies takes time! By setting goals and eliminating time stealers, you will have the extra time to accomplish those goals.

Where Does Your Time Go?

Have you ever wasted time? Time, although a cheap commodity, is our most valuable resource. There are some commonly identified time stealers, and individuals must recognize them to guard against them. At the heart of time management is an important shift in focus. Concentrate on results, not on being busy.

Doing Too Much. Do you try to do too much at once? At work, do you have three or four major projects going simultaneously? Are you a member of more than one organizational committee? Do you have to worry about what will be on the table for dinner while you are hanging an IV and planning a staff meeting? Have you ever completed a nursing intervention and realized that your mind was really somewhere else and you had ignored the patient? If you *think* you have too much to do, you probably do! Learn to have fewer projects running simultaneously and to concentrate your efforts on one thing at a time. The first step is to be realistic and limit major commitments, and then give each activity your full and undivided attention. Sometimes completing one task before starting another is the most efficient method for getting everything done. Prioritization of goals and activities each day is very helpful.

In the nursing profession, however, limiting commitments is not always possible. When you are feeling overwhelmed by the sheer volume of tasks to be completed, take the time to establish priorities for the day. Decide what must be done versus what would be nice to do. Do not let yourself get distracted from your priority tasks. Nursing is a balancing act; priorities are always changing.

Inability to Say "No." Sometimes the smallest and simplest words are the most difficult to learn. If you are suffering from overload, you probably have gotten there by not being able to say "no." Learning to say "no" to requests is difficult, and in the process, others may be displeased. If you do not say "no," however, you may end up spending much time on projects that are uninteresting or have no relationship to your personal goals and priorities. When someone asks you to do something, you need to stop and consider the request. Do you want to do the task now or sometime in the future? If not, then say so. If you wish to do the task but simply do not have the time, consider delegation. However, be honest with the requester—if you simply do not have the time, say so as politely as possible. If you wish to take on the task but at a later date, negotiate. Remember, accepting an assignment you will never be able to complete sheds an unfavourable light on you.

Procrastination. Do you put off important tasks because they are not enjoyable or because they may be difficult? Do you find excuses for not starting or completing tasks? Are you a procrastinator? By engaging in procrastination, or doing one thing when you should be doing something else, you give up time to complete your task and therefore limit the quality of the work you produce. There are techniques to help deal with procrastination. First, identify the reason for procrastinating. Then make that task your highest priority the next day. Reward yourself after you finish the task. Another technique is to select the least attractive element of the task to do first, and the rest will seem easy.

Some people find that they procrastinate when the task ahead is very large. The solution is to break the task down into manageable pieces and plan rewards for accomplishing each of the smaller tasks. Developing a *program evaluation and review technique* (PERT) chart or a Gantt chart may help in this process. PERT charts were originally developed as tools to assist in complex projects that require a series of activities, some of which must be performed sequentially and others that can be performed in parallel with other activities. Envisioned as a network diagram, a PERT chart (Figure 28-2) indicates dependent activities that must be completed before a new activity is undertaken. A Gantt chart (Figure 28-3) consists of a table of project task information and a bar chart that

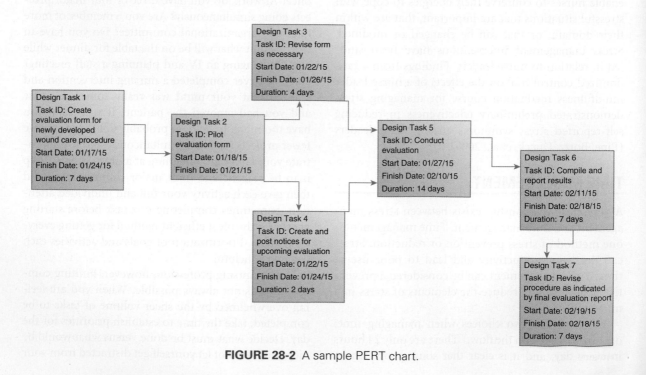

FIGURE 28-2 A sample PERT chart.

TASK	ACCOUNTABILITY	JAN	FEB	MAR	APR	MAY	JUNE
1. Conduct literature search	Unit clinical nurse specialist	———→					
2. Hold nursing practice committee meeting to review material	Chair, nursing practice committee		X				
3. Create a report for the medical staff	Chair, nursing practice committee			————→			
4. Disseminate findings to nursing and medical staff	Chair, nursing practice committee					————→	

FIGURE 28-3 A sample Gantt chart.

graphically displays the project schedule. This method of tracking project activities in relation to time is often used in planning and project management. Both chart techniques can be used to outline how you will approach a large project. The PERT chart clearly illustrates task dependencies but can be more difficult to interpret than the Gantt chart.

Complaining. *Complaining* is the act of expressing dissatisfaction ("Complain," 2004). Often, the time people spend complaining about a task or a particular situation is greater than the time needed to complete the task or to deal with the issue. If you find yourself complaining repeatedly about something, stop and ask yourself what would be the ideal solution and then take the risk to act on it. If the complaint is related to another person, either take the time to talk with the person and get the problem out in the open or write a letter to the person discussing your point of view (even if you do not mail it). If you find yourself complaining about something within the workplace, rethink the problem, generate some possible solutions, and then talk to your manager. Look for solutions that are very simple or "outside the box." Talk to your manager and be prepared to discuss solutions—not just your dissatisfaction or annoyance. In this way, your manager will see you as interested in contributing to the goals of the organization.

Perfectionism. Perfectionism is the uncompromising pursuit of perfection ("Perfectionism," 2004). Some perfectionists have a hard time completing tasks and projects if they are not yet perfect. A perfectionist approach tends to consume a lot of time, especially when the expected outcome is not attainable. Overcoming perfectionism takes considerable effort. However, this does not mean that you should do less

than your best. Being aware of perfectionism means that you occasionally need to give yourself permission to do slightly less than a perfect job, such as buying a takeout dinner rather than preparing a four-course meal after a day at work.

Interruptions. One common distraction from priority activities is interruptions. Some interruptions are integral to the positions that you hold, but others can be controlled. A home care nurse with a large caseload can expect to be paged at any time. More commonly, however, are the numerous small interruptions by individuals who want just a "minute of your time" and take 2 minutes getting to the point! Box 28-2 identifies some strategies to prevent and control interruptions. The two keys to dealing with interruptions are to resume "doing it now" so that an interruption does not destroy your schedule and to maintain the attitude that whatever the interruption, it is a part of your responsibility. When you make a conscious decision not to worry about the things you cannot control, you have more energy to maintain a positive perspective and to move projects forward.

Disorganization. One of the most serious time wasters of all is disorganization. Organization can be a great time saver. Remember that the guiding principle is that organization is a process rather than the product. You can spend so much time organizing that you will never get to the task at hand (procrastination). Simple organizing guidelines include eliminating clutter, keeping everything in its place, and doing similar tasks together. By contrast, Vohs, Redden, & Rahinel (2013) found that people in disorderly environments (e.g., a messy room) were more creative thinkers and produced stimulating new ideas as compared with those in orderly environments.

BOX 28-2 TIPS TO AVOID INTERRUPTIONS AND WORK MORE EFFECTIVELY

- Ask people to put their comments in writing—do not let them catch you "on the run."
- Let the office or unit administrative assistant or administrator know what information you need immediately.
- Conduct a conversation in the hall to help keep it short or in a separate room to keep from being interrupted.
- Do paper work away from your computer to maximize time spent on task.
- Be comfortable saying "no."
- When involved in a long procedure or home visit, ask someone else to cover your other responsibilities.
- Break projects into small, manageable pieces.
- Get yourself organized.
- Minimize interruptions—for example, allow voice mail to pick up the phone; shut the door.
- Set a specific time each day to read and respond to e-mails.
- Keep your work surface clear. Have available only those documents needed for the task at hand.
- Keep your manager informed of your goals.
- Plan to accomplish high-priority or difficult tasks early in the day.
- Develop a plan for the day and stick to it. Remember to schedule in some time for interruptions.
- Schedule time to meet regularly throughout the shift with staff members for whom you are responsible.
- Recognize that crises and interruptions are part of the position.
- Be cognizant of your personal time-waster habits, and try to avoid them.

Too Much Information. The newest time waster to evolve is data proliferation. The technology within our workplace forces us to receive huge amounts of data and to transform these data into useful information. The computer workstation, once touted as a time-saving device, has become the driving force behind care delivery. Nurses can view the computer either as a stress-producing slave driver or as a simple tool to assist them in their daily activities.

Information overload, or "data smog," is a state of stress brought about by the reception of too much information, too fast, and too often and not having adequate information-processing skills. Information literacy is a self-directed independent ability to access information efficiently and evaluate its quality as well as manage and organize the information while understanding the implications of doing so (Belcik, 2007).

In the information age, information literacy skills are imperative for reducing stress and improving productivity (Badke, 2010). Gaining a new appreciation of information is important. Information is simply a tool to use to plan action or make decisions. By learning what information is important, you can learn to use it to your advantage.

Time-Management Concepts

Table 28-3 presents a classification scheme for time-management techniques. The unifying theme is that each activity undertaken should lead to goal attainment and that goal should be the number-one priority at that time.

Goal Setting and Plan Development. The first steps in time management are goal setting and developing a plan to reach those goals. Set goals that are reasonable and achievable. Do not expect to reach long-term goals overnight—*long term* means just that. Give yourself time to meet the goals. Determine many short-term goals to reach the long-term goal, giving you a frequent sense of goal achievement. Give yourself flexibility. If the path you chose last year is no longer appropriate, change it. Write your goals, date the entry, keep it handy, and refer to it often to give yourself a progress report.

Setting Priorities. Once the goals are known, priorities are set. They may, however, shift throughout a

TABLE 28-3 CLASSIFICATION OF TIME-MANAGEMENT TECHNIQUES

TECHNIQUE	PURPOSE	ACTIONS
Organization	Designed to promote efficiency and productivity	Organize and systematize things, tasks, and people. Use basic time-management skills.
Keep focused on goals	Focuses on goal achievement	Assemble a prioritized "to do" list daily, based on goals.
Tool usage	Uses the right tool for planning and preparation	Use tools such as a smart phone.
Time-management plan	Helps to refocus, to gain control, and to use information	Develop a personal time-management plan appropriately.

given period in terms of goal attainment. For example, working on a budget may take precedence at certain times of the year, whereas new staff orientation is a high priority at other times. Knowing what your goals and priorities are helps shape the "to do" list. On a nursing unit or as you work in a community setting, you must know your personal goals and current priorities. How you organize work may depend on geographical considerations, patient acuity, or some other schema.

A particular strategy to assist in prioritization suggests that people generally focus on those things that are important and urgent. By placing the elements of importance and urgency in a grid (Figure 28-4), all activities can be classified as shown (Covey, Merrill, & Merrill, 1994).

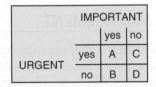

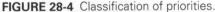

FIGURE 28-4 Classification of priorities.

Typically, we tend to focus on those items in cell A because they are both important and urgent and therefore command our attention. Making shift assignments is an A task because it is an important and urgent part of allocating work in a manner that is fair and practical while also matching patients to staffing competencies to ensure safe and effective patient care. Conversely, if something is neither important nor urgent (cell D), it may be considered a waste of time, at least in terms of personal goals. An example of a D activity might be reading "junk" e-mail. Even if something is urgent but not important (cell C), it contributes minimally to productivity and goal achievement. An example of a C activity might be responding to a memo that has a specific time line but is not important to goal attainment. The real key to setting priorities is to attend to the B tasks, those that are important but not urgent. Examples of B activities are reviewing the organization's strategic plan or participating on organizational committees.

Organization. A number of simple routines for organization can save many minutes over a day and enhance your efficiency. Keeping a workspace neat or arranging things in an orderly fashion may be a powerful time-management tool. Rather than a system of

"pile management," use "file management." Keep in mind the following organizing tips:
- Plan where things should go: your desk or your flash drive.
- Keep a clean workspace.
- Create a "to do" folder.
- Create a "to be filed" folder for any papers.
- Schedule time to work your way through the folders.
- Determine your priority goals for the next day, and have the materials ready to work on when you start the next morning.

Time Tools. Sometimes, the real problem is that the events of the day become the driving force, rather than a planned schedule. Days may become so tightly scheduled that any little interruption can become a crisis. If you do not plan the day, you may be responding to events rather than prioritized goals. If you think you are a reactor rather than a proactive time user, use a time log to list work-related activities for several days. You may not be able to plan well because you really do not have a good estimate of how long a particular activity actually takes or you do not know how many activities can be accomplished in a given time frame.

As the nurse's role in care management becomes more complex, the need for organizational tools increases. Tracking the care of groups of patients, either as the member of a care team or in a leadership capacity, can be overwhelming. Each nurse must devise a method for tracking care and organizing time, as well as delegating and monitoring care provided by others. Although some nurses depend on a shift flowsheet or a Kardex system, others have the benefit of computerized information tracking systems. Handheld computer devices such as PDAs or barcode scanners for medication administration are other methods to track information and increase safety and efficiency. However, the issue of patient confidentiality cannot be ignored when entering data into a PDA that you take home at the end of your shift. Chapter 12 provides further discussion about how technologies are used in the health care environment.

Managing Information. The first step in managing information is to assess the source. Once you have identified the sources of your data, you have a better idea of how to deal with the information. Track incoming information for a few days. Patterns will begin to emerge and will give clues as to how to deal with it.

By developing information-receiving skills, you can quickly interpret the data and convert them to useful information, discarding unneeded data. Initially, you should reduce or eliminate that which is useless. Delete the e-mail, or toss the memo in the garbage. Next, monitor the information flow and decide what to do with incoming data. Find and focus on the most important pieces, and then quickly narrow down the specific details you need. Identify resources that are most helpful, and have them readily available. Be able to build the "big picture" from the masses of data you receive. Finally, recognize when you have enough information to act.

Once you have mastered the receiving end of information, concentrate on information-sending skills. Remember, your information is simply another person's data! Try to keep your outflow short; make it a synthesis of the information. Finally, select the most appropriate mode of communication for your message from the technology available. You may be sending your information in written (memo or report) or verbal (face-to-face or presentation) form or via telephone, voice mail, e-mail, text, Twitter, or fax. Remember, the most important skill is to know when you have said enough. Chapter 29 provides a discussion of and guidelines on professional writing. Exercise 28-4 will help you consider how you have dealt with information.

EXERCISE 28-4

Think of the last time you were in a clinical area. How often did you record the same piece of data (e.g., a finding in your assessment of the patient)? Remember to include all steps, from your jotting down notes on a piece of paper or entering data into the computer to the final report of the day. What information-processing tools could decrease the number of steps?

Delegating

Delegation involves achieving performance of care outcomes for which you are accountable and responsible by sharing activities with other individuals who have the appropriate authority to accomplish the work. It is a critical component of self-management for nurse managers and care managers. Appropriate delegation not only increases time efficiency but also serves as a means of reducing stress. Delegation is discussed in depth in Chapter 26, but it is also appropriate

to discuss it briefly as a time-management strategy. Delegation works only when the delegator trusts the delegatee to accomplish the task and to report findings back to the delegator. The delegator wastes time if he or she checks and redoes everything someone else has done. Delegation requires empowerment of the delegatee to accomplish the task. If the nurse does not delegate appropriately, with clear expectations, the delegatee will constantly ask for assistance or direction. Delegation can be a means of reducing stress if used appropriately. However, if the nurse does not understand delegation and does not use it appropriately, it can be a major source of stress as the nurse assumes accountability and responsibility for care administered by others.

MEETING MANAGEMENT

Meeting management is a key time-management strategy. Even nurses who may not have extensive management responsibilities can benefit from learning to make the most of meetings, either as the leader or a group member.

Managing Meetings

Meetings serve various purposes, ranging from creating social networks to setting formal policy. Wodak, Kwon, and Clarke (2011) investigated the impact of leaders' communication strategies on the consensus-building process in meetings. They identified five discursive strategies that meeting chairs employed to drive decision making: bonding, encouraging, directing, modulating, and recommitting. During bonding, the leader uses the term *we* rather than *I* to cultivate group identity and promote consensus and shared decision making. Encouraging stimulates the participation of members to explore new ideas and/or develop synthesis with existing ideas related to the current topic. Directing occurs after encouraging and is used to bring about closure and resolution by reducing the equivocality of ideas that have been discussed. Modulating allows the leader to achieve a balance between encouraging and directing. Lastly, recommitting moves the group from a consensual understanding of the issue toward a commitment to action (Wodak et al., 2011). Critical findings from this research indicate that the meeting chair influences the outcome of the meetings in both negative and positive ways and that the specific meeting context mediates participation and the ability of the chair to control interactions within the committee (Wodak et al., 2011). Nurse leaders who embrace these techniques can make meetings more productive with tangible outcomes, leaving all members feeling a sense of empowerment and accomplishment.

Tips for Managing Meetings Effectively. Consider if the meeting is necessary. For example, a phone call, posted notice, e-mail, or brief "huddle" (a short, check-in meeting) might suffice. If the right people are not available, rescheduling may be a good option.

Schedule meetings right before lunch or at the end of the day. Participants will have an incentive to stick to the schedule. Set a start time and a stop time, and reward prompt members by starting on schedule. Avoid meetings lasting longer than 1½ to 2 hours. Select an appropriate setting in which the participants are not readily accessible to interruptions. If necessary, plan the seating arrangement to prevent inappropriate behaviours such as whispering or other interruptions. If the group meets over a period of time, have group members set rules for conduct and behaviour.

Distribute an **agenda**. Whenever possible, provide a written agenda to each member in advance of the meeting. Establish and make known the goal of the meeting. Attach all needed preparation reading to the agenda. The more advanced the reading or preparation that is required, the earlier members should receive agendas. Different types of agendas can be used for different purposes:

* *Structured agendas:* If a topic is particularly controversial, consider setting a rule that requires any negative comment to be preceded by a positive one.
* *Timed agendas:* Consider setting a specific amount of time to be dedicated to each item on the agenda. If you stick to the schedule, discussion will stay focused and you will be more likely to make it through the agenda. However, setting realistic times is critical to the success of this strategy.
* *Action agendas:* Consider submitting an agenda with a description of the needed or desired action, such as review proposals, approve minutes, or establish outcomes.

Keep the group on task. Use rules of order to facilitate meetings. Robert's Rules of Order (Robert, Evans, Honemann, et al., 2000) may seem overly structured; however, this structure is particularly helpful when diversity of opinion is likely or important. Specifically, these rules help the person chairing the meeting by setting limits on discussion and using a specific order of priorities to deal with concerns.

Keep minutes, and distribute them to participants. The minutes provide a record for reference if needed and convey contents to persons unable to attend.

Planning for the meeting is a group leader's best strategy for a satisfactory experience. Participants must also prepare for meetings. Reviewing the agenda (or requesting one in advance if not provided), reviewing preparatory materials, and thinking through agenda items are ways that group members may assist in accomplishing the meeting goals. Meeting participants should be on time for all meetings or communicate that they will be late or unable to attend. Participants should be prepared to leave on time as well. When a meeting is poorly chaired, a committee member could volunteer to ensure that the meeting agendas and minutes are distributed. It is important to recognize that some people deliberately avoid preparing agendas and distributing minutes in an attempt to control the meeting. Exercise 28-5 will help you understand the importance of well-run meetings.

EXERCISE 28-5

Have you ever sat in a meeting and wondered why you were there? Perhaps the purpose of the meeting, where the meeting was heading, or even who was in charge was unclear to you! Do the members often engage in lengthy discussion off of the main topic of discussion? Write down the three things about meetings you have attended that were most annoying, and then analyze how they could have been handled better.

CONCLUSION

Self-management is a means to achieve work–life balance, as well as a way of life to achieve personal goals within self-imposed priorities and deadlines. Time management is clock-oriented, and stress management is the control of external and internal stressors.

To achieve a balance in life and minimize stressors, nurses must learn to sit back and see their own personal "big picture" and examine their personal and professional goals. Personal priorities also must be established. Stressors and coping strategies need to be identified and used. By developing these techniques, nurses can gain a sense of control and become far better nurses in the process.

A SOLUTION

Denise sought advice from her co-workers, manager, and a counsellor on how to better handle stress. Denise feels that she handles the stress better than she used to. She takes better care of herself than she used to: she usually gets enough sleep; tries to eat a balanced diet; takes a multi-vitamin daily; exercises at least 15 to 30 minutes every other day; and tries not to procrastinate too much to avoid thinking about what she should be doing the whole time she is putting off doing it. Denise thinks becoming a part-time student has helped her be proactive with her to-do list.

Denise's partner is very supportive, and she has a good friend with whom she takes some exercise classes. She often takes herself out for lunch when work is becoming too stressful. She also meditates for 20 minutes each day and finds that doing so helps tremendously. Probably the most important thing she has learned to do is really be in the present moment. For example, when she plays with her kids or is out with friends, she does not fixate on happenings at work or

her next week's schedule. Denise has come to realize that how she handles stress is essential. She has learned that it is not the stress per se that can cause problems; it is her reaction to the stress that she must manage better. As a result, she has consciously reframed her thinking so that she only focuses on one thing at a time. Doing so has helped her reduce her stress level and be more productive because she is fully engaged in the task at hand. After completing a personal analysis of change exercise, Denise was able to create a list of stress-reduction strategies for different types of stressful events. She keeps this list on her smart phone so that she can quickly choose a strategy that will produce the greatest benefit in a particular situation.

Would this be a suitable approach for you? Why or why not?

THE EVIDENCE

Bogaert et al. (2010) investigated the impact of unit-level practice environment factors and burnout on nurse-assessed quality of care. A total of 546 staff nurses from four acute care hospitals were surveyed during the study, and the data were analyzed using a two-level random intercept model. The Nursing Work Index–Revised instrument was used to measure nurse practice environment dimensions, and the Maslach Burnout Inventory was used to measure burnout dimensions. The study found that emotional exhaustion is linked to job satisfaction, nurse turnover intentions, and assessed quality of care. The study concluded that widespread burnout merits special attention from all health care providers.

NEED TO KNOW NOW

- Choose to practise in an environment that works for you.
- Be alert to personal stress levels and how they affect your work.
- Create a list of stress management interventions that are helpful to you.
- Master information management skills.

CHAPTER CHECKLIST

Stress management and time management are two strategies for self-management. Balancing stress means caring for your emotional/spiritual, physical, and mental health needs. Delegating effectively, acquiring good information literacy skills, using schedules and calendars and other planners, using time-management principles, and managing meetings are key strategies to be integrated into the nurse leader role. By accomplishing self-management, managers, leaders, and followers will find themselves in control of work time and stressors, as well as more confident in achieving both personal and work-related goals. Effective leaders are responsible for creating an environment conducive to an excellent followership style (Gibbons & Bryant, 2013).

Stress and overwork are inherent in the nursing profession, and nurses can adapt and cope with stress and time pressures by learning effective ways to care for themselves and to manage time. By assessing and reducing specific stressors and time wasters, nurses

CHAPTER CHECKLIST—cont'd

can thrive in the health care challenges before them. Increasing skills in coping, organization, delegation, and effective time management is vital for effective leadership. A nurse manager who can be a role model and support his or her staff in turbulent times is a true leader.

- Self-management includes stress management, time management, and meeting management.
- Time management includes using tools and strategies to ensure that priority goals are achieved.

- Signs of excess stress must be heeded to prevent burnout or chronic health problems.
- Strategies to reduce stress include physical, mental, and emotional/spiritual approaches.
- Strategies to improve time management include identification of potential time wasters, use of time-management strategies, and appropriate delegation.
- Strategies to improve meeting management include effective organization, following an agenda, and using rules of order to facilitate the meeting.

TIPS FOR SELF-MANAGEMENT

- Know what your high-priority goals are, and use them to filter decisions.
- Know your personal response to stress, and self-evaluate frequently.
- Make your health a priority, and use strategies that keep yourself in control.

- Use organizational systems that meet your needs; the simpler, the better.
- Simplify.
- Refocus on your priorities whenever you begin to feel overwhelmed.

evolve WEBSITE

Visit the Evolve website for Suggested Readings, Internet Resources, and additional resources related to the content in this chapter: http://evolve.elsevier.com/Canada/Yoder-Wise/leading/.

REFERENCES

Applebaum, D., Fowler, S., Fiedler, N., et al. (2010). The impact of environmental factors on nursing stress, job satisfaction and turnover intention. *Journal of Nursing Administration, 40*(7/8), 323–328. doi:10.1097/NNA.0b013e3181e9393b

Badke, W. (2010). Why information literacy is invisible. *Communications in Information Literacy, 4*(2), 129–141.

Bailey, J. (2009). The challenge for today's nurse managers: How to be fiscally competent & efficient while nurturing the workforce and sustaining self. *Spinal Cord Injury, 29*(1), 25–28.

Beecroft, P. C., Dorey, F., & Wenten, M. (2008). Turnover intention in new graduate nurses: A multivariate analysis. *Journal of Advanced Nursing, 62*(1), 41–52. doi:10.1111/j.1365-2648.2007.04570.x

Belcik, K. (2007, July). *Information literacy: A pre-requisite to evidence-based nursing.* Paper presented at the 18th International Nursing Research Congress Focusing on Evidence-Based Practice. Vienna, Austria.

Bogaert, P., Clarke, S., Roelant, E., et al. (2010). Impacts of unit-level nurse practice environment and burnout on nurse reported outcomes: A multilevel model approach. *Journal of Clinical Nursing, 19*, 1664–1674. doi:10.1111/j.1365-2702.2009.03128.x

Bold, K. (2010, October). Stressing the positive. *ZotZine, 3*(2). Retrieved from http://zotzine.uci.edu/v03/2010_10/maddi.php.

Canadian Nurses Association. (n.d.). Competencies. Retrieved from http://cna-aiic.ca/en/becoming-an-rn/rn-exam/competencies.

Canadian Nurses Association. (2008). *Code of ethics for registered nurses (2008 centennial edition).* Toronto, ON: Author. http://www.cna-aiic.ca/~/media/cna/files/en/codeofethics.pdf.

Canadian Nurses Association. (2011). *2009 workforce profile of registered nurses in Canada.* Ottawa, ON: Author.

Complain. (2004). In K. Barber (Ed.), *Canadian Oxford Dictionary* (2nd ed.). Don Mills, ON: Oxford University Press.

Covey, S. R., Merrill, A. R., & Merrill, R. R. (1994). *First things first: To love, to learn, to leave a legacy.* New York, NY: Simon & Schuster.

Garrosa, E., Moreno-Jimenez, B., Rodriguez-Munoz, A., et al. (2011). Role stress and personal resources in nursing: A cross-sectional study of burnout and engagement. *International Journal of Nursing Studies, 48*, 479–489. doi:10.1016/j.ijnurstu.2010.08.004

Gibbons, A., & Bryant, D. (2013). Followership: The forgotten part of leadership. *Casebook, 21*(2), 12–13.

Guimond-Plourde, R. (2011). Stress care: Turning failure into triumph. *Canadian Nurse, 107*(1), 16–17.

Hargrove, M. B., Quick, J. C., Nelson, D. L., et al. (2011). The theory of preventative stress management: A 33-year review and evaluation. *Stress and Health, 27,* 182–193. doi:10.1002/smi.1417

LaMontagne, A. D., Keegel, T., Louie, A. M., et al. (2007). A systematic review of the job stress intervention evaluation literature: 1990–2005. *International Journal of Occupational and Environmental Health, 13*(3), 268–280.

Laschinger, H. K. S., Finegan, J., & Wilk, P. (2009). New graduate burnout: The impact of professional practice environment, workplace civility and empowerment. *Nursing Economic$, 27*(6), 377–383.

Lavoie-Tremblay, M., Leclerc, E., Marchionni, C., et al. (2010). The needs and expectations of generation Y nurses in the workplace. *Journal for Nurses in Staff Development, 26,* 2–8. doi:10.1097/NND.0b013e3181d21115

Limm, H., Gundel, H., Heinmuller, M., et al. (2011). Stress management interventions in the workplace improve stress reactivity: A randomised controlled trial. *Occupational and Environmental Medicine, 68,* 126–133. doi:10.1136/oem.2009.054148

Maddi, S. (2013). *Hardiness: Turning stressful circumstances into resilient growth.* New York, NY: Springer. doi:10.1007/978-94-007-5222-1_3

Maslach, C., & Jackson, S. E. (1981). *Maslach Burnout Inventory manual.* Palo Alto, CA: Consulting Psychologists Press.

Maslach, C., & Leiter, M. (2008). Early predictors of job burnout and engagement. *Journal of Applied Psychology, 93,* 498–512. doi:10.1037/0021-9010.93.3.498

Maslach, C., Schaufeli, W., & Leiter, M. (2000). Job burnout. *Annual Review of Psychology, 52,* 397–422. doi:10.1146/annurev.psych.52.1.397

Nash, S. (2009). *Stress, hardiness and leadership style: An examination of factors that foster nurse manager survival in the healthcare environment* (Unpublished master's thesis). San Diego State University, San Diego, CA. Retrieved from http://www.leadershipchallenge.com/Research-section-Others-Research-Detail/abstract-nash--stress-hardiness-and-leadership-style.aspx.

Perfectionism. (2004). In K. Barber (Ed.), *Canadian Oxford Dictionary* (2nd ed.). Don Mills, ON: Oxford University Press.

Pipe, T. B., Bortz, J. J., Dueck, A., et al. (2009). Nurse leader mindfulness meditation program for stress management: A randomized controlled trial. *Journal of Nursing Administration, 39,* 130–137. doi:10.1097/NNA.0b013e31819894a0

Poghosyan, L., Clarke, S. P., Finlayson, M., et al. (2010). Nurse burnout and quality of care: Cross-national investigation in six countries. *Research in Nursing and Health, 33,* 288–298. doi:10.1002/nur.20383

Post, G. (2010, August 30). Tend and befriend behavior in women. *Women's Issues.* Retrieved from http://www.goodtherapy.org/blog/women-stress-social-relationships-psychology/.

Rice, V. (Ed.). (2013). *Handbook of stress, coping and health* (2nd ed.). Washington, DC: Sage.

Ritter, D. (2011). The relationship between healthy work environments and retention of nurses in a hospital setting. *Journal of Nursing Management, 19,* 27–32. doi:10.1111/j.1365-2834.2010.01183.x

Robert, H., Evans, W., Honemann, D. H., et al. (Eds.). (2000). *Robert's rules of order newly revised.* Cambridge, MA: Perseus Book Group.

Rochlen, A., Good, G., & Carver, T. (2009). Predictors of gender-related barriers, work and life satisfaction among men in nursing. *Psychology of Men and Masculinity, 10,* 44–56. doi:10.1037/a0013291

Roy, C. (2008). *The Roy adaptation model* (3rd ed.). Upper Saddle River, NJ: Pearson-Prentice Hall.

Selye, H. (1956). *The stress of life.* New York, NY: McGraw-Hill.

Selye, H. (1965). The stress syndrome. *American Journal of Nursing, 65*(3), 97–99.

Shirey, M., McDaniel, A., Ebright, P., et al. (2010). Understanding nurse manager stress and work complexity. *Journal of Nursing Administration, 40*(2), 82–91.

Stuart, G. W., & Laraia, M. T. (2008). Self-modification assistance. In G. M. Bulechek, H. K. Butcher, & J. M. Dochterman (Eds.), *Nursing interventions classifications* (5th ed., pp. 644–645). St. Louis, MO: Mosby.

Taylor, S. E., Klein, L. C., Lewis, B. P., et al. (2000). Biobehavioral responses to stress in females: Tend-and-befriend, not fight-or-flight. *Psychological Review, 107,* 411–429.

Teng, C.-I., Hsiao, F.-J., & Chou, T.-A. (2010). Nurse-perceived time pressure and patient-perceived care quality. *Journal of Nursing Management, 18,* 275–284. doi:10.1111/j.1365-2834.2010.01073.x

Understanding the stress response. (2011). *Harvard Mental Health Letter, 27*(9), 4–6. Retrieved from http://www.health.harvard.edu.

Unruh, L., & Zhang, N. (2013). The role of work environment in keeping newly licensed RNs in nursing: A questionnaire survey. *International Journal of Nursing Studies, 50*(12), 1678–1688. doi:10.1016/j.ijnurstu.2013.04.002

Vohs, K. D., Redden, J. D., & Rahinel, R. (2013, August 6). Physical order produces healthy choices, generosity, and conventionality, whereas disorder produces creativity. *Psychological Science.* doi:10.1177/0956797613480186

Wang, X., Kunaviktikul, W., & Wichaikhum, O. A. (2013). Work empowerment and burnout among registered nurses in two tertiary general hospitals. *Journal of Clinical Nursing, 22*(19–20), 2896–2903. doi:10.1111/jocn.12083

Watson, S., Goh, Y., & Sawang, S. (2011) Gender influences on the work-related stress-coping process. *Journal of Individual Differences, 32*(1), 39–46. doi:10.1027/1614-0001/a000033

Wodak, R., Kwon, W., & Clarke, I. (2011). Getting people on board: Discursive leadership for consensus building in team meetings. *Discourse Society, 22,* 592. doi:10.1177/0957926511405410

Wolf, G., Triolo, P., & Ponte, P. (2008). Magnet recognition program: The next generation. *Journal of Nursing Administration, 38,* 200–204. doi:10.1097/01.NNA.0000312759.14536.a9

Wu, H., Chi, T. S., Chen, L., et al. (2010). Occupational stress among hospital nurses: Cross-sectional survey. *Journal of Advanced Nursing, 66,* 627–634. doi:10.1111/j.1365-2648.2009.05203.x

Zangaro, G. A., & Soeken, K. L. (2007). A meta-analysis of studies of nurse's job satisfaction. *Research in Nursing & Health, 30,* 445–458. doi:10.1002/nur.20202

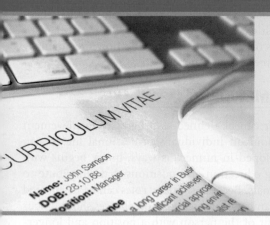

Managing Your Career

Debra Hagler
Adapted by Lyle G. Grant and Sarah E. Hanson

Successful people actively manage their careers rather than wait for "lucky breaks." Although trusted others may guide or influence career development, every individual must manage his or her own career. This chapter considers tools to document accomplishments and ways to extend career development beyond the work setting. Continuous lifelong learning and the ability to demonstrate and document competency are critical elements in effective career management.

OBJECTIVES

- Differentiate among career styles and how they influence career options.
- Analyze person–position fit.
- Develop a cover letter and résumé targeted for a specific position.
- Understand the critical elements of an interview.
- Be aware of the variety of professional development activities available to nurses, including academic and continuing education programs.
- Identify the contributions you could make and the benefits you could derive from active involvement in professional associations.

TERMS TO KNOW

career	curriculum vitae (CV)	professional association
certification	licensure	résumé
continuing education	portfolio	

❓ A CHALLENGE

Anne Marie has been nursing for 7 years on a rehabilitation unit. She recently completed her MScN and accepted a promotion to team leader of her unit. While she was excited about the leadership potential of this role, she was not prepared for some of the reactions and experiences that occurred over the first 3 months. She is amazed by how much of her time is taken up with paperwork, meetings, and trying to navigate through interdepartmental "mazes" as she tries to promote change. Also, no one told her how uncomfortable it would be addressing performance issues with nurses that "used to be" her friends.

Lately, Anne Marie has been coming home at the end of the day feeling discouraged, exhausted, missing direct patient care, and wondering if she made the right decision in accepting a formal leadership role.

If you were Anne Marie, what might you do in this situation? Who might you turn to for advice? What support or information might you seek?

INTRODUCTION

The number of career options and paths within nursing is staggering. Some of these options are the "traditional" and highly valued roles nurses have performed for years—providing direct care to patients, leading teams or organizations, teaching, researching, providing public health or school health services, or working in an occupational field. Other options have emerged over the past decade, and new options continue to emerge. Career choices include working with philanthropic organizations or insurance companies, working as a pharmaceutical company representative, assessing disability claims for government agencies, providing counselling, and taking on a political role. However, with career choices come challenges: how best to build a career, which education best serves the role, which experiences best prepare nurses for a specific field or role, and what new activities and roles need to be developed. Because a career extends over a lifetime and because nursing is defined by the discipline and by law, not by employing organizations, making choices can redirect a nurse's future. Some options build primarily on experience and others on education and experience; all, however, require that a nurse

engage in professional development and continue to advanced expertise to meet evolving challenges in health care. How nurses reach their career goals depends on the goals they set and how they manage their career development.

A FRAMEWORK

A career can be defined as progressive achievement throughout an individual's professional life. It can be developed in numerous ways, but it begins with selecting education and positions that contribute to career goals. Because so many roles can be performed in the name of nursing, position choices should focus on the fit of the person with a position and longer-term career goals. A good fit is built on strong, similar goals, and tolerable (or growth-producing) differences. The whole of any work situation comprises two elements—the person and position—interacting in an environment in which other elements influence both. The whole is symbolized by blending a person's talents with a position's expectations to create the productive whole. Analyzing positions and the required skills in light of individual talents can help applicants determine positions that fit with their strengths and define gaps to be addressed. When gaps occur, skills development might be needed to form a fit, or the position may not be a good fit (Center for Creative Leadership, 2010).

The person–position fit and how that fit evolves throughout a career are critical considerations in appreciating positions held throughout a career. Thus, when considering a career path, such as practitioner or administrator or educator, the person needs to recall prior positions held and the aspects of those positions that were most rewarding. As an example, if a nurse held multiple positions and then determined that the teaching and learning opportunities were the most rewarding aspects, the career plan of educator might emerge. Whatever career is pursued, key strategies include goal setting and planning to obtain the right education and experiences.

Different generations may view work, positions, and careers differently, yet many similarities exist across generations. For example, Deal (2007) reported that all generations prefer face-to-face coaching. Younger generations, however, seek more frequent feedback than do older generations.

In addition, Deal reported that almost everyone surveyed wanted to learn and thought learning was important. Learning was related to the work the person needed to do in the position, not to the generational group in which he or she was categorized. An important finding was related to the stereotype of younger generations wanting to learn everything via a computer; that was a wrong assumption. The key to applying these points about coaching and learning is that leaders and managers must listen to others to learn what others want and need. This strategy can apply to career development as well. Listening to what individuals tell others about their own interests and strengths can help them identify appropriate resources for personal and professional development and for creating effective networks. Speaking up and listening carefully are important skills that every nurse can use in being successful in a position and in pursuing a career path.

Another way to think about career development is to consider the work of Citrin and Smith (2003), who studied "extraordinary" careers. They identified three broad career phases: *promise*, *momentum*, and *harvest*. The names of these phases suggest progression from early to late career. Early in one's career, the focus is on developing skills, establishing credentials, and socializing into the role. Mid-career, the focus often shifts to honing specific areas of expertise (the things by which we will be known) and being more aware of the fit of positions within the broad array of opportunities that will enhance some goal. Finally, in a later career stage, many individuals focus on the profession (the broad view of the work) and how to leave it better off as a result of being a member of the profession. This movement through nursing life is predicated on having a vision of a career as opposed to a series of jobs.

Finally, Friss (1989) looks at careers from the perspective of career styles (Table 29-1). She describes four different career styles, with one being no better than another. *Steady state* (positional plateau) careers describe those individuals who select a role and stay in that role throughout their career. This type of career style is common in rural settings and for those individuals who commit their working life to a positional category such as staff nurse, clinic nurse, or nurse practitioner. The focus of this career style is to become increasingly competent in the role and

clinical area. *Linear* careers are those that represent vertical movement in the organizational hierarchy. This movement often creates more organizational knowledge and a more diversified view of what comprises nursing. This movement is characterized by changes in title; for example, moving from staff nurse to nurse manager to director represents this kind of career style. *Entrepreneurial and transient* style is appealing to nurses who wish to "see the world" or have a creative bent. The final style, *spiral*, focuses on one's career movement in and out and up and down. For example, nurses who move from within an organization as a staff nurse to nurse manager at another organization, then move in that organization to a nursing director role, and later leave for another opportunity exemplify this style.

It would be easy to label nurses' careers if they could each be described by a single style; however, the fluidity of the profession allows nurses to switch foci along a career path to gain a specific experience or meet a personal need. This dynamic suggests that it is difficult at best to label a nurse's style, career category, or generational attributes. The same dynamic makes leading and managing a group of nurses a challenge and provides for great diversity to meet organizational needs and nurses' career goals. The best opportunity for nurses to manage their careers and for a nurse manager to help nurses gain important experiences is for the individuals to know themselves.

Knowing Yourself

Being a professional holds both privileges and obligations. The legal privileges and expectations are codified in provincial or territorial nursing registration acts, regulations, and nursing practice standards and professional standards. These codified expectations are baseline (i.e., minimum) expectations of professional behaviour necessary for licensure (a right granted that gives the licensee permission to do something that he or she could not legally do absent of such permission) or registration and do not fully express expectations of leadership in improving the health of individuals and communities. The profession, through various professional associations, embraces the expectation that nurses will belong to professional associations and provide leadership in improving communities. For example, the International Council of Nurses has recognized

TABLE 29-1   CAREER STYLES

	EXAMPLE	DESCRIPTION	MOTIVATION AND CHARACTERISTICS	MANAGERIAL CONSIDERATIONS
Steady State	Staff nurse	Constancy in position with increasing professional skill	Increasing expertise High professional identity Obligation to serve Maintenance of standards Autonomy in performance of care Preference for action Personal accountability The work itself Stability	Hold work in high esteem Decentralize Use and recognize abilities Provide feedback about patient outcomes Reward competence and tenure Provide continuing education Provide permanent assignment
Linear	Nursing service administrator	Hierarchical orientation with steady climb	Requisite authority and power A challenging first job Guidance by internalized norms Money Recognition Opportunities for self-development	Provide management development Reward and value both education and competence Modify management selection and development systems Provide decreasing supervision
Entrepreneurial and transient	Nurse in private practice; nurse in temporary assignments	Desire to create new service; meeting own priorities	Limited organizational commitment Opportunism Novelty or creativity Other people Achievement	Use flexibility to organization's benefit Avoid burdening nurse with organizational and practice decisions Provide immediate feedback
Spiral	Nurse who returns after raising a family	Rational, independent responsibility for shaping career	Novelty Prestige Intense period of employment followed by nonemployment or a different employment Care for others Opportunities for self-development Typically well paid, service-oriented Recognition	Configure specific job that needs doing Be flexible about terms and length of commitment Find challenging initial assignment Negotiate Encourage creativity

Data from Friss, L. (1989). Strategic management of nurses: A policy oriented approach. Owings Mills, MD: AUPHA Press.

both the need and importance of nurses in shaping necessary health reforms through effective leadership and management roles by developing the Leadership for Change™ program (http://www.icn.ch/pillarsprograms/leadership-for-change/). Nurses also assume responsibility to provide services in the public interest as part of licensure or registration privileges. This creates responsibility to communities, other health care providers, and individuals that require nurses to assume leadership roles of varying types that may alter over time and with the circumstances. The challenge, of course, is how to incorporate leadership development and community leadership activities into a busy, committed life! It is often those "additional" activities and interests that enrich a career and provide for invaluable insight into clinical and professional issues. Knowing what is important to you, what is valued by both yourself and the organization, and the commitment needed form the basis for understanding one's self. It is also beneficial to understand your own goal orientation. The role of goal orientation in leadership development is considered in the Literature Perspective.

📖 LITERATURE PERSPECTIVE

Resource: DeGeest, D., & Brown, K. G. (2011). The role of goal orientation in leadership development. *Human Resource Development Quarterly, 22* (2). http://dx.doi.org/10.1002/hrdq.20072

Effective leaders and managers learn leadership competencies (e.g., knowledge, skills, and judgement). Job assignments can provide valuable workplace experiences that contribute to developing these competencies. Questions arise about why similar work experiences produce different leadership skills development in individuals. Goal orientation is likely an important factor. Goal orientation can be understood under theoretical constructs related to personal motivation of mastery or learning and achievement relative to others. Researchers constructed a model linking goal orientation to situational and an individual's characteristics to help explain the differential impact of situational learning on leadership development. Yet to be empirically tested, their theoretical framework lays the groundwork for such testing and for determining how important goal orientation may be to experiential learning of leadership skills. There is reason to believe that enhanced goal orientation improves leadership knowledge and skills building.

Implications for Practice

Goal orientation affects how managers develop leadership skills from experience. Moreover, individual and situational factors influence managers' experiential learning. The model proposed by the authors suggests how situations can be modified to enhance learning from work experiences.

Whether positions are plentiful or scarce, knowing one's self can focus the available work or selection process toward capitalizing on one's strengths. Even assessing one's strengths through a formal avenue (e.g., StrengthsFinder 2.0 at http://strengths.gallup.com/110659/Homepage.aspx or Buckingham's [2008] *The Truth About You: Your Secret to Success*) can provide insight. Therefore, the first steps in creating a person–position fit rests in understanding the person involved. Throughout schooling and during the initial experiences in nursing, insight begins to evolve that helps each of us determine our preferences for our life work. It is not that some positions are valueless; rather, it is that some positions add more to what we want to be able to achieve in the long term than other positions. As an example, any position that offers educational compensation or flexible scheduling might work well for the short term if the goal is to return to school and complete advanced education for a specialized role.

EXERCISE 29-1

Think about what you believe you should be doing in a career and what motivates you. Do you require movement to new types of challenges and learning, or do you value consistency and security? Do you like variety in your work, or do you value specialty skills to become an expert? Would you like to rapidly move upward in responsibility, or would you prefer to broaden your skills and knowledge base? How does thinking about these questions help you recognize your career style (Table 29-1)?

Being able to describe yourself from various perspectives is useful. First, knowing your strengths tells you what you bring to a position and on what you can rely. When you know your strengths, you can say what they are in a succinct manner and use them as a filter in reading position descriptions to find your fit and to learn the organizational language. An analysis of your competencies allows you to see what work needs to be done to meet required or desired standards and competencies. Finally, entering into such analyses can help you see the bigger picture of your career and how what you can learn from a particular position might contribute to your overall goals. The career styles described in Table 29-1 include the motivation and characteristics of each style. Seeing how your self-analysis fits with the descriptors in the third column may suggest how you see yourself approaching your career. The goal of all this work is to know yourself well so that your pursuit of a position or career path fits you and your strengths.

Knowing the Position

Few people assume a nursing or leadership position and remain in that position forever. Exceptions occur in rural areas and in highly specialized positions. Thus most nurses hold more than one position throughout their work life. Those positions can be selected by chance or by plan. Chance positions should not be ignored, but they should be evaluated in light of career goals and an assessment of the position and the organization. Managing a career actively allows for these chance opportunities to enrich a career rather than detract from it. Can a position contribute to increased skills and competencies? Does a position have the potential to recast one's professional profile so that others see the potential for greater contributions? Are the benefits of the position so enticing that they offset limitations of the position itself? These are the kinds of questions to ask yourself when considering a particular position.

Position assessment begins with understanding the basics of the organization and its vision and mission (see also Chapter 9 to improve understanding of organizations). Assessment also requires finding out specifics of the position, which may be available only through an interview. Bolles (2009) points out that most managers look first within the organization to promote someone rather than looking broadly at the talent available. This is in contrast to how many people seek jobs; they look broadly first. So one key strategy to use is selecting an organization where you want to work, even if the position is not exactly the right one. The potential for inside connections and networking, in addition to knowledge about management styles in the organization and future position openings, can lead you to the position that is the right fit for you.

CAREER DEVELOPMENT

A career extends beyond employment positions. A career includes the various ways in which an individual engages in activities that provide care to patients, support that care, educate for that care, support the providers of that care, study the ways in which to deliver the care, and engage in the broader perspective of professional and community service. Thinking broadly about a career in a rapidly changing field such as health care is critical to remaining competent and relevant.

In today's rapidly changing society, a position that was once "a fit" may no longer work. The position may have evolved as much as the person did. If the movement was in harmony, the fit remains, but if the position changes one way and the person another, the fit devolves.

Bolles (2009) also suggests that there are life-changing positions. These can best be described as changing positions and fields simultaneously (such as may occur with a spiral career style). For example, when a charge nurse in a critical care unit assumes the role of a chief nursing officer in a rural community hospital, a major shift has occurred. Nurses who follow a spiral career path, especially if they are second-career students (having a degree in another field or a career prior to nursing), may also experience this phenomenon. These individuals may have worked in another field and now are pursuing their passion. They may have become bored with a prior career that had few interactions with people, or they may have studied in fields such as science and realized that the best application

of knowledge could occur in patient care. Because of prior career successes, these individuals may craft career patterns that appear very different from the majority of the profession: they are using talents from two fields and are trying to capitalize on both.

Core career development strategies are important to success. Selecting professional peers and mentors to share in your development is crucial to gaining good, ongoing advice. Some important aspects of mentorship related to leadership were introduced in Chapter 3. Having a few well-chosen peers, mentors, and role models who respond openly from various perspectives can enrich career planning and development.

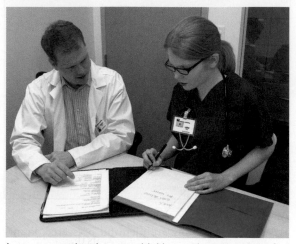

A mentor can inspire new thinking and new opportunities and steer you toward various roles and clinical areas.

EXERCISE 29-2

Think about an experienced nurse who serves as a role model to you. Would you want that person as a mentor? If so, consider how you would enlist that person's assistance in moulding your career.

Table 29-2 defines six key aspects of creating and managing a career. Although each aspect is important, one aspect that can be most useful to consider is the "who"—the mentor you choose. That person can inspire new thinking and new opportunities and steer you to various roles and clinical areas. That person can also create connections for you and help guide decisions related to timing and context. Mentors might even be able to create opportunities for you to test new

TABLE 29-2 **KEY ASPECTS OF CREATING AND MANAGING A CAREER**

Who	Mentor
What	Role and clinical options
When	"Timing is everything"; always remain open to opportunities; don't leave in the middle of a critical project
Where	Local or not; inpatient or outpatient
How	Proactive; your search is your job
Why	Seeking challenge and testing out ideas

approaches to clinical care or to new aspects of a position you thought of as boring.

CAREER MARKETING STRATEGIES

Even the steady-state or experienced nurse who is not seeking a new position needs to have a curriculum vitae (CV) or résumé that documents continued development of expertise. Interviewing, which is a two-way process, also contributes to successful position choices and career development.

Although professional data can be recorded in numerous ways, most people are not systematic about it. Therefore, when information about one's career is needed quickly, it is difficult to recall and then to hone the most pertinent information for a position. A goal of this chapter is to develop a systematic strategy for creating marketing documents that you can use throughout your professional career. Some organizations use an electronic form of professional records so that an individual can readily access and convert the information into various documents. The Canadian Nurses Association provides such a service through its NurseONE website (http://www.nurseone.ca—create an account to get started). Many position searches, even those internal to an organization, begin with a résumé. The key is to make information distinctive in telling your professional story and in establishing the appearance of a competent professional.

Data Collection

Depending on your unique background, the extent of data collection varies considerably. The first step is to collect all your professional career information. If you are fairly new in the profession, analyze anything special you did in school, such as electives, offices held, and special assignments, honours, and recognitions. If you are a second-career nurse, consider your previous work and how it relates to your profession now. If you have an employment history, start with your nursing positions. Include relevant information from volunteer roles, which can illustrate skills such as leadership, ability to balance budgets, communication, and political astuteness as well as professional commitment.

To begin data collection, begin with where you are and think back. If you have short experience or no difficulty recalling details, you are in great shape to start a systematic plan. If, however, you have a long history as a nurse or a prior relevant career, your task is more challenging because you have to actively think about what you did in the past and, for a prior career, determine how to translate those experiences into relevance for nursing. The important aspect of this phase is to begin the process and to save it electronically so that you can shape information for specific reasons using a cut-and-paste technique rather than creating an original document each time you need to provide information about yourself.

Compile as many facts as possible for each of the ten categories identified in Table 29-3. Even if you have no entry for a specific category, retain the heading as a reminder and think about what you would like to be able to list there in the future. If you do not have regular access to a computer, at least keep the information on a USB flash drive or a DVD so that you do not need to recreate it the next time. This is your private data bank for information to list on a curriculum vitae or to select for a résumé.

EXERCISE 29-3

Draft entries for your data bank. Using that information, go to the *Evolve* website (http://evolve.elsevier.com/Canada/Yoder-Wise/leading/) and refer to the supplied examples to draft a CV and a résumé for a position you are seeking. As a checkpoint for yourself, make a list of four or five key strengths or facts that you want others to know. Be sure they are listed in your CV and described in your résumé. Save the list for preparing for interviews.

Curriculum Vitae

A **curriculum vitae (CV)** is the documentation of one's professional life. It is designed to be all-inclusive and may be lengthy. A CV follows some designated flow

TABLE 29-3	DATA COLLECTION

TOPICS	FACTS NEEDED
1. Education	Name of school, address, phone numbers, website address, years of attendance, date of graduation, name of degree(s) received, minor earned, honours received (e.g., Dean's List)
2. Continuing education	Dates attended, academic institutions, topics and any special outcomes, type and amount of credit earned
3. Experience	Dates of employment, title of position, name of employer, location and phone numbers, website address, name of chief executive officer, chief nursing officer, immediate supervisor, typical duties (role description)
4. Community or institutional service	Dates of service, name of committee or task force and the parent organization (e.g., name of hospital or professional association), your role on the committee (e.g., chairperson, secretary, member), general description of committee's functions, any unique accomplishments
5. Publications	Articles: author(s) name(s), year of publication, title, journal, volume, issue, pages; books: author(s), year of publication, title, location, and name of publisher
6. Honours and awards	Date, description of award, special factors related to award (e.g., competitive, community-wide, national)
7. Research and funding awards	Date, title of research, role in research (e.g., principal investigator, co-investigator, team member), funded or unfunded; include related funding awards, source, and amounts
8. Speeches or presentations contributed to or given	Date, title of speech presented, place, name of sponsoring organization, nature of the presentation (e.g., keynote, concurrent session), your honorarium, indication of presenters (e.g., underlining indicates presenter)
9. Workshops or conferences presented	Date, title of workshop or conference presented, place, name of sponsoring group and nature of the presentation, brief description of the activity, your honorarium
10. Certification	Initial date of certification, expiration date, certifying body, area, and type of certification

of information reflective of the ten categories identified in Table 29-3. However, empty categories are not listed on a CV. A CV is often used to support academic or research positions and is an important record or portfolio summary.

Typically, a CV begins with your name and contact information. Your contact information should include address with postal code; phone numbers designated by work, home, and cell; fax number; e-mail address; and, if you have one, a website address. Use an e-mail account with a professional name and avoid usernames that are overly casual such as "sweetiepie@domain.com" or those that provide personal information such as "crabbynurse@domain.com." Centre the contact information on the CV or place a dividing line under it to help a prospective employer quickly locate that information. Information in the body of the CV should be presented in *reverse chronological order*. This approach allows a prospective employer to find the most recent (and, theoretically, most relevant) information quickly. By drawing attention to your most recent accomplishments, you give the reader a sense of where you are in your career.

> **EXERCISE 29-4**
> Create a CV from your data. Define a plan to keep your CV current, such as copying data facts from your collection system onto the CV each time you enter data into your files.

Résumé

A **résumé** is a customized document that presents the qualifications of an individual for a specific organizational position. Unlike a CV, a résumé allows more stylistic freedom. It is presented in sentences or phrases (not both) to share the value of the information. For example, rather than listing years of service in a position by title and organization, a résumé might include information that you served as the only nurse to provide some distinctive service. For the experienced nurse, a résumé could be used to reflect increasing skills and abilities; for the new nurse, it could focus on specific "extra" abilities (e.g., competencies) that are not normally expected of a new graduate.

The résumé is a better choice than a CV for advertising your skills, competencies, and talents to a prospective employer. Because a résumé is brief (typically no more than two pages) and tailored to the position being sought, the information is pointed toward specific position requirements. Details and action words help the reader view you as accomplishing work. Verbs that relate to outcomes (e.g., *produced, created*) are most powerful. Fox (2006) suggested that the purpose of the résumé is to elaborate on what you said during an interview, but often the interviewer will have read your résumé as a basis for scheduling the interview. Either way, it is a good idea to arrive for an interview with a copy of your résumé as a reminder of your capabilities. Bringing a résumé to an interview is especially useful if you were asked previously to provide a CV. This additional work of applying your talents to the specific position in the résumé helps the interviewer see how you would fit in the organization.

There are two basic ways to develop a résumé. One is *conventional*, and it provides information by positions and activities. The other approach is *functional*, and it combines multiple positions into role areas you are trying to highlight. So, rather than using "experience" as a heading (as in a conventional résumé), the functional résumé heading may relate to writing or patient education and describe how you achieved results across several positions. A functional approach is best if you are planning a sharp departure from your present position or if you have considerable experience before entering nursing. The focus is on experience in diverse roles or positions rather than the specific positions held.

As with the CV, your résumé should be error-free and grammatically correct, accurate, and logical. Both of these documents should be printed on high-quality paper, preferably 100% cotton bond. Electronic résumés are best sent as attachments in a PDF or commonly used image file like JPG so that they can easily be opened by the user and no distortion in the design or layout can occur.

Along with an electronic résumé, nurses and other professionals are creating e-portfolios, an electronic collection of a **portfolio** (a professional assemblage of materials that represent the work of the professional) that includes work samples or competencies acquisition. (Portfolios are discussed further, later in the chapter.) E-portfolios can include course work, multimedia, blog entries, and images, all organized to highlight your skills and competencies. The advantage of an e-portfolio is that it can be digitally attached to your résumé or brought on a USB flash drive or a DVD to prospective employers for them to

view. Should you decide to compile an e-portfolio, the following website provides guidelines on how to do so: http://slisweb.sjsu.edu/career-development/using-eportfolio-job-search/why-use-eportfolio. Keep in mind that an e-portfolio will utilize many of the same headings used for your résumé or CV (see Table 29-3) and can be modified to meet the requirements of the position or purpose for which you are writing.

Many nurses use professional social networking sites to communicate with others in the profession. While such social networking sites are useful and can connect you to others in your field, in order to be effective, your profile must remain active and current. Other professionals familiar with your profile may even point you toward job openings. It is important to remember, however, that your online profile is not a substitute for a complete job application. Some people simply try to link their online social network profile to a job posting only to be disappointed when busy executives and hiring committees pass by these applicants in favour of those who have appropriately provided a detailed résumé, application, and cover letter.

EXERCISE 29-5

Draft statements you could use in a résumé (conventional or functional, whichever would best serve your purpose) to describe one of your strengths or best outcomes. Consider whether you are expressing accomplishments, skills, and competencies of relevance to prospective employers of choice.

Professional Writing

During your career, you will need to communicate effectively through written communications including letters and electronic media like e-mails. Every written communication says something about you as a professional. The commonly used letters are a cover letter, a thank-you letter, and a resignation letter. You may also write letters declining positions that you have been offered or recommending others for positions.

All of these types of letters include your name and contact information and should match the comparable contact information on your résumé and CV. This is especially important for the cover letter because it accompanies another document. The same quality paper should be used for letters as is used for the CV and résumé. If any of these documents are sent by e-mail or fax, you may still choose to send a hard copy.

These letters should be no longer than one page. The date and an inside address with the name (and credentials) of the addressee, the person's title, the name of the organization, street address, city, province or territory, and postal code should be included. The next area of the letter is the greeting. The typical salutation (greeting) (e.g., "Dear Ms. Smith") is followed by a colon or comma. The end of the letter (closing) allows sufficient space for signing your name between the formal closing (e.g., *Sincerely*) and your printed name followed by credentials. If your address did not appear at the top of the letter, it should appear below your typed name. Between the greeting and the closing are paragraphs conveying the letter's main message. You may optionally include a reference line between the greeting and your first paragraph that may start with a "RE:" that clearly identifies the employment position and competition number, if any, to which you are applying. This line should be highlighted through bolding and underlining. As with all formal documents, the letters should be proofread for layout, typographical errors, spelling, and content. E-mail communication contains essentially the same information, although no inside address is used. A discussion of each of the major types of letter follows.

Cover Letter. The cover letter is your introduction to a prospective employer and key to getting your CV or résumé read. A cover letter is a brief and carefully written document that includes why you are writing, why you "fit" the position, and invites follow-up. Sometimes you will be asked to include specific details in your covering letter as part of the application processes, so do not forget to include these.

Numerous positions may be advertised by an organization simultaneously in multiple formats and media. Thus, immediately stating which position interests you and how you learned of it is helpful. Once you have stated your reason for writing, you should address the issue of "why you."

The second paragraph should indicate why someone should take time to read your attached résumé. This section should state how you see yourself fitting with the organization (by experience, by philosophy, by clinical focus, and so forth). Two or three examples are helpful to provide the details of any general statements. Be sure to address how you meet key qualifications highlighted as required in the advertisement. It is

also appropriate to refer to the attachment of your CV or résumé based on what the organization requested.

The final paragraph should convey your optimism—you anticipate being interviewed and restate the best method of contacting you for follow-up.

EXERCISE 29-6

Write a cover letter that highlights information from at least two items from your data bank. Select items that best market you and that will entice the reader to call you for an interview. For an example of a cover letter, go to the *Evolve* website (http://evolve.elsevier.com/Canada/Yoder-Wise/leading/)

Thank-You Letter or Note. The written thank-you letter or note is underutilized and can be a powerful business and professional tool that helps propel your career. Writing a thank-you letter after an interview is a good place to start. The business format described earlier can be used for a formal thank-you letter, expressing appreciation for the opportunity that you had to interview. A more personal approach is to hand-write a brief thank-you note. The thank-you letter is your last chance to provide information about your communication skills and values at this point in the process. A quick e-mail message to acknowledge the interview is not sufficient; if you send an immediate e-mail, a formal letter or note should follow.

The content should be brief and the lead paragraph of the thank-you letter may help the interviewer recall your interview. Identify which position you are seeking and perhaps a key statement that you discussed during the interview. If you discussed multiple positions, you should identify which of those positions most interested you. The next paragraph should reiterate one of your strengths and what you found most interesting in the interview. This paragraph could also answer any question that was left unanswered during the interview.

The closing paragraph should reference specific times when you expect to hear about the interview outcomes and confirm any follow-up you were expected to make. If you decided the position was not a fit, you should thank the person for the time devoted to the interview and wish him or her success in seeking the best candidate. Even the worst interview should be followed by a thank-you letter expressing your appreciation for the interviewer's taking time to talk with you and sending the organization your best wishes for the future. These actions create a positive impression both for the present and for future interactions. Finally, if the position is offered to you, another thank-you letter is appropriate and might include a statement related to your excitement about joining the organization, the date you expect to transition, and any key agreements that were made verbally but that are not yet in writing.

Resignation Letter. When you secure a new position, it is essential to resign effectively from your current position. Occasionally this is not applicable—for example, if you are transitioning from a student role or if you were terminated or laid off. Otherwise, being polite and diplomatic in your resignation process keeps communications open with your current employer so that you could return or seek support from the colleagues you left behind. The best approach to resigning is having a personal meeting with your manager and indicating that you will provide a formal letter of resignation. Your resignation should be given with adequate notice, which depends on your conditions of employment. Being flexible in your resignation date and negotiating that date with your manager creates a positive exit strategy. Do not show up at the last minute thrusting a hastily written note to your supervisor. Make an appointment and discuss your rationale for leaving and give some indication of what you have appreciated about the current position. Remember, how you leave a position speaks to your professionalism. Even if you are not planning to use your current boss as a reference, this does not mean that he or she may not speak casually to those in the unit or organization to which you are applying, and you want these discussions to reflect well on you.

The letter of resignation follows the format guidelines described for other professional letters and begins with an acknowledgement of your intent to resign. Your date of resignation should be stated, and you might include whether this date is negotiable. This paragraph should also reference the verbal discussion you had with your manager.

The second paragraph highlights aspects of the employment experience that enhanced your career development. Identifying any major contribution you made to the organization is also appropriate. The worst thing to do would be to offload any negative feelings you have for the organization, manager, or

co-workers in writing. Always say something positive about the position you have held.

The closing paragraph concludes by asking for a copy of your exit evaluation. It is important to learn your final standing as you leave an organization, and this appraisal for your own records may be valuable to you in the future.

E-mail and Social Networking Sites

E-mail communication is replacing many other forms of written or oral communication in business settings. Every e-mail you send reflects upon your professional image and can form a permanent record, so using it wisely is important. Always think of e-mail as business communication with rules of etiquette and avoid being too casual when using this form of communication. Some simple things to remember about e-mail communication are outlined in Box 29-1. A common and potentially dangerous issue with e-mails is misunderstanding the tone, meaning, and emphasis of the communication. Think before you write, and if you believe there is any room for misunderstanding, consider a richer form of communication that allows the recipient to interpret your message by hearing your voice or seeing your facial expression.

Social networking sites are used for personal and business communications. Be careful about how you build your profile and participate in social networking sites as they may follow you professionally in your career. Social networking sites can be viewed as public advertisements. What is said or posted on social networking sites may be seen as equivalent to posting the same thing in a national newspaper for everyone to read. The image you portray to any online community and the reach of these communities is often beyond an individual's comprehension. Would you like your boss or work colleagues to know what you post or what others post about you? Remember your audience may be your boss, your patient, a co-worker, or a potential employer. Never post anything on a social networking site that contains confidential information that you are restricted from disclosing under any employment or professional relationship or that you would not like everyone to know. Postings on social network sites containing confidential information, defamatory comments, or unprofessional conduct have been subject to professional disciplinary proceedings, employment terminations, and academic institution sanctions.

BOX 29-1	TEN TIPS FOR E-MAILS

1. **Think before you type:** Avoid being too casual in your communication. Take the time to organize your thoughts, decide the purpose of the communication, then be clear and polite. Check your e-mail again before sending. In situations requiring particular care, it may be useful to ask a trusted colleague to read the note for tone before you send it.

2. **Use a precise subject line:** The subject line reinforces your message and helps the receiver manage your request.

3. **Use a greeting and closing:** Avoid being too casual. Use formal greetings like "Dear Dr. Grant" or "Dear Sarah" and formal closings like "Sincerely," or "Regards," for communications outside of your organization. Even when communicating within your organization, use greetings like "Hello Jim," and closings that are more casual but do not imply overfamiliarity.

4. **Use standard punctuation, capitalization, spelling, and grammatical form:** Your work may look sloppy and your message may be misunderstood or ignored if difficult to read. Using good paragraph structure helps readability. When you change ideas, change paragraphs; one-sentence paragraphs are acceptable in e-mails.

5. **Avoid using words in all capital letters:** Words written in ALL CAPS are considered "yelled" in e-mail etiquette and should not be part of business communication.

6. **Copy only those necessary:** Most people now receive too much e-mail, so include only those necessary in any recipient list. Doing so will help ensure that your e-mail is preserved as important to read and not simply viewed as creating unnecessary work for others.

7. **Use "reply all" judiciously:** E-mail has created additional workload for almost all who use it, so be sure that those included in any communication *must* be included before using the "reply all" option.

8. **Never include confidential or embarrassing information:** E-mails can too easily be forwarded, with or without intent, and can be permanently stored.

9. **Avoid fancy fonts and formatting:** Not all fonts, formatting, or backgrounds are easily recognized by other systems or after an e-mail transmission. Avoid hard-to-read coloured or fancy fonts, background patterns, and pictures.

10. **If another form of communication is better suited or saves time, use it:** E-mail is not always the best form of communication. Know its limitations and disadvantages.

Based on Gaertner-Johnston, L. (n.d.). Email etiquette: 25 quick rules. Retrieved from http://www.syntaxtraining.com/PDF/Rules_of_Email_Etiquette.pdf.

DATA ASSEMBLY FOR PROFESSIONAL PORTFOLIOS

Finding ways to track your career-related data so that they can be easily maintained and assembled for presentation is important. See the Portfolio Checklist on the *Evolve* website for an example (http://evolve.elsevier.com/Canada/Yoder-Wise/leading/). In your portfolio, the inclusion of elements that support each entry in your CV ensures a comprehensive view of your professional contributions. Creating a professional portfolio can help organize one element of your professional life. Keeping notes of recognition, copies of evaluations, and pictures of your successes are examples that help round out the resource documents behind your CV data. Maintaining a portfolio takes time, but this work can pay off at times of evaluation, promotion, or alternative position-seeking. The information is always available, and it is easy to expand information in a given area or focus when required. In other words, this system of maintaining professional information provides a resource to respond promptly to new or emerging opportunities.

EXERCISE 29-7

Go to the *Evolve* website (http://evolve.elsevier.com/Canada/Yoder-Wise/leading/) and view the sample portfolio. Based on information in the portfolio, what types of positions in your community would you suggest might be the best fit for this nurse? What information in the portfolio supports your suggestions?

THE INTERVIEW

After your letters and résumé are effective in career marketing, the next step is participating in an interview. Interviewing is a two-way proposition; the interviewee should be gathering as much information as the interviewer is. Both should be making judgements throughout the process so that if a position is offered, the interviewee will be prepared to accept, decline, or explore further. Interviews may take place with one or more individuals and may include a range of activities. To be at ease, the interviewee should wear professional and comfortable clothing. Rehearse specific questions to ask and points to make so that you can feel more at ease during the interview. Be prepared to cite how you have faced challenges and dilemmas, because those types of questions are likely to be asked.

Even in times of a nursing shortage, employers are using behavioural interviewing techniques to identify the most appropriate applicant for the vacant position. Rather than being asked, "What are your weaknesses?" you may be asked, "Tell me how you handled a difficult situation" or "How did your educational program prepare you for critical care nursing?" Always listen carefully and ask for clarification if necessary. A quick online search will offer many of the most frequently asked behavioural questions. Five common questions are as follows:

1. Have you ever had to give an employee bad news?
2. Tell me about a time when you had difficulties with a team member. What, if anything, did you do to resolve the difficulties?
3. There are times in all jobs where we are under extreme pressure. Tell us about a time when you were under pressure and how you handled it.
4. On many occasions managers have to make difficult decisions. What was the most difficult decision you have had to make?
5. Tell us what has been your greatest workplace accomplishment.

It is worth your while to prepare for these types of questions with your own examples in mind, so that when asked you are prepared to not only share the situation you encountered but also describe in detail what actions you took and the results achieved. Try to learn keywords that describe the skills you applied in the situation posed by the behaviour question so that you can demonstrate the value of the skill set you bring to a potential employer. Some resources to help you in understanding the nature of these questions and how to prepare for them in an interview are provided in the *Evolve* online resources for this text.

Applicants in some organizations are screened and interviewed by a panel and then asked to participate in a series of interviews to allow fellow employees more say in the hiring process. In business and health care settings, many prospective employers administer basic skills tests. Researching the organization in advance can help prepare you for the interview.

Interview Topics and Questions of Concern

During interviews, employers should ask all applicants for a given position the same or similar questions. In addition to providing comparable information as the basis for a decision, the applicant's expectation for equal treatment is upheld. Only questions related to the position and its description are legitimate. Employers should not ask questions related to gender, age, sexual orientation, ethnicity, religion, disabilities, or child-rearing. Applicants should express appropriate concern if asked such inappropriate questions.

If the interviewer asks an inappropriate question, the applicant can choose not to answer the direct question but instead address the content area. For example, if asked about your spouse's employment, you might say, "The employment status of any of my family members will not affect my ability to accept this position or the fulfillment of its requirements."

The key to ensuring a fair interviewing process is being prepared, knowing what can be asked legitimately, and knowing how to respond to inappropriate questions.

If you have prepared well, you will know what the organization's stated beliefs are and whether they are compatible with yours. The challenge in an interview is to determine whether those stated beliefs are lived or are merely printed words. If numerous people can relate how the mission is translated into a specific role, the beliefs are likely lived ones.

EXERCISE 29-8

Select a partner and role-play an interview for a professional nursing position. The potential employer (manager) should focus on competencies of the prospective employee. Include questions and scenarios about common conflicts and challenges seen in the clinical setting. The interviewee (prospective employee) should highlight competencies, decision-making abilities, and critical-thinking abilities when responding to the situation-based questions. Debrief how well you did.

Plank (2010)*, in a *Wall Street Journal* article, identified five must-ask questions and, therefore, five must-be-prepared-to-answer questions:

1. In what ways will this role help you stretch your professional capabilities? (This question is designed to provide clues about weaknesses.)
2. What have been your greatest areas of improvement in your career? (This question identifies weaknesses again and this time identifies what action you took; just knowing one's weaknesses is not good enough.)
3. What's the toughest feedback you've ever received and how did you learn from it? (This question is

---

* Willa Plank, "Five Must-Ask Interview Questions." Reprinted with permission of Wall Street Journal, Copyright © 2010 Dow Jones & Company, Inc. All Rights Reserved Worldwide. License number 3440190585249 (print), 3440190733091 (eBook).

TABLE 29-4   INTERVIEW GOALS AND CONTENT

INTERVIEW GOALS	CONTENT
1. Personal characteristics	Describe the type of person you are, including personality traits. Be expected to cite examples of when these traits helped or hindered you in previous situations.
	List situations that characterize your energy, initiative, drive, ambition, and enthusiasm.
	Clarify your professional values.
	Have a story ready that illustrates how you see yourself.
2. The work itself	Emphasize what makes you distinctive. Describe how your education and experience prepared you for this position.
	Describe your skills as a member of a team and a leader of a team.
	Prepare to address hypothetical situations that display your problem solving, reasoning, self-confidence, knowledge, and critical thinking (creates an opportunity to evaluate you in action and under some stress).
	Ask intelligent questions that suggest you have prepared for this interview and know something about this organization.
3. The organizational fit	Be clear about what you believe to be distinctive about this organization and how it meets your expectations for a position.
	Articulate your "fit" with the organization's philosophy, mission, and vision.
4. The professional opportunities	Be clear about what you expect to obtain from any position you consider. Include advancement opportunities, educational support, and work–life balance.

designed to identify candidates who can be forthright and who are learners.)

4. What are people likely to misunderstand about you? (This question is all about how the candidate "reads" others and potentially adapts approaches.)

5. If you were giving your new staff a "user's manual" to you, what would you include in it to accelerate their "getting to know you" process? (This question reveals information about how the person will function in the team.)

The *Evolve* website contains a Checklist for Interviewing (http://evolve.elsevier.com/Canada/Yoder-Wise/leading/) that can be used in conjunction with "Interview Goals and Content" (Table 29-4) as a means of helping prepare for an interview. Using the thank-you letter described earlier in this chapter is an additional opportunity to market yourself, especially if you wish to correct or expand on an answer you provided during the interview.

PROFESSIONAL DEVELOPMENT

Active involvement in education, service, and scholarship opportunities can help prepare you to deal with new roles and challenges in your employment setting and the larger scope of nursing and health care. Engaging in service activities (both community and professional organizations) and sharing your knowledge through research, writing, and speaking (scholarship) allow you to influence others in the profession and through the profession (see the Research Perspective below).

RESEARCH PERSPECTIVE

Resource: Cummings, G., Lee, H., MacGregor, T., et al. (2008). Factors contributing to nursing leadership: A systematic review. *Journal of Health Services Research & Policy, 13*(4), 240–248.

Leadership practices contribute to outcomes in health care, so developing strong leaders in health care organizations is important to ensure effective health care. Through a systematic review of articles indexed in health care databases, authors identified 24 research studies about the development of nurse leaders. Several studies indicated that actively practising leadership styles, skills, and roles influenced nurses' development of leadership. In addition, after participating in formal leadership educational programs, nurses reported using leadership behaviours more frequently.

Implications for Nursing Practice

At the beginning of your career, you may not be applying for a leadership or management position. It is helpful to keep in mind that leaders and followers are roles, not people. In an interview, you may want to highlight the positive followership skills you have. For example, you can highlight situations in which you showed good judgement, reliability, loyalty, honesty, and a strong work ethic. Leaders are looking to hire people who demonstrate

RESEARCH PERSPECTIVE—cont'd

these skills and who are able to move the goals of the organization forward by working alongside.

Often those who are good followers—at first or at the right times—develop into good leaders. Leadership development is supported through attending educational activities, identifying role models, mentorship, and practising leadership behaviours. Look for opportunities to attend workshops, and read articles on leadership. Observe effective leaders in your workplace, and consider whether the ways that those leaders handle challenges might work well for you in similar situations. Volunteer to lead work groups, committees, and community organizations to practise the leadership behaviours that you have read about and observed.

In settings in which positions are scarce or when you are competing for a very desirable position, community and professional service experience and scholarly contributions to nursing may give you an advantage over other candidates.

One of the keys to maintaining competence and versatility is a commitment to lifelong learning. Nursing professional development begins with the basic nursing education programs but extends to include maintaining competencies, further career development, and education. NurseONE (http://www.nurseone.ca) can assist you with planning and tracking professional development. Learning can occur also through informal means: in a conversation with colleagues, by reading an article in the general literature, or sometimes in an "aha" reflective moment that provides sudden enlightenment.

ACADEMIC AND CONTINUING EDUCATION

A graduate degree opens the door to numerous career opportunities. Graduate education consists of either master's-level or doctorate-level study in a clinical specialty area, in preparation for a specific role, or a combination of both. A graduate degree has been suggested as the national standard for educational preparation for advanced nursing practice (Canadian Nurses Association [CNA], 2008).

Increasingly, employment situations or career specialties require advanced education. For example, nurse practitioner preparation requires graduate-level degree preparation as opposed to the earlier certificate programs. As health care has become more

complex, nurses recognized as independent practitioners need more education to meet health care demands.

Admission to graduate programs may require taking a test (often the Graduate Record Examination [GRE]), having an above-average grade point average (GPA), and graduating from a professionally accredited school of nursing.

EXERCISE 29-9

Analyze the academic and clinical preparation you received in your nursing program. Do you feel confident in your knowledge base and clinical skills? Can you effectively manage multiple roles? Based on these answers and your career goals, determine whether you should pursue graduate education immediately or wait until you have gained additional work experience.

Deciding to pursue graduate education may be very simple. Some applicants to baccalaureate degree programs already have a specific career focus requiring graduate preparation in mind. In the past, new graduates were often encouraged (or even required) to gain work experience before seeking a master's degree or doctorate. Although experience can enrich the learning process, the philosophy of delaying entry into graduate education is changing as nurse leaders have identified the profession's need for nurses who have completed graduate degrees earlier in their careers. Working while attending a graduate program may be difficult, but it is common among graduate students in nursing. Box 29-2 lists some factors to consider in selecting a graduate program.

Consider the following example of a nurse who has begun researching a graduate program that fits:

You know you want to work with elderly patients. Your library subscribes to the *Journal of Gerontological Nursing* and *Geriatric Nursing*. You review the most recent year's issues of both. You scan the masthead (i.e., the page with the editors and board members). Where are these individuals affiliated? Now you scan the articles. Are there some that are particularly intriguing? Where are the authors affiliated? Finally, look back over the lists. Are there any places emerging where the leaders in the field may be? What centres of excellence in geriatrics have related graduate programs? This is a good starting place.

Distance education provides an additional option for earning an advanced degree. Flexible scheduling

BOX 29-2	FACTORS TO CONSIDER WHEN SELECTING A GRADUATE PROGRAM

Accreditation and reputation	• Is the program offered by a private or public university?
	• If out-of-country, does the program have national nursing accreditation (master's and doctoral levels)?
	• Does the program or university have a strong international reputation?
	• Will the degree or qualification you attain be recognized internationally or where you intend its use?
Clinical and functional role	• How closely do the descriptions of clinical and functional courses of study meet career goals?
Credits	• How many graduate credits are required to complete the degree?
	• How many are devoted to clinical or practicum experiences?
	• How many relate to classroom experiences?
Thesis and research	• Is a thesis, dissertation, or capstone project required?
	• If not, what opportunities exist for research development?
	• What support is available for graduate students?
Faculty	• What credentials do faculty members hold?
	• Are they in leadership positions in the provincial, territorial, national, or international scenes?
	• Are they competent in your field of interest?
	• What is their reputation?
Current research	• What are the current research strengths of the institution?
Flexibility	• Do these strengths fit with your interests, or is there flexibility to create your own direction?
	• Is flexibility present in scheduling and progress through the program?
	• Is classroom attendance required or is online attendance an option?
Admission	• What is required?
	• Is the GRE used?
	• What is the minimum undergraduate GPA expected?
	• Is experience required? What kind? How much?
Costs	• What are the total projected costs?
	• What financial aid is available?

GPA, Grade point average; *GRE*, Graduate Record Examination.

and the convenience of online courses permit many individuals to participate who would not be able to attend traditional programs because of class times or geographical distance.

EXERCISE 29-10

Assume that you are interested in graduate education.
• Use the Internet or the library to locate information about graduate education and financial assistance.
• Determine what specialties exist at the master's and doctoral levels.
• Determine the location of programs nearby and access to distance programs.
• Evaluate the clinical interest of the programs of study.
• Decide if the diverse roles of the advanced practice registered nurse appeal.
• Consider doctoral programs, including those permitting entrance from the baccalaureate level.

Continuing education often comprises formal education that enhances practice knowledge and learning, contributes to professional growth, and supports new and continued competencies. The Canadian Nurses Association and Canadian Association of Schools of Nursing have issued a joint position statement regarding the importance of continuing education for nurses: "Continuing nursing education develops and enhances competencies significantly. Continuing nursing education consists of learning experiences organized by the nurse, a facility, employer or an educational institution and undertaken by a nurse to enhance his or her nursing competencies"(CNA, 2004, p. 2).

Opportunities for continuing education exist at local, provincial, territorial, national, and international levels and may be offered by not-for-profit or profit-generating organizations. Selecting among the numerous opportunities to pursue may be difficult. Box 29-3 lists some factors to consider in selecting a course, but depending on your particular goal, certain factors may be more influential than others. For example, if cost is a major factor, course length and instructor may be less influential factors.

BOX 29-3 FACTORS TO CONSIDER WHEN SELECTING A CONTINUING EDUCATION COURSE

- Is the course accredited and approved? If so, by whom?
- Is the amount of credit appropriate in terms of the expected outcomes?
- Is the instructor a known expert in the field? Highly experienced in the field?
- Is the content highly relevant to current practice requirements?
- Is the cost equitable with other similar courses? Is travel required?
- What is the expectation of your employer to use or share this knowledge with the rest of your team?

In addition to increasing your knowledge base, continuing education provides professional networking opportunities, contributes to meeting or maintaining certification and licensure requirements, and documents additional pursuits in maintaining or developing clinical expertise. Sponsors of continuing education include employers, professional associations, schools of nursing, and private entrepreneurial groups.

Both types of formal professional development (i.e., graduate education and continuing education) are valuable, and both can contribute to a specific area of career development—certification.

EXERCISE 29-11
Like an organization, you will develop a strategic plan for yourself. Imagine that you have decided to earn a master's or doctoral degree in nursing. This decision can be enhanced by a strategic plan.
- What values do you have that influence your plan?
- Are your interests in primary care, administration, research, or education?
- What is your target date for completion of the program?
- What factors might interfere with or affect your strategic plan?
- Do you have specific short-term goals or operational plans that must be attained before enrollment?

CERTIFICATION

Certification is a credential that confirms an individual has demonstrated competence in a particular specialty or area by having met predetermined standards (CNA, n.d.). The Canadian Nurses Association has long operated a nursing certification program that allows nurses to be certified under a number of different specialty areas. More recently, some provinces require special certification for certain nursing acts before they can be performed (such acts are called *certified practices*). For example, in British Columbia, the categories for certified practice are RN First Call, Contraceptive Management, Sexually Transmitted Infections, and Remote Nursing Practice. Certification allows RNs to independently conduct assessments and treatments within select areas beyond the usual scope of RN practice. Certification may be an expectation in some employment settings for career advancement.

Obtaining certification may require testing, continued education, and documented time in practice in a specific practice area. Recertification is a process of continued recognition of competence within a defined practice area, and may need to be undertaken every few years.

Certification plays an important part in the advancement of a career and the profession. The Canadian Nurses Association offers voluntary certification in various areas (see http://www.nurseone.ca). Certification recognizes competence of the nurse in a specialized area. Nurses, managers, and administrators value certification. Intrinsic rewards include indicating a level of competence, enhancing professional autonomy, and building personal confidence. Extrinsic rewards include recognition from peers and employers, the opportunity to participate in important practice development, increased patient confidence, university transfer credit toward a degree, and, in some settings, increased salary.

PROFESSIONAL ASSOCIATIONS

Belonging to a professional association not only demonstrates leadership but also provides numerous opportunities to meet other leaders, participate in policy formation, continue specialized education, and shape the future of the profession. A professional association is an alliance of practitioners within a profession that provides members with opportunities to meet leaders in the field, hone their own leadership skills, participate in policy formation, continue specialized education, and shape the future of the profession. Many nursing associations with regulatory responsibilities set standards and objectives to guide the profession and specialty practice. Standards can also serve as critical measurements for the profession and its practitioners.

In today's changing health care environment, increasing numbers of professional associations are serving unique health care interests in society. Although professional associations have different agendas and goals, many share the same motivation and long-term goal of uniting and advancing the profession.

Specialty nursing associations represent nurses in particular areas of the profession. Some are clinically focused, such as the Canadian Association of Critical-Care Nurses or the Canadian Association of Nurses in Oncology. Others may have more general membership or be role focused, such as the Canadian Hospice and Palliative Care Association. Still others represent specific groups in nursing, such as the Aboriginal Nurses Association of Canada. To attract future members, many specialty organizations offer reduced membership rates to students and new graduates, which include discounted meeting and convention rates, networking opportunities, and informative publications and mailings about the association.

An "umbrella organization" representing the most nurses in Canada is the Canadian Nurses Association (CNA), which comprises registered nurses throughout the country (http://www.cna-aiic.ca). The CNA advances the nursing profession by fostering high standards of nursing practice and nursing leadership. The work of the CNA is grounded in public policy, regulatory policy, nursing policy, and international policy and development (CNA, 2011).

EXERCISE 29-12

Research the CNA and your provincial or territorial professional association or regulatory body on the Internet. Find its mission and the legislative issues it focuses on. Obtain or download association or regulatory body brochures for further information.

Unlike most professional associations that are open memberships (i.e., if you meet the basic criteria, you are eligible to be a member), Sigma Theta Tau International is an invitational nursing association. Established in 1922, membership is available to nurses enrolled in baccalaureate, master's, and doctoral education programs and community leaders through a nomination process. Its mission is to create a global community of nurses who lead in using scholarship, knowledge, and technology to improve the health of the world's people (http://www.nursingsociety.org). This organization is one source for small grants to aid in beginning research and disseminates research and leadership information through various publications and international meetings.

A MODEL FOR INVOLVEMENT

Few nurses graduate from their basic nursing educational program and then immediately join and become involved in professional associations beyond those required for licensure. Upon graduation, nurses often are focused on key aspects of professional life, such as learning basic policies and the organizational culture, evaluating peers to determine who to trust and who to avoid, and resolving numerous transitional issues, such as where to live, how to afford housing, how to manage payment of student loans, how to network with old and new friends, and how to be safe practitioners. Few new graduates think about how they can benefit from professional association membership, and, unfortunately, many nurses never pursue membership in any professional association. Yoder-Wise (2006) describes the common path for development of professional involvement as movement from only a clinical focus (direct patient care) to a broader professional focus (policy level).

Connecting with a Professional Association

The size of a professional association is not as important as how the group is organized and who is leading it. Therefore, it is extremely important to do some online reading about the officers and membership composition of the association before making a commitment through membership. Most associations have a website that lists information regarding leader contact and biographical information, the location of the next meetings or activities, current policy issues and their positions, election information, and other valuable resource links. Some associations permit e-mail subscriptions so that you are notified on a regular basis about evolving events.

EXERCISE 29-13

Attend a local meeting of a professional association, observe the dynamics, and network with the members.

Expectations of Membership

Upon joining a professional association, you may receive information on its history, future meetings and current activities, officer contact information, and local contacts. One of the most important things that you can do is connect with your local association so that you can immediately begin networking. Decide how much time you can allocate to the association. There are several different ways to be involved, all of which carry different time commitments. Do not assume that a certain role or committee position entails a set amount of time. The fact remains that most associations consist of volunteers, all of whom have very busy schedules and different motivations for becoming involved. Taking time to talk to an officer or attend a local meeting and observe the group and the dynamics before deciding to make commitments will help ensure that you make an informed decision. Some members enter an association with unrealistic expectations and quickly become disenchanted and disappointed with the association, which leads them to completely pull away from the association. To maximize your experience, you owe it to yourself to do your homework, research the association, talk to the members, determine the sense of the group dynamics, and assess what you want to derive from the experience and how you can contribute to the association. Look at your strengths and talents to determine if there is a need or a fit within the association. Finally, remember that the association consists of people who are volunteering their time; therefore, you should not expect a "perfect" association. Every association has its struggles, but you can gain tremendous personal and professional benefits from your involvement.

EXERCISE 29-14

While you are at an association meeting, challenge yourself to speak to at least two members to learn about their work setting and their nursing role. Make sure to get contact information or a business card from at least two individuals whom you can call in the near future. On the back of the business card, write something about that person that will help you remember him or her for the future (e.g., long black hair, nurse manager on the neurology unit at General Hospital). It is also helpful to have a date and the name of the meeting so you can "place" the person in your mind. You may use these cards in the future when you are looking for a job or need a specific question answered.

Joining and Reasons for Involvement

Membership in a nursing professional association has become an integral part of nurses' career development. Nurses may hold membership in a variety of social and professional associations, devoting more time to one particular area of interest. Nurses who define themselves as leaders and who want to have influence beyond their workplaces should join at least one professional association. Some reasons for joining organizations include feeling a sense of responsibility to the profession, contributing to the greater good of the profession, enhancing résumé and marketability, supporting particular legislative interests, and social networking. A common belief among nurses is that their association can help improve conditions and care for their patients. In addition, some nurses choose to be active members by joining committee work, running for office, or taking on other leadership roles. These volunteer roles can benefit new graduates by offering leadership experiences and connecting with potential mentors. Associations need all types of members, both active and passive members, so that they can carry out their missions and conduct activities and business. Organizational involvement is a socialization process that can improve morale—being around others who take pride in and celebrate the nursing profession is contagious. Whatever your preferred level of involvement, you can contribute greatly to your profession by simply becoming a member of a professional association, and progressing to active involvement guarantees a world of opportunities.

Some nurses choose to belong to their provincial association or other nurses' association because they want to affect health care by influencing public policy. Others choose to belong because of specific benefits such as education and mentorship. Some individuals belong to professional associations because they are required to do so; for example, some employment contracts make it mandatory for the nurse to join a union and pay dues in order to receive a paycheque.

EXERCISE 29-15

Think about what motivates you to join a professional association. Make a list of your strengths (communication, organization, budgeting, legislative interests). Look at positions within the association that interest you. On a separate list, write out reasons why you would want to be a part of the association.

Personal and Professional Benefits. Some professional associations offer substantial scholarships for nurses who are pursuing higher education and certifications. Associations provide conferences, leadership materials, and networking opportunities; the Nursing Leadership Network of Ontario (http://www.nln.on.ca)

is one such organization. Occasionally, government agencies or provincial offices of the Chief Nursing Officer provide opportunities to more directly participate in internships or scholarly undertaking to learn about and influence public health policy. These opportunities typically offer nurses pursuing graduate studies more direct experiences with legislative issues, political processes, and health care advocacy from government perspectives.

With ever-increasing time demands on individuals, volunteering for activities outside of work and family has become more difficult. Associations are aware that traditional incentives for member participation may not be enough to draw new members; however, the most valuable benefits are often intangible. Networking and exposure to different opportunities within the nursing profession are two of the most valuable benefits of belonging to an association. Some nurses may stop working for a time because of family or educational priorities. Organizational membership can help these nurses stay connected to professional issues and colleagues through meetings and publications and smooth the transition back into practice.

Membership in associations can provide nurses with access to professional colleagues they can draw upon for advice and support. All nurses encounter ethical dilemmas and professional challenges. With a connection to the Internet, nurses working in rural or remote locations can also have timely access to professional associations and communities of practice for assistance. Members of nurses' organizations can be nonbiased, safe colleagues to ask for advice about your situation. They can provide feedback on options to handle a situation, based on their experience, especially when you may not want to discuss the matter with co-workers who could be directly involved. Also, they may be connected to experts in the field and serve as a link to further dialogue with them.

With abundant opportunities in nursing, chances are that most nurses will work in a variety of settings over the course of their career. Therefore today's nurse needs to socialize with nurses in different professional career paths. For example, nurse association conventions typically showcase nurses working from a variety of innovative positions within a field. The presentation and informal networking opportunities that come with convention attendance facilitate introduction to new information and connection to individuals with whom networks can be built. Associations can also provide

a training ground where nurses can build skills and gain valuable experiences. Examples of these skills can be found in Box 29-4. Nurses may also benefit from participating in non-nursing organizations that foster leadership development; for example, local business networks and peer-supported leadership development organizations that focus on public speaking, networking, and community leadership. Public service community organizations provide an opportunity to build strong communities while also providing opportunities for leadership skills training and practice, particularly if experiences include committee participation or acting as an officer in governance structures.

Professional association members can influence health care policy through opportunities to influence and educate policymakers. Members of nursing associations learn firsthand about diversity among the patient populations and clinical issues of fellow members, as well as diversity within the profession. On the most basic level, nurses can influence legislation for health care and the profession by simply becoming a member and adding political strength through numbers. Further, nurses can participate on a legislative committee and become involved in their local grassroots politics. Nurses' ability to advocate for their patients is not confined to the bedside; nurses must learn to use advocacy skills in the political arena as well. By being acquainted

---

BOX 29-4   **SKILLS DEVELOPED THROUGH INVOLVEMENT IN PROFESSIONAL ASSOCIATIONS**

- Conflict resolution
- Interpersonal communication
- Public speaking
- Mentoring
- Conducting meetings
- Creating agendas
- Facilitation
- Delegation
- Consensus building
- Strategic thinking
- Team building
- Political advocacy
- Legislative work or lobbying
- Problem solving
- Governance

with the key political figures in their area, nurses can ensure that they are at the table for discussions on health care and policymaking decisions. Consistently, polls and surveys rank public trust in nurses highly (Gordon, 2010). With this trust comes the responsibility for nurses to advocate for and influence patient care and health public policy, which reinforces the importance of their involvement in health care discussions and policy decision making.

CONCLUSION

Nurse leaders, managers, and followers manage their careers in a variety of ways and utilize different tools at different stages in their careers. Involvement in professional associations, participating in continuing education opportunities, networking, and documenting professional activities in a résumé or CV can enhance career management.

A SOLUTION

Anne Marie is undergoing professional growth and transition. She is developing changed professional relationships with front-line nurses that impact the personal relationships previously established. Previous support mechanisms are no longer available to Anne Marie, so she is focused on locating new supports. Education, networking, and mentoring will offer some support. Anne Marie has been approved by her nurse manager to attend a "women in leadership" conference and is looking forward to being with others in similar positions. She plans to take a leadership and management program at the local university and has asked her employer to support her in leadership development courses. An experienced team leader from outside her department is meeting her regularly as a mentor, and she is considering some team-building exercises on her unit to help restructure relationships with staff within her new role identity. Anne Marie has also decided to meet with her two closest friends on the unit and have a frank discussion about what the changes in her role mean to create shared understandings of which areas are perhaps now "off topic" and what new boundaries might look like.

Would this be a suitable approach for you? Why or why not?

THE EVIDENCE

A wise mentor can provide a safe learning environment for honest reflection and discussion about challenging issues while acting as a sounding board, an advisor, a role model, a bridge to connections with new colleagues, and a support structure for new responsibilities (Boldra, Landin, Repta, et al, (2008). Working with a helpful mentor provides support for career development by facilitating the learning of new roles and leadership skills. In addition to the benefits for those who work with a mentor, the mentoring relationship can benefit the mentor and the organization in improving organizational commitment. Organizations need to prepare future leaders at every level to take on positions of greater responsibility as other formal leaders retire or move to other positions in the organization. Some organizations offer structured mentoring programs as a path to leadership development.

NEED TO KNOW NOW

- Take responsibility for your own career. Make it what you want it to be.
- Identify colleagues who might serve as a mentor for you in considering strategies for career success.
- Keep track of your professional accomplishments in an organized way. Doing so will help you prepare position applications efficiently and quickly when opportunities are advertised.
- Network with colleagues through professional associations. Building relationships with other nurses can lead to many career opportunities.
- Familiarize yourself with the professional interview and application process to help build confidence and enhance your presentation to prospective employers.

CHAPTER CHECKLIST

- Nurses must make decisions about career goals and career development. Managing a career requires a set of planned strategies designed to lead systematically toward the desired goal. The use of each strategy should be geared toward finding a good person–position fit. Career planning and development is a lifelong process focused on continual competence. Continued professional development, whether via graduate education, continuing education, certification, or service in professional associations, is a crucial component of success as a nurse. Involvement in professional associations can open doors to opportunities and skills development that would never have been possible otherwise.

- Career styles contribute to the diversity of the nursing profession and reflect different ways of achieving success.

- The four career styles are as follows:
  - Steady state: characterized by constancy with increasing professional skills
  - Linear: characterized by a hierarchical orientation with a steady climb
  - Entrepreneurial or transient: focused on new services and personal priorities
  - Spiral: characterized by rational, independent responsibility for shaping the career

- Certain career strategies are effective with every career style:
  - Selecting professional peers, mentors, and role models helps shape professional development.
  - Designing personal and professional documents that open doors for further action includes the following:
    - The curriculum vitae (a listing of facts) (quantitative)
    - The résumé (a sampling of the most relevant facts, with details) (qualitative)
    - Appropriate business letters that market effectively

- A professional portfolio includes elements that support each entry in your CV, ensuring a comprehensive view of your professional contributions.

- Interviewing at its best is a two-way interaction that enables both people to determine whether there is a good person–position fit.

- Both graduate education and continuing education contribute to a nurse's ability to provide competent care.

- Certification is a credential that confirms an individual has demonstrated competence in a particular specialty or area and is a requirement in some employment settings. Being a professional carries additional obligations and privileges to ensure that the nurse remains competent, advances the profession, and improves health care.

- Numerous professional associations exist in health care:
  - The Canadian Nurses Association and numerous specialty associations focus on improving the profession and patient care.
  - Associations focused on communities of practice may offer involvement at local, provincial, territorial, national, or international levels.
  - Involvement varies based on one's personal situation.
  - Strengths and talents should guide involvement.
  - Involvement permits an opportunity for mentorship in areas of interest and leadership skills development and growth.

- Nurses can contribute to the profession through association involvement:
  - Networking is facilitated.
  - Knowledge dissemination is enhanced.
  - Associations provide the input to policymakers who determine policies and legislation affecting the practice of nursing and patient care.
  - Attendance at meetings provides valuable contacts and different points of view.

TIPS FOR A SUCCESSFUL CAREER

- Use an expanding file to organize hard copies of your accomplishments, such as continuing education certificates, by year so that you can report accurate data for licensure or certification.

- Update your CV at least once a year (6 months is better, and 3 months is ideal) so that you always have an accurate, current set of data to share with someone should a special opportunity appear.

Better yet, make these changes as you complete achievements.

- Stay connected with colleagues.
- Find a mentor; be a mentor; self-mentor.
- Learn from what you do each day: what to do differently, how to pre-empt errors, who to turn to for support.
- Focus on your strengths and build them into spectacular performances; hone the basics so that you are always prepared.
- Create an individual mission statement.
- Think about the future and what you need to do to be employable.

- Research and create a file of educational programs of interest.
- Join two professional associations; for example, your practice group of the Canadian Nurses Association (national focus) and a practice group or committee at your workplace (localized focus).
- Read professional journals and, on a regular basis, at least one other journal external to nursing to keep current with the world.
- Attend at least one professional meeting each year, especially outside of your geographical area, to network.
- Volunteer in your profession and your community.

℮volve WEBSITE

Visit the Evolve website for Suggested Readings, Internet Resources, and additional resources related to the content in this chapter: http://evolve.elsevier.com/Canada/Yoder-Wise/leading/.

REFERENCES

Boldra, J., Landin, C. W., Repta, K. R., et al. (2008). The value of leadership development through mentoring: More experienced colleagues can help protégés. *Health Progress, 89*(4), 33–36. Retrieved from http://www.chausa.org/home/.

Bolles, R. N. (2009). *What color is your parachute? A practical manual for job-seekers and career-changers.* Berkley, CA: Ten Speed Press.

Buckingham, M. (2008). *The truth about you: Your secret to success.* Nashville, TN: Thomas Nelson.

Canadian Nurses Association. (n.d.). What is certification? Retrieved from http://www.nurseone.ca/Default.aspx?portlet=StaticHtmlViewerPortlet&plang=1&ptnme=Specialty%20Certification%20What%20Is%20Certification.

Canadian Nurses Association. (2004). Joint position statement: Promoting continuing competence for registered nurses. Retrieved from http://www.cna-nurses.ca/CNA/documents/pdf/publications/PS77_promoting_competence_e.pdf.

Canadian Nurses Association. (2008). *Advanced nursing practice: A national framework.* Ottawa: Author. Retrieved from http://www.srna.org/images/stories/pdfs/nurse_resources/2009_advanced_NP.pdf.

Canadian Nurses Association. (2011). CNA's work. Retrieved from http://cna-aiic.ca.

Center for Creative Leadership. (2010). *Addressing the leadership gap in healthcare: What's needed when it comes to leader talent. A white paper.* Colorado Springs, CO: Author. Retrieved from http://www.ccl.org/leadership/pdf/research/addressingLeadershipGapHealthcare.pdf.

Citrin, J. M., & Smith, R. A. (2003). *The five patterns of extraordinary careers.* New York, NY: Crown Business Books.

Cummings, G., Lee, H., MacGregor, T., et al. (2008). Factors contributing to nursing leadership: A systematic review. *Journal of Health Services Research & Policy, 13*(4), 240–248. doi:10.1258/jhsrp.2008.007154

Deal, J. J. (2007). *Retiring the generation gap: How employees young and old can find common ground.* San Francisco, CA: John Wiley and Sons.

DeGeest, D., & Brown, K. G. (2011). The role of goal orientation in leadership development. *Human Resource Development Quarterly, 22*(2), 157–175. doi:10.1002/hrdq.20072

Fox, J. J. (2006). *How to land your dream job: No resume! And other secrets to get you in the door.* New York, NY: Hyperion.

Friss, L. (1989). *Strategic management of nurses: A policy oriented approach.* Owings Mills, MD: AUPHA Press.

Gaertner-Johnston, L. (n.d.). Email etiquette: 25 quick rules. Retrieved from http://www.syntaxtraining.com/PDF/Rules_of_Email_Etiquette.pdf.

Gordon, S. (2010, December 9). Nurses again win public trust [Web log message]. Retrieved from http://www.suzannegordon.com/?p=472.

Willa Plank, "Five Must-Ask Interview Questions." Reprinted with permission of *Wall Street Journal,* Copyright © 2010 Dow Jones & Company, Inc. All Rights Reserved Worldwide. License number 3440190585249 (print), 3440190733091 (eBook).

Yoder-Wise, P. S. (2006). Professional issues: Creating the challenge of engagement. *Annual Review of Nursing Education, 4,* 67–83. Retrieved from http://www.springerpub.com/products/series/Annual-Review-of-Nursing-Education.

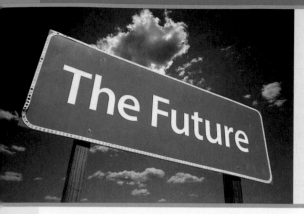

Thriving for the Future

Patricia S. Yoder-Wise
Adapted by Sandra Regan and Lyle G. Grant

Contemplating the future of nursing allows nurses to explore how the changes they will face can be maximized to benefit the profession and the public. This chapter presents the key leadership skills of visioning and forecasting. Projections for the future and their implications for nursing are also discussed.

OBJECTIVES

- Value the need to think about the future while meeting current expectations.
- Describe the six leadership strengths that will be essential in the future.
- Ponder two or three projections for the future and what they mean to the practice of nursing.
- Determine three projections for the future that have implications for individual nursing practice and nurse leadership.

TERMS TO KNOW

chaos	shared vision
complexity compression	vision

❓ A CHALLENGE

Janice, a student in the last year of her undergraduate nursing program, is beginning to plan her career in nursing. She knows that health care is changing to meet the complex needs of the population and that nurses have an important role in leading change to meet these needs. She is reflecting on what practice setting she would most like to work in, which roles she might work toward, and how she could be involved in the profession. She wonders what the future will bring.

What do you think you would do to better understand your future and that of nursing if you were Janice?

INTRODUCTION

Leading and managing in nursing are a consistent challenge. Even nurses who say they do not want to lead or manage find that new demands call for continuous leadership and increased self-management skills. More important, the work of the future is being accomplished in teams, with people working together to achieve a vision.

The first part of the twenty-first century brought new challenges and opportunities, some for which society was well prepared and others for which it struggled for some time. Think, for example, about concerns regarding the new millennium with the change to year 2000, or *Y2K* as it was called. There were predictions that computers could shut down everywhere because they might not be able to recognize that the number *2000* was a new century. Endless hours were spent in testing and fixing computers worldwide so that when the clock struck midnight throughout the world, people would still have computer access. We are an increasingly global community, and events occurring thousands of kilometres away might be felt locally. Consider the impact of the 2004 Indian Ocean earthquake and subsequent tsunami, or the more recent earthquake in Haiti. How did these disasters affect you and your community? The global health community responded and was instrumental in leading humanitarian efforts in these and other disaster events. Canadians have also experienced recent challenges, such as the floods in Calgary and the train derailment in Lac-Mégantic, Quebec. Consider how the SARS (Severe Acute Respiratory Syndrome) outbreak of 2003 has influenced health care delivery in your province and nationally. Pandemic plans have been implemented, infection control practices changed in hospitals, and the public health system was revitalized. Clearly, past events have shaped the present, and the present will influence the future. What role will you have in influencing health care, today and tomorrow?

In order for nurses to lead in health care, a number of present challenges need to be addressed. These include an aging nursing workforce, a current nurse shortage that is projected to worsen in the next decade, a shortage of nursing faculty to teach the next generations of nurses, and a lack of succession planning for future nurse leaders in administrative positions. In addition to these issues, societal issues such those related to current economies and changing population demographics will influence health service delivery. As Sister Elizabeth Davis noted:

> *We're in a new place; we're not on the edge of the old place. We're not pushing the envelope; we're in a totally new envelope. So the rules have changed. Every fundamental premise of the old way of thinking no longer applies.* (as cited in Villeneuve & MacDonald, 2006, p. 3)

LEADERSHIP DEMANDS FOR THE FUTURE

Nurse administrators and leaders consistently say that the characteristic they are most seeking in tomorrow's professional nurse is leadership. In probing what that means, we often find themes that relate to nursing activities that have serendipitous outcomes. Nurses shape the public's view of the profession, the organizations in which they work, and health care in general. Nurses influence interdisciplinary views of what it is to be a professional, and they create expectations for the profession's potential. All of these examples form some of the leadership potential that exists for the future.

If we think about the world as a loose web, we know that every element has the potential to influence every other element. This connectivity with one another, whether among those within our profession or within a team, means that we influence others all of the time, just as others influence us. This influence moulds our practices and beliefs as we move health care forward and changes how we influence others subsequently. Thus, even positions without formal leadership titles contain an element of leadership, and we must all be prepared and willing to lead whenever the need arises. In their book *The Starfish and the Spider*, Brafman and Beckstrom (2006) liken this type of decentralized leadership to the starfish and centralized leadership to the spider. A starfish has no head and its major organs exist in each arm, so if one arm is damaged or removed, the starfish can grow a new arm and will continue to thrive (which is what happens in a decentralized organization with members who take on leadership roles as needed). By contrast, if you remove the leg of a spider, it is crippled; if you remove its head, it dies (which is what happens in a centralized organization when the main leader is no longer in charge).

EXERCISE 30-1

Using the analogies of the starfish (decentralized) and the spider (centralized), analyze two or three community or health care organizations with which you are familiar. If the leader left, what do you think would happen to the organization? Would it flourish or diminish?

LEADERSHIP STRENGTHS FOR THE FUTURE

When Lipman-Blumen (2000) proposed her six strengths of connective leaders, she may have had no idea how important these strengths would be for the future (Box 30-1). Any one of these strengths is valuable to an organization or an individual, but in combination they make a leader invaluable. A nurse leader's ethical political savvy can be based on the *Code of Ethics for Registered Nurses* (Canadian Nurses Association [CNA], 2008a) and provincial or territorial nursing professional standards. Basing our actions on ethical

---

BOX 30-1 **SIX LEADERSHIP STRENGTHS FOR THE FUTURE**

Ethical political savvy: knowing how to effect change and use resources from an ethical, altruistic perspective

Authenticity and accountability: being committed to the group rather than self, which leads to credibility; being open in decisions

Politics of commonalities: ensuring an environment that allows as many stakeholders as possible to achieve at least a part of their respective agendas

Thinking long term, acting short term: committing to what is best for the future and acting in the present to move toward that goal, including developing the future leadership to succeed current leaders

Leadership through expectation: encouraging others through expectations rather than through micromanagement

Quest for meaning: leaving a legacy by guiding others

From Lipman-Blumen, J. (2000). The age of connective leadership. *Leader to Leader*, 17 (Summer), 39-45. Copyright © 2000 the Drucker Foundation.

---

principles to affect the political system that influences the availability of health care (and other) resources allows us to demonstrate the trust the public places in us. Most of us have capitalized on our authenticity and accountability to demonstrate our concern for others, whether through collective action, crying with families, or listening carefully to what our colleagues and patients say.

Because nursing work is relational, nursing leadership styles have been the focus of studies, particularly by Canadian nurse researchers. A growing body of literature suggests that leaders who are transformational, resonant, supportive, and considerate influence patient, nurse, and organizational outcomes (Cummings, MacGregor, Davey, et al., 2010; Wong & Cummings, 2007). Leadership styles that are relational in nature (rather than task oriented) promote and facilitate change, which is important to realizing a future vision.

When we are faced with the pressures of providing care to patients versus changing the system, we often remain focused on the individual patient, thus losing the opportunity to change an issue for many patients. To be effective in the future, we must embrace the opportunities to think longer term so that more people are affected by our actions. Perhaps because of our history of being attentive to the details, we may need to challenge ourselves to develop broader leadership skills. Moving from micromanaging to focusing on setting expectations for those who are accountable to us may feel uncomfortable at first. However, that movement reinforces our ability to deal with longer-term issues. In addition, the quest for meaning suggests that our actions today create the foundation on which future leaders will build. Thus, if we fail to capitalize on today's opportunities, we are diminishing the place at which future leaders will start their careers.

It is incumbent on nurses to raise expectations about what comprises good, safe, quality, patient-centred care and how nurses in leadership roles contribute to those expectations. Developing one's ability to lead occurs over time, but the key is that the foundation be present. As Gladwell (2008) suggested, it takes about 10 000 hours to be an expert at anything (see the Literature Perspective). Our foundation begins with our concern for and advocacy of patient care. That foundation is fairly well engrained in professional nurses' beliefs. The movement from focusing on the nurse–patient relationship to the "big picture" of nursing (politics and public or health policy activities) may take several years but is rewarding nonetheless. What we do in our professional lives is the legacy we leave for future generations.

LITERATURE PERSPECTIVE

Resource: Gladwell, M. (2008). *Outliers: The story of success.* New York, NY: Little, Brown.

Based on research findings in numerous fields, the author identified the characteristics of highly successful people. Some of those characteristics, such as the year an individual is born, are uncontrollable. Other characteristics, such as the amount of time spent mastering a strength, are within the control of the individual. Various characteristics, such as the generation in which an individual is born, family, socioeconomic status, and culture are explored. In addition to providing some insights into successful individuals' lives and cultures, Gladwell presents a compelling case for the 10 000-hour rule. The gist of the rule is that in a field in which people must think critically, they achieve mastery once they have reached around 10 000 hours of practice.

Implications for Practice
Developing as a leader occurs over time; it is not something that happens upon assuming a role. The 10 000 hours of practice equates to approximately 5 years of a full-time position that deals with complex decisions.

EXERCISE 30-2
Using the six strengths cited in Box 30-1, write a description of what you believe your strengths to be. Provide as much detail as possible so that the description helps you see your best strengths. What competencies have you gained in your nursing education program that align with the six strengths?

Nurses who seek leadership opportunities will find that many are available—in the employment setting, in professional associations, and in voluntary community organizations. Balancing multiple demands in an era of rapid changes and new expectations can be challenging. Merely being employed is no longer sufficient; an individual must be *employable*. This suggests that we must constantly be focused on competence, on learning, on what the future holds, and on what patients want and need. Failure to do so will make us unemployable and will make the profession

undesirable. To be valued in the future, we need to know what the future might encompass.

VISIONING

Whether you are a leader, a manager, or a follower, the ability to visualize in your mind what the ideal future is becomes a critical strategy. A **vision** is the articulated goals to which an individual, group, or an organization aspires. No matter how we engage in this visioning activity, we must be open and honest about what we think. Creating our own circle of advisors or brain trusts (those who do not necessarily think as we do, but who are creative thinkers) allows us to test ideas so that we enhance our own thinking and performance to higher levels. Senge (2006), author of *The Fifth Discipline: The Art and Practice of the Learning Organization*, said that all leadership is really about is people working at their best to create the future. And that, in reality, is what we do every day.

This chapter is designed to share some views about the future so that you can think about them in relation to what it means to lead and manage and your role in shaping the future. This "thinking about" the future, like visions, is further enriched through sharing in open dialogue with colleagues.

EXERCISE 30-3
Select a group of three or four peers and brainstorm what you think the future of nursing will be. Consider how technology will affect nursing; consider where our primary place of service will be and how we will deliver care. Think about the changes in society and the political pressures for effective health care and what those might mean for nursing. Think about how you would reform health care. Create a list of ideas to share with others.

Although no one knows the future for certain, many entities engage in formal predictions. These predictions arise from structured groups, such as the World Future Society (http://www.wfs.org), regular trend reports, and books. Although not everyone is a futurist, each of us needs to be aware of trends. Thinking about the future should be mind-expanding; it is the most nonstereotypical thinking you can do. In everyday practice, you can ask yourself and others "what if" questions. We take for granted that certain practices have remained unchanged. Yet, technology *and* creative thinkers and investigators prove us wrong on a regular basis. Our challenge is to think about the future in a way that does not necessarily rely on history and yet builds on today.

Because the future is about teams and collaborative work, many implications exist for nursing. Skills related to working with others and facilitating their work as well as reaching decisions about practice and the workplace will be crucial.

SHARED VISION

The concept of shared vision suggests that two or more people endorse a particular view. How society and we view the world as individuals is always evolving. Consider stability and chaos (a condition of disorder or confusion) as the opposite ends of a continuum (see figure below). Moving in some way between those two ends suggests that we live in a constant state of disequilibrium in which we strive toward stability while recognizing that we experience chaos. In times of great stability, society makes little progress (but life probably seems serene). In times of great chaos, by contrast, society may transform itself (and life may seem uncontrollable). Thus, it is even more important to think about projections for the future to have a sense of the direction we are heading on the continuum. Think about what you were doing, thinking, believing, and valuing on September 10, 2001. Then think about what you were doing, thinking, believing, and valuing on September 11, 2001 (9/11). Society moved from some point on that continuum closer to chaos, no matter where one was in the world.

Stability   Chaos

◄─────────────────────────────────►
                    Society

Consider the idea of a shared vision of health care. As we continue to move from "traditional" practices to evidence-informed ones and from a heavy focus on tertiary (hospital-based) care to one that includes community (including the home) and primary health care, we can assume that we might experience more chaos. The comfort of the known is gone; rather, practices are evaluated on a regular basis and changes are incorporated so that we are all doing the latest "best" for patients. In our efforts to do the best we can as soon as we can, we have experienced the phenomenon complexity compression. In essence, this term refers to the intensity of increasing functions and expectations without a change in resources, including time. This compression can be distracting or useful. Krichbaum, Diemert, Jacox, et al. (2007) studied nurses' experiences of complexity compression and identified common themes. For example, when nurses experienced rapid changes in practice (e.g., through the introduction of new technology) without the supports to learn or were given additional responsibilities without additional time, they expressed concern about patient safety. The authors suggested that nurses were frustrated with not being included in decisions about changes that affect their practice. They emphasized the importance of nurse involvement in decisions and control over their practice. As changes occur in health care, it is important for nurse leaders, managers, and followers to be involved in creating the shared vision.

Our ability to retrieve, analyze, and evaluate information influences our currency with practice expectations. We seem to value the need for a shared vision, which includes the idea of operating from a rich data-based approach. To be able to achieve a shared vision, however, we also need to hone our skills in projecting for the future so we know where practice is headed, we need to consider how we interact with our patients, and we need to consider how quickly we can elevate all nursing practitioners to a satisfactory level of working with an evidence-informed practice approach. Kouzes and Posner (2009)* have indicated how leaders can help create a shared vision:

> As counterintuitive as it might seem, then, the best way to lead people into the future is to connect with them deeply in the present. The only visions that take hold are shared visions—and you will create them only when you listen very, very closely to others, appreciate their hopes, and attend to their needs. The best leaders are able to bring their people into the future because they engage in the oldest form of research: They observe the human condition. (pp. 20-21)

PROJECTIONS FOR THE FUTURE

If you watch future reports on television or read *The Trend Letter* or *The Futurist* (The World Society publication) or books such as *The World Is Flat: A Brief History of the Twenty-First Century* (Friedman, 2005) or *Hot, Flat, and Crowded* (Friedman, 2008), you will find comparable themes about the future. The following are some forecasts for the future that will affect nursing; it is possible to ask "What if" questions about each.

Knowledge and Technology Influences

- Knowledge will change dramatically, requiring that we all be dedicated learners.
- Knowledge will evolve from the intensity of the current information evolution so that we will access content with meaning and applicability for our work.
- Leaders will continue to require the best evidence available to inform decisions.
- Technology will continue to revolutionize health care.
- A power shift will occur toward health care because of the intensity of the developing knowledge and its use in making cost-effective decisions about care.

Economic Influences

- The health care system will have to change to remain financially sustainable.
- Department and grocery stores will be either very small or huge; people will increasingly shop "online."
- Macromarketing (targeting masses) will be out; micromarketing (targeting specific populations) will be in.

Global Trends

- The world will be seen increasingly as a continuum without borders that prevent trade and inventions, including those related to health care.
- Increasing diversity will result in the following:
  - More people who are older
  - More people moving to different parts of the country or the world
  - A greater need for speaking two or three languages

- There will be increased violence and, simultaneously, an increased expectation for civility.
- Climate change will affect the social determinants of health.

Health Trends

- More older adults living longer will require innovations in care.
- More people will be living with chronic diseases.
- More people will be overweight and consequently experience various related diseases.
- Bioengineering will make possible interventions that currently do not exist.
- As genetics allows us to know more about how an individual would respond to treatment, a shift toward eliminating the current disparities is more likely.
- Emphasis on prevention will redirect health care efforts.

Work Trends

- Job security will be out; career options will be in.
- Competition will be out; cooperation will be in.
- Work will be sporadic.
- Work will be accomplished by teams.
- Everyone will need to be a leader.

Canadian Nurses Association's 20/20 Vision

Villeneuve and MacDonald (2006) conducted an extensive "visioning" consultation for the CNA to provide a starting place for discussions about nursing's role in shaping the Canadian health care system of the future. *Toward 20/20: Visions for Nursing* describes several "preferred futures" and various scenarios. For example, the authors suggested that patient-led care will increase; nurses will assist patients to navigate the system and coordinate care; a significant shift will occur to community-based care (see the Research Perspective) as opposed to hospital-based care; and care delivered by interprofessional teams will integrate a variety of health care workers, including assistive and support workers and those providing complementary and alternative health services. At the core of these envisioned changes is "nurses leading." The authors observed: "Nurses can be at the forefront of the coming changes, setting the agenda to create a health care system that truly serves and reflects the priorities of Canadians. But no one will appoint them to the task" (Villeneuve & Mac-Donald, 2006, p. 3).

Drawing on the work of Villeneuve and MacDonald, the Canadian Nurses Association (2008b) offered this vision for change:

- The health system can and must **revolutionize patient care**, redesigning delivery systems to focus on individuals, families, and communities and not just on providers and institutions.
- The system can and must use **innovative and emerging technology to achieve new benchmarks in efficiency and effectiveness.** We must rapidly accelerate the adoption of promising technologies wherever services are, or could be, delivered.
- The health system can and must **integrate nursing knowledge in the development of healthy public policy** across this country. (Canadian Nurses Association, 2008b, p. 1)

RESEARCH PERSPECTIVE

Resource: Schofield, R., Ganann, R., Brooks, S., et al. (2011). Community health nursing vision for 2020: Shaping the future. *Western Journal of Nursing Research, 33*(8), 1047–1068. http://dx.doi.org/10.1177/0193945910375819

The authors conducted a qualitative study to understand priority issues currently facing Canadian community health nurses related to education, practice, research, administration, and policy. The aim of the study was to develop a national vision for community health nursing to shape the future of the profession moving toward the year 2020. Focus groups and key informant interviews were conducted with 35 community health nurses across Canada. Five key themes were identified: community health nursing in crisis now, a flawed health care system, responding to the public, vision for the future, and community health nurses as solution makers. Study participants identified a number of key strategies, including developing a common definition and vision of community health nursing, collaborating on an aggressive plan to shift to a primary health care system, developing a comprehensive social marketing strategy, refocusing basic baccalaureate education, enhancing the capacity of community health researchers and knowledge in community health nursing, and establishing a community health nursing centre of excellence.

Implications for Practice
The nursing profession needs to continually look to the future to ensure its relevance and maintain its ability to respond to the changing context. Visioning exercises can be useful strategies to reflect on a preferred future and strategically plan to achieve it.

EXERCISE 30-4

Review the list of projections for the future, the CNA's vision for change, and some of the preferred futures and scenarios in *Towards 20/20: Visions for Nursing* and consider how each might affect how you envision your career. Make a note of one or two phrases that are the top implications. Look at the list of projections again, and evaluate each of the items to determine which ones you believe will be most important to you. Rank in order the top five. Compare your list with those of two or three colleagues and offer your rationale for your selection. After you hear their viewpoints, consider whether you would change your own rankings.

NURSING: PREPARING FOR THE FUTURE

A number of issues will influence nursing's direction in the future. For example:

- How will shared governance and interprofessional collaboration continue to enhance the role of staff nurse?
- How will increased public accountability of health care providers and health care services change nursing practices?
- How will changes to the practice environment affect nurse recruitment and retention?
- Will we have a dramatically richer set of evidence to describe the difference nurses make in patient care and health promotion and disease prevention?
- How will continuing competence and quality assurance be measured in the future?
- How will health care emerge over the next several years as a desirable place to work and as a source of help for health-related needs?

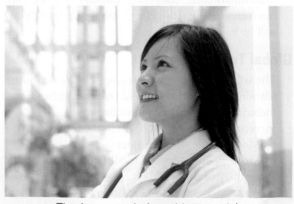

The future explodes with potential.

- Will nurses be paid by a salary, or will their economic worth be reflected in what they are paid?
- How will the increasing number of men in nursing change the "profile" of the profession? How can we achieve a diverse profession?
- What can health care organizations learn from other sectors and vice versa?
- Will increasing concern about terrorism, pandemics, and trade and mobility agreements affect the flow of nurses across borders?

How does nursing prepare itself for the future? One way is through how we prepare the future nursing workforce, and nursing education programs play a very important role. The nursing profession has identified that the knowledge, skills, attitudes, and judgement required to meet the demands of the health care system today and in the future are gained through baccalaureate education. All Canadian provinces and territories (with the exception of Quebec) require a baccalaureate education as the entry to the profession for registered nurses. This ensures that new registered nurses have the competencies required to navigate the complexity of health care and actively participate as advocates for change. Baccalaureate degrees are now also offered in psychiatric nursing, although not required for entry to practice, and practical nursing diploma programs are increasingly more comprehensive and lengthier than in the past. All point to the importance of enhanced education to support the future of nursing.

IMPLICATIONS

Should we be concerned with the forecasts for nursing? Are they likely to come true? Historically, Cornish (1997) analyzed the predictions from the February 1967 issue of *The Futurist*. Of the 34 forecasts that could be judged, 23 were accurate and 11 were not. However, some of the 11 were accurate trends that did not meet the targeted date, often because of shifting national priorities, such as funding. If this is true historically, we

might assume that forecasting, which becomes better refined each year, will continue to be a valuable tool for the future. We can see from the economic downturn of 2008 that continued movement toward expected changes occurred, but most time lines were altered.

CONCLUSION

Numerous changes will occur throughout our lifetimes. It is only a matter of time before we say (if we have not already), "When I was young . . ." Our description might be of something that today is considered fairly advanced. For those who want to thrive, the future forecasts are like the gold ring on the merry-go-round. If you risk and reach far enough, you can grasp it! Lead on . . . the future is now!

💡 A SOLUTION

Janice, like most students, is asking important questions, searching for meaning, and beginning the process of shaping her future as a nurse. She can use tools gained from this textbook and this chapter to reflect on and identify her role as a leader and follower in nursing and health care, examine trends that will influence nursing and health care, and look toward a future that she can help to shape. New graduate nurses often take on a follower role initially but, because of the competencies gained in their undergraduate nursing program, they often have the most "up-to-date" information that can help them lead evidence-informed practice initiatives. Their exposure to practice experiences from acute care to community settings, their knowledge of health promotion, and their exposure to interprofessional collaboration means they are well-prepared for changes in practice. Over the course of her career in nursing, Janice will apply the competencies gained in her educational program and in practice to lead in a variety of settings and with different populations. She has the tools to thrive in the future.

Would this be a suitable approach for you? Why or why not?

NEED TO KNOW NOW

- Ask "what if" when challenged by a problem in your work.

- Use the changes you have seen in health care in the past 6 months as a reminder that the future will be different from the past.

■ CHAPTER CHECKLIST

This chapter addresses the need to think about the future and what that means for current practice. Involvement by all nurses is needed to keep the profession relevant to the constantly emerging future.

- Six leadership strengths are needed for the future:
  - Ethical political savvy
  - Authenticity and accountability

- Politics of commonalities
- Thinking long term, acting short term
- Leadership through expectation
- Quest for meaning
- Shared visions are important.
- Numerous projections for the future can shape what our individual and collective practices will be.

■ TIPS FOR THE FUTURE

- At least monthly, read literature external to nursing and health care. Then ponder whether what you have read has implications for nursing.

- Talk with people outside of nursing about their view of the world and what is happening in their discipline.

⊘volve WEBSITE

Visit the Evolve website for Suggested Readings, Internet Resources, and additional resources related to the content in this chapter: http://evolve.elsevier.com/Canada/Yoder-Wise/leading/.

REFERENCES

Brafman, O., & Beckstrom, R. A. (2006). *The starfish and the spider: The unstoppable power of leaderless organizations.* New York, NY: Penguin.

Canadian Nurses Association. (2008a). *Code of ethics for registered nurses (2008 centennial edition).* Toronto, ON: Author. Retrieved from https://www.cna-aiic.ca/~/media/cna/files/en/codeofethics.pdf.

Canadian Nurses Association. (2008b). *Vision for change.* Retrieved from http://wapsrv2.acs.ucalgary.ca:4450/rid=1H28YFRJN-16H4D6V-1NR/Vision_of_Change_e%5B1%5D.pdf.

Cornish, E. (1997). The Futurist forecasts 30 years later. *The Futurist, 31*(January/February), 45–48.

Cummings, G. G., MacGregor, T., Davey, M., et al (2010). Leadership styles and outcome patterns for the nursing workforce and work environment: A systematic review. *International Journal of Nursing Studies, 47*(4), 363–385. doi:10.1016/j.bbr.2011.03.031

Friedman, T. L. (2005). The world is flat: A brief history of the twenty-first century. New York, NY: Farrar, Straus & Giroux.

Friedman, T. L. (2008). *Hot, flat, and crowded: Why we need a green revolution and how it can renew America.* New York, NY: Farrar, Straus & Giroux.

Gladwell, M. (2008). *Outliers: The story of success.* New York, NY: Little, Brown.

Krichbaum, K., Diemert, C., Jacox, L., et al. (2007). Complexity compression: Nurses under fire. *Nursing Forum, 42*(2), 86–94.

Lipman-Blumen, J. (2000). The age of connective leadership. *Leader to Leader, 17*(Summer), 39–45.

Schofield, R., Ganann, R., Brooks, S., et al. (2011). Community health nursing vision for 2020: Shaping the future. *Western Journal of Nursing Research, 33*(8), 1047–1068. doi:10.1177/0193945910375819

Senge, P. (2006). *The fifth discipline: The art and practice of the learning organization.* New York, NY: Doubleday Currency.

Villeneuve, M., & MacDonald, J. (2006). *Toward 20/20: Visions for nursing.* Ottawa: ON: Canadian Nurses Association. Retrieved from http://www.cna-nurses.ca/CNA/documents/pdf/publications/Toward-2020-e.pdf.

Wong, C. A., & Cummings, G. G. (2007). The relationship between nursing leadership and patient outcomes: A systematic review. *Journal of Nursing Management, 15*, 508–521. doi:10.1111/j.1365-2834.2007.00723.x

absenteeism   The rate at which an individual misses work on an unplanned basis. (Ch. 24)

accommodating   An approach to conflict resolution in which people neglect their own needs, goals, and concerns (unassertive) while trying to satisfy those of others (cooperative). (Ch. 23)

accountability   The obligation to account for one's actions. (Ch. 26)

accreditation   A process of assessing health care services against standards, to identify what is being done well and what needs to be improved. (Ch. 8)

active listening   Focusing completely on the speaker and listening without judgement to the essence of the conversation; an active listener should be able to repeat most of the speaker's intended meaning. (Ch. 19)

adverse event   An event that results in unintended harm to the patient and is related to the care and services provided to the patient rather than to the patient's underlying condition. (Ch. 2)

advocacy   Acting to support a cause or an interest; it is often embedded in nursing codes of ethics. (Ch. 20)

agenda   A written list of items to be covered in a meeting and the related materials that meeting participants should read beforehand or bring along. Types of agendas include structured agendas, timed agendas, and action agendas. (Ch. 28)

appreciative inquiry (AI)   An attribute associated with how we question and problem solve; it focuses on identifying what is working well and building on those strengths. (Ch. 1)

authentic leadership   Leadership where leaders are constantly re-aligning their actions to match their values and moral convictions. (Ch. 1)

autonomy   Personal freedom and the right to choose what will happen to one's own person. (Ch. 6)

availability bias   The tendency for people to base their judgement on a preceding and memorable event that is readily recalled rather than complete information on the present situation. (Ch. 7)

average daily census (ADC)   Average number of patients cared for per day in the unit for the reporting period. (Ch. 15)

average length of stay (ALOS)   Average number of days that a patient remained in an occupied bed. (Ch. 15)

avoiding   An approach to conflict resolution that is very unassertive and uncooperative because people who avoid neither pursue their own needs, goals, or concerns immediately nor assist others to pursue theirs. (Ch. 23)

barriers   Factors that can hinder the change process. (Ch. 18)

battery   When someone intentionally touches another without consent. (Ch. 5)

benchmarking   The process of comparing best practices, processes, or systems with the practice, process, or system under review. (Ch. 21)

beneficence   The principle that states that the actions one takes should "do good." (Ch. 6)

bioethics   A division of applied ethics rooted in biological research and medicine and increasingly concerned with questions related to health care; its major principles are autonomy, justice, beneficence, and nonmaleficence. (Ch. 6)

biomedical technology   Involves the use of equipment in the clinical setting for diagnosis, physiological monitoring, testing, and administering therapies to patients. (Ch. 12)

blog   A type of website, usually maintained by an individual, with regular entries of commentary, descriptions of events, images, and videos. (Ch. 12)

budget   A detailed financial plan for carrying out the activities an organization wants to accomplish for a certain period. (Ch. 13)

budgeting process   An ongoing activity in which plans are made and revenues and expenditures are managed to meet or exceed the goals of the plan. (Ch. 13)

bullying   A practice closely related to lateral or horizontal violence, but a real or perceived power differential between the instigator and recipient must be present in bullying. (Chs. 23, 25)

bureaucracy   Characterized by formality, low autonomy, a hierarchy of authority, an environment of rules, division of labour, specialization, centralization, and control. (Ch. 9)

burnout   A prolonged response to chronic emotional and interpersonal stressors on the job. (Ch. 28)

capital budget   A budget that reflects expenses related to the purchase of major capital items such as equipment and physical plant. (Ch. 13)

career   Progressive achievement throughout an individual's professional life. (Ch. 29)

case management model   A model of delivering patient care based on patient outcomes and cost containment. Components of case management are a case manager, clinical pathways/critical pathways, and unit-based managed care. (Ch. 14)

case manager   A master's degree–prepared clinical nurse specialist who coordinates patient care from preadmission through discharge. (Ch. 14)

case method   A model of nursing care delivery in which one nurse provides total care for a patient during an entire work period. (Ch. 14)

case mix groups (CMGs)   A patient classification system used to group the types of inpatients a hospital treats. (Ch. 13)

certification   A credential that confirms an individual has demonstrated competence in a particular specialty or area by having met predetermined standards. (Ch. 29)

chain of command   The hierarchy depicted in vertical dimensions of organizational charts. (Ch. 9)

change agent   An individual with formal or informal legitimate power whose purpose is to initiate, champion, and direct or guide change. (Ch. 18)

change fatigue   Fatigue that occurs when key leaders and staff get tired of new initiatives and the way they are implemented. (Ch. 18)

change management   The coordination of processes and strategies used to transition from situation A to situation B and achieve lasting results. (Ch. 18)

change process An ongoing effort applied to managing a change. (Ch. 18)

change situations The field comprising various factors and dynamics within which change is occurring. (Ch. 18)

chaos A condition of disorder or confusion. (Ch. 30)

chaos theory A theoretical construct defining the random-appearing yet deterministic characteristics of complex organizations. (Ch. 18)

charge nurse A registered nurse responsible for delegating and coordinating patient care and staff on a specific unit. (Ch. 14)

chemical dependency A psychophysiological state in which an individual requires a substance, such as medications or alcohol, to prevent the onset of symptoms of abstinence. (Ch. 24)

circle of care The individuals and institutions directly connected to an individual's health care. (Ch. 5)

clinical decision support (CDS) A clinical computer system, computer application, or process that helps health care providers make clinical decisions to enhance patient care. (Ch. 12)

clinical decision support systems (CDSSs) Interactive computer programs designed to assist health care providers with decision-making tasks by mimicking the inductive or deductive reasoning of a human expert. (Ch. 12)

clinical nurse leader (CNL) A highly skilled master's degree–prepared nurse who has completed advanced studies in clinical care with a focus on the improvement of quality outcomes for specific patient populations at the point of care. (Chs. 3, 14)

clinical pathway A patient-focused document that describes the clinical standards, necessary interventions, and expected outcomes for the patient at each stage of the treatment process or hospital stay. (Ch. 14)

clinical practice guidelines Systematically developed statements of practice that assist practitioners and patients in making appropriate clinical decisions. (Ch. 22)

coaching A process in which a manager helps others learn, think critically, and grow through communications about performance. (Ch. 16)

coalitions Groups of individuals or organizations that join together temporarily around a common goal. (Ch. 11)

code of ethics A statement of a set of values that help guide nurses in ethical practice. (Ch. 2)

collaborating A group of people working together to achieve a common goal. (Ch. 23)

collaboration A complex, voluntary, and dynamic process with underlying concepts of power, interdependency, sharing, partnership, and process. (Ch. 26)

collaborative practice An interprofessional process for communication and decision making that enables the separate and shared knowledge and skills of the care providers to synergistically influence the client/patient care provided. (Ch. 26)

collective action Activities that are undertaken by a group of people who have common interests or goals. (Ch. 20)

collective agreements A special type of employer–employee contract that governs employment arrangements including wages, benefit entitlement, job protection, and employee rights. (Ch. 5)

collective bargaining A mechanism for negotiating a labour contract between the employer and representatives of the employees. (Ch. 20)

common law Laws that have been derived from the system of courts that operate in Canada and are commonly referred to as "judge made." (Ch. 5)

communication technology An extension of wireless technology that enables hands-free communication among mobile hospital workers. (Ch. 12)

competing An approach to conflict resolution in which people pursue their own needs and goals at the expense of others. (Ch. 23)

complexity compression The intensity of increasing functions and expectations without a change in resources, including time. (Ch. 30)

complexity science The study of complex systems, including how they are related, sustained, and able to self-organize, as well as how outcomes emerge. (Ch. 1)

compromising An approach to conflict resolution that involves both assertiveness and cooperation on the part of everyone and requires maturity and confidence. (Ch. 23)

confidentiality The promise to hold in private any information provided and to prevent the release of information to those who are unauthorized. (Chs. 5, 6)

confirmation bias The tendency for people to seek information that reaffirms past experience and to discount information that contradicts past judgements. (Ch. 7)

conflict Two or more competing responses to a single event. (Ch. 19) Also, a disagreement in values or beliefs within oneself or between people that causes harm or has the potential to cause harm. (Ch. 23)

continuing education Formal education that enhances practice knowledge and learning, contributes to professional growth, and supports new and continued competencies. (Ch. 29)

coping The immediate response of a person to a threatening situation. (Ch. 28)

cost The amount spent on something. (Ch. 13)

cost centre An organizational unit for which costs can be identified and managed. (Chs. 13, 15)

creative decision making The generation of new and imaginative ideas that are critical for problem solving. (Ch. 7)

critical thinking The intellectually disciplined process of actively and skillfully conceptualizing, applying, analyzing, synthesizing, and/or evaluating information gathered from, or generated by, observation, experience, reflection, reasoning, or communication, as a guide to belief and action. (Ch. 7)

cross-culturalism Mediating between or among cultures. (Ch.10)

cultural competence The process of integrating values, beliefs, and attitudes different from one's own perspective in order to render effective nursing care. (Ch.10)

cultural diversity The variation between people in terms of a range of factors such as ethnicity, national origin, race, gender, ability, age, physical characteristics, religion, values, beliefs, sexual orientation, socioeconomic class, or life experiences. (Ch.10)

cultural imposition The tendency of an individual or group to impose their values, beliefs, and practices on another culture for varied reasons. (Ch.10)

cultural marginality Situations and feelings of passive betweenness when people exist between two different cultures and do not yet perceive themselves as centrally belonging to either one. (Ch.10)

cultural safety What is experienced by a patient when health care providers communicate in a respectful and inclusive way, empowering the patient in decision making and ensuring maximum effectiveness of care. (Ch.10)

cultural sensitivity The capacity to recognize that people from cultures other than our own are individuals who share similarities and differences. (Ch.10)

culture Shared patterns of learned behaviours and values transmitted over time, and that distinguish the members of one group from another. (Ch.10)

culture of safety A focus on effective systems and teamwork to accomplish the mutual goal of safe, high-quality performance. (Ch. 2)

curriculum vitae (CV) The documentation of one's professional life. It is designed to be all-inclusive and may be lengthy. (Ch. 29)

cybernetic theory The regulation of systems by managing communication and feedback mechanisms. (Ch. 18)

data Discrete entities that describe or measure something without interpretation. (Ch. 12)

database A collection of data elements organized and stored together. (Ch. 12)

decision bias An error in judgement, when relevant information is omitted. (Ch. 7)

decision making A process that chooses a preferred option or a course of actions from among a set of alternatives on the basis of given criteria or strategies. (Ch. 7)

delegation Achieving performance of care outcomes for which you are accountable and responsible by sharing activities with other individuals who have the appropriate authority to accomplish the work. (Chs. 26, 28)

differentiated nursing practice A model of clinical nursing practice that recognizes the difference in each nurse's level of education, expected clinical skills or competencies, job descriptions, pay scales, and participation in decision making. (Ch. 14)

diffusion of innovations The process by which an idea is spread through a culture. (Ch. 22)

direct care hours Paid time used for the care of patients. (Ch. 15)

disease management A model of care that coordinates health care interventions and communication for those individuals whose self-care needs are significant. (Ch. 14)

dualism An "either/or" way of conceptualizing reality in terms of two opposing sides or parts (right or wrong, yes or no), limiting the broad spectrum of possibilities that exists between. (Ch. 19)

electronic health record (EHR) A complete health record under the custodianship of a health care provider(s) that holds all relevant health information about a person over their lifetime. (Ch. 12)

electronic medical record (EMR) A partial health record under the custodianship of a health care provider(s) that holds a portion of the relevant health information about a person over their lifetime. (Ch. 12)

emerging workforce Employed persons who belong to Generation Y or Z. (Ch. 3)

emotional intelligence (EI) The ability to know one's own and others' feelings and emotions. (Ch. 1)

employee assistance program (EAP) A program designed to provide counselling and other services for employees through either in-house staff or by contract with a mental health counsellor. (Ch. 28)

empowerment The process of exercising one's own power; also the process by which we facilitate the participation of others in decision making and taking action so they are free to exercise power. (Chs. 11, 16)

entrenched workforce Employed persons who belong to the Baby Boomer generation or Generation X. (Ch. 3)

environmental assessment An assessment carried out to understand the specific internal and external forces that influence the health care setting. (Ch. 17)

ethical dilemma A situation in which equally compelling reasons exist for and against two or more possible courses of action, and when choosing one course of action means that something else is let go. (Ch. 6)

ethical (or moral) distress A type of distress that occurs when a person is faced with a situation in which two ethical principles compete. It also occurs when the nurse knows the right thing to do, but he or she cannot act on that insight. (Ch. 6)

ethical violation An action or failure to act that breaches fundamental duties to patients or to other health care providers. (Ch. 6)

ethics A branch of philosophy that deals with what is right and wrong. (Ch. 6)

ethnocentrism The belief that one's own ways are the best, most superior, or preferred ways to act, believe, or behave. (Ch.10)

evidence-based practice The integration of the best research evidence with clinical expertise and the patient's unique values and circumstances in making decisions about the care of individual patients. (Ch. 22)

evidence-informed practice A systematic approach to clinical decision making that provides the most consistent and best possible care to patients. It integrates current research findings that define best practices, clinical expertise, and patient values to optimize patient outcomes as well as their quality of life. It also involves acknowledging and considering the myriad factors beyond evidence, such as local indigenous knowledge, cultural and religious norms, and clinical judgement. (Ch. 12)

expected outcomes See *Patient outcomes.* (Ch. 14)

expenditures Money spent on goods and services. (Ch. 13)

facilitator Factors that can expedite the change process. (Ch. 18)

factor evaluation system A patient classification system that gives each task, thought process, and patient care activity a time or rating. These indicators are then summed to determine the hours of direct care required, or they are weighted for each patient. (Ch. 15)

fallacies Beliefs that appear to be correct but are found to be false when examined by logical reasoning rules. (Ch. 7)

fixed costs Costs that do not change as the volume of patients changes. (Ch. 13)

fixed full-time equivalent (FTE) A full-time equivalent position that does not fluctuate based on patient care demands. (Ch. 15)

flat organizational structure   A structure characterized by the decentralization of decision making to the level of personnel carrying out the work. (Ch. 9)

followership   Engaging with others who are leading or managing by contributing to the work that needs to be done. (Ch. 1)

forecast   The process of making decisions about the future based on multiple sources of data. (Ch. 15)

foreseeability   The concept that certain events may reasonably be expected to cause specific consequences; an element of negligence and malpractice. (Ch. 5)

full-time equivalent (FTE)   An employee who works full-time, typically 37.5 hours per week (1950 hours per year). (Chs. 13, 15)

functional nursing   A model for providing patient care in which each regulated and unregulated member of the care team performs specific tasks for a large group of patients. (Ch. 14)

functional structure   Arrangement of departments and services by specialty. (Ch. 9)

general adaptation syndrome (GAS)   A theory by Hans Selye that details a predictable multi-stage response to stress. (Ch. 28)

goal setting   The process of developing, negotiating, and formalizing the targets or objectives of an organization. (Ch. 17)

grievance   An allegation, usually by an individual (employee), but sometimes by the union or management, of misinterpretation or misapplication of a collective bargaining agreement or of traditional work practices. (Ch. 24)

group   A number of individuals assembled together or who have some unifying relationship. (Ch. 19)

group invulnerability   The perception of group members that the group cannot be wrong, which can lead the group to make overly optimistic or overly risky decisions. (Ch. 7)

group polarization   The tendency for groups to make decisions that are more extreme (risky or conservative) than the privately held beliefs of individual group members. (Ch. 7)

groupthink   A phenomenon in which group members are so concerned with avoiding conflict and supporting their leader and other members that important facts, concerns, and differing views are not raised that might indicate an alternative decision. (Ch. 7)

halo effect   A type of cognitive bias where our perception of one personality trait influences how we view a person's entire personality. (Ch. 16)

health care system   The sum total of all the organizations, institutions, and resources whose primary purpose is to improve health. (Ch. 8)

health equity   The absence of unfair or unjust differences in life circumstances and access to resources so that all persons have fair opportunities to achieve their full health potential to the extent possible. (Ch. 20)

healthy work environment   A practice setting that maximizes the health and well-being of nurses, quality patient outcomes, and organizational and system performance. (Ch. 4)

heuristics   Educated guesses or "rules of thumb" based on experience and general knowledge about how things work, as opposed to specific information about the situation at hand. (Ch. 7)

hierarchy   Chain of command that connotes lines of authority and responsibility. (Ch. 9)

high-complexity change   A complicated change situation characterized by the interactions of multiple variables of people, technology, and systems. (Ch. 18)

hindsight bias   The tendency for people to overestimate their ability to predict an event after the fact. (Ch. 7)

horizontal violence   An act of aggression that is perpetuated by one colleague toward another colleague. (Chs. 23, 25)

hybrid organizational structure   A structure that has characteristics of several types of organizational structures. (Ch. 9)

incivility   A wide range of behaviours from ignoring, to rolling one's eyes, to yelling, and eventually to personal attacks, both physical and psychological. (Ch. 25)

indirect care hours   Paid time used for other required unit activities, such as staff meetings or continuing education. (Ch. 15)

influence   The process of using power—from the punitive power of coercion to the interactive power of collaboration. (Ch. 11)

informatics   The use of technology and information systems to support improvements in patient care and health care administration. (Chs. 4, 12)

information   Knowledge consisting of interpreted, organized, or structured data. (Ch. 12)

information overload   A state of stress brought about by the reception of too much information, too fast, and too often and not having adequate information-processing skills. (Ch. 28)

information technology   The use of computer hardware and software to process data into information to solve problems. (Ch. 12)

informed consent   Authorization to undergo a proposed treatment by a patient who has fully understood and weighed the risks of that treatment. (Ch. 5)

interactional justice   The perceived fairness of the quality of interactions by people who are affected by decisions and subsequent outcomes. (Ch. 4)

interdisciplinary team   A team that comprises members from different clinical disciplines who have specialized knowledge, skills, and abilities. (Chs. 19, 26)

interpersonal conflict   Conflict that occurs between and among patients, family members, nurses, physicians, and members of other departments. (Chs. 23, 25)

interprofessional team   A team that comprises different health care disciplines working together toward common goals to meet the needs of a patient population. Team members divide the work based on their scope of practice; they share information to support one another's work and coordinate processes and interventions to provide a number of services and programs. (Chs. 19, 26)

intrapersonal conflict   Conflict that occurs within a person when confronted with the need to think or act in a way that seems at odds with one's sense of self. (Ch. 23)

intuition   A gut feeling; the subconscious integration of all the experiences, conditioning, and knowledge of a lifetime. (Ch. 7)

justice The principle that everyone should be treated equally and fairly. (Ch. 6)

knowledge Information that is combined or synthesized so that interrelationships are identified. (Ch. 12)

knowledge broker Go-betweens who facilitate communication and exchange between knowledge producers and users. (Ch. 12)

knowledge brokering A means of facilitating the exchange of knowledge between those who know and those who need to know. (Ch. 12)

knowledge technology The use of expert systems to assist clinicians in making decisions about patient care. (Ch. 12)

knowledge translation (KT) A dynamic and iterative process that includes synthesis, dissemination, exchange, and ethically sound application of knowledge to improve people's health, provide more effective health care services and products, and strengthen the health care system. (Ch. 22)

knowledge worker An individual who performs nonrepetitive, nonroutine work consuming considerable levels of cognitive activity and judgement. (Ch. 12)

labour cost per unit of service A measure that compares budgeted salary costs per budgeted volume of service (productivity target) with actual salary costs per actual volume of service (productivity performance). (Ch. 15)

lateral violence Psychological harassment evidenced by verbal abuse, intimidation, exclusion, unfair assignments, denial of access to opportunities, and withholding of information. (Chs. 23, 25)

leader A person who sets a direction, develops a vision, and communicates the new direction to staff. (Ch. 4)

leadership The process of engaging and influencing others. (Ch. 1) Also, the use of personal traits to constructively and ethically influence patients, families, and staff through a process in which clinical and organizational outcomes are achieved through collective efforts; the process of influencing others. (Ch. 3)

learning organization A type of organization that is continually expanding its capacity to create its future and provide opportunities and incentives for its members to learn continuously over time. (Chs. 3, 18)

liability One's responsibility for his or her own conduct; an obligation or duty to be performed; responsibility for an action or outcome. (Ch. 5)

licensure A right granted that gives the licensee permission to do something that he or she could not legally do absent of such permission; the minimum form of credentialing, providing baseline expectations for those in a particular field without identifying or obligating the practitioner to function in a professional manner as defined by the profession itself. (Chs. 5, 29)

line function A function that involves direct responsibility for accomplishing the objectives of a nursing department, service, or unit. (Ch. 9)

lobby A group of people who seek to influence government policymakers on a particular issue. (Ch. 11)

lobbying Seeking to influence. (Ch. 11)

low-complexity change An uncomplicated change situation characterized by the interactions of the limited influences of people, technology, and systems. (Ch. 18)

malpractice Failure of a professional person to act in accordance with the prevalent professional standards or failure to foresee potential consequences that a professional person, having the necessary skills and expertise to act in a professional manner, should foresee. (Ch. 5)

management Ensuring that the job gets done and providing people with the necessary resources to get the job done. The activities needed to plan, organize, motivate, and control the human and material resources required to achieve outcomes consistent with the organization's mission and purpose. (Chs. 1, 3)

manager A person who addresses complex issues by planning, budgeting, and setting target goals. (Ch. 4)

mandatory overtime The expectation that staff will stay on duty after their shift ends to fill staffing vacancies. (Ch. 15)

matrix structure An organizational structure influenced by dual authority, such as product line and discipline. (Ch. 9)

mediation A process using a trained third party to assist with conflict resolution. (Ch. 23)

mentor Someone who models behaviour, offers advice and criticism, and coaches the novice leader or mentee to develop a personal leadership style. (Ch. 3)

mentorship A formal supportive relationship between two, or more, health professionals that has the potential to result in professional growth and development for both mentors and mentees. (Ch. 27)

meta-analysis An analysis that statistically combines results of similar studies to determine whether the aggregated findings are significant. (Ch. 22)

mission Statement of an organization's reason for being. (Ch. 9)

moral uncertainty Feeling indecisive or unclear about a moral problem, while at the same time feeling uneasy or uncomfortable. (Ch. 6)

multiculturalism A society characterized by ethnic or cultural heterogeneity; it is an important part of Canadian identity that is recognized in the *Canadian Charter of Rights and Freedoms*. (Ch.10)

natural law A *higher* law that applies to all human beings and thus should override a human-made law. (Ch. 5)

near miss A clinical situation that resulted in no harm but highlights an imminent problem that must be corrected. (Ch. 21)

negligence Failure to exercise the degree of care that a person of ordinary prudence, based on the reasonable standard, would exercise under the same or similar circumstances. (Ch. 5)

negotiation Conferring with others to bring about a settlement of differences. (Ch. 23)

network The result of identifying, valuing, and maintaining relationships with a system of individuals who are sources of information, advice, and support. (Ch. 11)

never events Errors in medical care that are clearly identifiable, preventable, and serious in their consequences for patients and that indicate a real problem in the safety and credibility of a health care facility. (Ch. 21)

nominal group technique A technique that involves asking individual group members to respond to questions posed by a moderator and then asking participants to evaluate and prioritize the ideas of all group members. (Ch. 7)

nonlinear change Change occurring from self-organizing patterns, not human-induced ones, in complex, open-systems organizations. (Ch. 18)

nonmaleficence The principle that states that the actions one takes should "do no harm." (Ch. 6)

nonproductive hours Paid time that is not worked, such as vacation, statutory holidays, orientation, education, and sick time. (Chs. 13, 15)

nonpunitive discipline A disciplinary measure, usually verbal, describing existing standards and goals to which the parties agreed; pay is not withheld, and the employee agrees either to adhere to the standards in the future or to be terminated. (Ch. 24)

nurse outcomes The result of nursing work, including staff vacancy rate, nurse satisfaction, staff turnover rate, retention rate, and nurse burnout rate. (Ch. 15)

nursing care delivery model The method used to provide care to patients. (Ch. 14)

nursing case management The process of a nurse coordinating health care by planning, facilitating, and evaluating interventions across levels of care to achieve measurable cost and quality outcomes. (Ch. 14)

nursing governance The methodology or system by which a department of nursing controls and directs the formulation and administration of nursing policy. (Ch. 20)

nursing minimum data set (NMDS) A system that collects essential nursing data in a standardized manner. (Ch. 12)

nursing practice act Legislation that creates nursing regulatory authorities or regulatory bodies. (Ch. 5)

nursing productivity A formula-driven calculation that represents the ratio of required staff hours to actual provided staff hours. (Ch. 15)

nursing professional practice council A formal committee of nurses in a health care setting that identifies, reviews, and addresses issues that influence nursing professional practice. (Ch. 20)

nursing-sensitive outcomes Patient outcomes that are sensitive to nursing practice or interventions. (Chs. 2, 21)

open-systems theory A theory that views organizations as dynamic, interactive systems that are strongly influenced by internal and external forces. (Ch. 8)

operating budget The financial plan for the day-to-day activities of the organization. (Ch. 13)

optimizing decision Selecting the ideal solution or option to achieve goals. (Ch. 7)

organization A business structure designed to support specific business goals and processes; or a group of individuals working together to achieve a common purpose. (Ch. 9)

organizational chart A graphical representation of work units and reporting relationships. (Ch. 9)

organizational conflict Conflict that arises when discord exists about policies and procedures, personnel codes of conduct, or accepted norms of behaviour and patterns of communication. (Ch. 23)

organizational culture The implicit knowledge or values and beliefs within the organization that reflect the norms and traditions of the organization. (Chs. 4, 9, 20)

organizational structure How work is divided in an organization; it delineates points of authority, responsibility, accountability, and non–decision-making support. (Ch. 9)

organizational theory The systematic analysis of how organizations and their component parts act and interact. (Ch. 9)

outcome criteria The result of patient goals that are expected to be achieved through a combination of nursing and medical interventions. (Ch. 14)

overtime Time in excess of the standard amount per day. (Ch. 15)

overwork A situation in which employees are expected to become more productive without additional resources. (Ch. 28)

partnership model A method of providing patient care when a registered nurse is paired with another nurse (e.g., a technical assistant) to provide total care to a number of patients. (Ch. 14)

patient- or client-centred care An approach in which the patient is viewed as a whole person; it is not just about delivering services and involves advocacy, empowerment, and respecting the patient's autonomy, voice, self-determination, and participation in decision making. It includes patients and their family members in the design and delivery of health care at all levels. (Chs. 1, 2, 26)

patient-focused care model A team-based approach to care incorporating principles of patient-centred care with the goals of (1) improving patient satisfaction and other patient outcomes, (2) improving worker job satisfaction, and (3) increasing efficiencies and decreasing costs. (Ch. 14)

patient outcomes The result of patient goals that are achieved through a combination of medical and nursing interventions with patient participation. (Chs. 14, 15, 21)

patient safety The absence of preventable harm to a patient during the process of health care. (Chs. 2, 21)

percentage of occupancy The patient census divided by the number of beds in the unit. (Ch. 15)

perfectionism The uncompromising pursuit of perfection. (Ch. 28)

performance appraisal Individual evaluation of work performance. (Ch. 16)

performance improvement (PI) The application of quality improvement principles on an ongoing basis. (Ch. 21)

personal liability A person's responsibility at law for his or her own actions. (Ch. 5)

philosophy Values and beliefs regarding the nature of work derived from a mission and the rights and responsibilities of people involved. (Ch. 9)

Plan-Do-Study-Act (PDSA) cycle Shorthand for testing a change in the real-work setting—it involves *planning* the change to be implemented, *doing* (carrying out) the plan, *studying* the results, and then *acting* on what is learned to plan full implementation. (Ch. 18)

planned change Change expected and deliberately prepared in advance using systematic processes. (Ch. 18)

policy A specifically designated statement to guide decisions and actions. (Ch. 11)

policy process The process of developing, implementing, and evaluating policy on the basis of the best evidence available. (Ch. 11)

politics The use of power to influence, persuade, or otherwise change—it is the art of understanding relationships between groups in society and using that understanding to achieve particular outcomes. (Ch. 11)

portfolio A professional assemblage of materials that represent the work of the professional. These materials include elements such as evaluations, letters of recommendation or appreciation, certificates of accomplishment, copies of articles, documentation of projects (e.g., research, clinical changes, management projects), and additional educational achievements (continuing education and degree achievement). (Ch. 29)

position description A statement of the role and responsibilities of a specific position in an organization. It also describes the scope and duties of the work assignment, as well as to whom the individual reports. (Ch. 16)

power The ability to get things done, to mobilize resources, to get and use whatever it is that a person needs for the goals he or she is attempting to meet. (Ch. 11)

preceptorship A period of practical experience and training for a trainee supervised by an expert or specialist in a particular field. (Ch. 27)

price The rate that health care providers set for the services they deliver. (Ch. 13)

primary care The first point of entry in the Canadian health care system and deals with the majority of health issues. (Ch. 8)

primary health care (PHC) A community-based health care service philosophy that is focused on illness prevention, health promotion, treatment, rehabilitation, and identification of people at-risk. (Ch. 8)

primary nurse The registered nurse who is responsible for planning and delivering care to a consistent group of patients. Typically, the primary care nurse works with a team to deliver care. (Ch. 14)

primary nursing A model for organizing patient care delivery in which one nurse functions autonomously as the patient's primary nurse throughout the hospital stay. (Ch. 14)

privacy The right of the individual to determine when, how, and to what extent he or she will release personal information. (Ch. 5)

problem solving A comprehensive, sequential, cognitive process used to solve a problem by reducing the difference between current and desired conditions. (Ch. 7)

procrastination Doing one thing when you should be doing something else. (Ch. 28)

productive hours Paid time that is worked. (Chs. 13, 15)

productivity The ratio of outputs to inputs; that is, productivity equals output/input. (Ch. 13)

professional association An alliance of practitioners within a profession that provides members with opportunities to meet leaders in the field, hone their own leadership skills, participate in policy formation, continue specialized education, and shape the future of the profession. (Chs. 20, 29)

professional standard An authoritative statement that sets out the legal and professional basis of nursing practice. (Ch. 2)

progressive discipline A step-by-step process of increasing disciplinary measures, usually beginning with a verbal warning, followed by a written warning, suspension, allowing the employee to return with conditions, and termination (if necessary). (Ch. 24)

project management A framework for implementing changes. (Ch. 18)

prototype evaluation system A patient classification system that classifies patients into broad categories and uses these categories to predict patient care needs. (Ch. 15)

prudence trap The tendency for people to be too cautious and avoid risks that may be justified. (Ch. 7)

public policy A course of action that is anchored in a set of values regarding appropriate public goals and a set of beliefs about the best way of achieving those goals. (Ch. 11)

quality assurance (QA) The regular monitoring and evaluation of services and processes to ensure that they conform to standards of practice. (Ch. 21)

quality improvement (QI) An ongoing process of innovation, error prevention, and staff development that is used by organizations that adopt the quality management philosophy. (Ch. 21)

quality indicators Measurable elements of quality that specify the focus of evaluation and documentation. (Ch. 4)

quality management (QM) The philosophy of a health care culture that emphasizes patient satisfaction, innovation, and employee involvement. (Ch. 21)

quality work environment An environment that provides physical, cultural, psychosocial, and work design conditions that maximize health and well-being. (Ch. 1)

randomized controlled trial (RCT) A study involving at least two groups where study participants are randomly assigned to either the control group or the intervention group in order to test a treatment's effectiveness. The gold standard in RCT is the double-blind study, where participants and those who are evaluating the outcomes do not know who has received a particular treatment. (Ch. 22)

redesign A process of analyzing tasks to improve efficiency (e.g., identifying the most efficient flow of supplies to a nursing unit). (Ch. 9)

re-engineering A total overhaul of an organizational structure. It is a radical re-organization of the totality of an organization's structure and work processes. (Ch. 9)

Regional Health Authority (RHA) A regional body created by a provincial health ministry to be responsible for the delivery and administration of health care services in a specific geographical area. (Ch. 8)

regulatory body A body that controls who can be licensed, the types of actions that are regulated or reserved to nurses, and scope of practice; set out educational and examination requirements for registration and continuing competency requirements; and establish governing bodies and processes for monitoring professional conduct and acting on misconduct. (Ch. 5)

relational ethics   An ethical approach that focuses on the ethical action that takes place in relationships. Its core elements are engaged interactions, mutual respect, embodied knowledge, uncertainty and vulnerability, and interdependent environment. (Ch. 6)

research   The diligent, systematic inquiry or investigation to validate and refine existing knowledge and generate new knowledge. (Ch. 22)

research utilization   The process of synthesizing, disseminating, and using research-generated knowledge to influence or change existing practices. (Ch. 22)

restructuring   Fundamental changes to an organization to achieve greater efficiency or profit. (Chs. 1, 9)

résumé   A customized document that presents the qualifications of an individual for a specific organizational position. (Ch. 29)

revenue   Money received for providing goods or services. (Ch. 13)

risk management   The systematic identification, assessment, and prioritization of risks and the development and implementation of strategies to reduce adverse events and liability associated with these risks. (Chs. 5, 21)

role ambiguity   A situation in which individuals do not have a clear understanding of what is expected of their performance or how they will be evaluated. (Ch. 16)

role clarity   When an individual understands his or her own role and that of others and applies this understanding while performing the role, communicating within the role, collaborating with others, and delivering care. (Ch. 26)

role conflict   A condition in which individuals understand the role but are unwilling or unable to meet the requirements. (Ch. 16)

role discrepancy   The gap between role expectations and role performance. (Ch. 27)

role expectations   The attitudes and behaviours others anticipate that a person in the role will possess or demonstrate. (Ch. 27)

role integration   The process of adjusting perceptions of one's role and reconciling discrepancies between the previous understanding of the role and what it is. (Ch. 27)

role model   An individual who enacts a role, typically in a positive way, so that others can follow the example. (Ch. 20)

role negotiation   Resolving conflicting expectations about personal performance through communication. (Ch. 27)

role orientation   A formal employment process whereby the expectations of the role are clearly identified and the new employee is introduced to the organizational structure within which he or she will be working. (Ch. 27)

role preparation   Education and socialization to the professional role within postsecondary and/or health care systems. (Ch. 27)

role stabilization   When an individual matures in his or her performance of all facets of the role, to the point where he or she internalizes the role, performing it fluidly and with confidence. (Ch. 27)

role strain   The subjective feeling of discomfort experienced as a result of role stress; it may be reflected by (1) withdrawal from interaction, (2) reduced involvement with colleagues and the organization, (3) decreased commitment to the mission and the team, and (4) job dissatisfaction. (Chs. 24, 27)

role stress   A condition in which role demands are conflicting, irritating, or impossible to fulfill. (Chs. 24, 27, 28)

role theory   A framework used to understand how individuals perform within organizations. (Chs. 4, 16)

role transition   The process of moving from a role that is familiar (e.g., nursing student) to one that is unfamiliar (e.g., novice professional nurse). (Ch. 27)

root-cause analysis   A deeper review of an incident and the sequence of events that led to it with the goals of identifying and addressing the underlying causes to reduce the likelihood of reoccurrence. (Ch. 21)

satisficing decision   Selecting an option that is acceptable but not necessarily the best option. (Satisfy + suffice = satisfice.) (Ch. 7)

scheduling   The implementation of the staffing plan by assigning unit personnel to work specific hours and days of the week. (Ch. 15)

scope of practice   Defines the procedures, processes, and actions that are permitted for a person who is licensed. (Ch. 5) It is activities nurses are educated and authorized to perform, as established through legislated definitions of nursing practice complemented by standards, guidelines and policy positions issued by professional nursing bodies. (Ch. 26)

self-management   The ability of individuals to actively gain control of their lives; components include stress management, time management, meeting management, and the ability to delegate. (Ch. 28)

sentinel event   A serious, unexpected occurrence involving death or physical or psychological harm, such as inpatient suicide, infant abduction, or wrong-site surgery. (Ch. 21)

service-line structure   A type of structure in which the functions necessary to produce a specific service or product are brought together into an integrated organizational unit under the control of a single manager or executive. (Ch. 9)

shared governance   A flat type of organizational structure with decentralized decision making. It is also described as a democratic, an egalitarian, and a dynamic process resulting from shared decision making and accountability. (Chs. 9, 20)

shared vision   When two or more people endorse a particular view; it also describes concurrence on what the desired state in the future will be. (Ch. 30)

situational leadership   The premise is that no single "best" leadership style exists, but rather that effective leaders and managers adapt their behaviours based on the situation. (Ch. 4)

six thinking hats   A decision-making tool that can be used by groups to look at problems laterally from six different perspectives. (Ch. 7)

S.M.A.R.T. objectives   The key attributes of effective objectives; that is, objectives are Specific, Measurable, Agreed on (or some use the word Achievable), Realistic, and Time bound. (Ch. 17)

social determinants of health The conditions in which people are born, live, and work; these conditions are shaped by economics, social policies, and politics. (Ch. 8)

social justice The fair distribution of society's benefits, responsibilities, and consequences for all. (Ch. 6)

span of control The number of individuals a supervisor manages. For budgetary reasons, span of control is often a major focus for organizational restructuring. (Ch. 9)

speech recognition (SR) Refers to electronic devices and programs that permit data entry by human speech. (Ch. 12)

staff function Function that assists those in line positions in accomplishing primary objectives. (Ch. 9)

staff mix The proportion of regulated nurses and unregulated care providers in a specific setting. (Ch. 14)

staffing Planning for recruiting, hiring, deploying, and retaining qualified human resources to meet the needs of a group of patients. (Ch. 15)

staffing plan The conceptual approach of accomplishing the work to be done on a given unit. (Ch. 15)

stakeholders Individuals, groups, or organizations that are influenced by an issue or invested in policy related to an issue. (Ch. 11)

statute A rule/regulation created by elected legislative bodies. (Ch. 5)

strategic planning A process by which the guiding members of the organization envision their future and develop the necessary and appropriate procedures and operations to actualize that future. (Ch. 17)

strategies Approaches designed to achieve a particular purpose based on anticipation and consideration of myriad human, technological, and system responses. (Ch. 18)

strengths-based leadership The notion that people are more productive when they build on their strengths rather than focusing on addressing their weaknesses. (Ch. 1)

subculture A group within a main culture that differs from the main culture with respect to core values, goals, and relationships, including approaches to issues and conflicts. (Ch. 20)

SWOT analysis A study of an organization's internal strengths and weaknesses, as well as its external opportunities and threats. (Chs. 7, 17)

synergy A phenomenon in which teamwork produces extraordinary results that could not have been achieved by any one individual. (Ch. 19)

Synergy Model A model of care delivery adopted by the American Association of Critical-Care Nurses that matches the needs and characteristics of the patient with the competencies of the nurse. (Ch. 14)

system A group or organization working together as a unified whole. (Ch. 9)

systems theory An approach to consider how various independent parts interact to form a unified whole or to disrupt a unified whole; the construct related to the operation of the whole process or entity. (Ch. 9)

team A number of individuals who work closely together toward a common purpose and are accountable to one another. (Ch. 19)

team dynamics The way team members interact and react to changing circumstances. (Ch. 7)

team nursing A small group of regulated and unregulated personnel, with a team leader, responsible for providing patient care to a group of patients. (Ch. 14)

telehealth The use of telecommunications and information technologies for the provision of health care to individuals at a distance and the transmission of information to provide that care; involves use of two-way interactive video conferencing, high-speed telephone lines, fibre optic cable, and satellite transmissions. (Ch. 12)

time management The appropriate use of tools, techniques, and principles to control time spent on low-priority needs and to ensure that time is invested in activities leading toward achieving desired, high-priority goals. (Ch. 28)

tort A civil wrong or injury, not related to a contract, for which a court will provide a remedy (usually monetary damages). (Ch. 5)

total patient care See *Case method.* (Ch. 14)

toxic workplace An organization in which people feel devalued or dehumanized and in which disruptive behaviour often flourishes. (Ch. 25)

transactional leaders Similar to managers, they manage the status quo or day-to-day operations. (Ch. 1)

transactional leadership The act of using rewards and punishments as part of daily oversight of employees in seeking to get the group to accomplish a task. (Ch. 3)

transculturalism Bridging significant differences in cultural practices. (Ch.10)

transformational leadership A process whereby leaders and followers set higher goals and work together to achieve them. It involves leadership that encourages followers to follow the leader's style and change their interests into a group interest with concern for a broader goal. (Chs. 1, 3)

Transforming Care at the Bedside (TCAB) An initiative focused on redesigning the work environment and work processes of nurses to improve care for patients. (Ch. 14)

union An organization that undertakes collective action on issues such as nurses' working conditions, salaries, and benefits. (Ch. 20)

unit of service A measure of the work being produced by the organization; for example, patient days, clinic or home visits, hours of service, admissions, deliveries, or treatments. (Chs. 13, 15)

unregulated care providers (UCPs) Unregulated caregivers who perform a variety of nursing tasks. (Chs. 14, 26)

utilization The quantity or volume of services provided. (Ch. 13)

variable costs Costs that vary in direct proportion to patient volume or acuity. (Ch. 13)

variable full-time equivalent (FTE) A full-time equivalent position that depends on the demand for care, and is typically a staff position. (Ch. 15)

variance The difference between the projected budget and the actual performance for a particular account. Also, a deviation from the normal path. (Chs. 13, 14)

variance analysis The process of determining differences between projected and actual costs. (Ch. 13)

variance report A report defining the difference between the actual and projected staffing or budgeting. (Ch. 15)

vicarious liability Indirect liability of the employer for the actions of an employee acting within his or her scope of employment. (Ch. 5)

vision The articulated goals to which an individual, group, or an organization aspires. (Chs. 9, 30)

whistle-blowing Exposing negligence, abuses or dangers, professional misconduct, or incompetence that exists in the organization. (Ch. 20)

wisdom The appropriate use of knowledge to manage and solve human problems. (Ch. 12)

workload The amount of work distributed to a person or unit for a given time period. (Ch. 15)

workplace advocacy An umbrella term that encompasses advocacy activities within the practice setting. (Ch. 20)

CHAPTER 2

Unnumbered Figure 2-1: Lewis, et al. *Medical-surgical nursing*, 7th ed., 2007, St. Louis, Elsevier.

Figure 2-1: Baker, G. R. (2010). Effective Governance for Quality and Patient Safety [online toolkit]. Retrieved from Canadian Patient Safety Institute. http://www.patientsafetyinstitute.ca/English/toolsResources/GovernancePatientSafety/Pages/default.aspx.

CHAPTER 3

Figure 3-1: Essays on nursing leadership by FAGIN, CLAIRE M. Reproduced with permission of SPRINGER in the format Book via Copyright Clearance Center.

CHAPTER 4

Unnumbered Figure 4-2: © Can Stock Photo Inc. / michaeljung

CHAPTER 5

Unnumbered Figure 5-1: © Can Stock Photo Inc. / michelloiselle

CHAPTER 6

Unnumbered Figure 6-1: © Can Stock Photo Inc. / 4774344sean

CHAPTER 8

Unnumbered Figure 8-1: © Can Stock Photo Inc. / blondsteve

Figure 8-1: CIHI. (2013). Health spending in Canada. Retrieved from http://www.cihi.ca/CIHI-extportal/internet/en/document/spending+and+health+workforce/spending/release_29oct13_infogra1pg.

Figure 8-2: Marchildon, G. P. *Canada. Health system review.* Copenhagen, WHO Regional Office for Europe, 2013:22 (Health Systems in Transition, Vol. 15 No. 1 2013).

CHAPTER 10

Figure 10-1: Purnell Model for Cultural Competence. Used by permission of Dr. Larry Purnell.

CHAPTER 11

Unnumbered Figure 11-2: © Can Stock Photo Inc. / michaeljung

CHAPTER 12

Figure 12-1: From Graves, J. R., Amos, L. K., Huether, S., Lange, L. L., & Thompson, C. B. (1995). Description of a graduate program in clinical nursing informatics. *Computers in Nursing, 13*(2), 60–70.

CHAPTER 15

Figure 15-1: From Kane, R. L., Shamliyan, T. C., Duval, S., & Wilt, T. Nursing staffing and quality of patient care evidence report/technology assessment. No. 151, Rockville, MD. Agency for Healthcare Research and Quality, March, 2007.

Figure 15-2: The Canadian Nurses Association (CNA). (2012). Staff Mix Decision-making Framework for Quality Nursing Care. © Canadian Nurses Association. Reprinted with permission. Further reproduction prohibited.

CHAPTER 17

Unnumbered Figure 17-1: © Can Stock Photo Inc. / iqoncept

CHAPTER 19

Figure 19-1: Modified from St. Charles Medical Center. [1993]. People centered teams. Bend, OR: SCMC.

Figure 19-2: Modified from Satir, V. (1988). The new peoplemaking. Mountain View, CA. Science & Behavior Books; and Olen, D. (1993). Communicating speaking & listening to end misunderstanding and promote friendship. Germantown, WI: JODA Communications.

CHAPTER 20

Unnumbered Figure 20-1: Courtesy of Julie Fraser.
Figure 20-1: © Canadian Nurses Association. Reprinted with permission. Further reproduction prohibited.
Figure 20-2: Based on International Council of Nurses. (n.d.). Pillars & programmes. Retrieved from http://www.icn.ch/pillarsprograms/pillars-and-programmes/.

CHAPTER 22

Figure 22-1: Reprinted from *Nursing Outlook, 49,* From Stetler, C. B., "Updating the Stetler Model of Research Utilization to facilitate evidence-based practice," pages 272-279, Copyright (2001), with permission from Elsevier.
Figure 22-2: Graham, I. D., Logan, J., Harrison, M. B., Straus, S. E., Tetroe, J., Caswell, W., & Robinson, N. (2006). Lost in knowledge translation: time for a map? *Journal of Continuing Education in the Health Professions, 26,* 13-24. Copyright © 2006, Wiley Periodicals, Inc.
Figure 22-3: Campbell, B. (2010). Applying knowledge to generate action: A community-based knowledge translation framework. *Journal of Continuing Education in the Health Professions, 30*(1), 65–71. Copyright © 2010 The Alliance for Continuing Medical Education, the Society for Academic Continuing Medical Education, and the Council on CME, Association for Hospital Medical Education.
Unnumbered Figure 22-2: Courtesy of Cheryl Briggs, RN, Annapolis, MD
Figure 22-4: Adapted from Collins, S., Voth, T., DiCenso, A., & Guyatt, G. (2005). Finding the evidence. In A. DiCenso, G. Guyatt, & D. Ciliska (Eds.), *Evidence-based nursing: A guide to clinical practice* (pp. 20-43). St. Louis, MO: Elsevier.

CHAPTER 23

Figure 23-2: Joan Almost, "Conflict within nursing work environments: concept analysis," *Journal of Advanced Nursing, Volume 53,* Issue 4, pages 444–453. Copyright © 2006, John Wiley and Sons.

CHAPTER 26

Figure 26-1: Canadian Interprofessional Health Collaborative. (2010). A national interprofessional competency framework. p. 11. Retrieved from http://www.cihc.ca/files/CIHC_IPCompetencies_Feb1210.pdf.
Figure 26-2: Ruth Martin-Misener, Ruta Valaitis, Sabrina T. Wong, Marjorie MacDonald, Donna Meagher-Stewart, Janusz Kaczorowski, Linda O-Mara, Rachel Savage, and Patricia Austin, "A scoping literature review of collaboration between primary care and public health," Primary Health Care Research & Development, Volume 13, Issue 04, October 2012, pp 327-346, reproduced with permission.

CHAPTER 27

Unnumbered Figure 27-1: © Can Stock Photo Inc. / Andres
Figure 27-1: Boychuk Duchscher, J. (2008). A process of becoming: the stages of new nursing graduate professional role transition. *Journal of Continuing Education in Nursing, 39*(10), 441-450. Reprinted with permission from SLACK Incorporated.
Figure 27-2: Boychuk Duchscher, J. (2012). *From surviving to thriving: Navigating the first year of professional nursing practice* (2nd ed.). Calgary, AB: Nursing the Future. (Used with permission of Judy Boychuk Duchscher.)

CHAPTER 28

Unnumbered Figure 28-1: Courtesy of Shelley L. Cobbett
Figure 28-1: Modified from Selye, H. (1991). History and present status of the stress concept. In A. Monat & R. Lazarus (Eds.), *Stress and coping: An anthology* (pp. 21–36). New York, NY: Columbia University Press.
Figure 28-4: Modified from Covey, S. R., Merrill, A. R., & Merrill, R. R. (1994). First things first: To love, to learn, to leave a legacy. New York, NY: Simon & Schuster.

CHAPTER 29

Unnumbered Figure 29-1: © Can Stock Photo Inc. / barneyboogles

CHAPTER 30

Unnumbered Figure 30-1: © Can Stock Photo Inc. / Feverpitched
Unnumbered Figure 30-2: © Can Stock Photo Inc. / szefei

Page numbers followed by *f* indicate figures; *t*, tables; *b*, boxes.

A

ABF. *see* Activity-based funding (ABF)
Absenteeism, 458–460, 460f, 460b–461b, 462t
  evidence in, 470
  workplace violence and, 477
Abuse, emotional, in workplace, 201–202
Academic education, 549–551, 549b–550b
Access
  to health records, 84–85
  to opportunity, 190
  to resources, 190
  to support, 190
Accommodation, as conflict resolution strategy, 444–445, 446b
Accountability, 488–489
  as leadership strength, 560b
Accreditation
  in health care organization, 139
  of information systems, 216
Accreditation Canada, 216
  Governance Standards, 216
  in health care services, 288
  required organizational practices in patient safety, 405b
Acknowledgement, guidelines for, 364b
Action, in conflict, 443
Action agendas, 531
Active listening, 367–368, 368t
  guidelines for, 367b
Active participant, as follower characteristic, 16t
Activity, using of, in informing budget, 242, 242b
Activity-based funding (ABF), 241, 242b
Acute care, 133t
Adaptable, as quality of team member, 357
ADC. *see* Average daily census (ADC)
ADCs. *see* Automated Dispensing Cabinets (ADCs)
Addiction services, 133t
Additional health care services, 133t, 134
Advanced nursing practice (ANP), 269
Advanced practice nurses, 269
Adverse event, 26
Adverse patient outcomes, 30
Advocacy
  collective action and, 375–378, 376b, 377f, 378b
  definition of, 375–376
  inter-organizational, 382–383
  workplace. *see* Workplace advocacy
Agenda, 531
"Aggressive planning," 320
AGREE Collaboration, 427
Agreements, collective, 80
ALOS. *see* Average length of stay (ALOS)

Ambiguity, role, 304
Ambulatory care, 133t
American Association of Critical-Care Nurses, 271
American National Database of Nursing Quality Indicators®, 282–284, 283t
American Nurses Association (ANA), in staffing levels, 284
American Society of Health-System Pharmacists, 422–423
ANA. *see* American Nurses Association (ANA)
Anecdotal notes, 308, 308b
ANP. *see* Advanced nursing practice (ANP)
Apology Act, 85
Applied ethics, 91–92
Appraisal tools, 427
Appreciative inquiry (AI), 8
  5-D cycle of, 8
Assessment
  environmental, 321, 321f–322f
    external, 322, 322b
    internal, 322
  of position, 540
  team, 354t, 354b
  workplace, 508
Assignments, as characteristic of effective and ineffective team, 355t
Attitudes
  cultural, problem-solving communication in, 181b
  demonstrating hardiness, 518
  positive, of leader, 47
Attractors, 13
Attribution to blame, 365t
Authentic leadership, 10, 10b–11b
Authenticity, as leadership strength, 560b
Automated Dispensing Cabinets (ADCs), 210
Automated medication administration systems, 224
Autonomy, 93–95, 94b
Availability bias, 109
Average daily census (ADC), in inpatient setting, 296
Average length of stay (ALOS), 296b, 297
Avoidance, as conflict resolution strategy, 444, 446b
Awareness
  cultural, 176–178
  model, 363f

B

Baby Boomers, 45–46
Bar charts, 398
Bargaining, collective, 379
Barriers
  in change situations, 334, 334f
  of communication, 365–366

BARS. *see* Behaviourally anchored rating scales (BARS)
Basic nursing education, issues in, 430
Battery, 82
Behavioural change, model for, 460, 460f
Behaviourally anchored rating scales (BARS), 310–311, 311b
Behaviours
   disruptive, 517
   leader empowering, 192b
   multiple "stress-buffering," 521
   threatening, 475b
Being compassionate, in effective communication, 368
Being sued, 73
Benchmarking, 401–402
Beneficence, 95
Best Practice Guidelines
   evidence-informed, 402
   in preventing ventilator-associated pneumonia, 412–413
   through partnership among health care providers, 430b
Bioethics, 91–93
   principles of, 93–96
      autonomy, 93–95, 94b
      beneficence, 95
      justice, 95
      nonmaleficence, 96
Biological system, 136
Biomedical ethics. *see* Bioethics
Biomedical technology, 209–211, 211b
   for diagnostic testing, 210
   future trends and professional issues of, 226, 226f
   for intravenous fluid and medication dispensing and
      administration, 210
   for physiological monitoring, 209
   for therapeutic treatments, 210–211
Blame, attribution to, 365t
Blog, 229
Bounded rationality model, 113–114
   tools for, 114
Brainstorming, as decision support tool, 119
Breast cancer screening program, strategic planning of, 327b
Budgets, 63, 247–250
   capital, 249–250
   management of, 238–255, 239b
      evidence in, 253–254
      tips for, 254
   operating, 247–249, 249b
   revenue, 249
   using activity to inform, 242, 242b
Budgeting process, 247, 250–251, 250b
   developing unit and departmental budgets, 250–251
   gathering information and planning, 250
   negotiating and revising phase, 251, 251b
Bullying, 475–476
   management of, 452–453, 453b
   in workplace, 193, 201–202
Bureaucracy, 157–159, 157b, 159b
   organizational chart, 158f
Burnout, 522–523

C

CADTH. *see* Canadian Agency for Drugs and Technology in Health
   (CADTH)
Caffeine, 521
Campbell Collaboration, 199
Canada Health Act, 4, 70, 127, 138, 240
   key principles of, 144
   principles of universality and accessibility, 175
Canada Health Infoway, 226–227
Canada Occupational Health and Safety Act, 476
Canada's Privacy Act, 228
Canadian Adverse Events Study, 26–27
Canadian Agency for Drugs and Technology in Health
   (CADTH), 221, 226
Canadian Association of Schools of Nursing (CASN), 218–219
Canadian Charter of Rights and Freedoms (1982), 81
Canadian Classification of Health Interventions (CCI),
   database, 140
Canadian Council on Hospital Services Accreditation
   (CCHSA), 394
Canadian Diabetes Association, 141–142
Canadian Federation of Nurses Unions (CFNU), 49, 141, 379
Canadian HOBIC (C-HOBIC), 213
Canadian Institute for Health Information (CIHI), 142
   in health care organization cultural diversity, 173
   in nurse-sensitive outcomes, 31
   in patient safety, 27
Canadian Institutes of Health Research (CIHR), 412
Canadian Interprofessional Health Collaborative (CIHC), 489–490
Canadian Journal of Nursing Informatics, 218
Canadian National Association of Trained Nurses (CNATN), 379
Canadian National Nursing Quality Report, 284
Canadian Network for Environmental Scanning in Health
   (CNESH), 226
Canadian Nurses Association (CNA), 24, 95, 140–141, 413, 450,
   488, 552
   20/20 Vision, 563–564, 564b
   advocacy, 379
   Code of Ethics for Registered Nurses, 96, 96b, 476–477
   competencies for nurse managers, 58
   guide for evaluating impact of nursing staff mix
      decisions, 285, 286f
   leadership definition, 332
   in patient safety, 28, 29b
   in safe nursing care, 281–282
   safe workplace and, 476–477
   website for staffing decisions, 285
Canadian Nurses Protective Society (2009), 86
Canadian Nursing Informatics Association (CNIA), 218
Canadian Nursing Students' Association (CNSA), 49, 376–378
Canadian Patient Safety Institute (CPSI), 29–30, 30b, 142, 394, 405
   Effective Governance for Quality and Patient Safety: A Toolkit
      for Healthcare Board Members and Senior Leaders, 29, 30f
   patient safety competencies, 29b
   website of, 29
Canadian Root Cause Analysis Framework, for health care
   organizations, 142

Capital budget, 249–250
Capital expenses, 249
Care
    circle of, 77–78
    duty of, 83–84
    patient
        communication and, 175
        cultural diversity and, 175
        quality, predictors of, 62
Care delivery model, tips for selecting, 276
Care Delivery Model Redesign (CDMR), 306–307
Care delivery strategies, 256–278, 257b, 273b–275b
    case method, 257–258
    evidence in, 275
    functional nursing, 258–260, 259f
    nursing case management, 266–268, 266t
    primary nursing, 262–266, 263f
    team nursing, 260–262, 261f
Career
    definition of, 536
    development of, 540–541, 540f, 540b
    knowing yourself, 537–539, 539b
    linear, 537, 538t
    management, 535–557, 536b, 539b, 555b
        evidence in, 555–556
        framework of, 536–540
        key aspects of creating and, 540–541, 541t
    marketing strategies, 541–545, 541b
    phases of, 537
    positional plateau, 537
    spiral, 537, 538t
    steady state, 537, 538t
Career choices, 536
Career styles, 538t
Case management model, 266
Case manager, 266–267, 267f
Case method, 257–258
    model analysis in, 257, 258f
    nurse manager's role in, 257–258
    staff nurse's role in, 258, 258b
Case mix groups (CMGs), 242
CASN. see Canadian Association of Schools of Nursing (CASN)
Cause-and-effect diagram. see Fishbone diagrams
CCACs. see Ontario Community Care Access Centres (CCACs)
CCHSA. see Canadian Council on Hospital Services Accreditation (CCHSA)
CCI. see Canadian Classification of Health Interventions (CCI)
CDMR. see Care Delivery Model Redesign (CDMR)
CDS. see Clinical decision support (CDS)
CDSSs. see Clinical (diagnostic) decision support systems (CDSSs)
Center for American Nurses, 481
Centralization, 156
Certification, 71–72, 551
Certified practices, 551
CFNU. see Canadian Federation of Nurses Unions (CFNU)
Chain of command, 155

Change
    campaigns for, 339t
    definition of, 332
    experiencing, 335
    as external source of job stress, 516
    forces of, 334, 334f
    getting ready for, 347
    high-complexity, 344–345
    human side of, 340–341
    implementing, 347
    leading, 331–350, 332b, 347b–348b
        evidence in, 347–348
        tips for, 349
    linear approaches to, 333–334
    low-complexity, 344–345
    marketing, 339t
    military, 339t
    nonlinear, 333–334, 336–337
    personal analysis of, 521b
    political, 339t
    principles of, 346–347, 346b–347b
    processes and policies, unit-based decisions to, 341
    responses to, 340–342
    self-assessment for, 340t, 340b
    spreading, 347
    sustaining, 347
    systems and technological side of managing, 342
Change agents, 332
    in nonlinear changes, 333–334
    rewarding and recognizing, 346
    roles and functions of, 344–346, 345b–346b
    seeking feedback, 339
Change and innovate, willing to, as follower characteristic, 16t
Change environment, context of, 332–334, 333b
Change fatigue, 340
Change management, 337–338
    functions, 337–340, 338f, 338b
        evaluating, 338
        implementing, 338
        organizing, 338
        planning, 338
    systems and technological side of, 342
Change process, 334
Change situations, 332
Change theory, Lewin's, 334–335
Chaos, 562, 562f
Chaos theory, 137, 154, 336
    application of, 337
Charge nurse, 258–259
Chemical dependency, 465–467, 467b
Chronological order, reverse, curriculum vitae, 542
Churchill, Winston, 444
CIHC. see Canadian Interprofessional Health Collaborative (CIHC)
CIHI. see Canadian Institute for Health Information (CIHI)
CIHR. see Canadian Institutes of Health Research (CIHR)
Circle of care, 77–78

Civil liability, 73
Client-centred care. *see* Patient-centred care
Clinical decision support (CDS), 220
Clinical (diagnostic) decision support systems (CDSSs), 220–221
Clinical incompetence, 462t, 463–464
Clinical information systems, impact of, 223–225
Clinical Judgement Model, 114–115, 116b
   support tool for student, 115
Clinical nurse leader (CNL), 38, 270
   fundamental aspects of, 270b
Clinical nurse specialists (CNS)/nurse practitioners (NP), 269
Clinical pathways, 267–268
Clinical practice guidelines, 414
   environmental readiness assessment for implementation
     of, 429b
Clinical question, in evidence-informed practice, 221
Closed-loop electronic systems, 224–225
CMGs. *see* Case mix groups (CMGs)
CNA. *see* Canadian Nurses Association (CNA)
CNA (Canadian Nurses Association), 552
CNATN. *see* Canadian National Association of Trained Nurses
   (CNATN)
CNESH. *see* Canadian Network for Environmental Scanning in
   Health (CNESH)
CNIA. *see* Canadian Nursing Informatics Association (CNIA)
CNL. *see* Clinical nurse leader (CNL)
CNSA. *see* Canadian Nursing Students' Association (CNSA)
Coaching, 308–309, 308f, 309b
Coalitions, 195
   inter-organizational, 382, 382b
Coalition building, 195
Cochrane, Archie, 419
Cochrane Collaboration, 199, 199b, 419
Cochrane Library, 199
Code of ethics, 24, 25b
   for nurses, 96–97, 97b
Code of Ethics for Registered Nurses, 24, 25b, 64, 172,
   195, 413
Coercion, 344
Collaboration, 429–430, 488
   barriers to, 487
   as conflict resolution strategy, 448–449, 448b
   interprofessional, framework for, 489–490, 490f–491f, 490b
   public health, barriers and facilitators to primary care, 491f
   as quality of team member, 357
   in workplace advocacy, 385
Collaborative practice, 488
   moving forward in, 491–493, 491b–493b
Collection, data, 541, 542t
   quality improvement process, 398
Collective action, 374–390, 375b, 387b–388b
   and advocacy, 375–378, 376b, 377f, 378b
   definition of, 375–376
   nursing governance of, 383–387, 384b
   nursing organizations and, 378–383, 379b
   strategies used to achieve, 382
   tips for, 388

Collective agreements, 80
Collective bargaining, 379
Collective perceptions, of unit leadership, aspect of organizational
   culture, 153
Commitment, 518
   to project, 361
   quality of team member, 357
   to resolution, 362
Common laws, 70–71
Commonalities, politics of, 560b
Communication, 118, 337, 362–368
   barriers of, 365–366
   building team through, 351–373
   clinical information systems' impact on, 224
   during conflict, 364–365
   definition of, 362
   e-mail, 545, 546b
   education and, 342
   effective, 367b
     factors that hinder, 365–366
     guidelines for, 366–368, 367b
   importance of, in culturally diverse environment, 174
   linear approach of, 364–365
   networks, 214
   patient care and, 175
   patterns during stress, 365t
   pitfalls, 366, 366b
   problem-solving, in honoring cultural attitudes, 181b
   quality of team member, 357
   rhythms, 363f
   Situation-Background-Assessment-Recommendation
     (SBAR), 367b
   technology, 217–218, 228–231, 231b
   transactional approach of, 364–365
   wireless, 217
Communication model, positive, 363–364
Communicator, effective, as follower characteristic, 16t
Community care services, 133t, 135
Community Coalition Concerned about SARS, 195
Community mental health services, 133t
Competence, 24
   cultural, 172–173, 173b, 181b
   as dimension of empowerment, 191–192
   interpersonal, 459–460
   leading, following, and managing, 14–17
   quality of team member, 357
Competency
   entry-level, 24, 25b
   management, 14–15, 15t, 15b, 58
   skill checklists, 460, 462t
Competent, as follower characteristic, 16t
Competition, as conflict resolution strategy, 446, 447b
Complaining, 527
Complex change, Kotter's strategies for
   implementing, 336
Complexity, in organizational structures, 155
Complexity compression, 562

Complexity science, 12–14, 13b–14b, 19
  becoming leadership "tag," 13
  definition of, 12
  developing networks, 13–14
  encouraging non-hierarchical "bottom-up" interaction among
      workers, 13
  focusing on emergence, 13
  premise of, 12–13
  recognizing dynamic, complex, and interdependent nature of
      systems, 13–14
  thinking the "big picture," 13
Complexity theory, 333–334
Compression, complexity, 562
Compromise, as conflict resolution strategy, 447, 447b–448b
Computer-assisted ventilators, 210
Computer speech recognition. see Speech recognition (SR)
Computerized order entry, 223–224
Computerized systems, patient data, 211f
Conceptual knowledge translation framework, 416, 418f
Conceptualization, in conflict, 442–443
Conduct unbecoming a member of the profession, 73
Confidence, 370
Confidentiality, 77–79, 98, 98b
Confirmation bias, 109
Conflict, 440, 453b
  ability to handle, as characteristic of effective and ineffective
      team, 355t
  antecedents and consequences of, 451f
  aspects of, 362t
  categories of, 443–444
  communicating during, 364–365
  constructive, 443
  evidence of, 453–454
  goal, 443–444
  handling styles of, 447f, 449–450, 449b
  interpersonal, 441, 475–476
  intrapersonal, 441
  intraprofessional, 452–453
  management of, 360–361
  organizational, 441–442
  resolution of, 453
    approaches to, 444–449, 444b
    assessing degree of, 444b
  role, 304
    of leader in, 450–452, 450b
  self-assessment in, 445b
  stages of, 442–443, 442f
    action in, 443
    conceptualization in, 442–443
    frustration in, 442
    outcomes in, 443
  and teams, 360–362
  tips for addressing, 454–455
  types of, 441–442, 442b
  understanding and resolving, 437–456, 440b, 454b
Congruence, 365t
Connection power, 188b–189b

Consciousness, cultural, 176
Consent laws, 82
Constitution Act (1867), 70
Constructive conflict, 362t, 443
Consumers
  needs, identification of, 397–398, 397b
  in quality improvement, 395–396, 396b
Contemporary leader, 369–370
Contingent reward leaders, 10, 10b–11b
Continuing Care Act (1996), 84
Continuing care and rehabilitation, 133t
Continuing education, 550, 551b
  in dealing with cultural diversity, 180
Continuous dysrhythmia monitors, 209
Continuum of care, 164–165
Contract law, 85
Control, in team development, 356
Controlled acts model, 489
Controlled trial, randomized, 427–428
Conventional approach, for résumé development, 543
Cool-headedness, constrained, 365t
Cooperation, 118
  in team, 361
Cooptation, 344
Coordination, 118
Coping responses, 521
Co-primary nursing model. see Partnership model
Costs, 254b
  of health care, 239–240, 239t
  management of, 238–255, 239b
    evidence in, 253–254
    tips for, 254
Cost centre, 247, 292–293
Cost-conscious nursing practices, 243–247
  cost knowing and controlling, 243–244
  discussing cost of care with patients, 244–245, 245b
  evaluation of cost-effectiveness of new technologies, 245, 245b
  meeting patient rather than provider needs, 245
  predicting and using nursing resources efficiently, 245–246, 246b
  strategies for, 246b
  using research to evaluate standard nursing practices, 246–247,
      246b–247b
  using time efficiently, 244
Cost curve, bending of, 243
Cost-effectiveness, of new technologies, 245, 245b
Cost of care, 244–245, 245b
Counselling, 523–524
Cover letter, 544, 544b
CPSI. see Canadian Patient Safety Institute (CPSI)
Creative decision making, 108
Criminal act (actus reas), 72–73
Criminal Code (1985), 72–73
Criminal intent (mens rea), 72–73
Criminal liability, 72–73
Critical Care Unit setting, patient-care documentation and, 224
Critical social theory, 186
  empowerment and, 189–190, 189b–190b

Critical thinking, for problem solving and decision making, 107–108
Criticism, as characteristic of effective and ineffective team, 355t
Cross-culturalism, 178
Cultural attitudes, problem-solving communication in, 181b
Cultural awareness, 176–178
Cultural competence, 172–173, 173b, 181b
    model for, 176–178, 177f
Cultural consciousness, 176
Cultural desire, 176–178
Cultural diversity
    definition of, 172
    in health care, 170–184, 171b–172b, 179f, 182b
        concepts and principles of, 171–173
        dealing effectively with, 179–180, 180b, 183
        evidence in, 182
    in health care organizations, 173–175
    patient care and, 175
    prejudice and, 175–176, 176b
Cultural encounters, 176–178
Cultural imposition, 178
Cultural knowledge, 176–178
Cultural marginality, 173
Cultural safety, 173, 173b
Cultural sensitivity, 172, 178b
Culturally diverse environment, management of, 173–175, 174b
Culture, 171
    constructivist perspective of, 171
    essentialist perspective of, 171
    individual and societal factors in, 178–179, 179b
    organizational, 59, 152–154, 153b–154b
    of safety, 27–28
    theoretical models and, 176–178
Current health-care system, 412
Curriculum vitae (CV), 541–542, 542b
Custodians, of health information, 77
CV (curriculum vitae), 541–542, 542b
Cybernetic theory, 339
Cynicism-involvement dimension, 522–523

D

Data, 219
    privacy and security, 227–228
Data analysis, quality improvement process, 398
    bar charts, 398
    fishbone diagrams, 398, 401f
    flow charts, 398, 399f
    histograms, 398, 400f
    line graphs, 398, 400f
    Pareto chart, 398, 401f
Data collection, 541, 542t
    quality improvement process, 398
        bar charts, 398
        fishbone diagrams, 398, 401f
        flow charts, 398, 399f
        histograms, 398, 400f
        line graphs, 398, 400f
        Pareto chart, 398, 401f

"Data smog," 528
Database, 211
    Canadian Classification of Health Interventions
        (CCI), 140
    for nursing, 426b
Decentralized structure, 163
Decisions
    biases
        group, 109–110
        individual, 109
    factors affect the quality of, 109–110
        fallacies, 110
        group decision biases, 109–110
        individual decision biases, 109
        personal attributes, 110
    logistical, 244
    optimizing, 113–114
    satisficing, 113–114
    strategic, 244
    support for making and implementing, in workplace advocacy,
        385–386, 386b
    tactical, 244
Decision making, 106–107, 106b, 110b, 116b, 120b–122b
    as characteristic of effective and ineffective team, 355t
    clinical information systems, 223
    creative, 108
    definition of, 107
    difference between problem solving, 106
    ethical, 108
        model for, 100–101, 100b–101b
    evidence in, 121–122
    evidence-informed, of nurse manager, 58–59, 59b
    intellectual processing in, 107–109, 109f
    intuitive, 108–109
    leadership and team development for, 117–119
    participatory, in workplace advocacy, 385
    process, 108
    relationship between problem solving, 106–107
    tips for, 102, 123
Decision-making framework, nursing staff mix, 285t, 286f
Decision-making models, 112–115, 117b
    rational, 112–113
Declaration of Alma-Ata, 134b, 487
Delegation, 494–495, 530
Demands, leadership, for future, 559–560
Dependable, as quality of team member, 357
Dependency, chemical, 465–467, 467b
Desire, cultural, 176–178
Destructive conflict, 362t
Developing Workplace Violence and Harassment Policies and
    Programs: A Toolbox, 479
Differentiated nursing practice, 269–270
Diffusion, of innovations, 421–423, 421b–422b
Diffusion theory, 344
Direct billing, to consumer, 241, 242b
Direct care hours, 293
Direct research utilization, 424

Discipline
  distinct, rise of, 488
  nonpunitive, 460, 460f, 461b
  progressive, 468, 468b
  as quality of team member, 357
Discussion, as characteristic of effective and ineffective team, 355t
Disease management, 268–269
Disrespectful communications, 450
Disruptive behaviour, 517
Dissatisfaction, work, 459
Distractions, as communication barrier, 365
Distributive justice, 95
Divergent thinking, 108
Diversity, results of increasing, 563
Division of labour, in organizational structures, 155
DMAIC mnemonic, as steps methodology of
    quality management, 393b
Documentation, 458, 467–468, 467f
  of performance problems, 467b
  tips for, 471
Dominant logic, altering, guidelines for, 333b
Dorothy Wylie Nursing Leadership Institute, 48
Drug laws, 81–82
Dualism, 359
Duty of care, 83–84
"Duty to report" clause, 466

E

EAPs. *see* Employee assistance programs (EAPs)
Early adopters, 341
Early majority, 341
EBP. *see* Evidence-based practice (EBP)
Economic forces, influencing health care organizations, 138–139
Economic influences, 563
Education
  academic, 549–551, 549b–550b
  communication and, 342
  continuing, 180, 550, 551b
  in health care organizations, 143
Effective Governance for Quality and Patient Safety: A Toolkit for
    Healthcare Board Members and Senior Leaders, 29
Effective teams, 354–355
  characteristics of, 355t
EHRs. *see* Electronic health records (EHRs)
Electrocardiograms (ECGs), 209
Electronic health records (EHRs), 79, 140, 227
Electronic medical record (EMR), 62–63, 227
  adoption model, 214t
Electronic meetings, 119
Electronic patient care records, 227
Electronic résumés, 543
E-mail, 229, 545, 546b
  communication guidelines of, 230b
Emergence, in complexity science, 13
Emergency care, 133t
Emerging fluid relationships, in organization, 164–165, 165f, 165b
Emerging workforce, 45, 46b

Emotional abuse, in workplace, 201–202
Emotional intelligence (EI), 7–8, 8f
  underdevelopment, 463
Emotional problems, 464–465, 465b
Emotionally intelligent, as follower characteristic, 16t
Emotions
  as communication barrier, 366
  managing, 368–369
  suppressing, 369
Employee assistance programs (EAPs), 465, 524
Employees
  chemically dependent, 458
  immature, 463, 463b
  motivation, 460–461
  uncooperative or unproductive, 460–463
Employment Insurance Act (1996), 81
Employment law, 80–81
Employment ramifications, 74
Empowerment, 43, 189, 306
  critical social theories, 189–190, 189b–190b
  dimensions of, 191–192
  psychological, 191–192
  theories of, 48
    nursing and, 189–194
Engaged leadership, 37
Enthusiasm, 46
  quality of team member, 358
Entrenched workforce, 45–46, 46b
  challenges for, 46
Entrepreneurial/transient style, 537, 538t
Entry-level competencies, 24, 25b
Environmental assessment, 321, 321f–322f
  external, 322, 322b
  internal, 322
Environmental readiness assessment, for implementation of
    clinical practice guideline, 429b
E-portfolios, 543
Equity, health, 375
Ethics, 91–92
  applied, 91–92
  code of, for nurses, 96–97, 97b
  committees, 99–100, 100b
  law *vs.*, 85–86
  meta-, 91–92
  normative, 91–92
  relational, 92–93, 92b, 94b
  relational context of, 91–92
Ethical decision making, 108
Ethical dilemmas, 99
Ethical distress, 99
Ethical issues, 90–104, 91b, 101b–102b
  code of ethics, 97b
    for nurses, 96–97
  ethical decision making model, 100–101, 100b–101b
  ethics committees, 99–100, 100b
  evidence in, 101–102
  interdependent environment of nursing, 97–98

Ethical issues (*Continued*)
  for nurse managers, 98–99, 98b–99b
  principles of bioethics, 93–96
  relational context of ethics, 91–92
  relational ethics, 92–93, 92b
Ethical leadership, 7
Ethical political savvy, 560b
Ethical practice, 24
Ethical violation, 99
Ethnocentrism, 178
Evaluation
  as change management function, 338
  as strategic planning process phase, 326–329
Evidence-Based Nursing, 430
Evidence-based practice (EBP), 417–421, 419b–420b
  evaluation of, 425–428, 425b–426b
  hierarchy of, 427, 427f
  steps in, 425b
Evidence-informed decision making, of nurse manager,
      58–59, 59b
Evidence Informed Healthcare Renewal, 414
Evidence-informed nursing, resources for, 420b
Evidence-informed practice (EIP), 221–222
  acquire and appraise of, 221–222
  applying, 222
  asking clinical question, 221
  assessing outcomes in, 222
Excellent Care for All Act, 142
Exhaustion-energy dimension, 522–523
Expected outcomes, 267
Expenditures, 247
Experience, 43
Expert decision frame, for "give maximum dose of pain
      medication," 220b
Expert power, 188b–189b
External environmental assessment, 322, 322b
External sources, of job stress, 516–517

F

Facilitators, 334, 334f
Factor evaluation system, 282
Fallacies, 110
Fatigue, change, 340
Fayol, Henri, 157
Fear, 370
Federal funding, in health care services, 127–128, 127t
Fee-for-service, 242b
Feelings, as characteristic of effective and ineffective
      team, 355t
Firewall, 228
First-line nurse leaders, 17–18
Fishbone diagrams, 114, 114b, 115f, 398, 401f
Fixed costs, 245–246
Flat structures, 162–163, 162f
Flexibility, 334
  in effective communication, 368
  as follower characteristic, 16t

Flexible performance appraisal tools, 310–312, 310b
  behaviourally anchored rating scales, 310–311, 311b
  management by objectives, 311, 311b
  self-review, 312
Flow charts, 398, 399f
Focus
  on patient, 23–35, 24b, 32b–33b
  in quality improvement process, 396
  versus quality assurance process, 404t
Followers, 503t, 504
  characteristics of, 16t
Followership, 4b, 7b, 18b–19b
  competencies in, 15–17, 16t, 16b
  during complex times, 17–18
  definition of, 7
  evidence in, 19
  personal attributes to, 7–9, 8b
  theories of, 12
  theory development in, 9–12, 9b
  tips in, 20
Force field analysis, 334
Forecast, 292–293
Foreseeability, 82–83
Formal leaders, 369
Formal power, 190
Formalization, 156
"Framework for the Practice of Registered Nurses in Canada," 413
Freedom of Information and Protection of Privacy Act (FIPPA)
      (1990), 77
Front-line nurses, in patient outcomes, 31
Front-line nurse managers, 56
Frustration, in conflict, 442
FTEs. *see* Full-time equivalents (FTEs)
Full-time equivalents (FTEs), 248, 293
  calculation of, 293, 293b
  distribution of, 293–294
  fixed, 293–294
  variable, 294
Functional approach, for résumé development, 543
Functional nursing, 258–260, 259f
  model analysis in, 259, 259b, 260f
  nurse manager's role in, 259–260
  staff nurse's role in, 260, 260b
Functional status, 30
Functional structures, 159, 159f

G

Gantt chart, 526–527, 527f
GAS. *see* General adaptation syndrome (GAS)
Gender roles, as external source of job stress, 517
General adaptation syndrome (GAS), 518, 520f
Generation X, 45–46
Generation Y, 45
Generation Z, 45
Geographical dispersion, 156
Give-and-take relationship, in conflict resolution, 447
Global funding, 242b

Global trends, 563
Goal, quality improvement process, 395
    versus quality assurance process, 404t
Goal accomplishment, motivated to, as follower
        characteristic, 16t
Goal conflicts, 443–444
Goal setting, 319b, 323, 323b, 328b–329b
    and plan development, 528
Governance structure, of organization, 383
Graduate degree, 549
Graduate program, factors to consider when
        selecting a, 550b
Graphic rating scales, 310, 311f
Great Man Theory, 10b–11b
Grievance, 461b
Ground rules, in team development, 356, 357b
Group decision biases, 109–110
Group decision making, 115–120
    leadership and team development for, 117–119
    team decision support tools, 119–120
Group invulnerability, 109–110
Group polarization, 109–110
Group purchasing organizations (GPOs), 239
Groups, definition of, 352–355
Groupthink, 109–110
*Guidelines for Preventing Workplace Violence for Health Care and
        Social Service Workers*, 479

H

Hallmarks of culture, 13
Halo effect, 310
Hand-off protocol, 442
Handheld computer, 215f
Harassment, 475b
Hardiness, 518
Hardware, of information systems, 216–217
Hardy's role theory, 505b
Hasty generalization, 110
Havelock's model, for planning change, 335, 335b
HEAL. *see* Health Action Lobby (HEAL)
Health Action Lobby (HEAL), 195
Health Canada, 138, 142
Health care
    changing economic environment, 242–243,
        242b–243b
    in nursing practice, 243
    costs of, 239–240
        relationship of price and utilization rates to, 239t
    cultural diversity in, 170–184, 171b–172b, 182b
    financing of, 240–241, 241b
        approaches to, 241–242, 241b–242b
    quality management in, 392
    shared vision of, 562
Health care aides. *see* Unregulated care providers (UCPs)
Health care delivery, nurses in, 333
Health care facilities, risk factors for violence in, 478b
Health care informatics, 58–59

Health care organizations, 125–148, 126b, 144b–145b
    cultural diversity in, 173–175
    evidence in, 144–145
    external forces influencing, 137–142
    human resources, 142–144
    internal forces influencing, 137
    open-systems model of, 136b, 137f
Health Care Policy Directorate, 138
Health care services
    basic framework of, 132–134, 133t
    delivery of, 129–130, 130f
        approaches to, 130–131
    funding in, 127–129, 127t
        provincial and territorial, 128–129, 128f, 129t
    theoretical perspective in, 136–137
    types and classifications of, 132–136, 133t, 135b
Health care settings, management of, 60–62, 61b–62b
Health care system, 4–5, 126–127
    complexity of, 17
    organization of, 130f
Health care workers, regulation of, 71–72
Health care workforce, 450–451
Health equity, 375
Health human resources, 142–144
    education, 143
    scope of practice, 143–144, 144b
    type of practice, 143
Health Information: Nursing Components (HI:NC), 212
Health Information and Management Systems Society
        (HIMSS), 213–214
Health information technology, implementation of, 225–226,
        225b–226b
Health Outcomes for Better Information and Care (HOBIC), 213
Health Professions Act, 72, 74–75, 466
Health records, 84
Health-related websites, 229t
Health trends, 563
Healthy work environments, 57
Heart and Stroke Foundation of Canada, 141–142
Helping teammate advance the team, as quality of team member, 357
Heuristics, 109
Hierarchy, 155
High-complexity change, 344–345
HIMSS. *see* Health Information and Management Systems Society
        (HIMSS)
HI:NC. *see* Health Information: Nursing Components (HI:NC)
Hindsight bias, 109
Histograms, 398, 400f
HOBIC. *see* Health Outcomes for Better Information and Care
        (HOBIC)
Home care services, 133t
Home support workers. *see* Unregulated care providers (UCPs)
Horizontal violence, 452, 475–476, 480–482, 481b
Hospital-based violence, 478
Hospital care services, 133t, 135–136
Humour, as stress reducer, 521
Hybrid organizational structure, 163

I

ICN. *see* International Council of Nurses (ICN)
Identity, professional, empowering, 192–194, 192b, 193f
IHI. *see* Institute for Healthcare Improvement (IHI)
Immature employees, 463, 463b
Impact, as dimension of empowerment, 191–192
Implementation, 324
    as change management function, 338
Implementation Science, 430
Imposition, cultural, 178
"In" groups, in team development, 356
In Praise of Followers, 12
Inadequate staffing, absenteeism and, 458–459
Incident reports, 78
Incivility
    defining, 475–478
    workplace and, 474–485
Incompetence, 73
    clinical, 462t, 463–464
INCP®. *see* International Classification for Nursing Practice
    (INCP®)
Indirect care hours, 293
Indirect research utilization, 424
Individual decision biases, 109
Ineffective teams, 354
    characteristics of, 355t
Inefficacy-efficacy dimension, 522–523
Inferencing mechanism, 220
Influence, 185–204, 185b, 201b
    exercising, 195–199
    tips for using, 202
Informal leaders, 369
Informal power, 190
Informatics, 218–221
    future trends and professional issues of, 231–232
    health care, 58–59, 62–63, 63b
    nursing, 218, 219f
Information, 219
    managing, 529–530
    overload, 528
    tips for, 235
    triad of, 220b
Information management, 344
    skills, development of, 212b
Information systems, 213–217, 215b
    clinical, 223–225
    elements of, 216b
    in evidence-based practice, 417–419
    hardware of, 216–217
    quality and accreditation of, 216
Information technology, 209, 211–213, 213b
    future trends and professional issues of, 226–228
    for patient safety, 223
    for structured nursing terminologies, 212–213
Informed consent, 82, 82b
Infoways' Standards Collaborative, 227
Innovations, diffusion of, 421–423, 421b–422b

Innovation adopters, characteristics of, 422b
Innovators, 341
Institute for Healthcare Improvement (IHI), 341
Institute for Safe Medication Practices Canada
    (ISMP Canada), 210
Institute for Safe Medication Practices (ISMP), 142
Institute of Medicine (IOM), in patient safety, 26
Institutional liability, 84, 84b
Insurance, 75–76, 84, 84b
Insured risk, 75
Intake and output systems, 210
Integrated information systems, 224
Intellectual processing, 107–109, 109f
    creative decision making, 108
    critical thinking, 107–108
    decision-making process, 108
    ethical decision making, 108
    intuitive decision making, 108–109
    nursing process, 108
    problem-solving process, 107f, 108
    scientific method, 107
Intentional, as quality of team member, 358
Interactional justice, 59
Interdisciplinary settings
    concepts and definitions for, 487–488
    framework for interprofessional collaboration, 489–490
    leading interdisciplinary or interprofessional teams, 493–495,
        493f, 493b–495b
    moving forward in collaborative practice, 491–493, 491b–493b
    practising and leading in, 486–498, 487b, 496b
        tips for, 497
    rise of distinct disciplines, 488
    scope of practice, 488–489, 489b
    working "with" *versus* "alongside" others, 495
Interdisciplinary team, 353, 487–488
Intergenerational tensions, 450–451
Internal environmental assessment, 322
Internal sources, of job stress, 517–518
International Classification for Nursing Practice (INCP®), 212
International Council of Nurses (ICN), 537–538
    code of ethics, 93, 96–97, 97b
    leadership definition, 57
    in nursing diversity, 172
    three pillars essential to nursing and health
        improvement, 378, 378f
    workplace violence and, 476
Internet
    checklist for evaluation of sources, 230t
    in health care, 63
Interpersonal competence, 459–460
Interpersonal components, 496b
Interpersonal conflict, 441, 475–476
Interpersonal relationships, on team, 369
Interpersonal skills, 15
    as follower characteristic, 16t
Interprofessional collaboration, framework for, 489–490,
    490f–491f, 490b

Interprofessional team, 487–488
    leading interdisciplinary or, 493–495, 493f, 493b–495b
Interprofessional team, definition of, 353
Interruptions, 527, 528b
Interview, 546–548
    goals and content, 548t
    for performance appraisal, 312–313, 312b
    topics and questions of concern, 547–548, 547b
Intracranial pressure (ICP) monitoring systems, 209
Intramuscular injection technique, example of innovation
        diffusion, 423
Intrapersonal conflict, 441
Intraprofessional conflict, 452–453
Intravenous (IV) fluid, dispensing and administration of, 210
Intravenous (IV) smart pumps, 210
Intuition, 108–109
Intuitive decision making, 108–109
Involvement
    joining and reasons for, 553–555, 553b
    model for, 552–555, 552b
IOM. see Institute of Medicine (IOM)
Irrelevance, communication pattern during stress, 365t
ISMP. see Institute for Safe Medication Practices (ISMP)
ISMP Canada. see Institute for Safe Medication Practices Canada
        (ISMP Canada)

J

Joanna Briggs Institute, 419
Job interview, tips for conducting, 314
Job performance, dimensions of, 460–461
Job stress
    definition of, 516
    sources of, 516–519, 517b
        external, 516–517
        internal, 517–518
Joint, definition of, 284–285
Journal of the American Medical Association, 419
"Judge made," 70–71
Justice, 95
    distributive, 95
    interactional, 59
    social, 95

K

King, Martin Luther Jr., 37
Knowledge
    base, 220
    brokering, 232
    brokers, 232
    cultural, 176–178
    inadequate, as communication barrier, 365
"Knowledge navigators," 413
Knowledge technology, 209, 220–221, 220b, 232
Knowledge-to-action model, 415, 417f
Knowledge translation (KT), 412
    in policymaking, 196–197

Knowledge workers, nurses as, 208–209
Kotter's strategies, for implementing complex change, 336
KT. see Knowledge translation (KT)

L

Labour cost per unit of service, 297, 298b
Labour law, 80–81
Labour unions, in nursing organizations, 381
Laggards, 341
Lancaster, James, 423
Language clarity, 172
Laschinger, Heather, 191
Late majority, 341
Lateral violence, 475–476
    management of, 452–453, 453b
Laughter, as tension reducer, 521
Law
    contract, 85
    drug, 81–82
    ethics vs., 85–86
    mental health, 81
    and morality, interface of, 91f
    protective and reporting, 79–80
    sources of, 70–71
Leaders, 37–39, 37b, 503t, 504
    becoming, tips for, 52
    contingent reward, 10, 10b–11b
    definition of, 57
    effective, characteristics of, 37, 38b
    in emerging workforce, 44–46, 44b
    informal, 332
    management-by-exception active, 10b–11b
    management-by-exception passive, 10b–11b
    role of, 36–53, 51b
        in conflict, 450–452, 450b
        evidence in, 51
    surviving and thriving as, 46–47, 46b–47b
        building self-confidence, 47
        generating self-motivation, 46
        listening to constituents, 47
        maintaining balance, 46
        maintaining positive attitude, 47
    transactional, 10
Leader empowering behaviours (LEBs), 192, 192t, 192b
Leader-follower relationship, 15–17
Leadership, 4b, 7b, 18b–19b, 38
    approaches to, 39–42
    authentic, 10, 10b–11b
    barriers to, 42, 42b
        false assumptions, 42
        time constraints, 42
    challenge of, 50–51, 50b
    as characteristic of effective and ineffective team, 355t
    in community, 49
    competencies in, 14–15, 15t, 15b
    during complex times, 17–18
    definition of, 6

Leadership (Continued)
  demands, 559–560
  development of, 42–44, 42b, 50b
    acceptance of responsibility, 43
    clear vision, 43
    leading by example, 43, 43f
    mentor selection, 42–43
    and planning, 17–18, 18b
    sharing rewards, 43
    willingness to grow, 43–44
  engaged, 37
  ethical, 7
  evidence in, 19
  impact on productivity, 298
  as important concept for nurses, 38–39
  International Council of Nurses definition of, 57
  and management, 524–525
  nursing, 37
    core elements of relational ethics
      applied to, 94b
  patient-focused, tips for, 34
  personal attributes to, 7–9, 8b
  perspectives, 74–77
    documentation requirements, 76–77
    duty to report, 74–75
    insurance, 75–76
  practice of, 39–42
  as primary determinant of workplace
      satisfaction, 39, 39b
  in professional organizations and unions, 49
  resonant, 9b
  role in team success, 369–371, 370b
  strengths, 560–561, 560b–561b
    authenticity and accountability, 560, 560b
    ethical political savvy, 560b
    politics of commonalities, 560b
    quest for meaning, 560b
    thinking long term, acting short term, 560b
    through expectation, 560–561, 560b
  theories of, 10–11, 10b–11b
    development in, 9–12, 9b
  through appointed and elected office, 49–50
  tips for, 20
  transactional, 10b–11b
  transformational, 10, 10b–11b
  visionary and authentic, 50
  within the workplace, 47–49
Leadership Rounding Tool, 342
Leadership "tag," 13
Leadership training, lateral violence and, 453
Lean (managerial tool), 244
Learn, willing to, as follower characteristic, 16t
Learning organizations, 38, 165, 336–337
  theory, 336–337
    application of, 337
    disciplines of, 337
LEBs. see Leader empowering behaviours (LEBs)

Legal issues, 69–89, 70b, 86b–87b
  consent to treatment, 82
  distinguishing law and ethics, 85–86
  drug laws, 81–82
  evidence in, 86–87
  implications and liability, 72–74
  labour and employment, 80–81
  leadership perspectives, 74–77
  malpractice, 82–84, 83b
  privacy and confidentiality, 77–79
  protective and reporting laws, 79–80
  regulation of health care workers, 71–72
  risk management, 84–85
  sources of law, 70–71
Legal-political forces, influencing health care organizations, 138
Legislation, 70
  ratio, 195–196
Length of stay (LOS), 244
Letter
  cover, 544, 544b
  resignation, 545
Lewin's change theory, 334–335
Liability, 72
  civil, 73
  criminal, 72–73
  institutional, 84, 84b
  personal, 76
  vicarious, 76
Licensure, 71–72, 537–538
Lifestyle choices, effect on stress, 518
Line functions, 157–159, 158f
Line graphs, 398, 400f
Linear approaches, planned change using, 334–336, 335b
Linear careers, 537, 538t
Linear change, contrasting patterns of nonlinear and, 337f
Lippitt, Watson, Westley's model, for planning
    change, 335–336, 335b
Listening
  active, 367–368, 367b, 368t
  as characteristic of effective and ineffective team, 355t
  communication during conflict, 364
Listserv, 229
Lobby, 195
Lobbying, 187
Local Health Integration Networks (LHINs), 130–131
Logistical decisions, 244
LOS. see Length of stay (LOS)
Low-complexity change, 344–345
Low-dose heparin (Heparin) flush solution, example of innovation
    diffusion, 422–423

M

Macromarketing, 563
Malpractice, 82–84, 83t, 83b
Management, 4b, 7b, 18b–19b, 38
  of change in complex organizations, 60
  competencies in, 14–15, 15t, 15b, 58

Management *(Continued)*
    during complex times, 17–18
    day-to-day challenges in, 59–60, 60b
    definition of, 6
    evidence in, 19
    of health care settings, 60–62, 61b–62b
    meeting, 530–531
    personal attributes to, 7–9, 8b
    project, 333–334
    of resources, 62
    role of, 56–58, 57b
    self-, 514–534, 515b, 532b
        evidence in, 532
    of stress, 519–523, 520b, 522b
        strategies, 523t
    of symptom, 520–522
    theories of, 11–12, 186
        development in, 9–12, 9b
    time, 525–530
        concepts, 528–530, 530b
        techniques, 528t
    tips for, 20
Management-by-exception active leaders, 10b–11b
Management-by-exception passive leaders, 10b–11b
Management by objectives (MBO), 311, 311b
Manager, 503t, 504
    basic functions of, 56, 56t
    definition of, 57
    role of, 38, 54–68, 55b, 66b
        evidence in, 65–66
Manager-led team, 353
Mance, Jeanne, 187
Mandatory overtime, 287, 287b
Manipulation, 344
Marketing change, 339t
Maslach Burnout Inventory, 522–523
Matrix structures, 161–162, 161f
MBO. *see* Management by objectives (MBO)
Meaning, as dimension of empowerment, 191–192
Mechanical ventilators, 210
Mediation, 452
Mediator, 452
Medical charts, 76–77
Medical records, electronic, 62–63, 227
Medication, dispensing and administration of, 210
Medication administration processes, clinical information systems' impact on, 224–225
Medication-dosing calculators, 220
Meditation, as relaxation technique, 521
Meetings
    electronic, 119
    management of, 530–531
Membership, expectations of, 552–553, 553b
Mental health laws, 81
Mental models, 337
Mentor, selection of, 42–43
Mentoring, as role of nurse manager, 59

Mentorship, 509, 510b–511b
    programs, in dealing with cultural diversity, 180
Meta-analysis, 422–423
Meta-ethics, 91–92
Micromarketing, 563
Military change, 339t
Millennium Generation, 45
Mintzberg, Henry, 12
Miscommunications, 450
Misconduct, 73
Mission, 150–152, 151b
    statement, 323, 323b
    team, singleness of, 361
Mission conscious, as quality of team member, 358
Model analysis
    in case method, 257, 258f
    in functional nursing, 259, 259b, 260f
    in nursing case management, 268
    in primary nursing, 263–264, 264f, 264b
    in team nursing, 261, 261b
Moral distress, 99
Moral uncertainty, 98
Morality, 91–92, 91f
Mortality rates, 31
Mother Teresa, 37
Multiculturalism, 178
Multidisciplinary planning, 393
Multiple "stress-buffering" behaviours, 521
Murphy, Gail Tomblin, 197–198, 412
Mussallem, Helen K., 187

N

National Case Management Network of Canada (2009), 266
National Database of Nursing Quality Indicators (NDNQI), 63
National Interprofessional Competency Framework, 353–354, 489–490, 490f
National Quality Forum, 180
National System for Incident Reporting (NSIR), 27
Natural laws, 71
NDNQI. *see* National Database of Nursing Quality Indicators (NDNQI)
Near miss, in risk management, 406
Negligence, nursing, 82–83
Negotiation, as conflict resolution strategy, 447, 448b
Networks
    definition of, 194
    developing, in complexity science, 13–14
Networking, as power strategy, 194–195, 194t
Never events, errors in medical care, 406
Newborn nursery systems, 210–211
Nexters, 45
Nightingale, Florence, 37
NMDS. *see* Nursing minimum data set (NMDS)
"No-win" situation, 444
Nominal group technique, 120
Non-hierarchical "bottom-up" interaction among workers, 13

Nonlinear change, 333–334, 336–337
  contrasting patterns of linear and, 337f
  strategies for, 342–344
Nonmaleficence, 96
Nonproductive hours, 248, 293
Nonpunitive discipline, 460, 460f, 461b
Normative ethics, 91–92
Novice nurses, personal/personnel problems of, 458
NSIR. *see* National System for Incident Reporting (NSIR)
Nurses
  in administrative role, 25b
  code of ethics for, 96–97, 97b
  conflict-handling styles of, differences of, 447f, 449–450, 449b
  contract, 288
  "floating," 288
  as leader, 47–51
  leadership as an important concept for, 38–39
  new graduate, stress of, 523
  role in patient safety, 28
  self-scheduling of, 65b
  in translating research into practice, 412
  workplace violence and, 190
Nurse characteristics, definition of, 289
Nurse executive, as leader, 48
Nurse leaders
  issues for, 429–431
  powerful Canadian, 187
  from practising nurse to, 503–504, 503t
  role in conflict, 450
  tips for, 146
Nurse managers
  in assessing staff diversity, 174
  in balancing three sources of demand, 59–60
  in budgetary allocations, 63
  competencies for, 58
  in conflict, 451–452
  in creating healthy work environment, 57
  in day-to-day management challenges, 59–60, 60b
  in decentralized scheduling, 294
  as "environmentalist" of unit, 57
  evidence-informed decision making of, 58–59, 59b
  functions of, 56t
  issues for, 429–431
  as leader, 48
  leadership styles of, 41
  in leading ethical, value-based management, 61–62
  in managing health care settings, 60–62, 61b–62b
  in managing resources, 62
  in mentoring, 59
  in patient outcomes, 31
  from practising nurse to, 503–504, 503t
  professionalism of, 64, 64b–65b
  quality indicators and, 63
  role of
    in case method, 257–258
    in functional nursing, 259–260
    implementing, 66

Nurse managers (*Continued*)
    in nursing case management, 268
    in personal/personnel problems, 458
    in primary nursing, 264–265, 265f
    in team nursing, 261–262
  tips for, 146
  in understanding and value of cultural
      diversity, 174
  in understanding organizational culture, 59
  in using health care informatics, 62–63
  in workplace violence, 60
Nurse outcomes, 290
Nurse researchers, 415
Nurse staffing, 284–289
  model, 280–292, 281f
Nurse surveillance capacity, of hospital, 289, 290b
Nurse-to-patient ratios, 195–196, 285, 289
  mandated, 284
NurseONE, 549
Nursing, 5–7
  databases and search platforms for, 426b
  diversity in, 172
  empowerment theories and, 189–194
  in future
    implications, 565
    preparation for, 564–565
    projections for, 563–564, 564f, 564b
    thriving in, 558–566, 558b, 565b
  interdependent environment of, 97–98
  policy advocacy and, 199–201, 200b
  strategic priorities/goals, 151b
Nursing associations, provincial and territorial, 380t
Nursing care delivery model, 257, 273b–274b
Nursing case management, 266–268, 266t
  case manager, 266–267, 267f
  clinical pathways, 267–268
  model analysis in, 268
  nurse manager's role in, 268
  staff nurse's role in, 268
Nursing governance, 383–387, 384b
  shared, 384, 384b
  workplace advocacy, 385–387, 385b–386b
Nursing graduate, new
  mentoring, 510b–511b
  role transition for
    professional, 506b, 507f
    stages of, 502t
Nursing informatics, 218, 219f
Nursing leadership, 37
Nursing minimum data set (NMDS), 212, 212b
Nursing organizations
  and collective action, 378–383, 379b
  inter-organizational advocacy and coalitions, 382–383,
      382b–383b
  labour unions, 381
  professional associations, 379–381
  regulatory bodies, 382

Nursing practice
  differentiated, 269–270
  health care economic environment for, 243
  standards of, 83–84
  translating research into, 423–425, 424f
    tips for, 433
  using research in evaluating, 246–247, 246b–247b
Nursing practice acts, 72
Nursing process
  for problem solving and decision making, 108
  vs. strategic planning process, 327f
Nursing productivity, 297
Nursing professional practice council, 385
Nursing regulatory bodies, provincial and territorial, 32
Nursing research designs, 414
Nursing resources, predicting and using of, 245–246,
  246b
Nursing-sensitive indicators, 282–283, 283t
Nursing-sensitive outcomes, 30–31, 31b, 398–401
  definition of, 30
  uses of, 31
Nursing Services Department, structure and philosophy of,
  290–291
Nursing student
  as leader, 48–49, 48f
  to practising nurse, 501–503
Nursing the Future, 48–49

O

Objectives, 323–324
  as characteristic of effective and ineffective team, 355t
  S.M.A.R.T, 323–324, 324b
Occupational Health and Safety Act, 476
Occupational Safety and Health Association (OSHA),
  US-based, 478
Occupational stress, 516
OECD countries. see Organization for Economic Co-operation and
  Development (OECD) countries
Off-peak shifts, 285–286
Office, appointed and elected, leadership through, 49–50
Office of Nursing Policy, 138, 186–187
Oncology Nursing Society, 420
Online health record. see Personal health record (PHR)
Ontario Community Care Access Centres (CCACs), 223
Ontario Ministry of Labour, 479
Open-systems organizations, 136b
Open-systems theory, 136, 136b, 137f
Operating budget, 247–249, 249b
Opportunity, access to, 190
Oppressed groups, 189
Optimizing decision, 113–114
Organization, 150, 529
  learning, 165
Organization for Economic Co-operation and Development
  (OECD) countries
  health care spending in, 128–129, 129t
  rank of Canadian health care system, 4–5

Organizational chart, 155
  bureaucratic, 158f
Organizational components, 496b
Organizational conflict, 441–442
Organizational culture, 59, 152–154, 153b–154b, 165–166, 383
Organizational development, factors influencing, 154–155, 155b
Organizational processes, influence on delivery of care, 272t
Organizational size, 156
Organizational staffing policies, 291
Organizational strategies, in translating research into practice,
  428–429, 428b
Organizational structures
  analyzing, 164
  bureaucracy of, 157–159, 157b
  characteristics of, 155–157, 156b
  emerging fluid relationships, 164–165, 165f
  influence on delivery of care, 272t
  types of, 159–164
    flat, 162–163, 162f
    functional, 159, 159f
    matrix, 161–162, 161f
    service-line, 159–161, 160f
    shared governance, 163–164, 164b
  understanding and designing, 149–169, 150b, 165b–166b
    evidence in, 165–166
    tips for, 167
Organizational support systems, 291, 291b
Organizational theories, 150, 186
Organizing, as change management function, 338
OSHA. see Occupational Safety and Health Association (OSHA)
Ottawa Model of Research Use, 416, 418f
"Out" groups, in team development, 356
Out-of-pocket expenses, 240–241
Outcome criteria, 262–263
Overload, information, 528
Overstress, signs of, 519t
Overtime, 287
Overwork, 517

P

Pain medication, maximum dose of, expert decision frame for, 220b
Paper-based system, 215
Paradox, 175–176
Pareto chart, 398, 401f
Parliament of Quebec, 97
Partnerships, building team through, 351–373
Partnership model, 265, 265b
Path-goal theory, 10b–11b, 55
Patient-care documentation, clinical information systems'
  impact on, 224
Patient-care hand-offs, 224
Patient-centred care, 7, 25–26, 151b, 492
  governance and management activities for, 27b
  values of, 26b
Patient classification system, 282
  electronic, 62–63
  types of, 282

Patient-focused care model, 265–266
Patient-focused leadership, tips for, 34
Patient information, in electronic clinical information system, 223
Patient outcomes, 259–260, 280–281, 398–401
    nurse staffing and, conceptual framework of, 281f
Patient safety, 24, 26–30, 28b, 85, 222–223, 405
    Accreditation Canada's required organizational
        practices in, 405b
    Canadian Nurses Association in, 28, 29b
    Canadian Patient Safety Institute's competencies in, 29b
    drivers for effective governance for, 30f
    evidence in, 33
    in information technology, 223
    role of nurses in, 28
    WHO definition of, 27
Patient satisfaction, 31
Patient surveillance systems, 209
Pay-for-performance (P4P), 241, 242b
PDSA cycle. see Plan-Do-Study-Act (PDSA) cycle
Pension Act (1985), 81
Perceived power, 188b–189b
Percentage of occupancy, 296–297, 296f, 296b
Perceptions
    collective, of unit leadership, 153
    differences in, as communication barrier, 366
Perfectionism, 527
Performance appraisals, 307–309, 309b
    anecdotal note, 308, 308b
    coaching, 308–309, 308f
    interview environment, 312–313, 312b
    tools for, 309–313, 309b–310b, 312b
        flexible, 310–312, 310b
        structured, 310, 310b
Performance improvement (PI), 394–395
Performance problems, documentation of, 467b
Personal analysis of change, 521b
Personal attributes, 110
Personal Health Information Protection Act (2004), 77, 98
Personal health record (PHR), 227
Personal Information Protection and Electronic Documents Act
    (PIPEDA), 228
Personal liability, 76
Personal mastery, 337
Personal/personnel problems, 458–467, 458b, 469b–470b
    absenteeism, 458–460, 460f, 460b–461b, 462t
        evidence in, 470
    chemical dependency, 465–467, 467b
    clinical incompetence, 462t, 463–464
    documentation of, 467–468, 467f, 467b
        tips for, 471
    emotional problems, 464–465, 465b
    immature employees, 463, 463b
    progressive discipline in, 468, 468b
    termination and, 468–469, 469b
    uncooperative or unproductive employees, 460–463
Personal power, 188b–189b
Personal qualities, 15

Personal stress, 517–518
Personal support workers. see Unregulated care providers (UCPs)
Personality, as communication barrier, 366
Persuasive research utilization, 424
PERT chart. see Program evaluation and review technique
    (PERT) chart
Petrucka, Pammla, 412
Philosophy
    and mission statement, 323, 323b
    of organizations, 150, 151b–152b, 152
PHR. see Personal health record (PHR)
Physical attacks, 475b
Physical illnesses, linked to stress, 519
Physiological monitoring, 209
PI. see Performance improvement (PI)
PICOT format, 425, 425b
PIPEDA. see Personal Information Protection and Electronic
    Documents Act (PIPEDA)
Placation, 365t
Placing computers, 215
Plan development, and goal setting, 528
Plan-Do-Study-Act (PDSA) cycle, 272, 306–307, 341
Planned change
    definition of, 334
    Havelock's model for, 335, 335b
    Lippitt, Watson, Westley's model for, 335–336, 335b
    strategies for, 342–344
    theories for, 335b
    using linear approaches, 334–336
Planning
    "aggressive," 320
    as change management function, 338
    multidisciplinary, 393
    poor, as communication barrier, 365–366
    for quality management, 393
    strategic, 319b, 320–329, 326b, 328b–329b
        of breast cancer screening program, 327b
        evidence of, 329
        for orthopedic centre of excellence, 325t–326t
        process, 321–329, 321f–322f, 327f, 328b
        reasons for, 320–321
    succession, 39
Point-of-care documentation, 215f
Policy, 185–204
    implementation of, 198
Policy advocacy
    forms of, 199–200
    nursing and, 199–201, 200b
Policy inputs, in policymaking, 196–197
Policy process, 195
    politics and, 195–199, 196b, 198b
"Policy" stream, in policymaking, 197
Policymaking, 197, 197f
Political activism, model of, 200b
Political change, 339t
Political savvy, ethical, 560b
"Political" stream, in policymaking, 197

Politics, 185b, 187, 201b
  policy process and, 195–199, 196b, 198b
Portable computers, 215
Portfolio, 543
  professional, data assembly for, 546, 546b
POS. *see* Positive organizational scholarship (POS)
Position
  assessment of, 540
  description, 304, 304b
  as external source of stress, 517
  knowing the, 539–540
Position power, 188b–189b
Positional plateau careers, 537
Positive communication model, 363–364
Positive organizational scholarship (POS), 8
Power, 185–204, 185b, 201b
  definition of, 186
  exercising, 195–199
  strategies, 194–195
  in team development, 356
  types of, 187–189, 188b–189b
Practice-based evidence, 219
Practising nurse
  to nurse leader or manager, 503–504, 503t
  nursing student to, 501–503
Preceptorship, 509
Prejudice, cultural diversity and, 175–176, 176b
Preparation, quality of team member, 358
Preprocessed evidence, 426
  hierarchy of, 427, 427f
Prevention services, 133t, 134–135
Price, definition of, 239
Primary care, 132
Primary Care Toolkit, 413
Primary health care (PHC) services, 132, 133t
  from Declaration of ALMA-ATA, 134b
Primary nurse, 262
Primary nursing, 262–266, 263f
  model analysis in, 263–264, 264f, 264b
  nurse manager's role in, 264–265, 265f
  staff nurse's role in, 265
Principled negotiation, 452
Priorities
  classification of, 529f
  setting of, 528–529
Privacy, 77–79, 98b
  informational, 227–228
Proactive, definition of, 320
Problem solving, 106–107, 106b, 116b, 121b–122b
  decision *versus*, 106
  definition of, 106–107
  evidence in, 121–122
  group decision making, 115–120
  intellectual processing in, 107–109, 109f
  in nursing practice, 111–112, 112b
  relationship between decision-making and, 106–107
  tips for, 123

Problem-solving process, 107f, 108
  applying, 110–112
"Problem" stream, in policymaking, 197
Procrastination, 526–527
Product lines. *see* Service-line structures
Productive hours, 248, 293
  calculation of, 248b
Productivity, 252–253
  impact of leadership on, 298
  unit, evaluation of, 295–298, 296b
Productivity performance, 297
Productivity target, 297
Professional organizations, leadership in, 49
Professional portfolio, data assembly for, 546, 546b
Professional practice
  environments, conflict in, 440–441
  models, 163–164
Professional sanctions, 73–74, 74b
  conduct unbecoming a member of profession, 73
  incompetence, 73
  misconduct, 73
Professional standard, 24, 25b
Professional values, in workplace advocacy, 386–387, 387b
Professional writing, 543–545
Professional associations, 140–142, 379–381, 551–552, 552b, 554b
Professional development, 548–549, 548b–549b
Professional identity, empowering, 192–194, 192b, 193f
Professionalism, of nurse manager, 64–65, 64b–65b
Program evaluation and review technique (PERT) chart, 526–527, 526f
Progressive discipline, 468, 468b
Project management, 333–334
Protection for Persons in Care Act (2009), 79–80
Prototype evaluation system, 282
Provincial funding, in health care services, 128–129, 128f, 129t
Prudence trap, 109
Psychological empowerment, 191–192
Public health collaboration, barriers and facilitators to primary care, 491f
Public health services, 133t, 134–135
Public policy, 186
  decision making, 198
  evaluation of, 199
  politics and, 196
Public-private partnerships (P3s), 131
Publicly funded services, 240–241
PubMed Central Canada, 419
Purnell's Model for Cultural Competence, 176, 177f

Q

QA. *see* Quality assurance (QA)
QI. *see* Quality improvement (QI)
QM. *see* Quality management (QM)
Quality assurance (QA), 403–404
  versus quality improvement process, 404t

Quality improvement (QI), 142, 392
   principles of, 394–396, 394b, 396b
   process, 396–403
      assemble a team, 398, 398b, 404t
      collect and analyze data, 398
      discussing plans, 402–403, 402f
      establishing outcomes, 398–402, 404t
      evaluation, 403
      identifying consumers' needs, 397–398, 397b
      versus quality assurance process, 404t
   roles and responsibilities in, 395t
Quality indicators, 63–64, 64f
Quality management (QM), 391–410, 391b, 408b
   benefits of, 392
   evidence, 408
   evolution of, 393–394, 393b
   in health care, 392
   planning for, 393
   principles of, 394–396, 394b
   tips for, 409
Quality work environment, 9b
Quid pro quo style, 39–40

R

Randomized controlled trial (RCT), 427–428
Ratio legislation, 195–196
Rational choice model. *see* Rational decision-making model
Rational decision-making model, 112–113, 112b
   tool, 113
RCT. *see* Randomized controlled trial (RCT)
Real-time reports, 222
"Reality shock," 192–193
Reasonably foreseeable, 82–83
Recognition, in demonstrating employee value, 61–62
Redesign, in organizational development, 155
Re-engineering, in organizational development, 155
Reflective practice, 369
Reframing, 521
Refreezing, 335
Regional Health Administration, 130–131
Regional Health Authorities (RHAs), 129–131, 151
Regionalization, 243
Registered Nurses' Association of Ontario (RNAO), 141, 420, 428
   patient- or client-centred care, 26
Registration, 71–72
Regulatory bodies, 72, 378–379
   influencing health care organizations, 142
   in nursing organizations, 382
   provincial and territorial, 380t
Rejectors, 341
Relational aggression, 480
Relational ethics, 92–93
   core elements of, 92b, 94b
Relationship management, 344
Relationship-oriented team member, 358
Releasing Time to Care™, 306–307
Reliable, as follower characteristic, 16t

Report, duty to, leadership perspectives, 74–75
Research, 413
   evidence in, 431–432
   for nursing practice improvement, 414
   translation of, into practice, 412b, 414b, 423–425, 424f, 431b–432b
   tips for, 433
   utilization, 414–417
      direct, 424
      indirect, 424
      persuasive, 424
"Research to action" project, 382b
Resident aides. *see* Unregulated care providers (UCPs)
Residential care, 133t
Resignation letter, 545
Resolution, of conflict, 444b
   approaches to, 444–449
Resonant leadership, 9b
Resource intensity weights (RIWs), 242
Resources
   access to, 190
   management of, 62
   using, developing, and being appreciated for, 356
Responsibility, acceptance of, 43
Restructuring, 7–8
   in organizational development, 155
Résumé, 542–543, 543b
   electronic, 543
   ways to develop a, 543
Revenue, 247
   budget, 249
Reverse chronological order, curriculum vitae, 542
Rewards, sharing of, 43
RHAs. *see* Regional Health Authorities (RHAs)
Risk management, 84–85, 391–410, 391b, 407b–408b
   evaluating, 407, 407b
   evidence in, 408
RIWs. *see* Resource intensity weights (RIWs)
RNAO. *see* Registered Nurses' Association of Ontario (RNAO)
Rogers' diffusion of innovations theory, 421b
Role ambiguity, 304
Role clarity, 491–492
Role competence, 459–460
Role conflict, 304
Role discrepancy, 506b
Role expectations, 504–505, 505b
   steps to clarify, 461b
Role integration, 506b
   phase, 510b–511b
Role negotiation, 508, 508b–509b
Role orientation, 506b, 510b–511b
Role preparation, 506b, 510b–511b
Role stabilization, 506b
   phase, 510b–511b
Role strain, 459–460, 505
Role stress, 459–460, 517
   type of, 505

Role theory, 55, 303, 303b
Role transition, 499–513, 500b–501b, 510b–512b
    ABCs of understanding, 504–505, 504b
    phase, 510b–511b
    process, 505
    professional, for new nursing graduate, 506b, 507f
    stages of, 502t
    strategies to promote, 505–511, 507b
        assess the workplace, 508
        grow through preceptorship and mentorship, 509–511,
            510b–511b
        negotiate the role, 508–509, 508b–509b
        strengthen internal resources, 505–508
    tips for, 512
    types of, 501–504
    unexpected, 506b
"ROLES" acronym, 504b
Root-cause analysis, in risk management, 406
Routine intra-abdominal pressure (IAP) monitoring, 209
Roy's adaptation model, 518

S

Safer Healthcare Now!, 162–163, 405
Satisficing decision, 113–114
Schedules
    constructing, 294–295
    variables that affect staffing, 295, 295b
Scheduling, 279–301, 298b–299b
    centralized, 295
    decentralized, 294
    definition of, 280
    evidence, 299
    staff self-scheduling, 294–295
    tips for, 300
Scientific method, for problem solving, 107
Scope of practice, 72
Scurvy, 423
Search platforms, for nursing, 426b
Secondary health care services, 132–134, 133t
Self-care, 30
Self-confidence, building, for effective leader, 47
Self-determination, as dimension of empowerment,
    191–192
Self-directed team, 353
Self-esteem, 370
Self-governance structures, 163–164
Self-governing team, 353
Self-improvement, as quality of team member, 358
Self-management, 514–534, 515b, 532b
    evidence of, 532
Self-managing team, 353
Self-motivation, from leader, 46
Self-regulation, as characteristic of effective and ineffective team,
    355t
Self-review, 312
Selfless, as quality of team member, 358
Senior nurse managers, 56

Sentinel event, in risk management, 406
Service-line structures, 159–161, 160f
Shamian, Judith, 187
Shared governance, 163–164
    in nursing, 384, 384b
    structure evolution, 164b
Shared vision, 337, 562–563
    of health care, 562
Sigma Theta Tau International, 552
Situation-Background-Assessment-Recommendation (SBAR)
        communication, 366–367, 367b
Situational-contingency theories, 10b–11b
Situational leadership theories, 10b–11b, 55
Six Sigma, 244
Six thinking hats, 119–120
Skills, using, developing, and being appreciated for, 356
Smadu, Marlene, 413
S.M.A.R.T. objectives, 323–324, 324b
Smart Beds, 62–63
Smart syringe pumps, 210
Social, as external source of job stress, 516–517
Social determinants of health, 139, 139b
Social exchange theory, 9b
Social exclusion, and health, 4
Social justice, 95
Social media (Web 2.0), 229–231
Social networking
    in nursing, 6
    as power strategy, 194, 194t
    sites, 545
Social psychological theories, 186, 191–192
Social support, 523, 523f
Sociocultural forces, influencing health care
        organizations, 139, 140b
Socioeconomic welfare, pillar of, 379, 388b
Solution-oriented team member, 358
Span of control, 7–8, 155
Specialization, in organizational structures, 155
Speech recognition (SR), 217–218
Spiral careers, 537, 538t
Stability, of society, 562, 562f
Staff
    development of, 303b, 306–307, 313b
    functions, 157–159, 158f
    morale of, 282
    participation and involvement, in change process, 343
    selection of, 303b, 304–306, 313b
    variance between projected and actual, 297–298, 298b
Staff mix, 260–261
Staff nurse
    as leader, 47–48
    role of
        in case method, 258, 258b
        in functional nursing, 260, 260b
        in nursing case management, 268
        in primary nursing, 265
        in team nursing, 262

Staff positions, 157–159, 158f
Staff self-scheduling, 294–295
Staffing, 279–301, 280b, 298b–299b
    definition of, 280
    effectiveness indicators of, 284b
    evidence in, 299
    external factors influencing, 288–289
    float pools and agency staff, 287–288
    hospital factors in, 289–290, 290b
    inadequate, absenteeism and, 458–459
    nurse characteristics and, 289
    nurse outcomes and, 290
    overtime and, 287
    patient and family expectation in, 289
    patient factors in, 282–284
    plans, 284–285
    process, 280–292
    schedules, variables that affect, 295
    services offered on unit and, 291–292
    tips for, 300
    24-hour, 285–287
    unit requirements, forecasting, 292–294, 292b
Stakeholders, 186–187
Standards of practice, 83–84
Starfish and the Spider, The, 345
Statutes, 70
    relating to privacy, confidentiality, and information access in
        health care, 78t
Steady state careers, 537, 538t
Stetler-Marram model, 415, 416f
S-TLC acronym, 364
Stop, ability to, communication during conflict, 364
Strategic decisions, 244
Strategic planning, 319b, 320–329, 326b, 328b–329b
    of breast cancer screening program, 327b
    evidence in, 329
    for orthopedic centre of excellence, 325t–326t
    process, 321, 328b
        vs. nursing process, 327f
        phases of, 321–329, 321f–322f
    reasons for, 320–321
Strategic plans, 247
Strategic Policy Branch, 138
Strategies
    communication and education, 342
    facilitation and support, 343–344
    identification of, in strategic planning process,
        324, 324b
    Kotter's, for implementing complex change, 336
    negotiation and agreement, 344
    for nonlinear change, 342–344
    participation and involvement, 343
    for planned change, 342–344
    to situations, 343f
Strengths, leadership, for future, 560–561, 560b
Strengths-based nursing leadership, 5
    principles of, 5t

Stress
    buffering, 519, 521
    communication patterns during, 365t
    definition of, 515–516
    dynamics of, 518–519
    job
        definition of, 516
        sources of, 516–519, 517b
    management of, 519–523, 520b, 522b
        strategies, 523t
        symptom management, 520–522
        theory of preventive, 520b
    of new graduate nurse, 523
    over, signs of, 519t
    personal, 517–518
    prevention of, 519–520
    resolution of, 523–525
    role, 517
    successful management of conflict and, 441
    understanding, 515–516
Stress response model, 365
Structural empowerment theory, 190–191, 190b–191b
Structured agendas, 531
Structured nursing terminologies, 212–213
Structured performance appraisal tools, 310, 310b
    graphic rating scales, 310, 311f
Style theories, 10b–11b
Subcultures, 383
Succession planning, 39
Supply and expense budget, 249
Support, access to, 190
Supportive of others, as follower characteristic, 16t
Supremacy of Parliament, 70
SWOT (Strengths, Weaknesses, Opportunities, and Threats)
        analysis, 120, 120b, 121t, 320
Syllogism, 110
Symptom management, 30, 520–522
Synergy
    creating, 358–359
    definition of, 358
    properties of, 358
Synergy Model, 271
Synthesis of evidence, in policymaking, 196–197
System, definition of, 150
Systematic relaxation technique, 521b
Systemic components, 496b
Systems and technological side, of managing change, 342
Systems theory, 136–137, 150
Systems thinking, 337

T

Tactical decisions, 244
TCAB. *see* Transforming Care at the Bedside (TCAB)
Teams, 15–17
    assemble, quality improvement process, 398, 398b
        versus quality assurance process, 404t
    conflict and, 360–362

Teams *(Continued)*
definition of, 352–355
development of, 118, 355–357, 356b
effective and ineffective, characteristics of, 355t
interdisciplinary, 353–354
interprofessional, 353–354
key concepts related to, 354–355
success, leadership role in, 369–371
types of, 353
Team assessment exercise, 354t, 354b
Team building
questions to assess the need for, 360b
through communication and partnership, 351–373, 352b, 371b
tips for, 372
value of, 359–360, 360b
Team competencies, 118
Team decision support tools, 119–120
Team dynamics, 118–119
Team learning, 337
Team members
generational differences among, 359, 359f
qualities of, 357–358, 358b
Team nursing, 260–262, 261f
model analysis in, 261, 261b
nurse manager's role in, 261–262
staff nurse's role in, 262
Team performance dynamics, 118–119
Team player, as follower characteristic, 16t
Teamwork, 352
Technology, 234b
biomedical, 209–211, 211b, 226, 226f
caring, communicating, and managing with, 205–237, 208b
communication, 217–218, 228–231, 231b
evidence in, 233–234
influences of, 563
in health care organizations, 139–140
information, 211–213, 213b, 226–228
knowledge, 220–221, 220b, 232
new
cost-effectiveness of, 245, 245b
professional, ethical nursing practice and, 232–233, 232b
solution in, 233b
tips for, 235
types of, 209–213
voice, 217–218
TEIP. *see* Towards Evidence Informed Practice (TEIP)
Telecommunications, 228–231
Telehealth, 228
Telemetry, 217
Telemonitoring, 209
Teletriage, 209
Tenacious, being, as quality of team member, 358
"Tend and befriend" response, 518
Termination, 468–469, 469b
Territorial funding, in health care services, 128–129, 128f, 129t
Thank-you letter/note, 544–545

The Fifth Discipline: The Art and Practice of the Learning Organization, 561
The Neighborhood, web-based virtual community, 179
The Starfish and the Spider, 154, 559–560, 560b
Theory, role, 303, 303b
Theory of preventive stress management (TPSM), 520b
Theory X (authoritarian), in motivating employees, 65b
Theory Y (participative), in motivating employees, 65b
Therapeutic treatment systems, 210
Thinking
communication during conflict, 364
critical, for problem solving and decision making, 107–108
divergent, 108
systems, 337
Threatening behaviour, 475b
Time management, 525–530
concepts, 528–530, 530b
for effective leader, 46
techniques, 528t
Time tools, 529
Timed agendas, 531
Tort, 73
Total patient care method. *see* Case method
Total required patient-care hours, 248t
Towards Evidence Informed Practice (TEIP), 420
Toxic workplaces, 475–476
TPSM. *see* Theory of preventive stress management (TPSM)
Training, leadership, lateral violence and, 453
Trait theories, 10b–11b
Transactional leaders, 10
Transactional leadership, 39–40, 40b
theories, 10b–11b
Transcultural Assessment Model, 178
Transculturalism, 178
Transformational leadership, 40–42, 41b–42b
clinical leaders with, 41
goal of, 40
key practices in, 40
outcomes of, 41
theories, 10, 10b–11b
vs. transactional, 40b
Transforming Care at the Bedside (TCAB), 271–272, 271b–272b
Transition, role, 499–513, 500b–501b, 510b–512b
"Transition shock," 192–193
Translation, knowledge, 196–197, 412
Trudeau, Pierre Elliott, 37
Trust
change agents and, 345
defined, 357
in team development, 357
Truth, telling, 368
Truth About Nursing, 186
Twenty-first-century IV pumps, 210, 226f

U

Uberrima fides, 76
UCPs. *see* Unregulated care providers (UCPs)

"Umbrella organization," 552
UMHDS. *see* Uniform minimum health data set (UMHDS)
Uncooperative or unproductive employees, 460–463
Unfreezing, 334
Uniform minimum health data set (UMHDS), 212
Unions, 140–142
    influence on organizational structures, 141, 141b
    influence on policy, 140–141
    influence on practice and research, 141–142, 142b
    labour, 381
    leadership in, 49
    nursing, 379, 380t, 388b
Unit and departmental budgets, development of, 250–251
Unit-level budget, management of, 251–253, 252t, 252b–253b
Unit of service, 247, 292–293
Unit staffing, evaluation of, 295–298, 296b
University Health Network, vision, mission, strategic priorities/
    goals, and practice philosophy for nursing at, 151b
Unregulated care providers (UCPs), 257–258, 494–495
Unsatisfactory resolution, 443
USA Patriot Act (2001), 79
Users' Guides to the Medical Literature. *see* Journal of the
    American Medical Association
Utilization, 239
    research, 414–417
        conceptual structure of, 424

V

Variable costs, 245–246
Variance, 251, 267–268
Variance analysis, 251
Variance report, 297
Vicarious liability, 76
Violation, ethical, 99
Violence
    horizontal, 452, 475–476, 480–482, 481b
    hospital-based, 478
    lateral, 475–476
        management of, 452–453, 453b
    types of, 475b
    in workplace, 60
Violence in the Workplace Prevention Guide, 476, 479
Vision, 150, 151b, 152, 561
    for leadership development, 43
    shared, 562–563
Visioning, 344, 561–562, 561b
Voice recognition, 217–218
Voice technology, 217–218

W

Wall Street Journal article, 547
Weber, Max, 157
Weblog, 229

WebQuest, 228–229
Websites
    of Canadian Patient Safety Institute (CPSI), 29
    health-related, 229t
Weighted decision matrix, 113, 113f, 113b
Well-run meetings, importance of, 531b
Whistle-blowing, in workplace advocacy, 387, 387b
WHO. *see* World Health Organization (WHO)
Wireless communication, 217
Wireless systems, 217
Wisdom, 219
Work, trends in, 563
Work dissatisfaction, absenteeism and, 459
Work redesign, 246
Work-related stressors, 516
Workforce
    emerging, 45
    entrenched, 45–46
Working environment, as characteristic of effective and ineffective
    team, 355t
Workload, 292–293
    calculation of, 247, 248t
Workplace, assessment of, 508
Workplace advocacy
    in nursing governance, 385–387, 385b–386b
    participatory decision making and collaboration, 385
    professional values, 386–387, 387b
    support for making and implementing decisions,
        385–386, 386b
    whistle-blowing, 387, 387b
Workplace empowerment, aspect of organizational
    culture, 153
Workplace satisfaction, leadership as primary determinant
    of, 39, 39b
Workplace violence, 190
    cost of, 477
    defining, 475–478
    ensuring safe workplace and, 476–477
    evidence in, 482–483
    identifying risk factors of, 478–480, 478b–480b
    and incivility, 474–485, 475b, 482b–483b
    making a difference and, 478
    prevention strategies for, 478–480
    program checklists for, 479b
    scope of the problem, 476
    tips for preventing, 483
    types of, 475b
Workplace Violence Research Institute study, 477
Workstations on Wheels (WOWs), 216–217
World Health Organization (WHO), in social determinants
    of health, 139
Worldviews on Evidence-Based Nursing, 430
WOWs. *see* Workstations on Wheels (WOWs)